a LANGE medical book

ALLERGY AND ASTHMA
Practical Diagnosis and Management

Edited by

Massoud Mahmoudi, DO, PhD, RM (NRM), FASCMS, FACOI, FACP, FCCP, FAAAAI
Assistant Clinical Professor
Department of Medicine
Division of Allergy and Immunology
University of California, San Francisco
Chairman, Department of Medicine
Community Hospital of Los Gatos
Los Gatos, California
Past President, Allergy Association of Northern California
Clinical Assistant Professor
Department of Medicine
University of Medicine and Dentistry of New Jersey
College of Osteopathic Medicine
Stratford, New Jersey
Adjunct Assistant Clinical Professor
Department of Medicine
San Francisco College of Osteopathic Medicine
Touro University
Mere Island, California

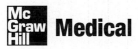
Medical

New York   Chicago   San Francisco   Lisbon   London   Madrid   Mexico City   Milan
New Delhi   San Juan   Seoul   Singapore   Sydney   Toronto

Allergy and Asthma: Practical Diagnosis and Management

1 2 3 4 5 6 7 8 9 0   DOC/DOC   0 9 8 7

ISBN 978-0-07-147173-2
MHID 0-07-147173-1

This book was set in Adobe Garamond by International Typesetting and Composition.
The editors were James Shanahan and Christie Naglieri.
The production supervisor was Cheryl Souffrance.
Project management was provided by International Typesetting and Composition.
The cover designer was Mary McKeon.
RR Donnelley was printer and binder.

This book is printed on acid-free paper.

Library of Congress Cataloging-in-Publication Data

Allergy and asthma : practical diagnosis and management / edited by Massoud Mahmoudi.—1st ed.
    p. ; cm.
Includes bibliographical references and index.
ISBN-13: 978-0-07-147173-2 (pbk. : alk. paper)
ISBN-10: 0-07-147173-1
    1. Allergy—Diagnosis.   2. Allergy—Treatment.   3. Asthma—Diagnosis.   4. Asthma—Treatment.
I. Mahmoudi, Massoud.
    [DNLM: 1. Hypersensitivity—diagnosis.   2. Hypersensitivity—therapy.   3. Anti-Allergic Agents—therapeutic use.
4. Asthma—diagnosis.   5. Asthma—therapy. WD 300 A432509   2007]
RC584.A394   2007
616.97—dc22

                                                                                    2007014242

To the memory of my father, Mohammad H. Mahmoudi, and
to my mother, Zohreh, my wife, Lily, and my son, Sam,
for their sincere support and encouragement.

Contents

1. Introduction to the Immune System 1
Massoud Mahmoudi, DO, PhD

2. The History and Physical Examination of the Allergic Patient 12
Mary Alice Murphy, MD, MPH

3. Prevalence of Allergic Diseases in Children, Adults, and the Elderly 18
Massoud Mahmoudi, DO, PhD

Authors

Mutasim Abu-Hasan, MD
Clinical Associate
Professor of Pediatrics
Pediatric Allergy and Pulmonary Division
University of Iowa
Iowa City, Iowa
Chapter 19

Pedro C. Avila, MD
Associate Professor
Division of Allergy-Immunology
Department of Medicine
Northwestern University's Feinberg School of Medicine
Chicago, Illinois
Chapter 32

Jonathan A. Bernstein, MD
Associate Professor of Clinical Medicine
Division of Immunology
Department of Internal Medicine
College of Medicine
University of Cincinnati
Cincinnati, Ohio
Chapter 17

Leonard Bielory, MD
Professor of Medicine, Pediatrics, and Ophthalmology
UMDNJ—New Jersey Medical School
Asthma and Allergy Research Center
Newark, New Jersey
Chapters 4, 34

Thomas B. Casale, MD
Assistant Dean for Clinical Research
Professor and Associate Chair of Medicine, Chief
Division of Allergy and Immunology
Department of Internal Medicine
Creighton University
Omaha, Nebraska
Chapter 41

Eric M. Chen, MD, FACP, FAAAAI, FACAAI
Assistant Clinical Professor
Department of Medicine
Division of Allergy and Immunology
University of California, San Francisco
San Francisco, California
Chapter 10

Paul Cheng, MD, PhD, FAAAAI
Associate Clinical Professor
Division of Allergy and Immunology
Department of Pediatrics
University of California, San Francisco
San Francisco, California
Chapter 31

Eric C. Chenworth, DO
Mayo Clinic College of Medicine
Department of Internal Medicine
Division of Allergic Diseases
Rochester, Minnesota
Chapter 15

Steven W. Cheung, MD
Associate Professor
Otology, Neurotology, and Skull Base Surgery
Department of Otolaryngology-Head and Neck Surgery
University of California, San Francisco
San Francisco, California
Chapter 9

Timothy J. Craig, DO
Professor of Medicine and Pediatrics
Division of Allergy
Department of Medicine
Penn State University
Hershey, Pennsylvania
Chapters 7, 16, 20, 37

Laura H. Fisher, MD
Section of Allergy
Asthma and Immunology
Penn State University
Allergy and Asthma Center
Lancaster, Pennsylvania
Chapter 16

Oscar L. Frick, MD, PhD
Professor Emeritus
Pediatrics and Attending Allergist
Pediatric Allergy Clinic
University of California, San Francisco
San Francisco, California
Chapter 24

Marianne Frieri, MD, PhD
Professor of Medicine and Pathology
State University of New York—Stonybrook
Director of Allergy Immunology
Nassau University Medical Center
East Meadow, New York
Chapters 23, 30

Donald F. German, MD, FAAAAI, FACAAI
Clinical Professor of Pediatrics
University of California Medical School
California Asthma and Allergy Clinic
   of Marin and San Francisco
San Francisco, California
Chapters 25, 26

Avraham Gianninni, MD
Clinical Professor of Pediatrics
University of California, San Francisco
San Francisco, California
Chapter 35

Joshua Gibbs, DO
Allergy/Immunology Fellow
Department of Pulmonary, Allergy and
   Critical Care Medicine
Penn State Milton S. Hershey Medical Center
Hershey, Pennsylvania
Chapter 20

Andrew N. Goldberg, MD, MSCE, FACS
Professor
Department of Otolaryngology-Head and Neck Surgery
Director of the Division of Rhinology and Sinus Surgery
University of California, San Francisco
San Francisco, California
Chapter 8

Sixto F. Guiang, MD
Assistant Clinical Professor
Department of Medicine
Division of Allergy and Immunology
University of California, San Francisco
San Francisco, California
Chapter 14

Jennifer Heimall, MD
Chief Medical Resident, Internal Medicine
UMDNJ—New Jersey Medical School
Newark, New Jersey
Chapter 34

Shuba Rajashri Iyengar, MD, MPH
Fellow; Allergy/Immunology
Division of Pulmonary and Pediatrics
Stanford University
Palo Alto, California
Chapter 36

Alexander Kapp, MD, PhD
Professor and Chairman
Department of Dermatology and Allergology
Hannover Medical University
Hannover, Germany
Chapter 11

Mitchell H. Katz, MD
Director of Health
Clinical Professor of Medicine, Epidemiology
   and Biostatistics
University of California, San Francisco
San Francisco, California
Chapter 33

Eric Kavosh, MD
Resident, Internal Medicine
UMDNJ—New Jersey Medical School
Newark, New Jersey
Chapter 4

Jennifer S. Kim, MD
Clinical Instructor of Pediatrics
Division of Allergy
Department of Pediatrics
Northwestern University's Feinberg School of Medicine
Attending Physician
Division of Allergy
Department of Pediatrics
Children's Memorial Hospital
Chicago, Illinois
Chapter 38

Dennis K. Ledford, MD
Professor of Medicine and Pediatrics
University of South Florida College of Medicine
James A. Haley V.A. Hospital
Tampa, Florida
Chapter 6

Sharon E. Leonard, MD
Fellow in Allergy and Immunology
Virginia Commonwealth University
Richmond, Virginia
Chapter 42

Doris Lin, MD
Chief Resident
Otolaryngology-Head and Neck Surgery
University of California, San Francisco
San Francisco, California
Chapter 9

Daniel E. Maddox, MD
Consultant
Allergic Diseases and Internal Medicine
Division of Allergic Diseases
Department of Internal Medicine
Mayo Clinic College of Medicine
Rochester, Minnesota
Chapter 15

Massoud Mahmoudi, DO, PhD, RM (NRM), FASCMS, FACOI, FACP, FCCP, FAAAAI
Assistant Clinical Professor
Department of Medicine
Division of Allergy and Immunology
University of California, San Francisco
Chairman, Department of Medicine
Community Hospital of Los Gatos
Los Gatos, California
Past President, Allergy Association of Northern California
Clinical Assistant Professor
Department of Medicine
University of Medicine and Dentistry of New Jersey
College of Osteopathic Medicine
Stratford, New Jersey
Adjunct Assistant Clinical Professor
Department of Medicine
San Francisco College of Osteopathic Medicine
Touro University
Mere Island, California
Chapters 1, 3, 5, 28, 29, 36

Giselle S. Mosnaim, MD, MS
Program Director
Division of Allergy/Immunology
Department of Immunology/Microbiology
Rush Medical College
Chicago, Illinois
Chapter 37

Mary Alice Murphy, MD, MPH
Private Practice; Associate Clinical Professor
Division of Allergy
Department of Pediatrics
University of California School of Medicine
San Francisco, California
Chapter 2

Kari C. Nadeau, MD, PhD
Faculty
Division of Allergy, Asthma, and Immunology
Department of Pediatrics
Stanford University
Stanford, California
Chapter 40

Michael R. Nelson, MD, PhD
Assistant Professor
Division of Allergy
Department of Medicine
Uniformed Services University of the Health Sciences
Chief of Clinical Laboratory Immunology Section
Division of Clinical Immunology
Department of Allergy-Immunology
Walter Reed Army Medical Center
Washington, DC
Chapter 22

Carah Santos, MS
College of Medicine
Department of Medicine
Penn State University
Hershey Medical Center
Hershey, Pennsylvania
Chapter 7

Lawrence Schwartz, MD, PhD
Charles and Evelyn Thomas Professor of Medicine
Division of Rheumatology, Allergy, and Immunology
Department of Internal Medicine
Virginia Commonwealth University
Richmond, Virginia
Chapter 42

Joseph D. Spahn, MD
Associate Professor of Pediatrics
Division of Allergy and Immunology
Department of Pediatrics
University of Colorado Health Sciences Center
National Jewish Medical and Research Center
Division of Allergy and Immunology
Department of Pediatrics
Denver, Colorado
Chapter 39

Jeffrey R. Stokes, MD
Assistant Professor
Division of Allergy/Immunology
Department of Medicine
Creighton University
Omaha, Nebraska
Chapter 41

Rachel E. Story, MD, MPH
Assistant Professor
Division of Allergy
Department of Pediatrics
Northwestern University's Feinberg School of Medicine
Attending Physician
Division of Allergy
Department of Pediatrics
Children's Memorial Hospital
Chicago, Illinois
Chapter 38

Peg Strub, MD
Assistant Clinical
Professor of Medicine
University of California Medical School
Chief of Allergy
Kaiser Permanente Medical Center
San Francisco, California
Chapter 18

Schuman Tam, MD, FACP, FAAAAI
Associate Clinical
Professor of Medicine/Allergy
Department of Medicine
University of California, San Francisco
San Francisco, California
Chapter 27

Haig Tcheurekdjian, MD
Clinical Instructor
Division of Allergy and Immunology
Department of Medicine
University of California, San Francisco
San Francisco, California
Chapter 28

Bettina Wedi, MD, PhD
Professor
Department of Dermatology and Allergology
Hannover Medical School
Hannover, Germany
Chapters 11, 13

Miles Weinberger, MD
Professor of Pediatrics and Director
Pediatric Allergy and Pulmonary Division
Department of Pediatrics
University of Iowa
Division of Director
Pediatric Allergy and Pulmonary Clinical Service
Department of Pediatrics
Children's Hospital of Iowa
Iowa City, Iowa
Chapter 19

Kevin C. Welch, MD
Chief Resident
Otorhinolaryngology-Head and Neck Surgery
University of Maryland School of Medicine
Baltimore, Maryland
Chapter 8

Jennifer Yoo, MD
Clinical Fellow
Division of Allergy/Immunology
Department of Internal Medicine
University of California, San Francisco
San Francisco, California
Chapter 5

Satoshi Yoshida, MD, PhD, FACP, FCCP, FAAAAI, FACAAI
Professor and Dean
School of Medical and Health Science
Clayton University
Honolulu, Hawaii
Vice President
Department of Medicine
Sakuragaoka Chuo Hospital
Yamato, Japan
Chapters 12, 21

Andrew R. Zolopa, MD
Associate Professor of Medicine
Division of Infectious Diseases and Geographic Medicine
Department of Medicine
Stanford University
Stanford, California
Chapter 33

Preface

Allergy is perhaps the most commonly used term in hospitals and ambulatory care settings. Inquiring about drug and latex allergy has become a routine part of the history taking of a new patient. *Hay fever, food allergy, poison ivy exposure, bee sting allergy*, and *asthma* are familiar terms to many individuals and important reasons for frequent visits to the doctor and emergency department.

Allergic diseases are the sixth leading cause of chronic diseases in the United States. Teaching the diagnosis and management of such important diseases was the reason for preparing this collection.

This book is a collaborative work by the knowledgeable experts in the field of allergy and clinical immunology. Teachers and expert clinicians share their expertise in an easy-to-follow Lange series format. What makes this book unique is the inclusion of uncommonly discussed but important topics such as pollution, cough, pseudoasthma, sick building syndrome, complementary and alternative therapy, and allergy in the elderly, among others.

Allergy and Asthma: Practical Diagnosis and Management consists of 42 chapters ranging from an introduction to immunology to the history and physical examination of the allergic patient, allergic diseases, diagnosis, and management. In addition, we have included six chapters on asthma, a common disease treated by allergists, and four separate chapters on medications. To keep readers up to date, we have added an evidence-based medicine section at the end of each chapter that discusses an important study or finding that has recently been published and has added to our knowledge and understanding of allergic diseases. These sections will be updated in future editions.

Our book is intended for all students of medicine, from medical students to interns, residents, fellows, primary care physicians and all medical specialists, nurses, allied health care providers, and finally, anyone who likes to learn and keep up to date in the field of allergy.

I am indebted to all the contributors who helped put this unique collection together. I am honored to have distinguished contributors such as Oscar L. Frick, MD, PhD, professor emeritus at the University of California, San Francisco, the 1972 president of the American Academy of Allergy Asthma and Immunology, and the upcoming president, Thomas Casale, MD. Finally, I am indebted to the editorial staff at McGraw-Hill: Jim Shanahan, who initially accepted my proposal; Maya Barahona, for her editorial help and coordination of the project; and the production team.

I look forward to receiving your feedback and hope to present an updated edition in the near future. I can be contacted at allergycure@sbcglobal.net.

Massoud Mahmoudi, DO, PhD, RM (NRM),
FASCMS, FACOI, FACP, FCCP, FAAAAI

Introduction to the Immune System

Massoud Mahmoudi, DO, PhD

THE IMMUNE SYSTEM

The human body is constantly exposed to a variety of external elements. These foreign materials find their way into the body via inhalation, ingestion, and penetration. As we inhale to get our required oxygen from the air, we also inhale fumes, smoke, dust, pollens, particles, molds, bacteria, viruses, and their by-products. Another way we expose our bodies to foreign invaders is through trauma and injury. The system responsible to defend us against these foreign substances is our **immune system**, and our protective status, natural or acquired, is known as **immunity**. The two types of immunity are **innate immunity** and **acquired or adaptive immunity**.

INNATE IMMUNITY

Innate immunity is a natural immunity against microbes and other nonmicrobial substances that exist before exposure to these substances. The various components of the innate immune system are primarily activated by the recognition of a small number of molecular patterns that are present on nearly all pathogens. This system consists of various defensive mechanisms that work collaboratively to eliminate foreign invaders (Table 1–1). The first defensive tool of this system is the skin, a physical barrier that protects the body from the invasion of organisms. Bodily secretions that moisturize the skin and mucous membranes also play a role in preventing colonization of bacteria, by washing them off or destroying them. For example, tears wash the eyes, remove the loose foreign bodies, and may destroy some organisms by enzymatic reactions; sweat contains lactic acid that has an acidic pH, creating an unsuitable environment for most organisms; and gastric juices are acidic and can destroy acid-labile organisms. In addition to skin and bodily secretions, several other defense strategies, such as coughing, sneezing, or ciliary movements of the respiratory epithelium, help remove foreign objects and organisms.

Another major mechanism of the innate immune system by which the body gets rid of organisms and foreign invaders is phagocytosis. This is an engulfing mechanism that host cells use to surround, engulf, and lyse materials with various hydrolyzing enzymes. The cells assigned to perform such activity are termed *phagocytes* and consist primarily of neutrophils and macrophages. Neutrophils are multilobed nucleated cells originating from the bone marrow, where they mature and stay for a short while before being released into the circulation. They contain various granules that carry destructive enzymes and chemical substances that can destroy engulfed organisms. Macrophages are derived from monocytes, which form in the bone marrow and are released into circulation. These kidney-shaped nucleated cells comprise 1% to 6% of all nucleated blood cells. After 1 day of circulation in the blood, they move to various tissues; in the tissues they are named macrophages or histiocytes. Macrophages of different tissues are named differently, although their basic mechanisms are the same. For example, the ones that reside in liver and lung tissues are known as Kupffer cells and alveolar macrophages, respectively.

Natural Killer Cells

Viruses can infect the host cells and replicate causing general infection. To prevent viral replication, the body needs to intervene and remove such infected cells. Natural killer (NK) cells are large granular lymphocytes that do just that; they are members of the innate immune system, and they function by recognizing and killing the infected cells. NK cells also activate macrophages to kill phagocytosed microbes. NK cells have granules that contain **perforin** and **granzymes**. Perforins create pores in target cells, and granzymes cause apoptosis of the target cells.

HOW ARE VIRUS-INFECTED CELLS RECOGNIZED?

Recognition of virus-infected cells relies on two sets of receptors, the **inhibitory** and **activating** receptors on

Table 1–1. Features of innate and adaptive immunity.

Features	Innate Immunity	Adaptive Immunity
Host memory to foreign antigens	–	+
Specificity	–	+
Barriers to foreign antigens: skin, mucous membranes, bodily secretions	+	–
B-cells and T-cell participation	–	+
Cell-mediated immunity	–	+
Antibody production	–	+
Natural killer (NK) cells	+	–
Phagocytosis	+	–

NK cells. Inhibitory receptors bind to class 1 major histocompatibility complex (MHC) receptors found on most normal cells; this inhibits activation of NK cells and therefore prevents the killing of normal host cells. But virus-infected cells decrease class 1 MHC expression, thereby eliminating the inhibitory signal sent to the NK cells. Because NK cell activation is now unopposed, the activating receptors can bind to and kill the virus-infected cells.

Complement System

The complements are a group of plasma proteins. They are an important part of the innate immune system and engage in the destruction of microbes via three different pathways: **classical, alternative,** and **lectin** pathways. Complement activation causes inflammation and lysis of invading microorganisms (see Chapter 23).

ADAPTIVE IMMUNITY

Adaptive immunity, also known as acquired immunity, serves as an organism-specific protective system. The components of this immunity retain memory of specific exposures to deter against subsequent invasion of the same organisms (Table 1–1).

There are two types of adaptive immunity: **humoral immunity** and **cell-mediated immunity**.

Humoral Immunity

This system is responsible for the production of antibodies against bacteria. The major players of this system are **B cells**, a class of lymphocyte.

B CELLS

B cells mature in the **bursa** of **Fabricius** in birds and in the fetal liver and bone marrow in humans. Pluripotent stem cells differentiate in the bone marrow and give rise to lymphocytes and other cells (Fig. 1–1). B cells comprise 10% to 15% of lymphocytes. The released mature B cells have a short lifespan of several days. Upon invasion of bacteria, these cells are activated and undergo several cycles of division and proliferation, and they give rise to two types of cells, **memory** B cells and **effector** B cells, or **plasma cells**. Memory B cells live for years. Their job is to remember the exposure to specific organisms and then in subsequent encounters to expedite the recognition of and antibody production against these organisms. The effector B cells are in charge of antibody or immunoglobulin production to fight against the invading bacteria. Mature B cells express immunoglobulins on their cell surface but do not secrete them, whereas effector B cells produce immunoglobulins in their cytoplasm and secrete them to their environments. The plasma cells survive for days to weeks to produce antibodies and die thereafter, whereas memory cells survive for many years.

Cell-Mediated Immunity

This system is responsible for recognizing and destroying intracellular microbes such as viruses, Mycobacteria, and Leishmania. The major players of this system are T cells. They encounter and destroy infected cells by either activation of macrophages that lead to destruction of phagocytosed microbes or by direct killing of the infected cells.

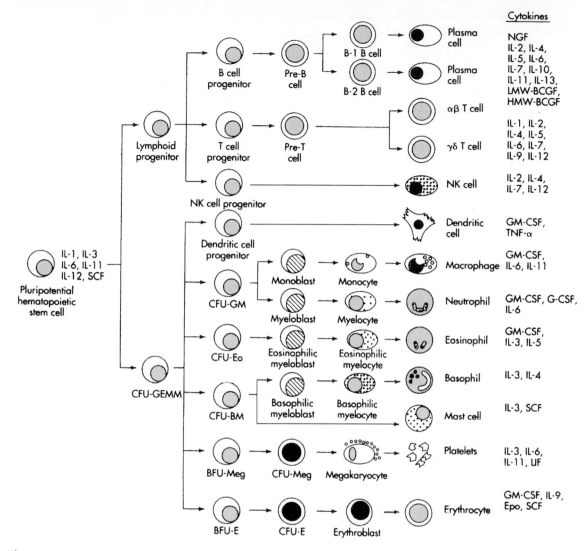

Figure 1–1. Schematic differentiation of hematopoietic cells. (Reproduced, with permission, from Lewis D, Harriman GR. Cells and tissues of the immune system. In: Rich RR. Fleisher TA, Schwartz BD, et al., eds. *Clinical Immunology Principles and Practice*. St. Louis, Mo: Mosby; 1996:18.)

T CELLS

These cells are "thymus-derived"; their precursors are originated from bone marrow but later they migrate to the thymus. In the thymus, T-cell precursor cells mature and learn to recognize self from nonself and are then released into the circulation as naive T cells. T cells represent 80% of the lymphocytes in peripheral blood circulation. Like B cells, on exposure to antigen, naive T cells differentiate and give rise to effector and memory cells. Those that do not confront antigens eventually die by programmed cell death known as **apoptosis**. The two major subsets of T cells are the T helper cells, designated as CD4+ T cells, and cytotoxic or cytolytic T cells, designated as CD8+ T cells. These cells are involved in interacting with intracellular organisms, for example infected cells (see type IV hypersensitivity). T cells express antigen-specific receptors known as T-cell receptors. There are two types of T cell receptors; one type has α and β chains, T$\alpha\beta$, and the other type has γ and δ chains, T$\gamma\delta$. These receptors are antigen specific, and T cells only recognize those antigens that are presented by **antigen-presenting cells**. Antigen-presenting cells have proteins on their surfaces known as the **major histocompatability complex (MHC)** that binds to the antigen. It is the combination of this complex and the antigen that is recognized by T cells.

In addition to T-cell receptors, many surface proteins are expressed on T lymphocytes with assigned functions. These receptors participate in various roles, such as antigen recognition and T-cell activation, among others.

INTERACTION OF ANTIGEN AND ANTIBODY

We are vulnerable to invasion by millions of different antigens. Is our body prepared to defend and fight against such vast numbers of structurally different antigens? We have clones of B and T lymphocytes that have unique antigen receptors for specific antigens; on exposure and contact to an antigen, the specific lymphocyte clones are recognized and selected, **clonal selection**, by the antigen and are activated. This activation stimulates the lymphocyte clones to proliferate, **clonal proliferation**, and produces high numbers of the same lymphocytes; this is called **clonal expansion**. In the next step, some of these lymphocytes differentiate to two groups of cells; one is the group capable of producing antibodies, the effector B cells, and the other group is cells that do not produce antibody but remember the antigen exposure and live for many years, also known as memory B cells. A similar process occurs with T cells. Some T cells become effector T cells and combat pathogens; others become memory T cells to remember the exposure in case of future infection. The nondifferentiated cells eventually end up dying (apoptosis).

B CELLS: RESPONSIBLE FOR THE PRODUCTION OF ANTIBODIES

Antibodies, also known as immunoglobulins, are glycoprotein molecules with a distinct structure (Fig. 1–2). Each molecule is made of an identical pair of heavy chain molecules held together by a disulfide bond and an identical pair of light chains. A disulfide bond also holds the light and heavy chains together. Each heavy and light chain contains a variable region (V) and a constant region (C). The variable regions of heavy and light chains form a unique antigen-binding site. Each antibody molecule has two such sites. Each antigen-binding site has three hypervariable regions that are complementary to the bound antigen. What makes each antibody unique is the structure of these hypervariable regions. These regions are also known as **complementarity-determining regions**, designated as CDR1, CDR2, and CDR3. The immunoglobulins are either membrane bound or secretory; the membrane-bound immunoglobulins act as receptors on B cells where they recognize a specific antigen. The secretory immunoglobulins are produced

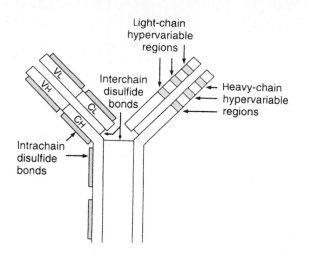

Figure 1–2. Schematic depiction of an IgG molecule showing the approximate locations of the hypervariable regions. (Reproduced, with permission, from Parslow TG. Immunoglobulins and immunoglobulin genes. In: Stites DP, Terr AI, Parslow TG, eds. *Medical Immunology.* 9th ed. New York: McGraw-Hill; 1997:95.)

by plasma cells, also known as effector B lymphocytes. Immunoglobulins are synthesized in the cytoplasm and stored in Golgi complexes. Immunoglobulin molecules are designated as **IgA, IgG, IgM, IgD,** and **IgE**. Each immunoglobulin molecule or isotype is unique in function and biological properties. The most common type of immunoglobulin, IgG, has subclasses of IgG1, IgG2, IgG3, and IgG4, each with unique biological properties. Immunoglobulin A also has two subclasses, designated as IgA1 and IgA2. Table 1–2 summarizes the features of immunoglobulins.

AUTOIMMUNITY

The role of our immune system is to defend against invading microorganisms and foreign antigens. The body is capable of differentiating between "self" and "nonself"; in other words, under normal conditions, the immune system does not react against self-antigens. This is the basis of **self-tolerance**. When self-tolerance is compromised, the immune system turns against itself; this response is the basis for autoimmune disease. Autoimmunity, such as in the case of Graves disease, is related to an antibody against thyrotropin receptors or T-cell autoreactivity. To maintain self-tolerance, the autoreactive T or B cells need to be controlled by elimination or suppression to spare autoreactivity against self. When there is a defect in such a control system, upon activation, autoreactive T or B cells can cause tissue injury.

Table 1–2. Immunoglobulins: features and characteristics.

Immunoglobulins (Ig)	Molecular Weight (d)	Serum Concentrations	Half-life (d)	Subclasses	Complement Fixation	Placenta Transfer	Immediate Hypersensitivity	Other Characteristics/ Functions
IgA	170,000 or 350,000 (secretory)	1.4–4 mg/mL	6	IgA 1, 2	–	–	–	Involved in mucosal immunity
IgD	160,000	0–0.4 mg/mL	3	–	–	–	–	Membrane-bound antigen receptor of B-cell surface
IgE	180,000	17–450 ng/mL	2.5	–	–	–	+	Immediate hypersensitivity, defense against parasitic infection
IgG	160,000	8–16 mg/mL	23	IgG 1, 2, 3, 4	IgG 1, 2, 3	+	–	Involved in type II hypersensitivity
IgM	900,000	0.5–2 mg/mL	5	–	+	–	–	Membrane-bound antigen receptor of B-cell surface; involved in type II hypersensitivity

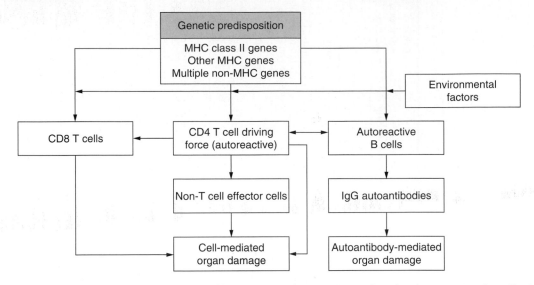

Figure 1–3. Steps involved in pathogenesis of autoimmune diseases. (Reproduced, with permission, from Kotzin BL. Mechanisms of autoimmunity. In: Rich RR, Fleisher TA, Shearer WT, et al., eds. *Clinical Immunology Principles and Practice.* 2nd ed. London: Mosby; 2001:section 58.1.)

Genetic predisposition plays an important role in the development of autoimmune diseases. The genes involved are MHC or non-MHC genes. In addition, environmental triggers, infectious agents, and noninfectious triggers such as drugs and loss of regulatory cells may contribute to autoreactivity. Figure 1–3 summarizes the steps proposed in the pathogenesis of autoimmune diseases. CD4 Th1 cells play the central role of T-cell tolerance. Activated autoreactive CD4 Th1 cells are able to cause cell-mediated tissue damage; they can also induce CD8 cells and lead to tissue injury.

T CELL–ANTIGEN INTERACTION

The steps leading to T cell–antigen interaction are as follows:

1. Antigen-presenting cells, such as monocytes, macrophages, dendritic cells, or B lymphocytes, process foreign antigens to form peptides.
2. Peptide antigens bind to a complex of protein known as major histocompatibility complex (MHC), either MHC I or II.
3. The complex is later expressed on the surface of antigen-presenting cells.
4. There are two subsets of T cells: T helper cells, designated as CD4+ T helper cells, and cytotoxic or cytolytic T cells, designated as CD8 T cells. CD4+T

cells recognize and bind to the antigen-MHC II complex, whereas CD8+ T cells recognize and bind to the antigen-MHC I complex of antigen-presenting cells.
5. The result of T cell–MHC I complex interaction is the destruction of infected cells. The result of T cell–MHC II complex interaction is activation of CD4+ T helper cells to promote further immune functions, such as providing stimulatory signals to B cells to produce immunoglobulins.

T HELPER CELL REGULATION

On exposure to antigens, naive T cells activate, proliferate, and then differentiate to T helper 1 (Th1) or T helper 2 (Th2) cells. Differentiation of activated cells to Th1 or Th2 effector cells depends on the presence of certain cytokines. For example, in the presence of interleukin 12 (IL-12), secreted by macrophages, activated T cells differentiate to Th1 cells, whereas in the presence of interleukin 4 (IL-4), produced by cells such as mast cells, activated cells differentiate to Th2 cells. When one pathway is under way, the other pathway is suppressed (Fig. 1–4). The cytokines involved in such regulations are interferon (IFN) γ and IL-10. IFN γ produced by Th1 cells not only promote Th1 differentiation but also inhibit the proliferation and production of Th2 cells. In contrast, IL-10 produced by Th2 cells blocks Th1 production.

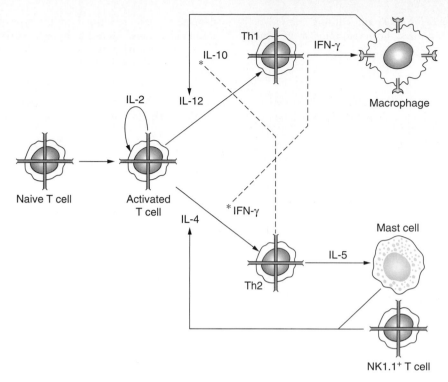

Figure 1–4. Cross-regulation of T helper cell responses. Stimulation of naive (Th0) T cells with antigen in the presence of IL-12 (macrophage produced) or IL-4 (produced by either NK1.1+ T cells or mast cells) leads to a Th1 or h2 response, respectively. IFN-γ production by Th1 cells inhibits the activity of IL-4, thereby limiting Th2 production. IL-10 production limits Th1 responses by blocking the production of IL-12 by macrophages. Thus the expression of Th1 and Th2 cytokines also serves to reinforce the production of similarly differentiated T cells. (Reproduced, with permission, from Eager TN, Tompkins SM, et al. Helper T-cell subsets and control of the inflammatory response. In: Rich RR, Fleisher TA, Schwartz BD, et al., eds. *Clinical Immunology Principles and Practice.* 2nd ed. St. Louis, Mo: Mosby; 2001:section 16.4.)

Differentiation of activated cells to Th1 or Th2 effector cells also depends on the types of presenting antigens. For instance, intracellular bacteria such as *Listeria monocytogenes* and *Mycobacterium tuberculosis* or certain parasites stimulate Th1 response, whereas allergens and helminths trigger Th2 response.

CELLS OF THE IMMUNE SYSTEM

Mast Cells

In addition to their role in defense against bacteria and parasitic invasion, mast cells play a role in allergic responses. These important effectors of hypersensitivity originate from bone marrow and mature in tissues. There are two types of mast cells: the connective and the mucosal type. They have prominent nuclei and cytoplasmic granules that contain various mediators, some

preformed and some newly synthesized. Mast cells carry high-affinity receptors on their surface, namely FcεRI. These receptors have high affinity for the Fc portion of IgE. The binding of Fc and FcεRI is needed for mast cell activation (see type I hypersensitivity). Based on their cytoplasmic granule contents, human mast cells are divided into those that contain tryptase only, known as MCt, and those that contain chymase, carboxypeptidase, and cathypsin G in addition to tryptase, known as MCtc. The MCt cells are abundant in intestinal mucosa, lung alveolar walls, and nasal mucosa, whereas MCtc are more abundant in the skin, intestinal submucosa, and blood vessels. MC cells are characterized as immune system–related and increased in allergic diseases, parasitic diseases, and chronic immune deficiency diseases and acquired immune deficiency syndrome (AIDS). The MCtc cells, in contrast, are non–immune system related, and their numbers do not increase in allergic or parasitic disease or in AIDS and chronic immune deficiency. Their numbers, however, increase in fibrotic diseases.

Basophils

These cells are also important effector cells in hypersensitivity and comprise less than 1% of white blood cells; they measure 8 to 10 μm and stain blue with Wright stain. The precursor cells of basophils are in bone marrow, where they mature before being releasing into the circulation. Like mast cells, they have a high-affinity receptor on their surfaces, FcεRI, that binds to the FC portion of IgE. Upon stimulation of basophils, the contents of granules are released; like mast cells, some mediators are preformed and some are newly synthesized.

Eosinophils

These cells are 12 to 17 μm, have bilobed nuclei, and cytoplasmic granules that are unique when stained or seen under an electron microscope. Eosinophils contain cytoplasmic primary granules that lack a core and a group of membrane-bound specific granules that contain electron-dense crystalline cores. These granules contain four major cationic proteins: major basic protein (MBP), eosinophil cationic protein (ECP), derived neurotoxin (EDN), and eosinophil peroxidase (EPO). The function of these proteins ranges from the destruction of parasites to the killing of microorganisms and tumor cells. In addition to granule cationic proteins, eosinophils have various lipid products, cytokines, and chemokines that participate in various functions. Eosinophils participate in various immune functions and are increased in parasitic infections and allergic diseases.

DEFECTIVE IMMUNE SYSTEM

Deficiencies and defects in any components of the immune system can result in immunodeficiency. The diagnosis of immunodeficiency starts with patients' complaints and a series of diagnostic evaluations. Some of these laboratory tests include a complete blood count with differentials, immunoglobulin concentration, human immunodeficiency virus (HIV) testing, evaluation of B- and T-cell function, NK cell evaluation, and analysis of gene defects, among others (see Chapter 32).

HYPERSENSITIVITY DISEASES

Repeated exposure of the body to an allergen makes susceptible individuals **sensitized** to that allergen. At some time, the body may overreact and become **hypersensitive** to the exposed allergen and cause tissue injury and damage. Diseases resulting from this type of reaction are immunologic and known as **hypersensitivity diseases.** The hypersensitivity diseases are traditionally classified in these four distinct types:

Type I: Immediate hypersensitivity or anaphylactic
Type II: Antibody-mediated hypersensitivity
Type III: Immune complex–mediated hypersensitivity
Type IV: Cell-mediated hypersensitivity

Table 1–3 summarizes the features of a hypersensitivity reaction.

Type I: Immediate Hypersensitivity or Anaphylactic

An immediate hypersensitivity reaction occurs within minutes of exposure to an allergen in a previously sensitized person. The reaction is a result of a chain of events that starts with exposure to an allergen (Fig. 1–5A). These steps are summarized as follows:

1. Initial encounter with the allergen
2. Binding of antigen-presenting cells (APCs) to the allergen
3. Antigen processing by antigen-presenting cells. The result of this process is antigen-bound MHC protein on the surface of APCs. Such cells then are capable of binding to T cells via T-cell receptors.
4. Activation of T helper cells after binding with APCs
5. Activation of B cells by activated T helper cells
6. Differentiation of B cells to plasma cells
7. Production of IgE by plasma cells
8. Binding of IgE to mast cells (sensitization step). This binding is a result of linking between Fc portions of IgE with the high-affinity Fc receptor, known as FcεRI on the surface of mast cells.
9. Subsequent exposure to the same allergen stimulates the sensitized mast cells to degranulate (i.e., opening the granules and releasing various mediators); the mediators so released cause the immediate hypersensitivity reaction.

Type II: Antibody-Mediated Hypersensitivity

This type of hypersensitivity reaction involves the interaction of non-IgE antibodies (i.e., IgM or IgG) with cell surface antigens or matrix-associated antigens. The mechanisms of tissue injury may involve opsonization of cells by antibody (i.e., binding of antibody to tissue antigen) that leads to complement activation and phagocytosis; leukocyte activations, in which their products cause the tissue injury (Fig. 1–5 B); or by **antibody-dependent cell-mediated cytotoxicity (ADCC).** In this

Table 1–3. Hypersensitivity diseases.

Type	Reactions	Mechanism	Onset of Action	Examples
Type I: Immediate hypersensitivity or anaphylactic	IgE mediated	Degranulation of mast cells and release of histamine and other mediators	Minutes to hours	Urticaria; allergic rhinitis; food allergy
Type II: Antibody-mediated hypersensitivity	Non-IgE (IgG or IgM) mediated	Interaction of antibody with cell surface antigens leading to complement activation and lysis or phagocytosis Autoimmune reactions Antibody-mediated cytotoxicity	Days	Hemolytic anemia; Hashimoto thyroiditis; transfusion reaction
Type-III: Immune complex–related hypersensitivity	Immune complex mediated	Formation of immune complex and deposition on various sites such as blood vessels	10–21 days	Serum sickness; systemic lupus erythematosus (SLE)
Type IV: Cell mediated	Cell mediated	Secreted cytokines from CD4+ and CD8+ cells activate macrophages leading to inflammation and tissue injury Direct killing of affected cells by CD8+ T cells	2–4 (or more) days	Mantoux reaction; allergic contact dermatitis

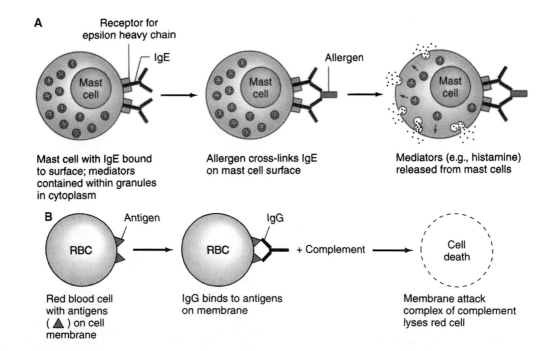

Figure 1–5. Four types of hypersensitivity diseases. **A:** Type I hypersensitivity (immediate or anaphylactic). **B:** Type II hypersensitivity (antibody mediated). **C:** Type III hypersensitivity (immune complex mediated). **D:** Type IV hypersensitivity (cell mediated). (Reproduced, with permission, from Levinson W. *Review of Medical Microbiology & Immunology.* New York: McGraw-Hill; 2006.)

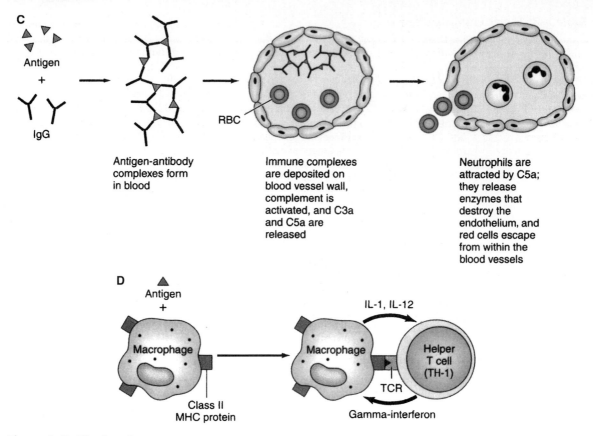

C

Antigen + IgG

Antigen-antibody complexes form in blood

RBC

Immune complexes are deposited on blood vessel wall, complement is activated, and C3a and C5a are released

Neutrophils are attracted by C5a; they release enzymes that destroy the endothelium, and red cells escape from within the blood vessels

D

Antigen +

Macrophage

Class II MHC protein

Macrophage

IL-1, IL-12

Helper T cell (TH-1)

TCR

Gamma-interferon

Figure 1–5. (*Continued*)

type of reaction, antibody binds to the infected cells. Then NK cells recognize and bind to the antibody-coated infected cells and destroy them. A known example of type II hypersensitivity, transfusion reaction, is briefly discussed later.

A transfusion reaction is a result of a blood transfusion from a noncompatible donor to a receiver. This reaction may occur as a result of ABO blood group or Rhesus (Rh) factor antigen incompatibility of donor and receiver. An example is blood transfusion from a donor with blood group A to a receiver with blood group B. Individuals with blood group A have antigen A and anti-B serum antibody, whereas individuals with blood group B have B antigen and anti-A serum antibody. Transfusion of blood from a donor with blood group A to a receiver with blood group B causes rapid hemolysis of donor blood cells. Rhesus (Rh) factor antigen is also a cause of hemolytic reactions; this occurs when an Rh-negative mother, who lacks the Rh antigen, carries an Rh-positive fetus. Blood crossing the placenta from the fetus to the mother can stimulate the mother to produce anti-Rh antibody. Maternal antibody crossing the placenta to the fetal circulation can destroy the fetal erythrocytes. Also, during a subsequent pregnancy, such anti-Rh antibody from a sensitized mother may cross the placenta and cause hemolysis of the fetal red blood cells, also known as **erythroblastosis fetalis.**

Autoimmune reactions in which the body produces antibody against self are also included in this type of immune reaction. Some examples include acute hemolytic anemia, myasthenia gravis, Graves disease, and Hashimoto's thyroiditis, to name a few.

Type III: Immune Complex–Mediated Hypersensitivity

The diseases caused by this type of hypersensitivity are based on deposition of the antigen-antibody complex in various anatomic sites. The ratio of antigen and antibody determines the amount of deposition. The deposition of antigen-antibody complex can occur in the presence of excess antigen (Fig. 1–5C).

The prototype of this category is "serum sickness" (see Chapter 22). The term *serum sickness* originated from the initial observation of diphtheria treatment. Antibody against diphtheria toxin was historically prepared in horses; thus subsequent administration of such horse serum containing antitoxin was noted to cause fever, rash, arthritis, vasculitis, and glomerulonephritis after 10 to 14 days. The depositions of antigen-antibody complexes activate complement and eventually cause tissue injury.

Type IV: Cell-Mediated Hypersensitivity

Type IV hypersensitivity includes diseases that are caused by T cell–mediated reactions. In delayed-type hypersensitivity, CD4+ T cells or CD8+ cells secrete cytokines that activate macrophages and result in inflammation and tissue injury. At times, CD8+ T cells directly kill the affected cells. The best known example of this type of hypersensitivity is the **Mantoux reaction,** which appears as an induration and erythema and is a result of the injection of tuberculin to a sensitized individual. The reaction appears in several hours and reaches a maximum in 24 to 48 hours. In this type of reaction, histological examination of the lesions reveals mononuclear phagocytes and lymphocytes (Fig. 1–5 D).

Allergic contact dermatitis is another example of this type of hypersensitivity. This type of reaction occurs as a result of contact with various allergens. Some common examples include reactions caused by contact with plants such as poison oak or poison ivy or with metals such as nickel sulfate found in jewelry. Chemicals used in various detergents, perfumes, hair dyes, and cosmetics may also cause this type of delayed hypersensitivity reaction. Delayed reaction may occur as early as 48 hours after initial contact and as late as 4 days or longer (see Chapter 13). Diagnosis of this type of allergy is by patch testing (see Chapter 31). Fig. 1–5 summarizes the four types of hypersensitivity reactions.

EVIDENCE-BASED MEDICINE

The world of immunology is constantly changing. As we learn and explore the unknowns, our understanding of the complex immune system changes. Discovery of new receptors, enzymes, and cytokines help us understand the once unexplainable immune puzzle. What we have learned about the human immune system in the last quarter of a century is astounding. A better understanding of the immune system helps us manage and treat allergic and immune diseases more effectively.

Thanks to continuous research in the field of allergy and immunology, we are learning more about our immune system. A combination of basic research, observational studies, and clinical trials helps us put together the pieces of the unknown.

As we learn about the immune system, we come up with newer and better explanations for the pathophysiology of allergic and immunologic diseases. For example, many studies have shed light on the pathophysiology of asthma; each study adds to our knowledge of evidence-based medicine in understanding the complicated nature of the disease. In their 2006 report, Bradding et al reviewed and discussed the recent advances in understanding the role of mast cells in the pathophysiology of asthma. Human mast cells localize in the airway smooth muscle, the airway mucous glands, and the bronchial epithelium of asthmatic subjects. This is likely caused by various chemoattractants produced by airway smooth muscles. The interaction of mast cells with structural airway cells via various mediators, such as histamine, prostaglandin D2, and leukotriene C4; proinflammatory cytokines, such as interleukin 4, 13 (IL-4, IL-13) and tumor necrosis factor alpha (TNF-α); and mediators, such as tryptase and many others, might lead to the bronchoconstriction, bronchial hyperresponsiveness, airway smooth muscle hyperplasia/hypertrophy, and tissue remodeling noted in patients with asthma. The authors of the report point to the complexity of the mechanisms involved in chronic activation of mast cells in the bronchial mucosa of asthmatics and remind us of the need for potent and specific drugs capable of inhibiting the release of mast cell mediators in asthmatic airways.

I refer you to the evidence-based medicine section of every chapter to learn more about the recent findings and investigations of the various topics.

BIBLIOGRAPHY

Abbas AK, Lichtman AH. *Cellular and Molecular Immunology.* 5th ed. Philadelphia: Elsevier Saunders; 2005.

Bradding P, Walls AF, Holgate ST. The role of mast cell in the pathophysiology of asthma. *J Allergy Clin Immunol.* 2006;117:1277.

Davidson A, Diamond B. Autoimmune diseases. *N Engl J Med.* 2001;5:340.

Eagar TN, Tompkins SM, Miller SD. Helper T-cell subsets and control of the inflammatory response. In: Rich RR, Fleisher TA, Shearer WT, et al., eds. *Clinical Immunology Principles and Practice.* 2nd ed. London: Mosby; 2001:section 16.1.

Fleisher TA, Oliveira JB. Functional and molecular evaluation of lymphocytes. *J Allergy Clin Immunol.* 2004;114:227.

Kotzin BL. Mechanism of autoimmunity. In: Rich RR, Fleisher TA, Shearer WT, et al., eds. *Clinical Immunology Principles and Practice.* 2nd ed. London: Mosby; 2001:section 58.1.

Rotenberg ME, Hogan PH. The eosinophil. *Annu Rev Immunol.* 2006;24:5.1.

Sell S. *Immunology, Immunopathology, and Immunity.* 6th ed. Washington, DC: ASM Press; 2001.

The History and Physical Examination of the Allergic Patient

2

Mary Alice Murphy, MD, MPH

THE PHYSICAL EXAMINATION

The medical history in a patient with allergies follows the standard model taught to all students of medicine. Therefore, only the major differences are emphasized in this chapter. These include a detailed focus on environmental exposures and seasonal variations in symptoms. References for the basic model are found at the end of the chapter.

Looking at the chapter topics in this text, it is apparent that allergic conditions involve many organ systems. Allergic individuals may have other medical conditions that affect both the allergic complaint as well as medications used to treat their allergies. Conversely, medications used in the general population can adversely affect allergic diseases (e.g., beta-blockers that are used to treat hypertension and arrhythmias).

A good allergy history involves detective work. This, in turn, takes time. It may also be necessary to explain to the patient that some details may be relevant to their problems or complaints. I tend to structure the history with a standard questionnaire. This is given to the patient to fill out in advance of the interview. It is then reviewed with the patient, allowing for clarification of details about their responses.

THE MEDICAL HISTORY

Chief Complaint

The chief complaint is the usual approach to beginning the medical history. This may be expressed in one or two sentences about the reason the person has sought a consultation with an allergist. (For example, "I am allergic to my grandmother's cat.") It may even be expressed in one or two words such as "sneezing," "a cough," "asthma," "sinus problems," or "I itch all over." I find it helpful to refer back to the patient's words at the end of the visit. This helps ensure that the treatment plan is perceived by the patient as pertinent to their initial concerns.

DETAILS ASSOCIATED WITH THE COMPLAINT (HISTORY OF THE CHIEF COMPLAINT)

This is the opportunity to describe in an organized fashion all of the symptoms relevant to the chief complaint as well as their duration, severity, location, and so on. This, plus pertinent negatives and our physical examination findings (both positive and negative), supports the conclusions that will form the diagnosis and treatment plan. In other words, we are "making our case." Often, in the specialty of allergy, we are dealing with what is called a differential diagnosis. This means we are listing possible causes for the patient's problems. By using a differential diagnosis, we are going from the most likely diagnosis (or cause) to the least likely consideration. This in turn prioritizes specific diagnostic studies and/or treatments. For example, when we suspect that the patient has asthma, we could use the criteria found in the National Institute of Health (NIH) guidelines to structure these details. Does the symptom occur daily or once a week? (The frequency is important.) Has the patient missed work or school? Does the symptom(s) interfere with sleep? Does the patient have any limitations of activity? The latter question often has to be asked creatively. For example, children with chronic asthma may have developed a sedentary pattern because of shortness of breath with exertion. However, they are not conscious of a cause and effect. Therefore, one must be very specific about their activity level (or lack thereof), rather than using the open-ended question that might be more appropriate for an adult with a recent onset of symptoms that interferes with a normally active lifestyle. Similarly, a sedentary adult tolerates more obstruction than an athlete.

Review of Systems

The review of systems is the checklist by physiologic systems that is essential to any complete medical history. I find it useful to cluster the more relevant areas for an allergic individual first before using a general review. For example, if a patient presents with complaints of asthma, it is important to find out if they have any symptoms of rhinitis, sinusitis, or dermatitis. I use a separate section in my questionnaire for this purpose. In this section I also ask about specific drug allergies, insect allergies, and adverse reactions to immunizations. If the review of systems is done via patient questionnaire, it is wise to use lay terminology (e.g., "high blood pressure" rather than "hypertension").

Medications

This is an important area to document carefully. The overall structure depends on personal preference. The following are some suggestions.

Drug Allergies

If drug allergies have not been covered in the previous section of system review, then this may be an appropriate place to document any history of adverse reactions to drugs. It is also important to document a negative history, that is, to document that the question was asked and the patient responded in the negative. The type of reaction should be noted (e.g., a rash or anaphylaxis). The patient's chart should be appropriately and prominently labelled with any drug allergies.

Current Medications

My initial focus is to list the name, dose, and frequency of medications being used for the presenting problem. This should include all prescription drugs as well as nonprescription (over-the-counter) medications; examples of the latter are decongestants, topical creams and ointments, nose sprays, and so on. A complete list of all the patient's medications is important. Drug interactions can adversely affect the patient's symptoms. Examples of such drug interactions are beta-blockers (prescribed for various cardiovascular conditions) that can exacerbate asthma and rhinitis; another is decongestant medications, such as pseudoephedrine, that can cause hypertension and tachycardia.

Past Medications

It is sometimes relevant to ask about medications used in the past for the chief complaint. The patient will appreciate not receiving prescriptions for products that were ineffectual or had adverse side effects. It is also a way to learn what class or category of medication might be most beneficial in formulating a treatment plan.

Hospitalizations

A separate section on hospitalizations often helps the patient's memory. A simple "yes" or "no" is a good way to start. If "yes", then the usual "when, where, and why?" should follow. Often when focusing on the current complaints, a previous hospitalization relating to this problem is forgotten. For example, patients with asthma may have had hospitalizations in the past that they forgot to mention. Another possibility is that an asthmatic was hospitalized with the diagnosis of bronchitis or pneumonia that was really a complication of the underlying problem, that is, their asthma. I also expand this section with specific questions about surgery, especially in this age of outpatient surgery centers. An adult who has had adenoid or tonsil surgery as a child most likely had conditions relevant to their current complaints about rhinitis and other upper respiratory symptoms.

The Clinic or Large Health Maintenance Organization Settings

In situations where medical care has been episodic or delivered by multiple providers, it may be useful to review the patient's medical records. For pediatric patients, a retrospective look at multiple visits may elicit a pattern of symptoms as well as a seasonal variation in the frequency of complaints. This is helpful not only in confirming the suspected diagnosis but also in assessing the severity of the symptoms. An example would be chronic asthma. A method I find useful in reviewing a rather large medical record is to use the date and diagnosis to create a table. This table can then be reviewed for recurrent symptoms and establishing any pattern that exists. For example, a child may have six clinic visits within 2 months with a diagnosis of an upper respiratory infection (URI). Further evaluation then establishes that all of these episodes occurred during grass pollen season (or the most significant pollen season in your region). Importantly, the vital signs reveal no febrile episodes. Likewise, physical examination details may make allergy more likely than infection.

Occupational History

The occupational history can be a simple notation of the person's occupation and duration of the same. The topic can be expanded if it seems relevant to the patient's presenting problem (see Chapter 17 on occupational asthma). Remember that children often spend the bulk of their day either in school, child care, or at a babysitter's home, which can often create significant exposures to allergens such as pets or even dust mites.

Social History

The section on social history might be used to explore hobbies, avocations, or volunteer activities that could be the occasion of an allergic exposure. The social history has other implications when HIV infection is suspected. In the elderly, their social situation may have environmental consequences. Once again, this data can be part of the detective work that results in an accurate diagnosis and successful treatment. For a child, teenager, or young adult, hobbies and sports are important pieces of data.

Environmental Exposures

Environmental exposures include the home, school, child-care center or work (see occupational history of the patient). My questionnaire dealing with the environment begins with an overview and works toward specific aspects of the environment. I start with the general area of residence (rural or urban), followed by asking if is it a house or an apartment, then what type of the heating system and lastly if there is a filter in the system. Also of interest is if there are problems with mold or water intrusions. It is also important to inquire about the floor coverings.

I ask about the patient's bedroom: specifically asking about the type of bed (mattress, box spring, etc.), pillows, and blankets. Floor coverings are again explored along with more questions about the room: including whether the bed is raised or on the floor, the number of beds in the room, and so on. Third, pets are an important topic in the allergic history. A caution here in regard to pets. As in other parts of the history, do not evaluate or prognosticate until you have gathered all your data, especially skin testing, because patients are often anxious about the fate of a pet. I include a question as to whether the patient (or parent) has noted specific symptoms on exposure to the pet in question.

Personal Habits

The section on personal habits is used to gather information about smoking (current as well as past history). Exposure to secondhand smoke should also be explored. If relevant, alcohol intake and other recreational drug use can be assessed. Another option is to cover alcohol intake with the food history. Caffeine intake can also be covered in a section on food.

Dietary (Food) History

Food intolerance and allergy symptoms associated with specific foods can be assessed in this section of the history. It can be formulated as specific yes-or-no questions or with a list of common foods that can be circled if associated with any symptoms. I use a combination of these techniques (see Chapter 24 on food allergies).

Geographic History

Discussing the different geographic locations where the patient has lived is also an important history to consider. This may be done with a series of blank lines indicating location, dates, and presence or absence of allergic symptoms. Again, this is a device for aiding the patient's recall for other details regarding environmental exposures in those different geographic areas. This includes indoor environmental exposures, such as pets.

Family History

The risk of inheriting allergies, especially rhinitis and asthma, is in a rather straightforward Mendelian fashion. Therefore, the family history is usually limited to first-degree relatives. A discussion of the complex polygenic factors involved in many allergic diseases is well beyond the scope of this chapter. However, it is helpful to know that as a practical matter, the immediate family history is the place to focus. It is important to note that the pattern of inheritance relates to the symptoms (e.g., Rhinitis, Asthma, etc.) not the specific allergen in question (e.g., cats and allergies).

Previous Allergy Diagnosis and Treatments

Skin testing, laboratory tests, imaging studies, immunotherapy, specific medications, and the response to past treatments are other vital components to the patient's medical history. Gathering this data is helpful in situations where the complaint is more complex. One particularly helpful reason for gathering data about previous immunotherapy (allergy shots) is that adults may experience recurrent symptoms after many years of remission. This can occur when the remission was the result of successful immunotherapy. It may be important to distinguish such a relapse of symptoms from new onset. Another benefit from taking a previous history of allergy treatment may be adverse events, such as anaphylaxis, associated with either skin testing or immunotherapy.

Although office-based spirometry is now available, it was not a commonly available test in the past. When available, such objective measurements are often indispensable for a definitive diagnosis of the complaint. Likewise it is an essential tool in assessing the course of a disease (National Institutes of Health, 2002).

THE PHYSICAL EXAMINATION OF THE ALLERGIC PATIENT

The physical examination, like the history, may be focused on one or more areas depending on the nature of the patient's complaints. The usual progression from observation to percussion, palpation, and auscultation should be followed. In the initial consultation, the examination should be appropriately complete. Subsequent or follow-up examinations may be more focused.

Vital Signs

The vital signs include the pulse, respiratory rate, and blood pressure. The height and weight should also be included. Temperature can be taken when symptoms indicate.

General Appearance

This includes an overview of whether the patient looks well or ill. If ill, does it seem to be an acute problem or a chronic one? In the field of allergy, there may be an abrupt change in the patient's status. For example, I have had a patient present at the desk for a new patient consultation looking well. While filling out the questionnaire, her status changed markedly. She became flushed, anxious, and uncomfortable. A rapid assessment revealed that she was having an anaphylactic reaction to a recently ingested food. Another common example in an allergy practice is a patient who begins to experience a systemic reaction to skin testing, immunotherapy, or a medication. These changes are abrupt and can signal a life-threatening emergency.

Skin

It is important to disrobe the patient for a complete dermatologic examination. Remember the patient's privacy and comfort level in doing this examination. I find it helpful to use a preprinted anatomic diagram to record my findings. Detailed descriptions of the lesion (e.g., color, size, texture, etc.) can be noted on that same page. Another useful adjunct can be a digital camera.

Sometimes it is useful to assess a patient for dermagraphism (Latin for "skin writing"). This is done by stroking the skin with the fingernail or the wooden end of a cotton swab. Choose a pattern such as a tic-tac-toe graph. Within minutes, the stroke pattern may raise in a red wheal. This is seen in some patients with urticaria. It also must be noted as a possible complication for the puncture skin testing (i.e., it produces a false-positive reaction). The examination of the skin is often the clue to a systemic diagnosis.

Face

Facial characteristic can offer important clues. In addition to conveying a clear nonverbal message about the patient's condition, chronic changes may be apparent. In hayfever (or allergic rhinitis), the patient may have shadows (allergic shiners) beneath their eyes. Children with adenoid and/or tonsillar hypertrophy may be mouth breathers. Sometimes there is a distinctive nasal quality in the voice of someone with marked nasal congestion or obstruction.

HEENT: Head, Eyes, Ears, Nose, and Throat

HEAD: The condition of the scalp and hair should be noted.

PARANASAL SINUSES: There is much disagreement about the accuracy of two of the different ways to assess for sinusitis by way of physical examination. One is called transillumination of the sinuses. The maxillary and frontal sinuses are the only ones accessible to the anterior skull. Transillumination is done with a light in a dark room (see references for details). In general, it is not felt to be accurate or useful. The second method is light percussion with the middle finger over the frontal and maxillary sinus cavities. In my experience, if this elicits a painful response, it indicates inflammation and pressure in the corresponding sinus cavity. However, the lack of a response does not correlate with absence of sinus disease (Ball J.W., Benedict G.W., Dains J.E., et al., 2003).

EYES: The examination of the allergic person is usually limited to the external eye. This includes the eyelids, conjunctivae, and sclera. If cataracts are suspected, then an ophthalmoscope must be used (see Chapter 4).

EARS: This examination should include the external ear (pinna), the canal, and the tympanic membrane.

NOSE: The nasal examination is often omitted from a general physical examination. Use the largest available speculum for this examination. This makes it easier to see the overall anatomy of each nostril. Assess the color of the mucous membranes. Are they normal in color, pale, or erythematous? Is there any discharge? If so, is it clear or purulent? Assess the turbinates. Are they normal or edematous? Look for polyps. Assess the nasal septum for irritation, erosions, and perforations. There may also be a marked septal deviation on your inspection. If done correctly, this is not uncomfortable for the patient.

THROAT: This is accomplished with a light and usually a tongue blade. (Some patients request omitting the tongue blade.) It is important to assess for the presence or absence of tonsillar tissue. If the tonsils are present, are they enlarged or infected? The oropharynx is assessed for evidence of postnasal mucous drainage. When this is chronic, there may be lymphatic proliferation along the posterior pharynx. This is often described as "cobblestoning."

During this assessment, you may notice a foul odor (halitosis, or bad breath). This is associated with sinusitis.

Neck

Palpate the neck for adenopathy. Enlargement along the anterior cervical chain of lymph nodes can be associated with both ear and sinus infections.

Chest

In observing the chest, look for any deformities such as an increased anteroposterior (AP) diameter, pectus excavatum. Although it is unusual to see an increased AP diameter in this day of asthma therapy, its presence indicates long-standing asthma that has not been well controlled. Splinting of the chest wall, raised shoulders, intercostal retractions, and labored breathing may all indicate respiratory distress and acute symptoms in an asthmatic.

Percussion of the chest is used to define masses, consolidation, and fluid levels. These are uncommon in asthma but may complicate the course of the disease. A positive finding may also indicate the necessity of further evaluation.

Auscultation of the chest is accomplished with the diaphragm of the stethoscope. It is important to listen carefully over the entire posterior chest wall as well as the upper anterior chest. Listening laterally, especially over the right middle lobe area, is very important in the evaluation of an asthmatic. Wheezing is not always present in an asthmatic. Obstruction must be sufficient to create wheezing. In severe asthma, wheezing may disappear because of diminished airflow. (This can be an ominous finding that may signal respiratory failure.)

The overall quality of breath sounds during inhalation and exhalation must be assessed. It is also important to assess for rhonchi and rales (also known as crackles). Rales occur with consolidation of the lung tissue, usually in pneumonia. This can often be heard before pneumonia is evident on a chest radiograph. Rhonchi are breath sounds caused by turbulent airflow in the bronchi. These may indicate bronchitis. The findings on the physical examination of the chest often dictate the treatment, as well as further diagnostic studies.

Cardiovascular

The cardiovascular examination includes the pulse and blood pressure, which are usually done with the vital signs. The cardiac examination should be performed in all initial consultations. In addition to assessing the heart sounds (S1 and S2), listen for extra heart sounds. Murmurs and rubs should be noted. The presence of any cardiac abnormality must be carefully assessed for two reasons: first, its physiologic effect on the pulmonary system and second, the possible cause of pseudoasthma (see Chapter 19).

Additional Examination (as Indicated by the Patient Complaint)

An abdominal examination is indicated when the history and physical examination lead the examiner to consider any condition that may lead to splenomegaly or hepatic abnormalities.

PROCEDURES

Skin Testing

Prick skin testing (or prick puncture testing) is used to assess sensitivity to aeroallergens as well as foods. A combination of prick skin testing and intradermal skin testing is used to assess venom allergy and penicillin allergy. This and radioallergosorbent (RAST) testing are discussed in the appropriate chapters that follow.

I mention it here at the end of the physical examination section because it is so integral to the assessment of the most common allergic disorders. It is often efficient to skin-test a patient after taking the history and examining them. By using a small number of screening aeroallergens, you can quickly and efficiently give the patient an indication about the cause of their symptoms. Is it just one allergen (e.g., Grandma's cat) or is it multiple sensitivities? These skin tests can be read in 15 minutes after application. This is in contrast to patch tests (see contact dermatitis), which are applied with a tape and must be read in 48 to 72 hours.

Spirometry and Peak Flow Meters

Spirometry and flow volume loops are well-standardized tests of pulmonary function. There are many new computer programs available to the office-based practitioner with which to do spirometry. This objective measure is essential to the accurate diagnosis of asthma. It can also be used to exclude this diagnosis. The use of spirometry in the treatment of asthma can be compared to measuring the blood sugar level in treating diabetes. The values for a patient are expressed as a percentage of the predicted values for height, weight, age, and sex. Their use can be seen in the NIH guidelines for the diagnosis and treatment of asthma.

Peak flow meters were introduced as an inexpensive and easy-to-use measure of expiratory force. There are many "action plans" used in asthma that have the patient assess their own peak flow. However, unlike spirometry, these values are not standardized. Furthermore, the meters themselves vary even within the same model from the same manufacturer. The variation between different models can be so great as to create confusion. Therefore, their usefulness must be assessed on an individual basis.

Pulse Oximetry

The technology for assessing oxygen saturation of the blood has gone from being an emergency department and intensive care technology to one that is available in an outpatient setting. It certainly has a role in situations when there are many visits from patients with acute severe asthma.

Nitrous Oxide Measurement

Nitrous oxide has been found to be a marker of inflammation in the airways. As the technology for measuring exhaled nitrous oxide becomes more accessible, its use in the diagnosis and treatment of asthma is likely to increase. Some preliminary research is also being done on its use in the diagnosis of sinusitis.

Endoscopy

Fiberoptic endoscopes are commonly used in otolaryngology practices to examine the nasal passages and the paranasal sinuses. In fact, endoscopic surgery for these areas is now routine, as opposed to the previous more invasive techniques. Allergists are learning to use these endoscopes as an extension of the physical examination in appropriate patients.

EVIDENCE-BASED MEDICINE

In recent years, assessments of sleep disorders and school performance in children have been linked to snoring and nasal inflammation. This has led to further studies by Gozal et al showing that adenotonsillectomy has a positive effect on neurocognitive dysfunction. Antiinflammatory medications may also be effectual according to studies by the same group.

As we ponder these links, it brings us back to a good history and the physical examination. Enlarged tonsils or marked nasal edema found in the physical examination can lead to an expanded history about snoring and behavior in a child. The appropriate diagnostic studies and treatment can have profound benefits for that child.

CONCLUSION

In this high-tech era, it is tempting to rush to use new technologies in medicine. This may result in not taking enough time with the patient or doing too brief an examination. The satisfaction derived from good detective work leading to a positive outcome cannot be understated.

BIBLIOGRAPHY

Adkinson NF Jr, Bochner BS, Busse WW, et al. *Middleton's Allergy Principles & Practice.* Vols. 1 and 2. Philadelphia: Mosby; 2003.

American Academy of Allergy, Asthma, and Immunology, American College of Physicians. *Allergy & Immunology Medical Knowledge Self-Assessment Program.* 3rd ed. Milwaukee: American Academy of Allergy, Asthma, and Immunology; 2003.

American Academy of Allergy, Asthma, and Immunology. *Pediatric Asthma: Guide for Managing Asthma in Children.* Rochester: Academic Services Consortium; 1999.

Ausillo D, Goldman L Cecil RL, et al., eds. *Cecil Textbook of Medicine.* 22nd ed. Vols. 1 and 2. Philadelphia: Elsevier Health Sciences; 2003.

Ball JW, Benedict GW, Dains JE, et al. *Mosby's Guide to Physical Examination.* 5th ed. Philadelphia: Mosby; 2003.

Bates B. *A Guide to Physical Examination and History Taking.* 6th ed. Philadelphia: J. B. Lippincott; 1995.

Behrman RE, Jenson HB, Kliegman RM, et al. *Nelson Textbook of Pediatrics.* 17th ed. Philadelphia: Elsevier Health Sciences; 2004.

Goldbart AD, Gozal D, Krishna J, et al. Inflammatory mediators in exhaled breath condensate of children with obstructive sleep apnea syndrome. *Chest.* 2006;130:142.

Gozal D. Sleep apnea in children—treatment considerations. *Paediatr Respir Rev.* 2006;7.1:S58.

Gozal D, Kheirandish L. Neurocognitive dysfunction in children with sleep disorders. *Dev Sci.* 2006;9:388.

Imboden JB, Parslow TG, Sites DP, et al. *Medical Immunology.* 10th ed. New York: McGraw-Hill; 2001.

National Institutes of Health. *Global Initiative for Asthma.* Bethesda, Md: National Institutes of Health Publication No. 95–3659; 1995.

National Institutes of Health. *Practical Guide for the Diagnosis and Management of Asthma.* Bethesda, Md: National Institutes of Health Publication No. 97–4053; 1997.

National Institutes of Health. *Guidelines for the Diagnosis and Management of Asthma: Expert Panel Report 2, Clinical Practice Guidelines.* Bethesda, Md: National Institutes of Health Publication No. 97–4051; 1997.

National Institutes of Health. *Guidelines for the Diagnosis and Management of Asthma: Expert Panel Report 2, Clinical Practice Guidelines—Update on Selected Topics 2002.* Bethesda, Md: National Institutes of Health Publication No. 02–5075; 2002.

Prevalence of Allergic Diseases in Children, Adults, and the Elderly

Massoud Mahmoudi, DO, PhD

Allergic diseases affect individuals of all ages from infancy to old age. The incidence and prevalence of the specific disease, however, changes as the allergic individual approaches late adulthood. Factors affecting the natural history of allergic diseases include genetic predisposition, environmental exposure, occupational exposure, climate, infection, socioeconomic status, and, most importantly, physiologic changes during aging (Table 3–1).

Theoretically, the same allergic disease may present in different age groups; yet the prevalence of a specific allergic disease may be higher in one age group than another. An allergic disease in adults or the elderly, 65 years and older, is either an extension of childhood disease, or less commonly, a new incidence. Table 3–2 summarizes the prevalence of common allergies and correlated age groups.

ALLERGIC RHINITIS

Every year in the United States, 40 million people are affected by allergic rhinitis, some 10% to 30% of adults and up to 40% of the children in the population (see Chapter 6). According to the 2005 report of the National Center for Health Statistics, 7.8% of adults 18 to 44 years, 10.7% of those 45 to 64 years, 7.8% of those 65 to 74 years, and 5.4% of those 75 years and older are affected in the United States.

In early childhood (i.e., younger than 5 years), allergic rhinitis symptoms are mainly caused by indoor allergens such as pet danders, dust mites, molds, and cockroaches. Seasonal allergies start at 3 to 4 years of age; this is because of the time needed, usually two to three seasonal exposures, from sensitization to expression of the symptoms. As people reach late adulthood, allergic rhinitis becomes a less common problem.

The incidence and remission of self-reported allergic rhinitis symptoms in an adult Swedish population was a subject of an investigation. The researchers mailed two sets of questionnaires, one in 1992 and the other in 2000. Responders, 4280 individuals, were in the 20- to 59-year-old age group. Analysis of the responses indicated an increase in prevalence of allergic rhinitis from 12.4% in 1992 to 15% in 2000. The incidence of allergic rhinitis from 1992 to 2000 was 4.8%. In 2000, 23.1% had a remission. The highest incidence was in the 20- to 29-year-old age group, and the highest remission was in the 50- to 59-year-old age group.

RESPIRATORY ALLERGY-ALLERGIC ASTHMA

Asthma affects 10 million adults and approximately 5 million children in the United States alone. Only a portion of wheezers in early life becomes asthmatics as adults. In a 2002 report by the Behavioral Risk Factor Surveillance System (BRFSS), lifetime asthma prevalence and prevalence of current asthma within 50 U.S. states and the District of Columbia were 11.8% and 7.5%, respectively. Current prevalence of asthma in the same report, using analysis of data regarding racial/ethnic population in selected areas (19 states), was highest in the non-Hispanic multiracial population (15.6%), followed by the non-Hispanic American Indian/Alaska Native (11.6%), non-Hispanic blacks (9.3%), non-Hispanic whites (7.6%), non-Hispanic persons of "other" race/ethnicity (7.2%), Hispanics (5.0%), non-Hispanic Asians (2.9%), and non-Hispanic native Hawaiian/Pacific Islander (1.3%).

According to the early release of selected estimates based on data from the January–March 2006 National Health Interview Survey of National Center for Health Statistics, in early 2006, the percentage of persons of all ages who experienced an asthma episode in the past 12 months was 4.3%. The prevalence of asthma (both sexes combined) was higher among children 0 to 14 years of age than among adults age 35 years or older. The sex-adjusted prevalence of current asthma was higher

Table 3–1. Various factors affecting prevalence of allergic diseases.

Factors	Examples
Genetic predisposition	Family history of allergic disease (e.g., allergic rhinitis)
Environmental exposure	Dust mites, molds, pollens, bee stings
Infection	Viruses: upper respiratory infections (asthma exacerbations)
Physiologic changes	Atopic dermatitis (less common in elderly) Food allergy (more common in children)
Occupational exposure	Latex allergy (e.g., in health care professionals)
Climate	Cool, dry, and humid climate affects growth of certain organisms (e.g., humidity and dust mites)
Socioeconomic status	Asthma: more prevalent in people with low socioeconomic status

among non-Hispanic black children under 15 years of age than among non-Hispanic white children of the same age group. For individuals older than 15 years of age, the prevalence of current asthma was similar among Hispanics, whites, and blacks).

To understand the natural history of asthma, patients must be followed over a long period of time. In a study reported by Lombardi and colleagues, 99 patients (mean age, 31 years) with allergic rhinitis alone (44), allergic asthma alone (12), and allergic asthma and allergic rhinitis (43) were followed for a period of 10 years. The report found that after 10 years of follow-up, 31.8% of allergic rhinitis patients had developed allergic asthma and 50% of patients with allergic asthma had developed allergic rhinitis. The study showed that the outcome of the disease progression was not the same for all the individuals.

Uncontrolled asthma in young adults leads to future airway remodeling later in adulthood. In addition, often elderly asthmatics present with a picture of asthma/chronic obstructive pulmonary disease (COPD); such

patients have a poorer prognosis and are more difficult to manage and treat than those with asthma alone (see Chapter 30).

FOOD ALLERGY

Food allergy is the most common in infants and children. By 2 to 3 years of age, most food allergies resolve, although some extend to adulthood. Cow's milk allergy is the most common food allergy in infancy with an incidence of 2% to 3% in the first year of life. Fortunately, there is an approximately 40% to 50% remission at 1 year of age, and the number increases to 60% to 75% at 2 years and to 85% to 90% at 3 years of age. In some children, complete remission may take 8 to 10 years.

Allergies to certain food groups such as tree nuts, peanuts, fish, and shellfish usually persist for life. Although 20% of children outgrow a peanut allergy by 5 years of age, tree nut allergy in one study was reported to have remission in 9% of patients.

Table 3–2. Prevalence of allergic diseases in various age groups.

Allergic Disease	Infancy–5 y	5–20 y	20–65 y	≥65 y
Atopic dermatitis	+++	++	+	+ or −
Allergic rhinitis	++	++	++	+
Allergic asthma	+ or −	+	++	++
Food allergy	++	+	+ or −	+ or −
Occupational allergy	−	+ or −	++	+

−, none; +–+++, increase of prevalence; + or −, rare occurrence.

In adults and the elderly, a food allergy is usually an extension of a childhood allergy, and a new food reaction is mostly a result of a food-adverse reaction and intolerance.

ATOPIC DERMATITIS

Atopic dermatitis is a common form of allergy in children. In the first few months of life, the motor skills of infants are not fully developed, and as a result, they are unable to scratch themselves and cause eczematous lesions. Williams and Strachan, using the National Child Developmental Study (NCDS), a database of 6877 children born in England, Wales, and Scotland during the one week in March 1958, analyzed the age of onset and clearance rate for examined and/or reported eczema at ages 7, 11, 16, and 23 years. Of the 571 children with reported or examined eczema, 65% had clearance at the age of 11 years and 74% at the age of 16 years.

In adults, atopic dermatitis is usually an extension of childhood onset, but adult-onset atopic dermatitis has also been reported. In a report by Ozkaya, the files of 376 patients with atopic dermatitis between June 1996 and June 2003 were analyzed. Of the patients studied, 16.8% (63 patients) had adult onset at age 18 to 71 years. Of the affected patients who developed atopic dermatitis, a majority (73%) were 18 to 29 years, followed by 30 to 39 years (14.3%), 50 to 59 years (6.3%), 40 to 49 years (4.8%), and 70 to 79 years (1.6%). In the study, flexural involvement was the main involved sites (88.9%), whereas trunk and extremities were the main nonflexural involved areas. For the complete discussion of atopic dermatitis, see Chapter 12.

OCCUPATIONAL ALLERGY

As individuals age, occupational allergies become prevalent. This is because younger adults may occupy their time with school and part-time jobs. Older adults, however, participate in various jobs in industry, manufacturing plants, and office settings, which increases the chance of developing sensitivity and finally allergy because of day-to-day exposure to occupational allergens. One example is a latex allergy in those with frequent exposure to latex products. This is seen in health care providers, workers at toy manufacturing plants, and others who are in frequent contact with latex products.

Older adults retire and are no longer in contact with potential occupational allergens. Occupational allergy during active employment will likely subside after retirement.

EVIDENCE-BASED MEDICINE

Many studies have enlightened us about the natural history of allergic diseases. One in particular is a longitudinal, population-based cohort study of childhood asthma in New Zealand children. The study followed a group of children born in New Zealand between 1972 and 1973 at 3 years of age, then every 2 years between 3 and 15 years of age, and then at 18, 21, and 26 years of age. The assessment included spirometry, methacholine test, prick skin testing to some indoor and outdoor allergens, and questionnaires regarding health, symptoms, and treatment history. According to the outcome, at age 26 years among 613 study members who provided respiratory data at every assessment, 14.5% had persistent wheezing from onset to 26 years of age, 12.4% had relapse, 15% were free of wheezing at 26 years of age, 9.5% had intermittent wheezing, 12.4% had transient wheezing, and 27.4% had a remission. The study identified sensitization to house dust mites, airway hyperresponsiveness, female sex, smoking, and early age at onset as risk factors predicting persistence or relapse of the wheezing. Thus by proper recognition of risk factors in affected children, one may be able to change the outcome of asthma in adulthood.

BIBLIOGRAPHY

American Academy of Allergy Asthma and Immunology. *The Allergy Report.* Vol. 1. Milwaukee: American Academy of Allergy Asthma and Immunology; 2000.

Centers for Disease Control and Prevention. Asthma prevalence and control characteristics by race/ethnicity—United States, 2002. *MMWR.* 2004;53:145.

Fleischer DM, Conover-Walker MK, Matsui EC, et al. The natural history of tree nut allergy. *J Allergy Clin Immunol.* 2005;116:1087.

Host A. Frequency of cow's milk allergy in childhood. *Ann Allergy Asthma Immunol.* 2002;89(suppl 1):33.

Lombardi C, Passalacqua G, Gargioni S, et al. The natural history of respiratory allergy: a follow-up study of 99 patients up to 10 years. *Respir Med.* 2001;95:9.

National Center for Health Statistics. *Early Release of Selected Estimates Based on Data from January–March 2006 National Health Interview Survey.* Bethesda, Md: CDC; 2006.

National Center for Health Statistics. *Summary Health Statistics for U.S. Adults: National Health Interview Survey.* Bethesda, Md: CDC; 2006.

Nihlen U, Greiff L, Montnemerry P, et al. Incidence and remission of self-reported allergic rhinitis symptoms in adults. *Allergy.* 2006;61:1299.

Ozkaya E, Adult-onset atopic dermatitis. *J Am Acad Dermatol.* 2005;52:579.

Sears MR, Greene JM, Willan AR, et al. A longitudinal, population-based, cohort study of childhood asthma followed to adulthood. *N Engl J Med.* 2003;349:1414.

Williams HC, Strachan DP. The natural history of childhood eczema: observations from the British 1958 birth cohort study. *Br J Dermatol.* 1998;139:834.

Wood R. The natural history of food allergy. *Pediatrics.* 2003; 111:1631.

Allergic Diseases of the Eye

Eric Kavosh MD, and Leonard Bielory, MD

Physicians in all specialties frequently encounter various forms of inflammatory diseases of the eye that present as red eyes in their general practice. However, the eye is rarely the only target for an immediate allergic-type response (less than 5% of allergic patients). Typically, patients have other atopic manifestations, such as rhinoconjunctivitis, rhinosinusitis, asthma, urticaria, or eczema. However, ocular signs and symptoms may be the initial and the most prominent feature of the entire allergic response that patients present to their physician.

The prevalence of allergies ranges as high as 30% to 50% of the U.S. population. Industrialized countries report greater allergy prevalence, correlating with the original reports of vernal catarrh in Great Britain after the Industrial Revolution. Many theories abound about the increasing prevalence of allergies in the United States, such as increased industrialization, pollution, urbanization, and the hygiene theory. The combination of allergic nasal and ocular symptoms (rhinoconjunctivitis) is extremely common, but it is not clear whether the two are equal (i.e., whether rhinitis is more common than conjunctivitis or vice versa). In studies of allergic rhinitis, allergic conjunctivitis is reported in more than 75% of patients, whereas asthma is reported in the range of 10% to 20%. However, in some studies that report a high prevalence of seasonal allergic rhinitis in the United States, the ratio of ocular to nasal symptoms appears clearly to double throughout all sections of the country.

The eye is probably the most common site for the development of allergic inflammatory disorders because it has no mechanical barrier to prevent the impact of allergens such as pollen on its surface. Allergic inflammatory disorders are commonly found in conjunction with allergic rhinitis, which is considered the most common allergic disorder. Although the nasal and ocular symptoms more appropriately called *conjunctivorhinitis* may be perceived as a mere nuisance, their consequences can profoundly affect the patient's quality of life. Seasonal allergic rhinitis and conjunctivitis have been associated with headache and fatigue, impaired concentration and

learning, loss of sleep, and reduced productivity. Patients may also suffer from somnolence, functional impairment, and increased occupational risks for accidents or injuries secondary to sedating oral antihistamine therapy, especially those sold over the counter. In 70% of patients with seasonal allergies, conjunctivitis symptoms are at least as severe as rhinitis symptoms.

THE OCULAR SURFACE

The surface of the eye easily attracts many deposits such as allergens and other ocular irritants. These agents are concentrated in tears, absorbed systematically, and can cause allergic conjunctivitis as well as irritant conjunctivitis. Overuse of vasoconstrictive agents used to alleviate allergic conjunctivitis can cause conjunctivitis medicamentosa. Uveitis, scleritis, or other systemic autoimmune disorders may also be a cause of red eye. Allergic inflammatory disorders are not limited to the eye and can affect the local ocular skin and tissue, mucosa, and sinuses. These effects are due to the inflammatory response, which is mediated by the release of histamine, leukotrienes, and neuropeptides.

CLINICAL EXAMINATION

The clinical examination of the eyes for ocular allergy should include an examination of the periorbital tissue as well as the eye itself. The eyelids and eyelashes are examined for the presence of erythema on the lid margin, telangiectasias, scaling, thickening, swelling, collarettes of debris at the base of the eyelashes, periorbital discoloration, blepharospasm, and ptosis that are seen in blepharoconjunctivitis and dermatoconjunctivitis. Next, the conjunctivae are examined for hyperemia (injection), cicatrization (scarring), and chemosis (clear swelling). The presence or absence of discharge from the eye is noted, as are its amount, duration, location, and color. Differentiation between scleral and conjunctival injection must be made in the clinical examination. Scleral injection (scleritis) tends to develop over several days and is associated with moderate or severe ocular pain on motion. Conjunctivitis is associated with discomfort but not *pain*. Scleritis commonly develops in patients with systemic autoimmune disorders, such as systemic lupus erythematosus, rheumatoid arthritis, and Wegener granulomatosis, but it has been known to occur in the absence of any other obvious clinical disorders. Another form of ocular injection is described as a ring of erythema around the limbal junction of the cornea (ciliary flush) that is a clinical sign for intraocular inflammation such as uveitis. The conjunctival surface should also be closely examined for the presence of inflammatory follicles or papillae involving the bulbar and tarsal conjunctivae. Follicles may be distinguished as grayish, clear, or yellow bumps, varying in size from pinpoint to 2 mm in diameter with conjunctival vessels on their surface, whereas papillae contain a centrally located tuft of blood vessels. The cornea is rarely involved in acute forms of allergic conjunctivitis, whereas in the chronic forms of ocular allergy, such as vernal keratoconjunctivitis and atopic keratoconjunctivitis, the prefix kerato- reflects the common involvement of the cornea.

The optimum examination of the cornea is with the slit-lamp biomicroscope. However, many important clinical features may be seen with the naked eye or a handheld direct ophthalmoscope. The direct ophthalmoscope can provide the desired magnification by "plus" (convex) and "minus" (concave) lenses. The cobalt blue filter on the new handheld ophthalmoscopic heads assists in highlighting anatomic anomalies affecting the cornea or the conjunctiva, which has been stained with fluorescein. The cornea should be perfectly smooth and transparent. Mucus adhering to the corneal or conjunctival surfaces is considered pathologic. Dusting of the cornea may indicate punctate epithelial keratitis. A localized corneal defect may develop into erosion or a larger ulcer. A corneal plaque may be present if the surface appears dry and white or yellow. The limbus is the zone immediately surrounding the cornea and normally invisible to the naked eye, but when inflamed this area becomes visible as a pale or pink swelling. Some case reports of limbal allergy exist. Conjunctival erythema can be measured objectively with a spectroradiometer, which measures the chromaticity of reflected light. Erythema and edema are graded by observation using a 0 to 4 scale. Itching is also graded on a 0 to 4 scale. Edema can be measured objectively by using a fractional millimeter reticule in the eyepiece of a slit-lamp microscope. Discrete swellings with small white dots (Horner-Trantas dots) are indicative of degenerating cellular debris, which are commonly seen in chronic forms of conjunctivitis. In addition, because the eye has thin layers of tissue surrounding it, there is an increased tendency to develop secondary infections that can further complicate the clinical presentation.

Direct signs of inflammation such as conjunctival injection and edema significantly correlate with the severity of corneal complications. The height of papillae and the amount of mucous discharge do not necessarily correlate with the severity of corneal complications.

IMMUNOPATHOPHYSIOLOGY OF OCULAR ALLERGY

Allergic diseases affecting the eyes constitute a heterogeneous group of clinicopathologic conditions with a vast array of clinical manifestations that range from simple intermittent symptoms of itching, tearing, or redness to severe sight-threatening corneal impairment (Table 4–1). Inflammation of the conjunctiva rather than mechanical factors play a greater role in the formation of corneal damage in chronic allergic eye disease. These conditions may be considered part of an immunologic spectrum that affects the anterior surface of the eye with a variety of disorders that may overlap and include seasonal and perennial allergic conjunctivitis (SAC, PAC), vernal and atopic keratoconjunctivitis (VKC, AKC), and giant papillary conjunctivitis (GPC). In addition, tear film dysfunction, also known as dry-eye syndrome, commonly complicates ocular allergy and its treatments, especially as the age of the patient increases. Tear film dysfunction is also included in the spectrum of IgE-mast cell hypersensitivity conditions to mixtures of mast cell and cell-mediated disorders that involve different mechanisms, cytokines, and cellular population. For example, mast cell degranulation, histamine release, and eosinophils play key roles in the common forms of seasonal and perennial conjunctivitis. In contrast, AKC and VKC are characterized by more chronic, inflammatory cellular infiltrates, primarily composed of CD8+ lymphocytes with minimal interplay with mast cells. Tear film dysfunction, which is a CD4+ mediated disorder, commonly complicates ocular allergy syndromes.

Mast cell mediators, such as histamine, tryptase, leukotrienes, and prostaglandins in the tear fluid, have diverse and overlapping biologic effects, all of which contribute to the characteristic itching, redness, watering, and mucous discharge associated with both acute and chronic allergic eye disease. Histamine alone is involved in regulation of vascular permeability, smooth muscle contraction, mucus secretion, inflammatory cell migration, cellular activation, and modulation of T-cell function. Histamine is a principal mediator involved in ocular allergy and inflammation. It is estimated that human conjunctival tissue contains approximately 10,000 mast cells per cubic millimeter. Large amounts of histamine are present in several mammalian ocular structures, including the retina, choroid, and optic nerve. Histamine receptors have been found on the conjunctiva, cornea, and ophthalmic arteries. Most ocular allergic reactions are mediated through the effects of

Table 4–1. Differential diagnosis of conjunctival inflammatory disorders.

Criteria	AC	VKC	AKC	GPC	DCS	BACT	VIR	CHLMD	DES	BC
Signs										
Predominant cell types	MC/eos	L/eos	L/eos	L/eos	L	PMN	PMN/M/L	M/L	M/L	M/L
Chemosis	+	+/–	+/–	+/–	–	+/–	+/–	+/–	–	+/–
Lymph node	–	–	–	–	–	+	++	+/–	–	–
Cobblestoning	–	++	++	++	–	–	+/–	+	–	–
Discharge	Clear mucoid	Stringy mucoid	Stringy mucoid	Clear white	+/–	++ mucopurulent	Clear mucoid	++ mucopurulent	+/– mucoid	++ mucopurulent
Lid involvement	–	+	+	–	++	+ (glue lids)	–	–	–	++
Symptoms										
Pruritus	+	+++	++	++	+	–	–	–	–	+
Burning	–	+	+	–	–	–	++	+	+	–
Gritty sensation	+/–	+/–	+/–	+	+	+	+	+	+++	++
Seasonal variation	+	+	+/–	+/–	–	+/–	+/–	+/–	–	–

The differential diagnosis of the red eye includes various inflammatory conditions that involve the outside and the inside of the eye. The list here focuses on the signs and symptoms of external causes of the red eye, which include the predominant cell type found in the conjunctival scraping and the presence or absence of chemosis, lymph node involvement, cobblestoning of the conjunctival surface, discharge, lid involvement, pruritus, gritty sensation, and seasonal variation.

AC, allergic conjunctivitis; AKC, atopic keratoconjunctivitis; BACT, bacterial; BC, blepharoconjunctivitis; CHLMD, chlamydial infection; DCS, dermatoconjunctivitis; DES, dry-eye syndrome; eos, eosinophil; GPC, giant papillary conjunctivitis; L, lymphocyte; M, monocyte; MC, mast cell; PMN, polymorphonuclear cell; VC, vernal conjunctivitis; VIR, viral; VKC, vernal keratoconjunctivitis.

histamine on H1 receptors. Histamine can induce changes in the eye similar to those seen in other parts of the body. These include capillary dilation leading to conjunctival redness, increased vascular permeability leading to chemosis, and smooth-muscle contraction.

In more severe chronic allergy-related conditions, T cells are the key components in ocular-surface impairment. Two predominant inflammatory pathways are differentiated by the CD4+ and CD8+ cell markers, which involve different cytokines and are crudely considered as antagonistic of each other when activated. In previous reports based on conjunctival biopsies in allergic patients, cytokine profiling displayed that Th2 activation occurred in VKC, whereas both CD4+ and CD8+ activation were found in AKC. Historically, studies using conjunctival biopsies or brush cytology specimens have demonstrated increased CD8+ cytokines in SAC: IL-4 and IL-13. However, in more recent tear studies, the only cytokine found to be significantly increased in SAC was IL-13. In addition, it is not rare for a patient treated for typical seasonal allergic conjunctivitis also to develop dry eye, tear film disturbance, meibomian dysfunction, adverse effects from the repeated use of toxic preservative-containing topical drugs, or contact cell-mediated conjunctival or eyelid hypersensitivity: conditions linked to the CD4+ cascade.

The four major ocular allergies, SAC/PAC, AKC, VKC, and GPC, exhibit increased levels of conjunctival cell adhesion molecules (CAMs) and eosinophils in conjunctival scrapings. The tears of patients challenged with high-dose allergens have been found to exhibit eosinophil cationic protein (ECP), which correlates with their symptomatology. Eosinophils found in the conjunctiva of patients with VKC are considered to be the "histologic hallmark" of the disease. It has been suggested that because the quantity of eosinophils correlate highly with the allergic signs, symptoms, and severity of VKC patients, their clinical status could be represented by tear ECP levels, which also correlate highly with the number of eosinophils. A large amount of major basic protein (MBP) has also been found in the tears of patients with VKC. The MBP is associated with the corneal ulcerations found in patients with VKC. In vitro experiments have shown that MBP exhibits corneal toxicity and retards wound repair in corneal epithelial cells. The number of eosinophils is higher in patients with corneal erosions and ulcers as opposed to those with superficial keratopathy, which suggests that eotaxin causes corneal damage in AKC. Interestingly, patients with GPC have higher levels of eosinophilic infiltrate than both VKC and AKC; however, tear ECP levels in these patients are significantly lower than tears from patients with VKC and AKC. Neutrophils as well as neutrophil-derived mediators (neutrophil myeloperoxidase, elastase) are also increased in the tears of both AKC and VKC. However, IL-8, which is a neutrophil

chemoattractant, is increased in tears from AKC but not in tears from VKC. IL-8 still plays a role in the pathogenesis of VKC, but the response of IL-8 is enhanced in AKC. Colonization of *Staphylococcus aureus* is a possible explanation for the enhancement of IL-8 in AKC. Peptidoglycan from *S. aureus* has been shown to stimulate IL-8 release from conjunctival epithelial cells and is enhanced in the presence of interferon (IFN). AKC is a manifestation of atopic dermatitis, and 67% of atopic dermatitis patients have colonization with *S. aureus* within conjunctival sacs and eyelid margins.

ACUTE ALLERGIC CONJUNCTIVITIS

Allergic conjunctivitis (AC) is a bilateral, self-limiting conjunctival inflammatory process. AC occurs in sensitized patients with no sex difference. The most common target organ for the mast cell IgE hypersensitivity-mediated reaction may actually be the eye. The allergic reaction in allergic conjunctivitis is caused by direct exposure of the ocular mucosal surfaces to environmental allergens such as pollens from trees, grasses, and weeds. These allergens interact with the pollen-specific IgE found on the mast cells of the eye. Of all the various pollens, ragweed has been identified as the most common cause of conjunctivorhinitis in the United States. Ragweed attributes for approximately 75% of all cases of hay fever with prevalence varying among different age groups in various regions of the world. Early allergy testing revealed timothy grass as one of the most potent ocular allergy-inducing allergens. There are two forms of AC seasonal allergic conjunctivitis (SAC) and perennial allergic conjunctivitis (PAC), which are defined by whether the inflammation is associated with seasonal change (spring, fall) or perennially. Both entities share the same inflammatory symptoms. However, seasonal allergic conjunctivitis is related to atmospheric pollens such as grass, trees, and ragweed that appear during specific seasons, whereas perennial allergic conjunctivitis is related to animal dander, dust mites, or other allergens that are present in the environment continuously. A major distinguishing feature between AC and VKC/AKC is that AC is self-limited, not causing ocular or visual damage, and VKC/AKC involves the cornea causing visual damage. Common conjunctival symptoms in AC include itching, tearing, and often burning. Involvement of the cornea is rare; however, blurring of vision can occur. Clinical signs include a milky or pale pink conjunctiva with vascular congestion that may progress to conjunctival swelling (chemosis). A white exudate may form during the acute state, becoming stringy in the chronic form. Ocular signs are typically mild; the conjunctiva frequently takes on a pale, boggy appearance that evolves into diffuse areas of papillae (small vascularized nodules), which tend to be most prominent on the superior palpebral conjunctiva.

Occasionally, dark circles beneath the eyes (allergic shiners) are present, which are formed as a result of localized venous congestion. The ocular reaction seen in both seasonal AC and perennial AC often resolves quickly when the offending allergen is removed. A detailed history from the patient or family members can expedite the diagnosis of AC. A family history of atopy or hay fever is often elicited. Both SAC and PAC are treated with agents that combine both antihistamines and mast cell stabilizers. The rationale for the dual treatment is rapid symptomatic relief with the antihistamine and long-term disease-modifying benefits with mast cell stabilization.

VERNAL KERATOCONJUNCTIVITIS

VKC is defined as a chronic allergic disorder of the conjunctiva mediated by mast cells and lymphocytes. There are three major forms of the disease: palpebral, limbal, and mixed. VKC is most prevalent in the spring (vernal). Symptoms include vehement bilateral ocular pruritus, which is often induced by nonspecific stimuli: dust, wind, bright light, hot weather, or physical exertion. VKC is more common in prepubescent boys; however, after puberty the sexes are equally afflicted. It is also noted that the symptoms of the disease cease in the third decade of life. The most remarkable physical finding in VKC is giant papillae present on the tarsal conjunctiva, measuring 7 to 8 mm in diameter of the upper tarsal plate, which result in the cobblestone appearance seen on examination. Horner points and Horner-Trantas dots, thin, copious, mild-white fibrinous secretions or yellowish-white points, may be present. Other physical findings include an extra eyelid crease (Dennie line), corneal ulcers, or a pseudomembrane formation of the upper lid when everted and exposed to heat (Maxwell-Lyon sign). VKC is most often bilateral; however, 5% of patients are affected more in one eye with severe cases causing blindness. The use of a cobalt blue light with the application of topical fluorescein dye can reveal diffuse areas of punctate corneal epithelial defects. These defects may progress into shield ulcers, which are areas of desquamation of epithelial cells caused by the release of major basic protein from eosinophilic infiltrate. More than 50% of patients with VKC have negative skin tests and radioallergosorbent tests to allergens despite the fact that VKC is an ocular allergy. Approximately 50% of patients with VKC do not report a history of atopic disease and do not show IgE sensitization, which proposes that VKC is not entirely mediated by IgE. VKC is characterized by infiltration of the conjunctiva by eosinophils, basophils, mast cells, CD4+ Th2, monocytes, macrophages, dendritic cells, plasma cells, and B lymphocytes organized as small lymphoid follicles. It is these infiltrates that cause the corneal involvement, photophobia, foreign body sensation, and lacrimation that are present in VKC. Conjunctival epithelium serves not only as an anatomic barrier, but they are also capable of synthesizing chemokines, most notably eotaxin, a potent CC chemokine, and RANTES (regulated on activation, normal T-cell expressed and secreted) that can modulate inflammation. It has been noted that tarsal and bulbar conjunctival biopsy specimens with VKC have stained positive for estrogen and progesterone receptors. Thus implicating that eosinophilic infiltrate in VKC may be influenced by these hormones.

The treatment of VKC includes cold compress, natural tears, avoidance of any known triggers, topical antihistamines, topical mast cell stabilizers, and periodic use of corticosteroids for acute exacerbations. The use of FK-506 has also shown favorable responses in VKC. In comparison to 2% cyclosporine, FK-506 was shown to decrease symptoms of VKC up to 26% from baseline, and FK-506 was not associated with the persistent burning sensation described with 2% cyclosporine. Montelukast treatment of asthma patients with coexisting VKC resulted in decreased hyperemia, secretion, chemosis, burning, tearing, and photophobia. The benefits persisted 15 days after discontinuation of treatment; thus suggesting a role for leukotrienes in VKC with coexisting asthma. The plaques associated with VKC, caused by eosinophilic infiltrate, may be removed by superficial keratectomy with possible reepithelialization of the cornea. Potential future treatments for VKC are targeting chemokine receptor antagonists to inhibit inflammation of the conjunctiva.

ATOPIC KERATOCONJUNCTIVITIS

AKC is a bilateral, chronic mast cell and lymphocyte mediated allergic disorder involving the conjunctiva, eyelids, and periorbital tissue often associated with a family history of atopy, eczema, and asthma. Approximately 15% to 40% of patients with atopic dermatitis also have ocular involvement due to AKC. Patients often have atopic dermatitis and or eczema from childhood and develop the ocular symptoms of AKC later in life. Primary care physicians should expect to see approximately 25% of their elderly patients who have eczema to develop some components of AKC. It usually presents in individuals older than 50 years. However, onset can occur as early as the late teens. There is no racial or geographical preference. AKC can cause disabling symptoms including blindness when the cornea is involved. Ocular symptoms of AKC are similar to the cutaneous symptoms of eczema, including intense pruritus and edematous, coarse, and thickened eyelids. Severe AKC is associated with complications such as blepharoconjunctivitis, cataract, corneal disease, and ocular herpes simplex, ropelike mucus discharge, tylosis, and meibomian gland dysfunction. The symptoms of AKC commonly include itching, burning, and tearing that are more severe than those seen in allergic conjunctivitis or perennial allergic conjunctivitis. The symptoms of AKC also tend to be present throughout the year. But it is also associated with seasonal exacerbations, especially in the winter and summer months. AKC can be exacerbated by exposure to animal dander, dust, and certain foods. The chronicity of AKC and corneal infiltration are due to T-cell involvement. However, unlike vernal keratoconjunctivitis, which has a T helper-cell type 2 profile, AKC is associated with a T helper-cell type 1 profile. Of note, mast cells and eosinophils are found in conjunctival epithelium of AKC patients but not in patients not afflicted with VKC. Ocular disease activity in AKC correlates with exacerbations and remissions of the dermatitis. AKC-associated cataracts occur in approximately 10% of patients with the severe forms of atopic dermatitis but are especially prone to occur in young adults approximately 10 years after the onset of the atopic dermatitis. A unique feature of AKC cataracts is that they predominantly involve the anterior portion of the lens and may evolve rapidly into complete opacification within 6 months. AKC patients may also develop posterior polar-type cataracts due to the prolonged use of topical or oral corticosteroid therapy. A small percentage of patients with atopic dermatitis also develop keratoconus, a conical protrusion of the cornea caused by thinning of the stroma. Retinal detachment is increased in patients with AKC; however, it is also increased in patients with atopic dermatitis in general. An association has been found between specific microorganisms such as *S. aureus* and keratoconjunctivitis. Staphylococcal enterotoxin-specific IgE antibody in tears of patients with VKC and AKC have been found. Staphylococcal enterotoxin may be an exacerbating factor and cause a type I allergic reaction as well as VKC and AKC. Treatment for AKC involves corticosteroids, antihistamines, mast cell stabilizers as well as treatment of any features of atopic dermatitis. The clinician should use antihistamines with caution in elderly patients because they cause drying of the conjunctival surface.

GIANT PAPILLARY CONJUNCTIVITIS

GPC is not a true ocular allergy. It is the result of chronic mechanical irritation. Many of the features of GPC mimic other ocular hypersensitivity syndromes. GPC is even noted to have an increase in symptoms during the spring pollen season. Therefore, it is included in the differential diagnosis of ocular allergy. GPC has an association with extended-wear soft contact lenses and other foreign bodies, such as suture materials and ocular prosthetics. Lens-induced papillary conjunctivitis may develop 3 weeks after using soft contact lenses. Patients who wear rigid or hard contacts may develop symptoms of GPC in 14 months from the onset of

wear. The pathogenesis of GPC is due to mechanical trauma followed by repeat immunologic presentation of foreign antigens, most often surface deposits or environmental agents. The signs of GPC include a white or clear exudate on awakening, which chronically becomes thick and stringy. The patient may develop papillary hypertrophy (cobblestoning), especially in the tarsal conjunctiva of the upper lid, which is more common in patients that wear soft contact lenses than hard contact lenses, 5% to 10% versus 4%, respectively. The contact lens polymer preservatives, such as thimerosal, and proteinaceous deposits on the surface of the lens have all been implicated in the cause of GPC. Common symptoms include intense itching, decreased tolerance to contact lens wear, blurred vision, conjunctival injection, and increased mucus production. Patients wearing contact lenses produce local antigenic factors that can trigger eotaxin production, which acts as a chemoattractant for eosinophils. The eosinophils then release major basic protein and toxic mediators causing the papilla formation. The treatment for GPC involves corticosteroids, antihistamines, mast cell stabilizers, and frequent enzymatic cleaning of the lenses or changing of the lens polymers. Disposable contact lenses have been proposed as an alternative treatment. GPC usually resolves when the patient stops wearing contact lenses or when the foreign body is removed from the eye.

DRY-EYE SYNDROME (TEAR FILM DYSFUNCTION)

Dry-eye syndrome (DES), also known as tear film dysfunction, develops from decreased tear production, increased tear evaporation, or an abnormality in specific components of the aqueous, lipid, or mucin layers that compose the tear film. DES is associated with atopy, female gender, and chronic medication use, including hormone replacement therapy. DES affects over 14 million people in the United States. Symptoms of DES are typically vague and include foreign body sensation, easily fatigued eyes, dryness, burning, ocular pain photophobia, and blurry vision. Upon the onset of DES, patients complain of a mildly injected eye with excessive mucus production and gritty sensation, as compared with the itching and burning feeling that many patients report with allergy-associated histamine release onto conjunctiva. Symptoms tend to be worse late in the day, after prolonged use of the eyes or exposure to adverse environmental conditions. DES has significant economic implications, including costs associated with increased health care utilization, missed school and work, and leisure and quality-of-life issues. Although dry eye may occur as a distinct disorder resulting from intrinsic tear pathology, it is more frequently associated with other ocular and systemic disorders, including ocular allergy, chronic blepharitis, fifth or seventh nerve palsies, vitamin A deficiency, pemphigoid, and trauma. DES is a frequent confounding disorder that may complicate ocular allergic disease with several overlapping signs and symptoms, such as tearing; injection, and exacerbation. As the cornea becomes involved, the symptoms, progress to include photophobia as well as more scratchy and painful sensations. DES and ocular allergy conditions are not exclusive; as patients age, the likelihood of tear film dysfunction complicating ocular allergy increases. A more systemic form of DES, associated with systemic immune diseases such as Sjögren syndrome, rheumatoid arthritis, and HIV infection, is commonly known as keratoconjunctivitis sicca and can be a symptom in postmenopausal women. The most common cause of DES is associated with the use of anticholinergic medications, which decrease lacrimation. Drugs with antimuscarinic properties include the first-generation antihistamines and even newer agents, such as loratadine and cetirizine, phenothiazines, tricyclic antidepressants, atropine, and scopolamine. Other agents associated with a sicca syndrome include the retinoids, β-blockers, and chemotherapeutic agents. Tear film dysfunction is also associated with several pharmacologic agents, including antihistamines, anticholinergics, and certain psychotropic agents. Patients often note that their symptoms are exacerbated in the winter when heating systems decrease the relative humidity in the household to less than 25%. The Schirmer test is used to diagnose DES. The test demonstrates decreased tearing (0 to 1 mm of wetting at 1 minute and 2 to 3 mm at 5 minutes). Normal values for the Schirmer test are more than 4 mm at 1 minute and 10 mm at 5 minutes. Treatments for DES include addressing the underlying pathology, discontinuing the offending drug (if possible), and making generous use of artificial tears or ocular lubricants. Topical cyclosporine (Restasis) has been approved by the U.S. Food and Drug Administration for the treatment of DES. For severe symptoms, insertion of punctual plugs may be indicated.

CONTACT DERMATITIS OF THE EYELIDS

Contact dermatoconjunctivitis is a delayed type of lymphocytic hypersensitivity reaction involving the eyelids and the conjunctiva as opposed to an ocular allergy, which activates the IgE mast cell. The eyelid skin is extremely thin, soft, and pliable and is capable of developing significant swelling and redness with minor degrees of inflammation or irritation. As a result, the patient frequently seeks medical attention for a cutaneous reaction that elsewhere on the skin would normally be less of a concern. Two predominant forms of contact dermatitis are attributed to cosmetics of the eye. These include contact dermatoconjunctivitis and

irritant (toxic) contact dermatitis. Contact dermatoconjunctivitis is commonly associated with cosmetics to the hair, face, or fingernails (e.g., hair dye, nail polish) or with topical ocular medications (e.g., neomycin). Certain preservatives, such as thimerosal, which is in contact lens cleaning solutions, and benzalkonium chloride, which is in many topical ocular therapeutic agents have both been shown by patch testing to be causes of contact dermatitis. The most common complaints associated with contact dermatitis are stinging, burning, and itching of the eyes and lids. The symptoms are subjective and are usually transitory if there is no evidence of objective signs of irritation. The patch test can assist in pinpointing the causative antigen, but interpretation of patch test results may be difficult. Patch testing is also associated with high false-positive reactions when associated with irritants. Patch tests performed with patients' own topical ophthalmic products are often negative. However, pretreatment with sodium lauryl sulfate increases patch test sensitivity.

BLEPHAROCONJUNCTIVITIS

Blepharitis is a primary inflammation of the eyelid margins that is most often misdiagnosed as an ocular allergy because it commonly causes conjunctivitis secondary to a blepharitis. The most common causes are seborrhea and infection; the most common organism is *S. aureus*. The signs of staphylococcal blepharitis are dilated blood vessels, erythema, scales, collarettes of exudative material around the eyelash bases, and foamy exudates in the tear film. Antigenic products play the primary role in the induction of chronic eczema of the eyelid margins. Certain lipophilic organisms such as *Malassezia* yeast may be highly antigenic and induce chronic inflammatory reactions. Symptoms include persistent burning, itching, tearing, and a feeling of dryness. Blepharitis differs from dry-eye syndrome in that the symptoms of blepharitis are more persistent in the morning. The symptoms of dry-eye syndrome are more persistent in the evening. Crusted exudate develops with blepharitis that may prevent the eye from opening when the patient awakens in the morning. Blepharitis may be controlled with proper eyelid hygiene: using detergents (e.g., nonstinging baby shampoos) and steroid ointments applied to the lid margin with a cotton tip applicator that are used to loosen scales and exudate.

OCULAR ALLERGY TREATMENT

A variety of treatment approaches have been used to manage allergic symptoms, foremost among them the avoidance of triggering allergens. In addition, pharmacotherapies with antihistamines, decongestants, nasal corticosteroids, mast cell stabilizers, and anticholinergics have all proven effective, as has immunotherapy. Primary treatment of any allergy, including ocular allergy, focuses on the avoidance of allergens. This strategy primarily involves the use of environmental interventions, from removal of the offending allergen source to a change of occupational venue. However, this is not often practical because it could mean attempting to avoid the outdoors or family pets. Lubrication is a form of avoidance, in that it has a dilutional effect on allergens and released mediators that interact with the conjunctival surface. Cold compresses provide considerable symptomatic relief, especially from ocular pruritus. All ocular medications should be refrigerated to provide additional subjective relief when applied to the conjunctival surface. Systemic agents can cause ocular drying that can alter the ocular tear film's ability to act as a protective barrier against external matter such as airborne allergens. This decreased tear production may decrease the eye's ability to wash allergens from the ocular surface, allowing them to remain there longer and possibly worsen allergic signs and symptoms. Secondary treatment regimens include the symptomatic use of topical agents, as well as oral decongestants, antihistamines, mast cell stabilizing agents, and antiinflammatory agents. Topical decongestants primarily act as vasoconstrictors, which are highly effective in reducing the erythema and are widely used in combination with topical antihistamines. Adverse effects of topical vasoconstrictors include burning and stinging on instillation, mydriasis, especially in patients with lighter irises, and rebound hyperemia or conjunctivitis medicamentosa with chronic use. In the conjunctiva, H1 stimulation principally mediates the symptom of pruritus, as seen in various binding studies, whereas the H2 receptor has been inferred to be clinically involved in the vasodilation of the ocular allergic response. Although topical antihistamines may be used alone to treat AC, combined use of an antihistamine and a vasoconstricting agent is more effective than either agent alone.

As monotherapy, oral or systemic-antihistamines are an excellent choice when attempting to control multiple early-phase and some late-phase allergic symptoms in the eyes, nose, and pharynx. Despite their efficacy in relief of allergic symptoms, systemic antihistamines may result in unwanted side effects, such as drowsiness and dry mouth. Newer, second-generation antihistamines are preferred to avoid the sedative and anticholinergic effects associated with first-generation agents. SAC and PAC are ideally treated with combination antihistamine/mast cell stabilizers. These combination therapies have the advantage of giving immediate symptomatic relief via the antihistamine effect as well as having long-term modifying effects on the disease with mast cell stabilization.

When the allergic symptom or complaint is isolated, such as ocular pruritus, focused therapy with topical antihistaminic agents is often efficacious and clearly

superior, either as monotherapy or in conjunction with an oral or nasal agent. Topical antihistaminic agents provide faster and better relief than systemic antihistamines. Topical antihistaminic agents also have a longer duration of action than other classes of topical agents. However, their duration of action may not be as long as that of systemic agents. Some of these agents have been found to have merits as topical multiple-action agents possessing unique properties, including H1-receptor antagonism, low antimuscarinic properties, and H2-receptor antagonism; these maximize the symptomatic treatment of seasonal AC and are now widely used as first-line pharmacotherapy for ocular allergy (Table 4–2). Many of the selective H1-receptor antagonists have also demonstrated several antiinflammatory components that may have an impact on the ocular late-phase reaction seen in more than 50% of patients and may explain the persistent qualities of the acute allergic ocular reaction. For example, some of these newer antihistamines can block intercellular adhesion molecule-1 (ICAM-1) expression in epithelial cells, effectively reducing inflammatory cell mucosal infiltration.

The use of mast cell stabilizers such as cromolyn was originally approved for more severe forms of conjunctivitis (i.e., GPC, AKC, VKC), but many physicians have used it for the treatment of acute seasonal and perennial AC with an excellent safety record. Mast cell stabilizers inhibit degranulation and block the release of preformed mediators within the mast cell. For mast cell stabilizers to be effective, the mast cell has to be deactivated before the allergic reaction is triggered. However, mast cell stabilizers require a loading period and must be applied for several weeks before antigen exposure to fully decrease the allergic response. Compliance is important with the use of mast cell stabilizers because they require frequent, regular dosing. Some of the studies reflecting their clinical efficacy for seasonal and perennial AC found marginal efficacy when compared with placebo in clinical settings and some animal models. After many years of clinical use, the mechanisms of cromolyn are still unclear. Olopatadine is a selective long-acting antiallergic medication that combines both mast cell stabilization and antihistamine effects. Olopatadine has limited interaction with membrane phospholipids, which limits membrane disturbance. This limits the release of intracellular contents including histamine.

Ketorolac is a nonsteroidal antiinflammatory drug (NSAID) that inhibits the prostaglandin production involved in mediating ocular allergy. Ketorolac is indicated for itchiness associated with AC. Clinical studies have shown that topical NSAIDs significantly diminish the ocular itching and conjunctival hyperemia associated with seasonal antigen-induced AC and VKC. These agents, unlike topical corticosteroids, do not mask ocular infections, affect wound healing, increase intraocular pressure, or contribute to cataract formation. Some of

Table 4-2. Topical (ophthalmic) agents for allergic conjunctivitis.

Topical Ophthalmic Agents Generic (Trade) Name	Mechanism of Action	Dosage	Most Common Side Effects
Olopatadine (Patanol)	Selective H1 receptor antagonist and inhibitor of histamine release from mast cell	≥3 y: 1–2 drops up to four times daily	Headache (7%)
Ketotifen (Zaditor)	Noncompetitive H1 receptor antagonist and mast cell stabilizer	≥3 y: 1 drop up to three times daily	Conjunctival injection, headache, rhinitis (10–25%)
Azelastine (Optivar)	Competes with H1 receptor sites on effector cells and inhibits release of histamine and other mediators involved in allergic response	≥3 y: 1 drop twice daily	Ocular burning (~30%), headache (~15%), bitter taste (~10%)
Epinastine (Elestat)	Direct H1 receptor antagonist. Does not penetrate the blood-brain barrier and therefore should not induce CNS side effects	≥3 y: 1 drop twice daily	Upper respiratory infection/cold symptoms (10%)
Emedastine difumarate (Emadine)	Relatively selective histamine receptor antagonist	≥3 y: 1 drop up to four times daily	Headache (11%)
Levocabastine (Livostin)	Selective H1 receptor antagonist	≥12 y: 1 drop up to four times daily	Ocular burning, stinging, itching (10%)
Lodoxamide tromethamine (Alomide)	Mast cell stabilizer	≥2 y: 1–2 drops up to four times daily	Ocular burning, stinging, itching (10%)
Nedocromil (Alocril)	Interferes with mast cell degranulation, especially release of leukotrienes and platelet-activating factor	≥3 y: 1–2 drops twice daily	Headache (10%), bitter taste (10%), ocular burning (10%), nasal congestion (10%)
Loteprednol etabonate (Lotemax, Alrex)	Decreases inflammation by suppressing migration of polymorphonuclear leukocytes and reversing capillary permeability	≥3 y: 1–2 drops twice up to four times daily	Headache (10%), pharyngitis (10%), rhinitis (10%)
Ketorolac tromethamine (Acular)	Pyrrolo-pyrrole NSAIDs; inhibits prostaglandin synthesis	≥12 y: 1 drop up to four times daily	Ocular burning, stinging, itching (10%)

CNS, central nervous system; H1, histamine 1; NSAID, nonsteroidal antiinflammatory drug; y, years old.

the studies reflecting their clinical efficacy for seasonal and perennial AC showed marginal efficacy when compared with placebo in clinical settings and in some animal models.

Tertiary treatment of ocular allergy using more potent immunomodulatory properties may be considered when topically administered medications, such as antihistamines, vasoconstrictors, or cromolyn sodium, are ineffective. However, the local administration of topical steroids may be associated with localized ocular complications, including increased intraocular pressure, viral infections, and cataract formation. Two modified steroids, rimexolone and loteprednol, have recently been investigated for their efficacy in AC. Rimexolone is a derivative of prednisolone that is quickly inactivated in the anterior chamber. Loteprednol is another modified corticosteroid that is highly effective in the acute and prophylactic treatment of AC.

Immunotherapy has been used for the primary treatment of allergies, once known as spring catarrh before the discovery of antihistamines and other pharmacologic agents. In fact, in the original report on allergy immunotherapy in the early 1900s, it was used to "measure the patient's resistance during experiments of pollen extracts to excite a conjunctival reaction." Immunotherapy involves the application of the suspected proteins in various formulations to the mucosa of the conjunctiva, gastrointestinal tract, and nose.

Although initial studies of allergen immunotherapy did not specifically address ocular symptoms, more recent clinical studies have started to identify improvement in ocular signs and symptoms in a separate domain of assessment outcomes. Additional physiologic studies have demonstrated a logarithmic increase (10- to 100-fold) in the tolerance to the allergen in the conjunctival provocation test or improvement of ocular symptoms. Interestingly, when specific allergen immunotherapy was instituted in adults and children with multiple allergies, the treatment was both effective and specific to the allergens in their season. Subcutaneous administrations of allergen solutions are not convenient for all patients.

Experimentally, AC has been suppressed by the oral administration of the offending allergen in animal models, with the concomitant decrease in the development of allergen-specific IgE. Recent experimental studies on the use of sublingual immunotherapy have also shown statistical improvement in the nasal and ocular symptom scores, which are also associated with an increase in the threshold dose for the conjunctival allergen provocation tests. Experimental topical application of allergen or immunostimulatory sequence oligodeoxynucleotides has predominantly shown a decrease in the late-phase response. Alternative forms of immunotherapy, such as sublingual swallow therapy, have also been attempted in the treatment of seasonal and perennial rhinitis with a statistical decrease in ocular symptoms. Some produce no changes in the rhinitis symptoms, suggesting that ocular symptoms may be more sensitive to treatment with allergen immunotherapy. Future treatments for ocular allergy may concentrate on decreasing eosinophil recruitment by inhibiting CCR-3.

VASOMOTOR CONJUNCTIVITIS OR PERENNIAL CHRONIC CONJUNCTIVITIS

The identification of vasomotor conjunctivitis (VMC) or perennial chronic conjunctivitis (PerCC) is not commonly included in the differential diagnosis of allergic conjunctivitis, although it may occur in as many as 25% of patients complaining of ocular symptoms that are commonly confused with allergy. These patients are by definition skin test negative, but they react to environmental stimulants such as weather, pollution, and/or wind. These disorders need to be better defined, categorized, and classified to determine the best treatment modalities.

CONCLUSION

The prevalence of ocular allergy is clearly underappreciated; it has been an underdiagnosed and undertreated area in primary care medicine. The ocular symptoms associated with the most common ocular allergy conditions, such as SAC and PAC, are intricately linked to allergic rhinitis in more than 80% of cases. The emergence of new medications for the specific treatment of ocular symptoms over the course of the past 15 years offers a new field for improved patient care by the primary and subspecialty health care providers.

EVIDENCE-BASED MEDICINE

The principal mediator in ocular allergy and inflammation is histamine. There are large amounts of histamine in the retina, choroid, and optic nerve. Histamine receptors have been found on the conjunctiva, cornea, and ophthalmic arteries, and two separate histamine receptors, H1 and H2, have been identified in the conjunctiva. Most ocular allergic reactions are mediated through the effects of histamine on H1 receptors. Histamine concentration in tears of patients who have allergic conjunctivitis can reach values greater than 100 µg/mL, as compared with values of 5 to 15 µg/mL in controls. Histamine can stimulate capillary dilation, causing conjunctival redness, increased vascular permeability leading to chemosis, and smooth-muscle contraction.

In AKC and VKC, T cells are the predominant inflammatory cells. Two inflammatory pathways are differentiated by the TH1 and TH2 cell markers, which involve different cytokines that are antagonistic of each other when activated. Cytokine profiling displayed that

TH2 activation occurred in VKC; both TH1 and TH2 activation were found in AKC.

Many of the selective H1-receptor antagonists, olopatadine, ketotifen, azelastine, and epinastine, have also demonstrated several antiinflammatory components that may have an impact on the ocular late-phase reaction seen in more than 50% of patients and may explain the persistent qualities of the acute allergic ocular reaction. For example, some of these newer antihistamines can block ICAM-1 expression in epithelial cells, effectively reducing inflammatory cell mucosal infiltration.

Although initial studies of allergen immunotherapy did not specifically address ocular symptoms, more recent clinical studies have started to identify improvement in ocular signs and symptoms in a separate domain of assessment outcomes. Additional physiologic studies have demonstrated a logarithmic increase (10- to 100-fold) in the tolerance to the allergen in the conjunctival provocation test or improvement of ocular symptoms. Interestingly, when specific allergen immunotherapy was instituted in adults and children with multiple allergies, the treatment was both effective and specific to the allergens in their season. Subcutaneous administrations of allergen solutions are not convenient for all patients.

BIBLIOGRAPHY

Bielory L. Allergic diseases of the eye. *Med Clin North Am.* 2006;90(1):129.

Bielory L. Ocular allergy and dry eye syndrome. *Curr Opin Allergy Clin Immunol.* 2004;4(5):421.

Bielory L. Update on ocular allergy treatment. *Expert Opin Pharmacother.* 2002;3(5):541.

Bielory L, Lien KW, Bigelsen S. Efficacy and tolerability of newer antihistamines in the treatment of allergic conjunctivitis. *Drugs.* 2005;65(2):215.

Calonge M. Ocular allergies: association with immune dermatitis. *Acta Ophthalmol Scand Suppl.* 2000(230):69.

Chambless SL, Trocme S. Developments in ocular allergy. *Curr Opin Allergy Clin Immunol.* 2004;4(5):431.

Cook EB, Stahl JL, Esnault S, et al. Toll-like receptor 2 expression on human conjunctival epithelial cells: a pathway for *Staphylococcus aureus* involvement in chronic ocular proinflammatory responses. *Ann Allergy Asthma Immunol.* 2005;94(4):486.

Leonardi M, Leuenberger P, Bertrand D, et al. First steps toward noninvasive intraocular pressure monitoring with a sensing contact lens. *Invest Ophthalmol Vis Sci.* 2004;45(9): 3113.

McGill J. Conjunctival cytokines in ocular allergy. *Clin Exp Allergy.* 2000;30(10):1355.

Ono SJ, Abelson MB. Allergic conjunctivitis: update on pathophysiology and prospects for future treatment. *J Allergy Clin Immunol.* 2005;115(1):118.

Rosenwasser LJ, O'Brien T, Weyne J. Mast cell stabilization and anti-histamine effects of olopatadine ophthalmic solution: a review of pre-clinical and clinical research. *Curr Med Res Opin.* 2005;21(9):1377.

Shoji J, Kato H, Kitazawa M, et al. Evaluation of staphylococcal enterotoxin-specific IgE antibody in tears in allergic keratoconjunctival disorders. *Jpn J Ophthalmol.* 2003;47(6):609.

Srivastava A, Sur S, Trocme SD. The role of eosinophils in ocular allergy. *Int Ophthalmol Clin.* 2003;43(1):9.

Stahl JL, Barney NP. Ocular allergic disease. *Curr Opin Allergy Clin Immunol.* 2004;4(5):455.

Prevalence of Pollens in the United States and Elsewhere

5

Jennifer Yoo, MD, and Massoud Mahmoudi, DO, PhD

Sensitization to pollens is associated with significant morbidity caused by symptoms of seasonal allergic rhinitis and seasonal asthma. Understanding patterns of pollen prevalence is useful for both the diagnosis and management of patients with seasonal respiratory disease due to pollens.

Pollen grains are male gametophytes of gymnosperms and angiosperms, or higher plants. Most pollens range in size from 10 to 60 μm in diameter, the small size allowing exposure through wind carriage and contact with the respiratory mucosa and conjunctiva. Pollens are composed of an outer wall with an external layer (exine) and internal layer (intine) that enclose cytoplasm. Immediate hypersensitivity reactions can occur when pollen contacts mucosal surfaces, triggering proteins stored in the exine and intine to be released through apertures (pores or furrows) of the outer wall. Most clinically relevant pollens are windborne, or anemophilous, rather than being from entomophilous plants, which pollinate via insect carriers. Pollens vary in morphologic structure by size, number, and form of pores, thickness of the exine, and other features of the cell wall. For example, ragweed pollen is about 20 μm in diameter and has characteristic short spines, whereas grass pollens range from 30 to 40 μm, have a smooth surface, and are monoporate.

Tree Pollen

Tree pollen allergens range from 20 to 60 μm in diameter. Prevalence of different types of tree pollens mainly depends on geography. The pollen from each tree genus is morphologically distinct and shows marked variation in terms of allergenicity, duration, and seasonal pattern of pollination. Cross-reactivity among species is uncommon. Thus there is higher specificity to skin testing with individual tree pollen extracts compared with grass pollens, which do have significant cross-reactivity.

Tree pollination season varies significantly between different regions but usually occurs during the springtime. The tree season is generally brief and rather distinct because pollination occurs before, during, or shortly after leaves develop in deciduous trees. Most tree pollen characterization has been studied using birch, hazel, alder, white oak, olive, and Japanese cedar allergens. Bet v 1, a birch pollen allergen, has been studied closely; it is a commonly known allergen in the oral allergy syndrome, which is due to cross-sensitizations between food proteins and certain pollens.

Grass Pollen

Worldwide, grass pollen sensitivity is the most common cause of allergic disease, due to the wide distribution of wind-pollinated grasses. Grass pollen is the second most common cause of allergic rhinitis and seasonal asthma in the United States, following ragweed. The season generally occurs in the spring and summer. Grass pollen is typically released in the afternoon. Concentrations of grass pollen are generally low at high altitudes.

Grasses are of the family Poaceae. Most grass pollens range from 30 to 40 μm in diameter, each grain having one pore or furrow, and a thick intine. Currently, immunochemical methods have identified between 20 and 40 different grass pollen antigens. It is difficult to distinguish different types of grass pollen from each other by morphology. There is also significant cross-reactivity among the grass species, with the exception of Bermuda grass. Therefore, the relative importance of a grass species in a given region is usually determined by its regional presence.

Weed Pollen

Weeds are small annual plants that grow without cultivation and tend to have relatively inconspicuous flowers. Weed pollens range from 20 to 40 μm in diameter.

Release of weed pollen depends on seasonal daylight variation and is released typically in the morning.

The most important allergenic weed group is the Compositae family, which includes the ragweed tribe (Tribe Ambrosieae). Ragweed is the single most important cause of seasonal allergic rhinitis and asthma in North America. In the United States, the highest concentrations of ragweed are found in the central plains and eastern agricultural regions.

Ragweed pollen season occurs in the fall, generally between late August and early October. Ragweed is a prodigious plant, with a single plant being able to release 1 million pollen grains in a single day. It also has a long travel range, having been detected even 400 miles out at sea. The first studies of ragweed pollen revealed two major allergens, Amb a 1 (antigen E) and Amb a 2 (antigen K). Now, eight other intermediate or minor allergens of ragweed have also been identified.

METHODS OF POLLEN COLLECTION

Various methods exist for quantifying pollen grains. There are three main types of air samplers: passive samplers, rotary-impact samplers, and slit-type volumetric spore traps.

Passive/gravitational samplers are placed in an exposed environment, where particles are allowed to collect on the surface, which can be a microscope slide or plate. These samplers tend to overestimate larger particles, which fall more rapidly. An example of this device is the Durham sampler.

Rotary-impact samplers are made of a collection surface that collects particles as it spins through ambient air. These devices are efficient for trapping larger particles but less efficient for particles less than 5 μm in diameter. Rotorod samplers that employ plastic rods as a collection surface are a common example of a rotary-impact device.

Slit-lamp samplers contain a vacuum pump that draws air in to a chamber in which a collection surface sits. This type of device can also convert observed pollen counts to actual volumetric counts in the ambient air. It has greater efficiency in collection compared to rotary devices. An example of a slit-lamp sampler is the Burkhard trap.

WORLDWIDE PREVALENCE OF POLLENS

Clinically relevant pollens vary from region to region. Several factors may influence the pollen count in a particular region. For example, preseasonal rainfall influences vegetative growth, which then determines abundance of pollen. Also, the release of pollen from anthers is promoted by low humidity and increased winds.

The collection of dependable pollen count data is slowly being accomplished worldwide (Table 5–1).

North America

In most climates in North America, the allergy season begins with tree pollination. This usually occurs during late February through April but may start as early as December in regions with cedar trees. The main tree pollens present in North America include oak, alder, cedar, elm, birch, ash, hickory, poplar, sycamore, cypress, and walnut.

Grass pollen season overlaps with the end of tree pollen season, starting approximately in May and lasting through July. The main North American grass pollens include timothy, Bermuda, orchard, sweet vernal, and red top and blue grasses.

In the late summer through October, weed pollination occurs. The most prominent weed causing allergic symptoms is ragweed, which is the single most important cause of seasonal allergic rhinitis in the United States. Other weeds include pigweed, marsh elder, dock/sorrel, plantain, Lamb's quarters, and Russian thistle.

Africa

The most common pollens in Africa are grass pollens. South Africa, for example, has a very extensive grassland comprising more than 957 (10%) of the known grass species worldwide. African grasses belong largely to the subfamilies Chloridoideae and Panicoideae; Northern Hemisphere grasses are predominantly members of the Pooideae (Potter). There are an estimated 947 indigenous and 115 naturalized grass species. Common grass pollens include rye grass, Bermuda grass, kikuyu grass, and eragrostis. The grass season lasts through a majority of the year, stretching from August through April.

The tree season is comparatively shorter than the grass season, ranging from August through November. Common tree pollens include acacia, willow, cypress, oak, eucalyptus, plane, and poplar. Weeds are not a highly prevalent source of pollen in Africa. However, plantain is a common weed.

Asia

JAPAN

The pollen responsible for a majority of seasonal allergic disease in Japan is Japanese cedar (*Cryptomeria japonica*). The Japanese cedar pollen is present from January through May. Another significant tree pollen is cypress. Weeds play a lesser role than tree pollens in Japan. Ragweed pollen is present in August and September.

INDIA

Pollen counts vary in the different regions of India. In Northern India, tree pollens including Holoptelea, Eucalyptus, and Casuarina are highly prevalent, as well as Cassia grass.

Table 5–1. World pollen calendar.

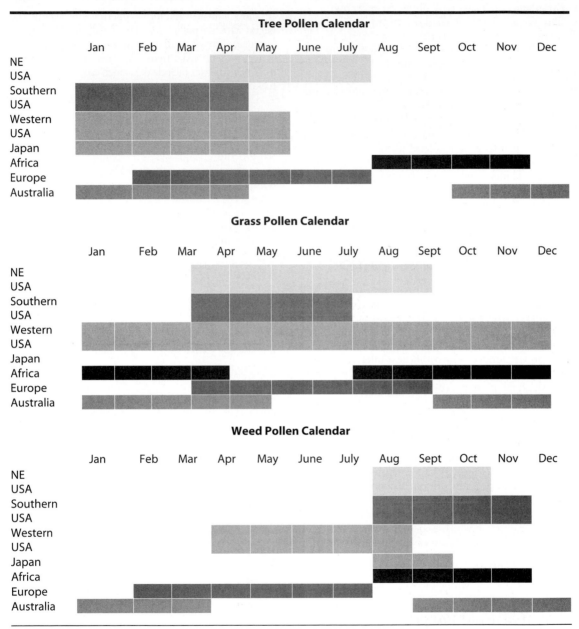

In Central India, dominant pollen types include Partheniam and Cheno/Amaranth weeds. Trees include Casuarina and Spathodia.

AUSTRALIA

The most prevalent pollens in Australia are grass species, including rye, Bermuda, annual and Kentucky blue grass, Paspalum, and prairie grass. The southeastern area is the worst affected area because of its widespread grasslands and north winds. The grass season occurs during October through June.

The dominant tree pollens include the indigenous wattle and ti-tree, as well as birch, maple, olive, poplar, ash, and oak. Plantain is the most prevalent type of weed pollen.

Table 5–2. U.S. regional pollens.

Type of Pollen	Genus and Species
Northeast Region of United States	
Trees	
Oak (white, red)	*Quercus alba, rubra*
Birch (yellow)	*Betula alleghaniensis*
Elm (white)	*Ulmus Americana*
Cottonwood	*Populus deltoids*
Beech	*Fagus grandifolia*
Ash (white)	*Fraxinus Americana*
Juniper	*Juniperus* spp.
Alder	*Alnus* spp.
Maple (sugar, red)	*Acer saccharum, rubrum*
Hickory	*Carya ovata*
Mulberry (red, black)	*Morus rubrum, nigra*
Red cedar	*Juniperus virginiana*
Sycamore	*Platanus* spp.
Walnut (black)	*Juniperus nigra*
Sweet gum	*Liquidambar styraciflua*
Grasses	
June/blue	*Poa pratensis*
Orchard	*Dactylis glomerata*
Timothy	*Phleum pretense*
Sweet vernal	*Anthoxanthum odoratum*
Red top	*Agrostis alba*
Rye	*Lolium* spp.
Weeds	
Ragweed	*Ambrosia* spp.
Lambs quarters	*Chenopodium album*
Sorrel	*Rumex* sp
Plantain	*Plantago lanceolata*
Pigweed	*Amaranthus* spp.
Mugwort	*Artemisia vulgaris*
Cocklebur	*Xanthium strumarium*
Southeast Region of United States	
Trees	
Oak (red, white)	*Quercus* spp.
Hickory (pecan)	*Carya* spp.
Maple (red)	*Acer rubrum*
Juniper/cedar	*Juniperus* spp.
Ash (white, green)	*Fraxinus americana*
Cottonwood	*Populus deltoids*
Sugar (hack) berry	*Celtis occidentalis*
Australian pine	*Casuarina* spp.
Mulberry (red, white)	*Morus* spp.
Sweet gum	*Liquidambar styraciflua*
Elm	*Ulmus* spp.
River birch	*Betula nigra*

Type of Pollen	Genus and Species
Southeast Region of United States (*Continued*)	
Grasses	
June/blue	*Poa pratensis*
Timothy	*Phleum pretense*
Bermuda	*Cynodon dactylon*
Orchard	*Dactyis glomerata*
Johnson	*Sorghum halepense*
Red top	*Agrostis alba*
Rye	*Lolium* spp.
Bahia	*Paspalum notatum*
Weeds	
Ragweed	*Ambrosia* spp.
Sorrel	*Rumex* spp
Plantain	*Plantago lanceolata*
Pigweed	*Amaranthus* spp.
Burning bush	*Kochia scoparia*
Marsh elder	*Iva* spp.
Western water hemp	*Acnida tamarascina*
Russian thistle	*Salsola pestifer*
Midwest Region of United States	
Trees	
Oak (red, white, bur)	*Quercus* spp.
Elm (white, slippery)	*Ulmus* spp.
Box elder	*Acer negundo*
Hickory (pecan)	*Carya* spp.
Juniper/cedar	*Juniperus* spp.
Maple	*Acer* spp.
Birch	*Betula* spp.
Ash	*Fraxinus* spp.
Walnut	*Juglans* spp.
Cottonwood	*Populus* spp.
Willow	*Salix* spp.
Sycamore (eastern)	*Platanus occidentalis*
Grasses	
June/blue	*Poa* spp.
Orchard	*Dactylis glomerata*
Bermuda	*Cynodon dactylon*
Timothy	*Phleum pretense*
Rye	*Lolium* spp.
Red top	*Agrostis alba*
Weeds	
Ragweed	*Ambrosia* spp.
Russian thistle	*Salsola pestifer*
Burning bush	*Kochia scoparia*
Burweed marsh elder	*Iva xanthifolia*
Plantain	*Plantago lanceolata*
Pigweed	*Amaranthus* spp.

(Continued)

Table 5–2. U.S. regional pollens. (Continued)

Type of Pollen	Genus and Species
Pacific Northwest region of the United States	
Trees	
Alder	*Alnus* spp.
Juniper/cedar	*Juniperus* spp.
Birch	*Betula* spp.
Cottonwood	*Populus* spp.
Walnut	*Juglans* spp.
Ash	*Fraxinus* spp.
Willow	*Salix* spp.
Elm	*Ulmus* spp.
Oak	*Quercus* spp.
Grasses	
June/blue	*Poa pratensis*
Timothy	*Phleum pretense*
Rye	*Lolium* spp.
Brome	*Bromus* spp.
Red top	*Agrostis alba*
Weeds	
Sage	*Artemisia* spp.
Sorrel	*Rumex* spp.
Nettle	*Urticaceae* spp.
Pigweed	*Amaranthus* spp.

Type of Pollen	Genus and Species
Southwest Region of United States	
Trees	
Juniper/cedar	*Juniperus* spp.
Elm	*Ulmus* spp.
Olive	*Olea europaea*
Ash	*Fraxinus* spp.
Mulberry	*Morus* spp.
Oak	*Quercus* spp.
Cottonwood	*Populus* spp.
Mesquite	*Prosopis* spp.
Box elder	*Acer negundo*
Grasses	
Bermuda	*Cynodon dactylon*
Johnson	*Sorghum halepense*
June/blue	*Poa* spp.
Weeds	
Ragweed	Ambrosia spp.
Sage	Artemisia spp.
Russian thistle	*Salsola kali*
Scales	*Atriplex* spp.

Europe

Europe is a geographically complex continent with a diverse climate and wide spectrum of vegetation, resulting in much variation in the types of pollens found in different areas.

By far, the most prevalent allergen in Europe is grass. Timothy, orchard, meadow foxtail, and rye grasses are highly prevalent. The grass season occurs during May through July in northern, central, and eastern Europe. In Mediterranean regions, grass begins and ends a month earlier. In general, grass flowering notoriously peaks in June.

Going northward, the tree season starts from April to late May and lasts generally through July. Pollens include birch, olive, hazel, alder, ash, and cypress. In Northern Europe, birch is a major cause of pollinosis, having the greatest allergenic potency. In Europe, the percentage of positive skin prick test to birch ranges from 5% in the Netherlands to 54% in Zurich, Switzerland. In Spain, southern Italy, and Greece, olive pollen is one of the main causes of pollinosis, with its pollination season occurring from April to June.

Weed season occurs during February through October, and pollens include ragweed, mugwort, pellitory, nettles, and less commonly ragweed.

EVIDENCE-BASED MEDICINE

As discussed, several different methods for identification of pollen have been developed. Traditional measurements of exposure to pollen grains involve collection of an air sample and identification of the pollen sources on the basis of the morphologic characteristics of the particles viewed under a microscope. Durham and Burkhard methods are commonly used worldwide.

However, newer methods are being developed in hopes of obtaining more accurate pollen count readings. For example, under certain circumstances, a significant amount of airborne allergen is not associated with intact pollen grains because some are carried on paucimicronic particles.

In the last several years, new methods of detection and morphologic identification of pollen sources have been studied. In Japan, use of imaging pollen particles by means of methods including laser scattering and also use of a photoacoustic microscope are being studied. An Australian group has also reported a new method for simultaneous immunodetection and morphologic identification of sources of pollen allergens by use of staining pollen grains with polyclonal and monoclonal antibodies, revealing not only intact pollen grains but also paucimicronic particles seen surrounding them.

BIBLIOGRAPHY

Allergy Net Australia. Available at: http://www.allergynet.com.au.

Allergy Research Group, Jikei University School of Medicine. Available at: http://www.tky.3web.ne.jp/~imaitoru/English.html.

D'Amato G, Speksma FT, Liccardi G, et al. Pollen-related allergy in Europe. *Allergy.* 1998;53:567.

Kaneko Y, Motohashi Y, Nakamura H, et al. Increasing prevalence of Japanese cedar pollinosis: a meta-regression analysis. *Inter Arch Allergy Immunol.* 2005;136:365.

Miyamoto K, Hoshimiya T. Measurement of the amount and number of pollen particles of *Cryptomeria japonica* (Taxodiaceae) by imaging with a photoacoustic microscope. *IEEE Transactions of Ultrasonics, Ferroelectrics, and Frequency Control.* 2006;53:586.

Potter PC, Cadman A. Pollen allergy in South Africa. *Clin Exp Allergy.* 1996;26:1347.

Razmovski V, O'Meara T, Taylor D, et al. A new method for simultaneous immunodetection and morphologic identification of individual sources of pollen allergens. *J Allergy Clin Immunol.* 2000;105:725.

Singh A, Kumar P. Aeroallergens in clinical practice of allergy in India, an overview. *Ann Agric Environ Med.* 2003;10:131.

Solomon W. Airborne pollen prevalence in the United States. In: Grammer L, Greenberger P, eds. *Patterson's Allergic Diseases.* 6th ed. Philadelphia: Lippincott Williams and Wilkins; 2002:131.

Weber R. Pollen identification. *Ann Allergy Asthma Immunol.* 1998;80:141.

White J, Bernstein D. Key pollen allergens in North America. *Ann Allergy Asthma Immunol.* 2003;91:425.

Allergic Rhinitis: Diagnosis and Treatment

Dennis K. Ledford, MD

Rhinitis is a syndrome defined by the symptoms of nasal congestion, postnasal drip, rhinorrhea, sneezing, and nasal itching, usually with physical findings of turbinate edema and increased secretions. The term implies inflammation as an essential component of the pathophysiology, but inflammation may not always be evident or confirmed in the pathophysiology of all rhinitis syndromes. Nevertheless, rhinitis is generally used to describe the constellation of symptoms listed. Classification of severity is generally based on symptom intensity and duration rather than physical examination or laboratory findings. Rhinitis may be subdivided into more than nine groups based on probable etiology or associations. These include allergic, idiopathic perennial nonallergic (sometimes referred to as vasomotor rhinitis), infectious, medication related (medicamentosa), hormonal, atrophic, polypoid or hyperplastic rhinitis, and rhinitis associated with systemic diseases (Table 6–1). Some authorities divide nonallergic rhinitis into subgroups based on triggers (e.g., weather, odor, alcohol ingestion or irritants), but the symptoms and physical findings of these rhinitis subgroups tend to be more alike than dissimilar, prompting others to classify all into one category. Occupational rhinitis is a classification sometimes used, referring to irritant, nonallergic rhinitis or allergic rhinitis related to work environments. This chapter focuses on allergic rhinitis and includes the differential diagnosis of other rhinitis syndromes (Table 6–1).

PATHOPHYSIOLOGY AND SPECIFIC IgE

The pathophysiology of rhinitis is well defined for allergic, infectious, some medication related, and select systemic disease–associated rhinitis syndromes. The pathophysiology of allergic rhinitis stems from the degranulation of mast cells and the subsequent mucosal recruitment of inflammatory cells, particularly eosinophils (Table 6–2). Mast cell degranulation has been established by nasal allergen challenge, nasal lavage with analysis of mediators, nasal cytology, and nasal biopsy. Inflammation, characterized by recruitment of eosinophils into the nasal mucosa, is an essential component of the pathology of allergic rhinitis.

The symptoms of allergic rhinitis are a composite of the effects of mediators on receptors, for example, histamine with H1 receptor or leukotrienes (LTD$_4$ specifically) with cysteinyl-leukotriene receptor 1, and of cell recruitment with inflammation. The mediators released from mast cells are responsible for the acute symptoms of allergic rhinitis, primarily itching and sneezing (Table 6–3; Fig. 6–1). The inflammation is primarily a result of eosinophil immigration, activation, and persistence, due largely to factors released by the mast cell. The mast cell degranulates when high-affinity IgE receptors are cross-linked by antigen (allergen). IgE specific for a causal allergen is bound to the mast cell, enabling the triggering of degranulation on exposure to the allergen. The production of specific IgE is a result of the complex interaction of genetic predisposition and the environment. Exposure to environmental allergens, which is a risk factor for sensitization, does not result in uniform immune responses, even in subjects with similar, or even identical, genetic backgrounds. Modulation of the IgE response depends on variables such as the type of allergen, the route and dose of exposure, the timing of exposure (e.g., childhood versus adulthood), and concomitant or preceding exposure to infectious organisms or adjuvants, such as endotoxin. Genetic factors affect the epitope or specific portion of the antigen to which the individual responds (some epitopes are more likely to evoke an IgE response) as well as the immunologic regulation that modulates the tendency to produce IgE. Interaction between antigen-presenting cells, such as dendritic cells and B-lymphocytes, T-regulatory cells and Th1- and Th2-like cells (types of helper T cells) affect the probability of IgG antibody formation versus IgE antibody formation versus tolerance to a specific allergen. To further complicate the understanding of

Table 6–1. Differential diagnosis of rhinitis.

Allergic Rhinitis	Other Forms of Rhinitis
Seasonal or intermittent	Atrophic rhinitis
Perennial or persistent	Perennial nonallergic rhinitis (vasomotor rhinitis)
Infectious Rhinitis	Nonallergic rhinitis with eosinophilia syndrome (NARES with or without polyps)

Viral
    Adenovirus   *Respiratory syncytial virus*
    Influenza virus   *Rhinovirus*
    Parainfluenza virus
	Rhinitis medicamentosa
	    Topical decongestants
	        Oxymetazoline
	        Cocaine
	        Neo-Synephrine
	    Systemic therapies
	        β-blockers
	        α antagonists
	        Estrogen supplements or oral contraceptives
	        Nonsteroidal antiinflammatory drugs

Bacterial
    Streptococcus
    Haemophilus	

Structural Nasal Disorders	

Nasal septal deviation	Systemic diseases
	    Endocrine/hormonal
	        Hypothyroidism
	        Pregnancy or breast feeding
	        Diabetes mellitus
	    Inflammatory
	        Sarcoidosis
	        Wegener granulomatosis
	        Relapsing polychondritis
	        Reticular histiocytosis (lethal midline granuloma)
	    Infiltrative
	        Amyloidosis

Nasal polyps (Fig. 6–4)	
Adenoid hyperplasia or cyst	
Concha bullosa (Fig. 6–5)	
Choanal atresia	

Neoplasm
    Squamous cell carcinoma (more common in cigarette smokers)
    Angiofibroma (more common in adolescent boys)
    Esthesioneuroblastoma (resembles a benign nasal polyp)
    Lymphoma
    Sarcoma
    Inverted papilloma
	Irritant rhinitis

Foreign body	Gastroesophageal reflux
Encephalocele	Fungal hypersensitivity sinusitis
Ciliary defects	
Cerebrospinal rhinorrhea	

this process, individuals may simultaneously be sensitized and tolerant to different allergens, for example, dust mite and cat, emphasizing that antigen properties and genetic factors regulate individual antigen responses. Finally, the blood concentration of specific IgE for a selected allergen or the magnitude of a skin test response with allergen does not generally correlate with the severity of symptoms on exposure to that allergen. Thus a simple, unifying explanation of the allergic response or a measurable parameter that will consistently predict symptoms is not available.

The importance of specific IgE in the development of allergic rhinitis is confirmed by nasal challenge with allergen in subjects with specific IgE, correlation of symptoms with the level of allergen exposure, the predictive value of specific IgE in determining response to specific allergen immunotherapy, evidence of mast cell degranulation with allergen contact, and the improvement of allergic rhinitis with anti-IgE monoclonal therapy. Local production of IgE, which would not be recognized by blood or skin tests, and non-IgE mechanisms of mast cell degranulation are hypotheses offered

Table 6–2. Mast cell mediators of allergy.

Mediator	Action
Preformed	
Histamine	Increases vascular permeability; increases mucus production; antiinflammatory effects via H2 receptors

Neutral proteases
    Tryptase(s)
    Chymotryptase(s)
    Carboxypeptidase(s)
	Protein degradation and activation of protein precursors

Synthesized During Cellular Activation	
Leukotriene C4, D4 (LTC4, LTD4)	Increases vascular permeability; increases mucus production
Leukotriene B4 (LTB4)	Increases neutrophil chemotaxis
Prostaglandin D2 (PgD2)	Smooth-muscle contraction
Thromboxane A2	Platelet aggregation, vasoconstriction
Platelet-activating factor (PAF)	Platelet aggregation; increases neutrophil and eosinophil chemotaxis and activation; increases vascular permeability, smooth-muscle contraction
Cytokines	
Interleukin-4 (IL-4)	Increases endothelial expression of VCAM-4; increases IgE production; stimulates Th2 and inhibits Th1 lymphocytes
Tumor necrosis factor (TNF)	Increases endothelial ICAM-1 expression
Interleukin-5 (IL-5)	Activates eosinophils and basophils
Interleukin-3 (IL-3)	Activates eosinophils and basophils; growth factor for mast cells
Granulocyte-macrophage colony-stimulating factor (GM-CSF)	Activates eosinophils and basophils; growth factor for mast cells
Select chemokines	Neutrophil, eosinophil. and basophil chemotaxis; enhanced mast cell and basophil mediator release

to explain allergic-like rhinitis in subjects without measurable specific IgE.

EPIDEMIOLOGY

The prevalence of atopic disease in general and of allergic rhinitis in particular has increased during the past century. Currently, the prevalence of allergic rhinitis is approximately 30%, increased from approximately 10% to 15% at the midpoint of the twentieth century. The increase is more apparent in affluent socioeconomic circumstances, particularly Western Europe, North America, Australia, and New Zealand. Explanation for this increase remains elusive, with a variety of hypotheses summarized in Table 6–4. The hygiene hypothesis, as first suggested by Salzman and colleagues in 1979, is

Table 6–3. Allergy symptoms and responsible mediators.

Symptom	Mediator
Itching/sneezing	Histamine Prostaglandins
Nasal blockage/ microvascular leakage	Histamine Prostaglandins Leukotrienes Platelet-activating factor (PAF) Kinins Chymase Substance P
Mucus secretion	Histamine Leukotrienes Platelet-activating factor (PAF) Kinins

probably the most widely accepted explanation. This hypothesis proposes that reduced infections and endotoxin exposure in infancy diminish the stimuli to convert the Th2-like immune response (allergic-like with a predominance of interleukin 4 [IL-4] and IgE production) present at birth to a Th1-like response (nonallergic with gamma interferon production and reduced IgE). The endotoxin association suggests that the innate immune system and Toll-like receptors are important in the conversion of Th2- to Th1-like immune responses. The data supporting this is found both in epidemiologic studies as well as experimental work. For example, urban children with similar ethnic and genetic backgrounds to those in rural farming areas have a higher occurrence of allergic rhinitis. Furthermore, the occurrence of allergic rhinitis correlates inversely with exposure to farm animals and to endotoxin in early childhood. Conflicting data are a reminder that the hygiene hypothesis is not proven, and additional explanations for the increased prevalence of allergic rhinitis are likely.

There is a bimodal variation with age in the prevalence of allergic rhinitis; one peak occurring in either the mid to late teenage years or late childhood and the second peak occurring in the mid-20s. Most affected subjects initially develop symptoms prior to adulthood. However, approximately 20% of people with allergic rhinitis report symptom onset after the age of 30 years. The prevalence of allergic rhinitis diminishes progressively as the population ages. However, an individual may develop allergic rhinitis at any age.

The importance of allergic rhinitis is its prevalence and impact on the quality of life of affected subjects. Individuals with symptomatic allergic rhinitis do not learn or process information as well as those unaffected.

Sleep quality and sense of vitality are also commonly adversely affected. The treatments used, particularly sedating or first-generation antihistamines, may compound these problems. Allergic rhinitis is also associated with a variety of other airway diseases or symptoms, including otitis media, sinusitis, cough, and asthma, and with other allergic conditions, including atopic dermatitis and food allergy. Treatment of allergic rhinitis improves asthma and may reduce the development of asthma in those predisposed. Treatment of rhinitis may also decrease other associated conditions, including sinusitis, otitis media, and sleep disturbance. Thus the importance of diagnosing and treating allergic rhinitis extends beyond the simple relief of nasal complaints.

CLASSIFICATION OF ALLERGIC RHINITIS

Traditionally, allergic rhinitis has been separated into perennial allergic rhinitis (responsible allergens found indoors, such as dust mites, dogs, and cats) with year-round symptoms or seasonal allergic rhinitis (responsible pollen allergens found seasonally outdoors, such as trees in the spring, grass in the summer, and weeds in the fall in temperate climates in the Northern Hemisphere). The Allergic Rhinitis and its Impact on Asthma (ARIA) Workshop, in collaboration with the World Health Organization, recommended a different classification, using the terms *intermittent* and *persistence* and the severity classifications of mild, moderate, and severe. Intermittent is defined as having symptoms for less than 4 weeks of the year. Mild is defined as not affecting quality of life. Most subjects who seek medical care are expected to be in the moderate to severe persistent category because over-the-counter products are available for treatment of less severe disease. Published studies report that the ARIA classification is more useful in clinical assessments than the seasonal and perennial terminology, suggesting that persistent rhinitis as defined is not equivalent to perennial rhinitis and intermittent is not equivalent to seasonal. Both classifications are used clinically and in the medical literature.

DIFFERENTIAL DIAGNOSIS OF ALLERGIC RHINITIS

Allergic Rhinitis

Allergic rhinitis is the most prevalent form of rhinitis and should be considered in any individual presenting with nasal complaints. Other possible diagnoses are listed in Table 6–1. The principal factors used in distinguishing allergic rhinitis from the other conditions are summarized in Tables 6–5 and 6–6, with history being the most important. The diagnosis of allergic rhinitis is presumptive until specific allergic sensitivity is identified

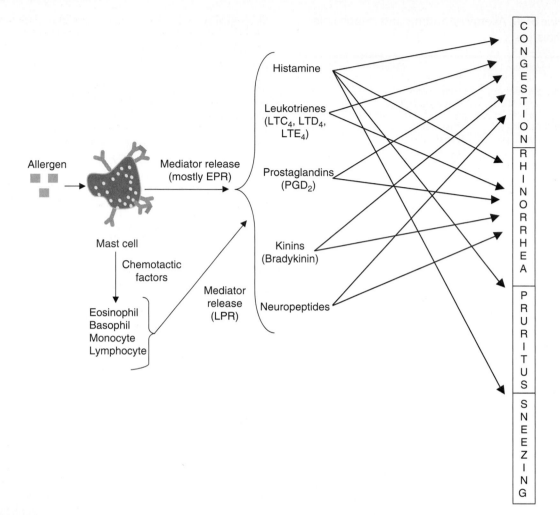

Figure 6–1. Mediators responsible for symptoms of allergic rhinitis. Symptoms result from a variety of mediators and the inflammatory effects of cell recruitment from *chemotactic factors*. The redundancy of causal mediators and mechanisms is one explanation for the failure of single mediator inhibitors, such as antihistamine therapy, to control the complex symptoms of allergic rhinitis, particularly congestion and rhinorrhea that result from multiple mediators. In contrast, pruritus and sneezing are more dependent on histamine, and therefore antihistamine therapy is more effective for these symptoms. EPR, early-phase reaction; LPR, late-phase reaction.

by epicutaneous or percutaneous testing or in vitro specific IgE testing. Immediate wheal and flare skin tests remain the most cost-effective means of identifying specific IgE. The value of intradermal allergy testing is primarily to exclude the diagnosis with negative results, with positive intradermal results providing only tenuous support of a diagnosis of allergic rhinitis. The evidence of specific IgE should be correlated with exposure and symptoms to support the diagnosis. Identifying environmental factors that trigger nasal symptoms is important in distinguishing allergic rhinitis from nonallergic or mixed rhinitis (components of both allergic and nonallergic rhinitis). For example, worsening symptoms from odor would be attributed to nonallergic rhinitis, rather than allergic. If odor affects symptoms in a subject with allergic rhinitis, the individual has mixed rhinitis (i.e., coexistence of two rhinitis syndromes).

Congestion is the most common symptom prompting physician evaluation of nasal complaints but is nonspecific (Fig. 6–1; Table 6–6). Itching, particularly with rubbing of

Table 6–4. Proposed explanations for the increase in atopic disease during the 20th century.

- Reduction in family size with fewer older siblings
- Urbanization with reduced exposure to farm animals and endotoxin
- Fewer serious infectious illnesses in infancy due to cleanliness, antibiotics, and vaccinations
- Change in enteric bacterial colonization due to diet or urbanization
- Modification of diet with either increase in calories or decrease in protective nutrients
- Increased exposure to diesel particles or other pollutants common in urban environs
- Stress
- Increased time indoors with greater exposure to potent indoor allergens
- Increased exposure to prenatal and/or postnatal passive cigarette smoke
- Reduced breastfeeding and earlier age of introduction of solid foods
- Obesity

the nose vertically, is typical of allergic disease. The repetitive rubbing results in the characteristic "nasal crease" of allergic rhinitis (Fig. 6–2). Additional supportive historical features for allergic rhinitis include rubbing the tongue on the roof of the mouth, producing a "clucking" sound, and paroxysmal or episodic sneezing, particularly four or more in succession. Itching and sneezing are more common

Table 6–5. Factors used in identifying and diagnosing allergic rhinitis.

- History of seasonal or situational environments with suspected allergens triggering symptoms
- Positive family history of atopic disease in first-degree relatives
- Personal history of atopic dermatitis or asthma or food allergy
- Onset prior to adult middle age
- Evidence or history of allergic conjunctivitis
- Predominance of itching and sneezing, particularly vertical rubbing of face and cluster sneezing (four or more)
- Clear nasal discharge, often copious, and usually watery
- Nasal mucosa pale or at least nonerythematous
- Nasal crease reflecting the constant rubbing of the face (Fig. 6–3)
- Identification of specific IgE for allergens associated with symptoms (skin testing or in vitro IgE testing)

with intermittent or seasonal than persistent or perennial allergic rhinitis. The less frequent discriminating symptoms of itching and sneezing in perennial or chronic allergic rhinitis result in more difficulty in distinguishing persistent allergic rhinitis from other nasal disorders.

The secretions in allergic disease typically are clear or white, but severe disease may result in cloudy mucus. Allergic rhinitis symptoms should be bilateral, with lateralizing complaints or findings suggesting an alternative diagnosis or a complication. The presence of other allergic diseases, particularly allergic conjunctivitis or atopic dermatitis, would also be strong support for the diagnosis of allergic rhinitis. Finally, family history is important because one immediate family member increases the likelihood of allergic rhinitis to approximately 40% to 50%. Having two affected immediate family members makes the probability of having allergic rhinitis greater than 60%.

Treatment of allergic rhinitis is reviewed in the next section.

Perennial Nonallergic Rhinitis

Perennial nonallergic rhinitis (PNAR) is a term used to designate a heterogeneous group of disorders that share clinical features. The pathophysiology is not completely defined, and nasal histology does not correlate with symptoms. PNAR is common, representing 30% to 60% of subjects referred to an allergy/immunology or otolaryngology clinic for evaluation. PNAR coexists with allergic rhinitis in more than 50% of adults with allergic rhinitis, a condition referred to as mixed rhinitis. Mucosal inflammation is less evident in PNAR than allergic rhinitis, making the term *rhinitis* sometimes a misnomer. However, the symptoms are consistent with other inflammatory nasal disease, and inflammation may be present in a subset of PNAR.

The typical presentation of PNAR is complaints of nasal obstruction, with or without rhinorrhea or postnasal drip, exacerbated by physical stimuli such as odor (particularly floral smells), air temperature changes, air movement, body position change, food, beverage (particularly alcoholic drinks such as wine), or exposure to airborne irritants such as cigarette smoke. Paroxysmal sneezing and itching are less common in PNAR than allergic rhinitis. A variant of PNAR, with copious rhinorrhea associated with eating or preparation for eating, is termed *gustatory rhinitis.* Exercise often improves the symptoms of PNAR, contrasting with allergic rhinitis.

Non-IgE degranulation of nasal mast cells, by physical stimuli, such as cold, dry air and hyperosmolar mucosal fluid, is not likely a critical part of the pathophysiology of PNAR because the symptoms of itching and sneezing paroxysms and mucosal eosinophilia are typically absent. However, mast cell degranulation has been demonstrated

Table 6–6. Distinguishing allergic rhinitis from nonallergic rhinitis.

Feature	Allergic Rhinitis	Nonallergic Rhinitis
Age of onset	Usually prior to 20 y (20% after age 30 y)	Usually after 30 y
Family history	Positive for atopic disease	May or may not be positive for "sinus"; negative for asthma and allergic rhinitis
Seasonal pattern	Variable but may be related to major seasonal changes; particularly dependent on predominant pollinating plants	No specific seasonal pattern but weather change or barometric pressure changes may affect symptoms, which may be confused with seasonal pattern
Primary triggers	Allergen exposure	Odor, irritants, body position change, weather change, alcohol ingestion
Primary symptoms	Sneezing paroxysms (four or more in succession), itching, congestion, clear rhinorrhea	Congestion, mucoid to watery nasal discharge, postnasal drip, facial pressure, sneezing two to three in succession (not more than four)
Other atopic features	Allergic conjunctivitis, atopic dermatitis or history of same	None, although dry eye or blepharitis may be reported and confused with allergic conjunctivitis; nonspecific dry skin confused with atopic dermatitis
Physical examination	Transverse nasal crease, mucosa variable but classically pale and watery or boggy	Erythematous with turbinate edema and mucoid or watery secretions
Confirmatory tests	Nasal eosinophilia, specific IgE for allergens that correlate with symptoms, blood eosinophilia, increased blood IgE (normal in 20–30% of affected subjects)	Negative tests for specific IgE or no correlation with positive tests and symptoms, eosinophilia only in nonallergic rhinitis with eosinophilia syndrome (NARES)

with cold air challenge of the nose in PNAR. Neurogenic mechanisms may play a pathophysiologic role in PNAR because some affected subjects hyperrespond with nasal congestion following nasal challenge with cholinergic agents, suggesting a type of nasal hyperreactivity similar to that occurring in the bronchial airway with asthma.

The diagnosis of PNAR is suggested by the symptom history, the nature of provoking stimuli, and absence of a family history of allergy. The nasal mucosa is variable in appearance but generally is congested with normal to erythematous color. The secretions are usually clear and do not contain a significant number of eosinophils or neutrophils. Other causes of nasal symptoms should be excluded because of the lack of a confirmatory diagnostic test for PNAR. The exclusion of perennial allergic rhinitis is particularly important because the symptoms of the two are similar, and some subjects have both conditions (Table 6–6). Sinusitis should also be considered because many symptoms are common to both.

The treatment of PNAR is symptomatic because the pathophysiology is usually unknown. The physician should focus the therapy on the primary symptom. Decongestants, nasal saline to lavage irritants from the mucosa or dilute secretions, and topical ipratropium bromide 0.03% (Atrovent Nasal™) for rhinorrhea are often helpful. Oral antihistamine therapy offers limited benefits, although the anticholinergic effects of first-generation, sedating antihistamines may be helpful for rhinorrhea. Topical antihistamine therapy with azelastine is efficacious and approved for treatment of PNAR, contrasting with the lack of approval for any oral antihistamines. Topical nasal corticosteroid therapy relieves

Nonallergic Rhinitis with Eosinophilia

Nonallergic rhinitis with eosinophilia (NARES) is a syndrome generally distinguished from PNAR by the presence of eosinophils in the nasal secretions or mucosa. The symptoms cannot be distinguished from PNAR, and the family history is generally negative, increasing the clinical confusion between NARES and PNAR. Affected subjects suffer from perennial nasal congestion, rhinorrhea, sneezing, and pruritus but do not have specific IgE for allergens, an increase in total IgE, or a personal or family history of atopy. The nasal secretions contain eosinophils, which distinguishes this condition from other forms of PNAR. The lack of an atopic personal and family history in NARES makes an undefined allergy unlikely as the cause. The condition may be part of the spectrum of eosinophilic rhinitis and nasal polyposis. Subjects with the aspirin triad (nasal polyps with eosinophils, asthma, aspirin sensitivity) experience eosinophilic rhinorrhea and nasal congestion prior to the development of nasal polyps, suggesting a spectrum of eosinophilic nasal disease (Fig. 6–3). However, most subjects with NARES do not develop the aspirin triad.

Allergic rhinitis and nasal polyposis are the principal diagnoses to be excluded when assessing a subject with NARES. Treatment is symptomatic with topical nasal corticosteroid therapy generally the most effective

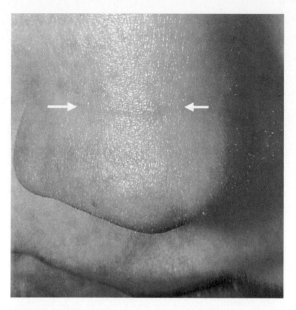

Figure 6–2. Transverse nasal crease of allergic rhinitis. This photograph shows the transverse nasal crease (arrows) that is characteristic of allergic rhinitis. This linear change occurs from repetitive rubbing of the nose vertically, pushing the tip of the nose cephalad. Identifying such a crease in a family member of a patient is a useful feature supporting a positive family history of allergy.

symptoms of PNAR, probably by reducing glandular secretion and blood flow to the nose because mucosal inflammation is not consistently present. The response to topical nasal corticosteroids is variable and not as predictable as with allergic rhinitis. Although only select nasal corticosteroids have a Food and Drug Administration (FDA) indication for nonallergic rhinitis, most likely all work and all are generally used. Nasal corticosteroids with a detectable odor, for example, beclomethasone (Vancenase AQ™) or fluticasone (Flonase™), may aggravate symptoms, suggesting a preference for sprays without smell. Regular aerobic exercise, 20 to 30 minutes two to three times a week, may help reduce symptoms, at least temporarily, and is good for general health. Nasal congestion and sinus pressure are often the most bothersome symptoms, so emphasis on avoidance of regular topical decongestants is important because this may lead to rhinitis medicamentosa. Oral lozenges containing menthol may affect the perception of nasal congestion but have no measurable effect on congestion. Finally, affected subjects need reassurance and sensitive care to reduce "doctor shopping", unnecessary surgery, overuse of antibiotics, and overinterpretation of allergy tests.

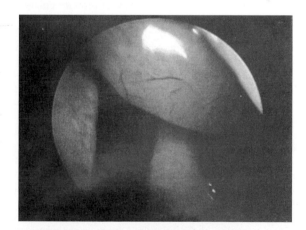

Figure 6–3. Nasal polyp. This is a view from the rhinoscope in the left nostril. The septum is on the left and the polyp is the pale soft tissue between the middle and inferior turbinate. Nasal polyps are associated with chronic inflammatory sinus disease, usually eosinophilic. Nasal polyps are not consistently found in subjects with allergic rhinitis but could explain persistent congestion. Cystic fibrosis is also associated with nasal polyps although not generally with eosinophilic inflammation.

pharmacologic agent. Symptom relief may require a higher dosage of nasal corticosteroid than generally required for allergic rhinitis. Titrating the dose of nasal corticosteroid against the presence of nasal eosinophils may be of clinical value in determining the appropriate dose. Azelastine reduces eosinophil chemotaxis in vitro but has not been studied in NARES.

Rhinitis Induced by Drugs or Hormones (Rhinitis Medicamentosa)

Topical use of α-adrenergic decongestant sprays for more than 5 to 7 days in succession may result in a rebound nasal congestion on discontinuation of treatment or after the immediate effects have waned. Continued use of the decongestant to control withdrawal congestion can lead to an erythematous, congested nasal mucosa termed *rhinitis medicamentosa*. Regular intranasal cocaine use will have the same effect and should be considered in the differential diagnosis. Other systemic medications or hormone changes may also be associated with nasal symptoms, although the nasal mucosa may not always appear the same with each medication.

The mechanisms responsible for nasal symptoms associated with medications or hormones are variable. Antihypertensive therapies with β-blockers and α-adrenergic antagonists probably affect regulation of nasal blood flow. Oral α-adrenergic antagonists are also commonly used for symptom relief of prostate enlargement. Topical ophthalmic β-blocker therapy may also result in nasal congestion by the same mechanism. Nasal congestion and/or rhinorrhea may also result from changes in estrogen, and possibly progesterone, either from exogenous administration, pregnancy, or menstrual cycle variations. Hypothyroidism is associated with nasal congestion, rhinorrhea, and a pale, allergic-like nasal mucosa. Aspirin and other nonsteroidal anti-inflammatory drugs (NSAIDs) may result in congestion and rhinorrhea, primarily in subjects with aspirin triad. Subjects with intermittent symptoms associated with aspirin or NSAIDs may be part of the evolving spectrum of chronic eosinophilic rhinosinusitis with nasal polyps (see NARES).

The primary treatment of rhinitis medicamentosa is discontinuation of the offending agent or correction of the hormonal imbalance, if possible. Symptomatic treatment may be helpful. Treatment of rebound nasal congestion associated with topical decongestant use may require 5 to 7 days of oral prednisone or equivalent, 20 to 30 mg per day, followed by topical intranasal corticosteroid therapy. Reassurance that the nasal symptoms are the result of the medications or hormonal changes may be sufficient to discourage other unnecessary investigations if the medical treatments causing the rhinitis are essential.

Atrophic Rhinitis

Atrophic rhinitis usually occurs in late-middle-age to elderly patients. The cause of atrophic rhinitis is unknown with the leading theory being age-related mucosal atrophy, sometimes complicated by secondary bacterial infection. Primary atrophic rhinitis resembles the rhinitis associated with Sjögren syndrome or previous nasal surgery, particularly extensive turbinectomy. Examination generally reveals a patent nasal airway with atrophic erythematous turbinates, despite the symptoms of congestion.

Some subjects with atrophic rhinitis report crusting of the nasal airway and a bad smell (ozena). Ozena is associated with bacterial overgrowth of the mucosa, particularly *Klebsiella ozaenae* and *Pseudomonas aeruginosa*. The appearance of ozena may resemble chronic granulomatous disease, such as Wegener granulomatosis or sarcoidosis, or the effects of previous local irradiation. The prevalence of ozena is variable with a greater occurrence in select geographic areas, such as southeastern Europe, China, Egypt, or India, rather than Northern Europe or the United States.

Symptomatic treatment of atrophic rhinitis with low-dose decongestants and nasal saline lavage is minimally effective. Individuals with confirmed sicca complex or Sjögren syndrome (Table 6–7) may benefit from oral cevimeline, 30 mg three times daily, keeping in mind that bronchospasm and arrhythmias are potential side effects. Oral antibiotic therapy is necessary for ozena. Topical antibiotic therapy, such as gentamicin or tobramycin, 15 mg/mL, or ciprofloxacin, 0.15 mg/mL in saline, may offer some benefit for subjects with atrophic rhinitis and recurrent mucosal infections or sinusitis, although no studies are available to validate this treatment. An over-the-counter topical treatment reported to reduce bacterial colonization, SinoFresh™, is another consideration. No clinical trials support this agent in atrophic rhinitis; thus a treatment trial is in reality a trial of one, and benefits may be the result of the lavage, at a much greater cost than saline. The addition of propylene glycol, 3% to 15%, or glycerin to nasal saline may prolong the benefits of topical moisturization by reducing the water's surface tension or reducing the irritation from irrigation. Application of petrolatum or petrolatum with eucalyptus/menthol (Vicks™ ointment) to the nasal mucosa at night may help reduce nasal bleeding. Topical shea butter (Butter Bar Moisture Therapy), an over-the-counter herbal therapy, also may be of some benefit but likewise is unproven.

Rhinitis Associated with Systemic Diseases or Anatomic Defects

The presence of systemic findings or the persistence of nasal symptoms despite treatment should prompt

Table 6–7. Laboratory tests for systemic diseases associated with nasal symptoms.

Test	Diagnosis
Erythrocyte sedimentation rate	Wegener granulomatosis Relapsing polychondritis Sarcoidosis
Delayed-type hypersensitivity testing	Tuberculosis Sarcoidosis
VDRL	Syphilis
Sweat chloride	Cystic fibrosis
CFTR genotyping	Cystic fibrosis
Antineutrophil cytoplasmic antibody	Wegener granulomatosis Churg-Strauss vasculitis
Angiotensin-converting enzyme level	Sarcoidosis
Quantitative immunoglobulins	Common variable immunodeficiency IgA deficiency
Thyroid-stimulating hormone	Hypothyroidism
ANA, anti-Ro (SSA), anti-La (SSB)	Sjögren syndrome
Schirmer tear test[†]	Sjögren syndrome
Saccharine taste test [*]	Immotile cilia syndrome

[*]Saccharine is placed with a cotton swab on the inferior turbinate, at the junction of the anterior and middle thirds of the turbinate. The time required for tasting is recorded, with normal usually less than 20 minutes. Greater than 30 minutes before tasting is considered indicative of dysfunction of ciliary motility. The patient must be instructed not to sniff, blow the nose, or use any topical nasal therapies during the test. (Stanley P, MacWilliam L, Greenstone M, et al. Efficacy of a saccharine test for screening to detect abnormal mucociliary clearance. *Br J Dis Chest*. 1984;78:62; Corbo GM, Foresi A, Bonfitto P, et al. Measurement of nasal mucociliary clearance. *Arch Dis Child*. 1989;64:546).

[†]A 5×35 mm piece of sterile filter paper is folded 5 mm from the end and inserted over the inferior eyelid at the junction of the middle and lateral third. The eye is gently closed for 5 minutes, and the length of wetting is measured after removal. Less than 5 mm indicates significant dryness; normal is more than 15 mm. (Available from Alcon Laboratories, Fort Worth, TX.)

ANA, antinuclear antibody; CFTR, cystic fibrosis transmembrane conductance register; VDRL, Venereal Disease Research Laboratory (test).

consideration of systemic diseases or anatomic problems resulting in nasal symptoms. Structural problems typically present with a predominance of unilateral symptoms or initially unilateral symptoms. Nasopharyngoscopy, paranasal computed tomography, and/or otolaryngologic consultation are major considerations with lateralizing nasal complaints, bleeding noted from one nasal airway or unremitting congestion. Nasal septal deviations are the most common anatomic nasal variants noted; but often septal deviation is not primarily responsible for the symptoms, unless very severe or coupled with mucosal disease such as allergic rhinitis or PNAR. A concha bullosa is an anatomic variant in which an air cell or cells occur within the turbinate, often resulting in enlargement of the turbinate with congestion (Fig. 6–4). Profuse rhinorrhea should prompt testing of the secretions for glucose or for β-2 transferrin (β-trace protein) to exclude cerebral spinal fluid (CSF) rhinorrhea.

Wegener granulomatosis may present initially with upper airway complaints, particularly hearing loss, intractable sinusitis, and persistent nasal congestion associated with purulent or bloody nasal discharge. Sarcoidosis of the nasal airway may appear similarly although not usually as necrotizing. Persistent

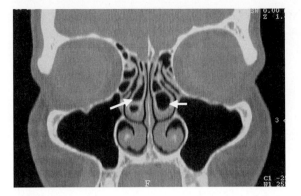

Figure 6–4. Concha bullosa. This figure shows a coronal computed tomography scan image of the paranasal sinuses. The arrows point to the concha bullosa in each middle turbinate. In this case, septae divide the concha bullosa into more than one air space. The usual result of the concha bullosa is enlargement of the turbinate, usually resulting in chronic nasal congestion. Infection may occur in the concha bullosa. Frequently the septum is deviated away from a unilateral concha bullosa. Therefore, this entity should be considered in a patient complaining of chronic congestion.

sinusitis or recurring infectious complications should prompt consideration of cystic fibrosis, partially cleft or submucosal cleft palate, humoral immunodeficiency, or ciliary dysfunction. Table 6–7 lists potentially useful tests to discriminate among the systemic possibilities.

TREATMENT OF ALLERGIC RHINITIS

The treatment of allergic rhinitis is three pronged—allergen exposure modification or avoidance, allergen immunotherapy (allergy shots), and/or pharmacotherapy (Fig. 6–5; Table 6–8). Clinical studies confirming efficacy of various therapies use symptoms as primary outcome variables. More objective means of assessing allergic rhinitis have been somewhat useful but have not supplanted symptom scores in clinical trials. These other methods include acoustic rhinometry, rhinomanometry, nasal peak flow, nitric oxide levels in exhaled air, concentration of mediators in nasal lavage, nasal cytology, and nasal histology. These objective methods show promise, but difficulties with reproducibility, necessity of patient cooperation or mastering the technique, sampling error, and cost combine to reduce their utility. Using symptom scores as the primary outcome variable limit the ability to compare treatments because the magnitude of response is not always consistent from study to study.

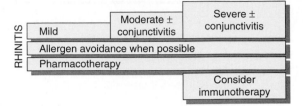

When to consider immunotherapy

Figure 6–5. Treatment strategies for allergic rhinitis based on severity of rhinitis. This approach is suggested by the World Health Organization ARIA (**A**llergic **R**hinitis and **I**ts Effect on **A**sthma) report. Pharmacotherapy and allergen avoidance are the initial approach to allergic rhinitis, with the severity of the rhinitis usually modifying the pharmacotherapy. Oral antihistamine therapy is used for mild disease; topical nasal corticosteroid therapy, with or without oral antihistamine therapy, in moderate to severe disease. Topical azelastine, oral montelukast or oral decongestants are considered either as add-on treatment or occasionally as monotherapy in the case of azelastine. Specific immunotherapy is generally reserved for more severe, persistent disease. (Adapted from WAO ARIA report.)

Allergen Avoidance

Avoidance is primarily helpful for indoor domestic allergens, although occasionally modifiable occupational exposures, such as animal contact or colophony fumes during soldering, may be effective. Indoor avoidance focuses primarily on dust mite allergen reduction (encasing the pillow, mattress, and box springs with a material that does not allow dust mite migration) and washing all bedding in water at a temperature greater than 130°F (Table 6–9). Washing removes the allergen, which is primarily digestive enzymes present in dust mite excrement. The hot water is essential to control dust mite populations, the source of the allergen. Studies to show benefit of dust avoidance have failed when hot water washing was not assured. Air filter systems probably do not have a significant role in allergen avoidance, although high-efficiency particulate air (HEPA) filters may be helpful for homes with animals and possibly help with indoor mold spore reduction. Very little data support the use of filtration.

Allergen Immunotherapy

Specific allergen immunotherapy provides a 50% reduction in medication and symptoms if sufficient doses of the major allergens are administered to significantly (epicutaneous or percutaneous positive skin tests) allergic subjects. This improvement is confirmed by the

Table 6–8. Stepwise approach to the treatment of seasonal allergic rhinitis.

Allergen Avoidance	
Pharmacologic Therapy	
Mild disease or with occasional symptoms	• Oral nonsedating H1 antihistamine when symptomatic (desloratadine, fexofenadine, loratadine, or possibly cetirizine)[*] OR • Topical nasal azelastine when symptomatic or sodium cromoglycate to eyes, nose, or both; alternative for intermittent eye symptoms is topical ocular antihistamine or topical nonsteroidal antiinflammatory (ketorolac tromethamine)[†]
Moderate disease with prominent nasal symptoms	• Intranasal corticosteroid daily (start early in season) PLUS • Antihistamine or topical eye therapy with sodium cromoglycate or lodoxamide tromethamine or olopatadine hydrochloride[†]
Moderate disease with prominent eye symptoms	• Oral nonsedating H1 antihistamine daily[*] OR • Intranasal corticosteroid and topical eye therapy with sodium cromoglycate or lodoxamide tromethamine or olopatadine hydrochloride/ topical nonsteroidal antiinflammatory (ketorolac tromethamine) additional therapy for exacerbations[†]
If above Ineffective	
• Review possibility of coexisting disease or complications (e.g., sinusitis). • Consider immunotherapy. • Try systemic corticosteroid therapy for a few days for severe symptoms. • Prescribe topical ipratropium bromide if rhinorrhea a major problem.	
Perennial Allergic Rhinitis in Adults	
• Allergen avoidance • Intranasal corticosteroids if long-term exposure	
Intermittent Disease	
• Oral nonsedating H1 antihistamine therapy[*] • Oral decongestants	

[*]Sedating, traditional (first-generation) antihistamine therapy is a consideration because of cost of second-generation antihistamines. However, functional impairment occurs with first-generation antihistamine therapy even if treated subjects do not perceive impairment. Therefore, it is difficult to evaluate the risk-benefit ratio, and a treating physician may be at legal risk if any accident occurs while a patient is being treated with a sedating antihistamine without first trying nonsedating antihistamine therapy. Fexofenadine, loratadine, and desloratadine are safe, effective nonsedating antihistamine therapies that have almost no side effects. There is no concern with combining these treatments with other therapies, including macrolide antibiotics and azole antifungals. Cetirizine is mildly sedating with clinical trial results variable as to the importance of this sedation. Oral antihistamine therapy achieves approximately 30% improvement in 50% of treated subjects. Azelastine (a topical antihistamine therapy for rhinitis) is also mildly sedating, but some authorities debate the clinical significance of this effect. Azelastine topical is indicated for nonallergic rhinitis, an indication not shared by any oral antihistamine. This point supports a mechanism of action that may be unique for azelastine topical.

[†]Topical ocular therapy is not recommended with contact lens use.

Table 6–9. Allergen avoidance measures.

Avoidance Measures for Mite Allergen

Bedrooms
- Cover mattresses and pillows with impermeable covers.
- Wash bedding regularly at 130°F.
- Remove carpets, stuffed animals, and clutter from bedrooms.
- Eliminate wall-to-wall carpet.
- Vacuum clean weekly (wearing a mask or using a HEPA [high-efficiency particulate air] filtered vacuum cleaner).

Rest of house
- Minimize carpets and upholstered furniture (particularly in basements or overlying concrete).
- Reduce humidity below 45% relative humidity or 6 g/kg (may not be feasible in many climates).
- Consider treatment of carpets with benzyl benzoate powder or tannic acid spray (questionable efficacy).

Avoidance Measures for Cat Allergen

Remove cat from the house (allergen reduction sufficient to affect symptoms may take ≥12–16 wk)

Measures to reduce cat allergen if cat remains in home
- Minimize cat contact with carpets, upholstered furniture, and bedding.
- Use vacuum cleaners with an effective filtration system.
- Increase ventilation.
- Consider a HEPA filter to remove small airborne particles.
- Consider washing cat every 2 weeks.

---

majority of controlled trials with immunotherapy in both seasonal and perennial allergic rhinitis. Laboratory tests and challenge studies, in general, correlate with the clinical findings. The most consistent humoral change is an increase in specific IgG, with some studies showing a switch from specific IgG1 to IgG4 (Table 6–10). However, the many exceptions indicate that there is not a specific confirmatory test to demonstrate clinical benefit. Symptom improvement remains the standard response variable.

Advantages of allergen immunotherapy, in addition to symptom improvement, are that the treatment may reduce the future development of additional sensitivities and minimize the occurrence of asthma in subjects with allergic rhinitis. Pharmacotherapy is not likely to achieve these goals. Finally, immunotherapy offers the potential of treating allergic airway disease beyond the nose with improvement in allergic conjunctivitis and/or asthma. Duration of allergen immunotherapy is based on clinical experience and limited evidence. In general, 3 to 5 years of maintenance treatment, usually administered every 3 to 4 weeks, is necessary to minimize reoccurrence of symptoms after discontinuation.

The major impediments to allergen immunotherapy are the inconvenience and cost of the therapy and risk of anaphylaxis. Analyses have shown that high-dose allergen immunotherapy is cost effective because of the reduction of regular medication use. Anaphylaxis following immunotherapy occurs in 0.1% to 3% of treated subjects. This risk, which is minimized by identification and treatment of anaphylaxis, requires that allergen immunotherapy be administered under the immediate supervision of a physician or provider trained in the treatment of anaphylaxis. Treated subjects should remain under observation for 30 minutes after receiving subcutaneous allergen immunotherapy to minimize risk of reaction after departure. The indications for allergen immunotherapy include severe symptoms, poor response to medications, intolerance to or side effects from medications, or reluctance to take medications (Fig. 6–5). Relative contraindications include uncontrolled asthma, β-blocker therapy, autoimmune disease, and malignancy. Immunotherapy

Table 6–10. Mechanisms of action of immunotherapy.

- Increase in T-suppressor activity
- Modulation of T regulatory cells
- Decrease in histamine-releasing factors
- Increase in specific IgG
- Decrease in specific IgE
- Decrease in mediator release from basophils

should be initiated and supervised by a trained specialist but can be administered by any physician who is prepared to treat anaphylaxis, the most serious adverse effect of the treatment.

The risk and inconvenience of allergen immunotherapy have stimulated the study of oral allergen immunotherapy. This technique has been used in the past, but the dose of allergen administered was inadequate for double-blind controlled trials to demonstrate efficacy. In the past 10 years, a series of investigations have shown clinical improvement with high-dose oral immunotherapy. Side effects do occur, but these tend to be less severe than with injection immunotherapy and usually localized to the mouth and gastrointestinal tract. The advantages of home administration, the minimized risk of anaphylaxis, and the relatively rapid attainment of the maintenance dose make this treatment attractive. The disadvantages are the requirement for a very large dose of allergen vaccine, reduced efficacy compared to injection treatment, less evidence of efficacy in children, and limited evidence for long-term disease modification. Nevertheless, sublingual allergen immunotherapy may be a consideration for select patients at risk for anaphylaxis or in circumstances not permitting regular visitation with a physician to administer immunotherapy. This treatment is not currently approved in the United States.

Pharmacotherapy

Pharmacotherapy may be divided into two broad classes—topical or oral (Table 6–8). Advantages of topical therapy are greater efficacy for nasal complaints and limited toxicity or side-effects. Patient acceptance due to nasal irritation or taste is the major objection. Advantages of oral therapy include the potential to address the systemic nature of the allergic response and greater patient acceptance compared to sprays.

TOPICAL THERAPY OF ALLERGIC RHINITIS

Topical corticosteroids offer 70% improvement in approximately three fourths of treated subjects with allergic rhinitis, making this option statistically the most efficacious (Table 6–8). In addition, topical nasal corticosteroids improve nonallergic rhinitis and subjects with nasal polyps, conditions that typically do not respond to oral therapy, other than corticosteroids and decongestants. Response with topical corticosteroids may occur within 7 to 12 hours, but maximum effect requires days to weeks. Differences among the various products are minimal, although the newer agents (fluticasone, mometasone) have a greater first-pass clearance of swallowed drug, making these treatments inherently safer. Almost 80% of a nasally administered drug is swallowed, but the relatively low dosage used in nasal therapy limits potential systemic side effects. However, a study with

beclomethasone dipropionate (Vancenase™ AQ or Beconase AQ) at recommended dosage demonstrated a reduction in 1-year growth of children. This is a reminder that systemic side effects may occur with topically applied medications. Mometasone has the youngest, approved age indication, 2 years of age, and budesonide has the safest FDA classification for pregnancy, Class B, with other agents Class C. The most common side effect with nasal corticosteroid therapy is nasal bleeding. Bleeding is minimized by instructing the patient to administer the spray in a lateral direction or toward the ipsilateral ear, to minimize septal deposition. Mucosal atrophy does not occur with topical corticosteroids, but the anterior nasal septum has a squamous epithelium, with a possibility of irritation, ischemia, and rarely perforation with topical corticosteroid application.

Other topical nasal treatments include azelastine, ipratropium, and cromolyn sodium. Topical nasal olopatadine, an antihistamine that reduces mast cell degranulation, will likely be approved in the United States in the near future. Azelastine is an antihistamine that seems to have antiinflammatory properties when applied topically. These effects include inhibition of mast cell degranulation, inhibition of inflammatory cell recruitment, and reduction of adhesion receptors necessary for cell trafficking. Azelastine nasal spray is approved for both seasonal allergic rhinitis and non-allergic rhinitis. Presumably, the antiinflammatory effects, rather than antihistamine properties, are important in the improvement of nonallergic disease because histamine does not seem to be an important mediator in nonallergic rhinitis. Thus oral antihistamine therapy is ineffective for nonallergic rhinitis. Topical azelastine may provide symptom improvement within 30 minutes to an hour in allergic rhinitis, making this an ideal therapy for intermittent or as-needed use. Ipratropium nasal spray minimizes rhinorrhea by inhibiting muscarinic receptors. The indication is for both allergic and non-allergic rhinitis, but the treatment is not as effective for mucoid secretions as it is for watery secretions. Nasal sodium cromolyn is available over- the- counter. This product must be used every 4 to 6 hours to be significantly effective because sodium cromolyn does not treat existing symptoms but rather reduces subsequent symptoms from mast cell mediator release. Nasal sodium cromolyn is likely to be useful in circumstances in which the affected subject can predict exposure to a known allergen and use the product before exposure. For example, an animal allergic individual could use topical sodium cromolyn to suppress allergic rhinitis if the medication were applied prior to visitation of the home with the animal and if the sodium cromolyn is reapplied every 4 to 6 hours. The requirement for regular administration makes sodium cromolyn relatively ineffective for chronic disease.

ORAL THERAPY OF ALLERGIC RHINITIS

Oral antihistamines, with or without decongestants, are the most commonly utilized approach in allergic rhinitis (Table 6–8). The newer second- and third-generation antihistamines offer excellent relief of itching and sneezing without the side effects of excessive sedation, dryness, constipation, or bladder dysfunction. Thirty percent improvement in 50% of treated subjects is the approximate expected clinical response. The explanation for the reduced magnitude of response with oral antihistamine therapy, compared to topical nasal corticosteroids, is the general lack of improvement in congestion and limited, if any, effect on nonallergic rhinitis. Nonallergic rhinitis may coexist with allergic rhinitis in up to 50% of affected adults. In addition, symptoms of allergic rhinitis are the result of a variety of mediators, limiting the benefits of a single inhibitor (Table 6–3; Fig. 6–1).

Selecting a non- or less-sedating antihistamine is often predicated on formulary coverage, previous therapeutic trials, or personal bias. Cetirizine, desloratadine, fexofenadine, and loratadine are the second- and third-generation oral antihistamines available in the United States. Levocetirizine, the active stereoisomer of cetirizine, will be approved in 2007. Distinguishing these agents is somewhat of a challenge and subject to individual opinion more than evidence. Loratadine, which is available without prescription, probably is the least potent of these and may not be effective for a full 24 hours. Fexofenadine has the least potential for sedation, but absorption is most affected by food. Cetirizine may have mild somnolence as a side effect but is considered to be the "strongest" antihistamine by many physicians. This is based on little clinical evidence but on experience, which could be clouded by the mild sedating effect of cetirizine. Desloratadine and cetirizine have an indication for both seasonal and perennial allergic rhinitis. Loratadine and cetirizine have a Class B rating in pregnancy; fexofenadine and desloratadine are Class C. Cetirizine, desloratadine, and loratadine have the youngest approved age indication, 6 months. One study shows some benefit in 50% of subjects after changing oral antihistamine therapy in individuals who have noted declining benefit with chronic antihistamine treatment. This supports the commonly reported phenomenon of "resistance" to oral antihistamine therapy, without evidence of measurable change in the histamine receptor. Cetirizine is unique in minimizing the development of asthma due to dust mite or grass allergens following chronic cetirizine therapy of atopic dermatitis in children. A similar study is currently under way using levocetirizine.

The first-generation antihistamines are equal or superior in efficacy compared to the newer agents but result in a variety of side effects due to central nervous system and anticholinergic complications. These result from the first-generation antihistamines readily crossing the blood-brain barrier and interfering with other receptors, such as the serotonin, acetylcholine, and dopamine receptors, among others.

Adding an oral decongestant to an antihistamine may improve the clinical response, particularly by reducing nasal congestion, but also may result in side effects of nervousness, sleep disturbance, increase in blood pressure, and bladder dysfunction. This is a popular alternative due to the primal importance of nasal congestion among affected subjects.

Oral montelukast is also effective for seasonal and perennial allergic rhinitis and associated with minimal side effects. The degree of improvement is difficult to compare to oral antihistamine therapy but is probably equivalent to slightly less effective. An advantage of oral montelukast is a greater effect on asthma than current oral antihistamines. Montelukast may be particularly useful in a subject with cough, attributed to upper airway disease, but who may have a component of asthma as well. Combining oral antihistamines and montelukast may or may not offer any clinical advantages but from a theoretical standpoint is appealing. The combination of oral second- or third-generation antihistamine and montelukast may increase treatment costs significantly.

Oral corticosteroid therapy of relatively short duration is effective for severe rhinitis associated with such congestion that topical therapy is limited by the inability to deliver the treatment to the affected mucosa. Oral corticosteroid therapy is also helpful for nasal polyps and rhinitis medicamentosa. Treatment is generally limited to 5 to 7 days to minimize side effects, and the dose is generally 0.5 mg/kg/d of prednisone or equivalent.

Future Therapeutic Options for Allergic Rhinitis

Future therapies for allergic rhinitis may include immunomodulators such as monoclonal anti-IgE (omalizumab), inhibitors of inflammatory cell immigration into the nasal mucosa, and antiinflammatory therapies. Omalizumab binds to soluble IgE and also results in a reduction in the high-affinity receptor for IgE on mast cells and basophils, and possibly on select dendritic cells. If dosed according to the recommendation of 0.16 mg/kg/IU IgE, the free plasma IgE concentration is reduced to approximately 15 IU/mL. This results in reduced allergic rhinitis symptoms and improvement in asthma. The necessity for injecting this compound and the cost are the major limitations on the eventual application of omalizumab for allergic rhinitis. A variety of antiinflammatory therapies or immunomodulators have been considered or tried for rhinitis. Syk-kinase inhibitor is an example of such therapeutic approaches. Syk-kinase is a signaling protein important for mast cell and basophil degranulation. By applying a topical inhibitor of syk-kinase to the nasal mucosa, allergic rhinitis symptoms are improved. Other similar targets of intervention are being explored as bench research is applied to the inflammation of allergic rhinitis. The potential of more rapid application of this cutting-edge science to allergic rhinitis is greater than other diseases due to the relative ease of applying these therapeutics to the nasal mucosa.

CONCLUSION

Allergic rhinitis is a common condition that significantly impacts the quality of life of affected subjects and occurs coincidentally with a variety of other airway, systemic, or allergic conditions. The application of an appropriate differential diagnosis and targeting therapy to the predominant symptom of the patient will allow the physician to make a major difference in the lives of affected subjects. Nasal disease is complex in scope, but the two most common, allergic rhinitis and perennial nonallergic rhinitis, can be assessed with a modest degree of investigation. As with most medical conditions, the history is paramount because the physical findings in rhinitis are somewhat limited or nonspecific. Consideration should always be given to systemic diseases other than allergy, particularly if the clinical data are inconsistent. Appropriate allergy testing is essential to confirm the diagnosis of allergic rhinitis. Knowledge of the environment and the important allergens in a particular area are critical to understanding the results of allergy testing. Many of the "panels" offered by commercial laboratories are not targeted to specific environments. Allergists/immunologists have a unique advantage in the assessment of affected subjects because their training encompasses the immunologic and environmental factors that affect the upper airway.

EVIDENCE-BASED MEDICINE

Pnagos M, Compalati E, Trantini F, et al. Efficacy of sublingual immunotherapy in the treatment of allergic rhinitis in pediatric patients 3 to 18 years of age: a meta-analysis of randomized, placebo-controlled, double-blind trials. *Ann Allergy Asthma Immunol.* 2006;97:141.

Cox LS, Linnemann DL, Nolte H, et al. Sublingual immunotherapy: a comprehensive review. *J Allergy Clin Immunol.* 2006;117:1021.

There is an ongoing debate concerning the role of sublingual immunotherapy in the treatment of allergic disease, with the bulk of evidence suggesting that the treatment is less effective than injection therapy but safer. Certainly additional information is needed, as emphasized by the article in the *Journal of Allergy and Clinical Immunology.* Treatment of young children with immunotherapy is an attractive alternative because there may be potential benefit in reducing need for medications and in altering the clinical course of disease. The

safety and acceptability of sublingual immunotherapy makes this a very attractive option in atopic young children. However, we do not have sufficient evidence showing long-term benefits of sublingual immunotherapy or modification of disease development. The lack of consistent immunologic changes in subjects, both adults and children, treated with sublingual immunotherapy is also a concern. There is most likely a significant dose effect, reminding us that we cannot use standard injection doses for sublingual immunotherapy because of antigen degradation by the oral and gastrointestinal mucosal contact. Finally, sublingual immunotherapy is not FDA approved. Monitoring of the literature related to this topic is essential.

Casale TB, Busse WW, Line JN, et al. Omalizumab pretreatment decreases acute reactions after rush immunotherapy for ragweed-induced seasonal allergic rhinitis. *J Allergy Clin Immunol.* 2006;117:134.

The possibility of combining anti-IgE with allergen immunotherapy is a potential synergistic strategy potentially allowing a more rapid achievement of maintenance dose and possibly a more effective maintenance dose. The proven long-term benefits of immunotherapy would complement the more rapid benefits of omalizumab. This article confirms these observations, although the degree of protection from anaphylaxis and the magnitude of symptom improvement were perhaps less than expected.

BIBLIOGRAPHY

Akerlund A, Andersson M, Leflein J, et al. Clinical trial design, nasal allergen challenge models, and considerations of relevance to pediatrics, nasal polyposis, and different classes of medication. *J Allergy Clin Immunol.* 2005;115:S460.

Bachert C. Persistent rhinitis-allergic or nonallergic. *Allergy.* 2004;59(suppl 76):11.

Bauchau V, Durham SR. Epidemiological characterization of the intermittent and persistent types of allergic rhinitis. *Allergy.* 2005;60:350.

Bousquet J, van Cauwenberge P, Khaltaev N, et al. Allergic rhinitis and its impact on asthma. *J Allergy Clin Immunol.* 2001;108:S147.

Gelfand EW. Inflammatory mediators in allergic rhinitis. *J Allergy Clin Immunol.* 2005;116:463.

Golightly LK, Greos LS. Second-generation antihistamines: actions and efficacy in the management of allergic disorders. *Drugs.* 2005;65:341.

Holgate ST, Djukanovic R, Casale T, et al. Anti-immunoglobulin E treatment with omalizumab in allergic diseases: an update on anti-inflammatory activity and clinical efficacy. *Clin Exp Allergy.* 2005;35:408.

Howarth PH, Persson CGA, Meltzer EO, et al. Objective monitoring of nasal airway inflammation in rhinitis. *J Allergy Clin Immunol.* 2005;115:S414.

Juniper EF, Stahl E, Doty RL, et al. Clinical outcomes and adverse effect monitoring in allergic rhinitis. *J Allergy Clin Immunol.* 2005;115:S390.

Nathan RA, Eccles R, Howarth PH, et al. Objective monitoring of nasal patency and nasal physiology in rhinitis. *J Allergy Clin Immunol.* 2005;115:S442.

Nielsen LP, Dahl R. Comparison of intranasal corticosteroids and antihistamines in allergic rhinitis: a review of randomized, controlled trials. *Am J Respir Med.* 2003;2:55.

Peters-Golden M, Henderson WR Jr. The role of leukotrienes in allergic rhinitis. *Ann Allergy Asthma Immunol.* 2005;94:609.

Portnoy JM, Van Osdol T, Williams PB. Evidence-based strategies for treatment of allergic rhinitis. *Curr Allergy Asthma Rep.* 2004;4:439.

Sanico AM. Latest developments in the management of allergic rhinitis. *Clin Rev Allergy Immunol.* 2004;27:181.

Taramarcaz P, Gibson PG. The effectiveness of intranasal corticosteroids in combined allergic rhinitis and asthma syndrome. *Clin Exp Allergy.* 2004;34:1883.

Till SJ, Francis JN, Nours-Aria K, et al. Mechanisms of immunotherapy. *J Allergy Clin Immunol.* 2004;113:1025.

Wilson DR, Lima MT, Durham SR. Sublingual immunotherapy for allergic rhinitis: systematic review and meta-analysis. *Allergy.* 2005;60:1.

The Effect of Rhinitis on Sleep, Quality of Life, Daytime Somnolence, and Fatigue

7

Carah Santos, MS and Timothy J. Craig, DO

Patients with allergic rhinitis, one of several inflammatory disorders of the upper respiratory tract, often suffer from impaired sleep. A recent survey of allergic rhinitis patients revealed that 68% of respondents with perennial allergic rhinitis (PAR) and 48% with seasonal allergic rhinitis (SAR) reported that their condition causes significant sleep disturbances. One of the major symptoms of the disorder, nasal congestion, in addition to such underlying disease processes as the release of inflammatory mediators, can cause the sleep impairment associated with allergic rhinitis.

The symptoms of allergic rhinitis include rhinorrhea, sneezing, pruritus of the eyes, nose, and throat, and nasal congestion. Nasal congestion stands as one of the most prominent and bothersome symptoms of the disorder, especially because it is linked to sleep-related problems associated with allergic rhinitis, such as sleep-disordered breathing, sleep apnea, and snoring.

The prevalence of inflammatory disorders of the upper respiratory tract make the sleep impairment associated with many of these disorders a common problem. Allergic rhinitis alone reportedly affects approximately 25% of the world's population, and its prevalence has continued to climb. It has been estimated that the disorder affects 20 to 40 million people in the United States, which includes approximately 40% of the nation's children. In Europe, the prevalence of allergic rhinitis is estimated as 23%.

Those who suffer from allergic rhinitis often cannot escape the socioeconomic burdens associated with living with the disorder. In 2000, patients spent over $6 billion on prescription medications for allergic rhinitis. Along with this overwhelming cost of treatment, patients must face the secondary cost of poor productivity, which stems from the negative impact of the disorder's symptoms on patients' lives, as well as the use of inappropriate therapies. The detrimental effect of allergic rhinitis on patients' quality of life has been demonstrated by generic health-related quality of life questionnaires, such as the Medical Outcomes Study Short Form Health Survey (SF-36), and disease-specific measures, such as the Rhinoconjunctivitis Quality of Life Questionnaire (RQLQ). This adverse impact on patients may result from the sleep impairment associated with the disorder.

Although studies have shown that treatments for allergic rhinitis, particularly those that improve symptoms of nasal congestion, can improve patients' sleep and quality of life, further research is needed to elaborate this limited existing data. This chapter explores the sleep impairment associated with allergic rhinitis and the adverse effects of disturbed sleep on patients' quality of life. This chapter also examines how these effects are impacted by therapies that target the disorder's underlying problems influencing sleep.

EVIDENCE FOR SLEEP IMPAIRMENT IN ALLERGIC RHINITIS

Allergic rhinitis and other inflammatory disorders of the upper respiratory tract are generally associated with sleep impairment, daytime somnolence, and fatigue. Of the multiple symptoms of allergic rhinitis, nasal congestion, in particular, detrimentally affects sleep. The Allergic Rhinitis and its Impact on Asthma (ARIA) guidelines (Table 7–1) serve to classify allergic rhinitis severity and provide a measure for this degree of sleep impairment. The sleep disturbances allergic rhinitis patients suffer from include microarousals and sleep-disordered breathing, which includes snoring to obstructive sleep apnea and/or hypopnea. Chronic excessive daytime sleepiness or fatigue has been demonstrated

Table 7–1. ARIA guidelines for the classification of allergic rhinitis.

Symptoms	
Intermittent	Present <4 d/wk and <4 wk
Persistent	Present 4 d/wk and >4 wk
Severity	
Mild	No impairment of sleep, daily activities, leisure or sport, or school or work No troublesome symptoms
Moderate–severe	One of more of the following are present: Impairment of sleep Impairment of daily activities, leisure, or sport Impairment of school or work Troublesome symptoms

as more likely disturbances in patients with frequent nighttime symptoms than in those with rare or no such symptoms. Further examples illustrating that sleep impairment stands as a major concern for allergic rhinitis patients include a study showing that allergic rhinitis leads to snoring in children, and another study demonstrating that concomitant allergic rhinitis independently relates to difficulty sleeping and daytime sleepiness in bronchial asthma patients.

MECHANISMS OF SLEEP IMPAIRMENT

To alleviate the symptom of sleep impairment in patients with allergic rhinitis, the mechanisms involved in this problematic issue must first be identified. Recent studies have proposed that the reduced sleep quality and daytime fatigue characteristic in allergic rhinitis patients may consequently arise from sleep impairment secondary to symptoms of the disorder, particularly nasal congestion, or to the effects of the disorder itself, such as the underlying pathophysiologic changes associated with allergic rhinitis leading to the release of cytokines and other inflammatory mediators.

Nasal Congestion

Nasal congestion, which results when the cavernous tissues of the nasal turbinates swell following dilation of the capacitance vessels, is a common and bothersome symptom that affects numerous allergic rhinitis patients. Its mechanism involves the reduction in the internal nasal diameter and the increase in airway resistance to nasal airflow, and the symptom can also cause nasal

obstruction. Subjective clinical assessments of nasal congestion severity exist, as well as objective measures of nasal airflow, such as peak nasal inspiratory flow (PNIF), assessments of airway resistance and conductance (rhinomanometry), and acoustic rhinometry, which assesses the volume and area of the nasal cavity by analyzing reflected sound waves.

The symptom of nasal congestion worsens at night and first thing in the morning, peaking at 6 AM, presumptively due to the posture change when an individual first lies down and to the normal decrease in serum cortisol levels overnight. The lower cortisol levels lead to greater nocturnal airway obstruction and may partially explain the large-amplitude circadian variation (Fig. 7–1). These changes and others noted in Table 7–2 may serve to explain why patients with inflammatory nasal conditions and nasal congestion often suffer from sleep impairment and daytime fatigue.

Results from an Internet survey of 2355 individuals with allergic rhinitis or the parents of children with allergic rhinitis further reinforced the complaints of those suffering from the disorder. Eighty-five percent of the respondents or their children reported experiencing nasal congestion, and 40% of all respondents, the greatest proportion of participants who rated the severity of various symptoms, considered their nasal congestion severe (Fig. 7–2).

Approximately 50% of the respondents reported that nasal congestion was their most bothersome symptom and that it woke them during the night and made it difficult to fall asleep (Fig. 7–3). Twenty percent of adult respondents claimed that their bed partner's sleep was adversely affected by their nasal congestion, and the

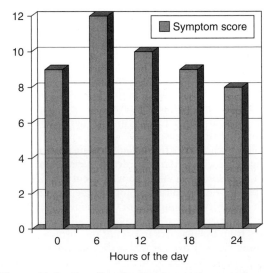

Figure 7–1. Circadian rhythms in nasal congestion.

Table 7–2. Changes in early morning that may account for the circadian variation seen in allergic rhinitis.

Increased vagal tone
Accumulation of secretions overnight
Cortisol at lowest level
Adrenaline and norepinephrine both low
Increased tryptase, histamine, and eosinophilic cationic protein (ECP) in nasal secretion
Mite and other indoor allergen exposure high

degree of sleep impairment correlated with the severity of their congestion. Moreover, the survey revealed that nasal congestion negatively impacted the individuals' or their children's emotions and ability to perform daily activities, all of which may result from the detrimental effects of nasal congestion on sleep.

Studies on treatments for the nasal congestion associated with allergic rhinitis, such as one by Craig et al. on treatment with topical nasal corticosteroids, propose that the poor sleep and daytime somnolence characteristic of the disorder is predominantly attributed to the symptom of nasal congestion. Increased sleep apnea and transient arousals even occur when subjecting healthy individuals to nasal occlusion with a nose clip. Previous studies that objectively assessed the sleep patterns of allergic rhinitis patients demonstrated that their symptoms of nasal congestion led to increased microarousals and episodes of apnea at night. Subjective instruments, such as Juniper's Nocturnal Rhinoconjunctivitis Quality of Life Questionnaire (NRQLQ), correlate with the objective findings noted on polysomnography. Allergic rhinoconjunctivitis patients who complained of impaired sleep due to nighttime symptoms found nasal and sinus congestion to be among their most bothersome and troublesome symptoms.

A population-based study on the role of acute and chronic nasal congestion in sleep-disordered breathing, which used 4927 subjects with a history of nasal congestion and impaired sleep, showed that patients with frequent nocturnal rhinitis symptoms, compared to those with rare or no symptoms, were more likely to complain of habitual snoring, chronic nonrestorative sleep, and excessive daytime fatigue. Additionally, the study illustrated that subjects with allergic rhinitis—associated nasal congestion were 1.8 times more likely to suffer from moderate-to-severe sleep-disordered breathing, compared to subjects with allergic rhinitis

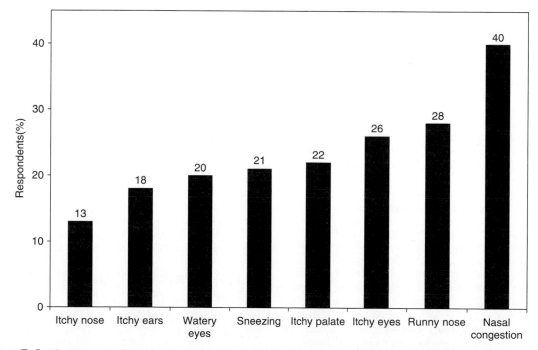

Figure 7–2. The severity of nasal congestion in individuals with allergic rhinitis. Results are expressed as a proportion of all survey respondents who experienced a particular symptom who rated it as severe (9 or 10 on a 10-point scale with 1 being mild and 10 severe).

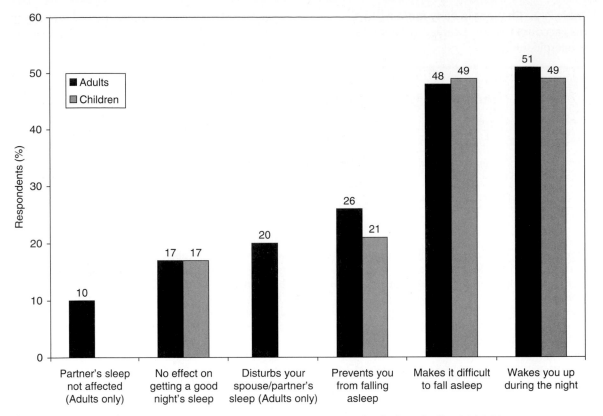

Figure 7–3. The effect of nasal congestion on sleep by a survey in individuals with allergic rhinitis.

and no reported nasal congestion. Rhinitis and other forms of nasal obstruction must be considered and treated in patients with primary sleep-associated breathing disorders as an adjunct to surgical and nonsurgical treatment. Topical nasal steroids may enhance compliance and effectiveness of continuous positive airway pressure (CPAP) especially, but not limited, to those patients with allergic rhinitis.

Immune Response Mediators

Histamine and cytokines are examples of inflammatory mediators released in the process of an allergic reaction, and such mediators may directly influence the central nervous system and result in the disturbed sleep daytime somnolence characteristic of allergic rhinitis. Histamine helps regulate the sleep-wake cycle and arousal; the higher levels of the cytokines interleukin (IL)-1β, IL-4, and IL-10 seen in patients with allergies, compared with healthy individuals, correlate with increased latency to rapid eye movement (REM) sleep, decreased time in REM sleep, and decreased latency to sleep onset. It is postulated that any such disruptions in REM sleep may

cause daytime fatigue, difficulty concentrating, and poor performance in allergic rhinitis patients. Inflammatory cells and mediators exhibit evident circadian variation, with its highest levels in the early morning hours, thus possibly explaining why the peak of allergic rhinitis symptoms frequently occurs upon waking and why nighttime sleep is detrimentally affected in the disorder. In addition, TNF, IL-1 and IL-6 are cytokines increased in allergic rhinitis and may cause fatigue and other nonspecific generalized symptoms typical of a flulike condition. Table 7–3 provides a list of inflammatory mediators in rhinitis that can account for the symptoms of daytime somnolence and fatigue.

SLEEP IMPAIRMENT AND QUALITY OF LIFE

The Effects of Sleep Impairment

Patients with allergic rhinitis often must face adverse consequences of sleep disturbances, such as impaired cognitive function and decreased productivity and performance in the workplace. In children with allergic

Table 7–3. List of mediators contributing to daytime somnolence and fatigue (allergic rhinitis vs. severe sleep apnea).

Mediator	Obese male with severe sleep apnea	Young female with allergic rhinitis
IL-1	Increased	Increased
IL-4	Increased	Increased
IL-6	Increased	Increased
Histamine	Abnormal	Abnormal
Bradykinin	Increased	Increased
IL-2	Decreased	Decreased

rhinitis, learning ability and school performance are afflicted. Although symptoms of the disorder may lead to these consequences, the sleep impairment caused by allergic rhinitis is the likely cause of aggravation. Sleep-disordered breathing and sleep impairment have been known to correlate with decreased quality of life in the general population. Specifically, experimentally induced sleep fragmentation in healthy subjects leads to impaired mental flexibility and attention, increased daytime fatigue, and impaired mood. Children and adolescents with allergic rhinitis also suffer from impaired sleep, which results in problems doing schoolwork and poor school performance, compared to controls.

A survey across five European countries using patients suffering from allergic rhinitis or urticaria showed that a considerable proportion of respondents reported snoring or poor sleep and not feeling rested in the morning. Of these respondents, 29% to 79%, and 28% to 56%, respectively, depending on the country, considered these problems either disruptive or extremely disruptive. Results from an Internet survey of 1322 individuals with rhinitis showed that both perennial and seasonal rhinitis interfered with sleep (68% and 51% of respondents, respectively) and daily routine (58% and 48%, respectively). Additionally, the sleep impairment suffered by allergic rhinitis patients has been linked to reduced psychological well-being, daytime fatigue, difficulty concentrating, and impaired psychomotor performance.

MEASURING SLEEP IMPAIRMENT AND IMPACT ON QUALITY OF LIFE

Studies on the subjective and objective measurements of sleep impairment and its influence on patients' quality of life particularly emphasize the major impact of this problem in patients with such inflammatory nasal

conditions as allergic rhinitis. In patients with this disorder, the majority of studies have used subjective measures, such as questionnaires (Table 7–4) or daily scoring of symptoms, sleep problems, daytime somnolence, and fatigue. Juniper's Rhinoconjunctivitis Quality of Life Questionnaire (RQLQ) uses quality of life measures that are disease specific and includes a domain that assesses the effects of disease and/or treatment on patients' sleep. Such questionnaires emphasize the problems and symptoms patients commonly complain of and seek help for and are thus more sensitive to alterations in patients' quality of life than generic health-status questionnaires. The Nocturnal Rhinoconjunctivitis Quality of Life Questionnaire (NRQLQ) focuses on the functional impairments of patients with nighttime symptoms and assesses problems and symptoms during sleep time, as well as upon waking hours. The Epworth Sleepiness Scale, Pittsburgh Sleep Quality Index, Calgary Sleep Apnea Quality of Life Index, and the University of Pennsylvania Functional Outcomes of Sleep Questionnaire serve as general questionnaires that examine quality of sleep and daytime somnolence. However, the latter four questionnaires may be inadequate in their analysis of the mild-to-moderate sleep impairment characteristic of allergic rhinitis because they have less sensitivity.

Studies on allergic rhinitis that objectively assess sleep by using polysomnography are small in number. One such study observed 25 patients with SAR and 25 healthy volunteers, all of whom underwent two consecutive nights of polysomnography before and during the pollen season, and results showed statistically significant differences between the two groups in sleep parameters, which included increases in the apnea index

Table 7–4. Disease-specific quality of life questionnaires and general measures of sleep quality.

Disease-specific questionnaires
Rhinoconjunctivitis Quality of Life Questionnaire (RQLQ)
Nocturnal Rhinoconjunctivitis Quality of Life Questionnaire (NRQLQ)

General sleep measures
Epworth Sleepiness Scale
Pittsburgh Sleep Quality Index
Calgary Sleep Apnea Quality of Life Index
University of Pennsylvania Functional Outcomes of Sleep Questionnaire

(number of apneas per hour), hypopnea index (number of hypopneas per hour), apnea–hypopnea index, snoring time, amount of REM sleep, and sleep latency. However, parameter values fell within normal limits, preventing the changes from showing clinical relevance. Statistical significance was also reported in daytime sleepiness, which was subjectively measured using the Epworth Sleepiness Scale, in SAR patients compared to healthy subjects. These results thus point toward a weak correlation between subjective and objective measures of sleep impairment.

EFFECTS OF THERAPY

Treatments aimed at reducing nasal congestion may alleviate sleep disturbances and daytime somnolence and consequently improve the quality of life in those who suffer from allergic rhinitis. However, the multiple treatments for the disorder vary in their efficacies.

Sedating antihistamines are contraindicated in patients who complain of daytime sedation, fatigue, and functional impairment; such treatment is also not recommended for most patients with allergic rhinitis. Common treatment for allergic rhinitis includes nonsedating oral antihistamines, which alleviate nasal symptoms such as rhinorrhea, sneezing, and pruritus but may be less effective in reducing nasal congestion. Two studies by Murray et al. and Golden et al. suggest that treatment using oral or topical antihistamines result in improved sleep and quality of life. Oral decongestants are successful in improving nasal congestion but may impact sleep detrimentally because of their stimulatory effects and, additionally, may result in systemic side effects, such as tachycardia and urinary retention. Topical decongestants improve sleep in patients with nasal obstruction but should not be used for more than a few days, due to the risk of rhinitis medicamentosa, or "rebound" congestion. Data, although very limited, show that the anticholinergic agent ipratropium bromide may improve sleep and quality of life. However, ipratropium bromide appears to be unsuccessful in the relief of nasal congestion. Studies have shown that either leukotriene receptor antagonists as monotherapy or in combination with an antihistamine effectively improves sleep and quality of life in allergic rhinitis patients and in those who suffer from sleep-disordered breathing. Intranasal corticosteroids alleviate congestion and other nasal symptoms of allergic rhinitis and are used as first-line therapy when nasal obstruction is a predominant symptom in patients.

The Role of Intranasal Corticosteroids

Intranasal corticosteroids have been shown to relieve all the nasal symptoms of allergic rhinitis effectively including congestion. The effectiveness of intranasal corticosteroids in relieving nasal congestion may have a positive impact on sleep, daytime somnolence, and quality of life in patients who suffer from allergic rhinitis. Studies on adults and children with PAR support the hypothesis that intranasal corticosteroids decrease nasal congestion and subjective daytime sleepiness and fatigue, and improve sleep and quality of life. Further studies displayed efficacy in the improvement of nasal symptoms and quality of life, as well as verbal memory. Treatment was also proven to alleviate allergic rhinitis associated with Obstructive Sleep Apnea Syndrome (OSAS) and consequently to lead to both significantly lower frequencies of apnea/hypopnea episodes and subjective improvements in nasal congestion and daytime alertness, although snoring noise was unchanged.

Studies in allergic rhinitis patients using the RQLQ, NRQLQ, and the Pittsburgh Sleep Quality Index revealed that intranasal corticosteroid improves both nasal congestion and health-related quality of life, including sleep. These studies therefore support the notion that treatments focusing on the nasal symptoms of allergic rhinitis may reduce sleep impairment and improve patients' quality of life.

CONCLUSION

The quality of life in patients with allergic rhinitis is detrimentally impacted by the sleep impairment associated with the disorder. One of the key causes leading to sleep disruptions and sleep-disordered breathing is nasal congestion, one of the most common and bothersome symptoms of allergic rhinitis. Recent research has led to the use of therapeutic agents that specifically target the nasal congestion associated with sleep impairment.

Intranasal corticosteroids stand as effective treatment that significantly reduces nasal congestion in allergic rhinitis. Clinical trials using this treatment suggest that this reduction in nasal congestion correlates with decreased sleep impairment, reduced daytime somnolence, and improved quality of life.

Further research is necessary to conclude definitively that intranasal corticosteroids hold the ability to improve sleep and quality of life in patients with allergic rhinitis. These studies should use sleep-related measures as primary endpoints and assess sleep parameters both subjectively and objectively, thus serving to identify the most effective therapies for alleviating the detrimental effects of sleep impairment associated with allergic rhinitis.

EVIDENCE-BASED MEDICINE

The hypothesis is that sleep and the consequences of poor sleep has been supported primarily by subjective assessments in studies where sleep-related outcomes stood as secondary endpoints. No controlled study has shown definitively that the reduction of nasal congestion, as measured by an objective instrument, correlates with improvement in daytime somnolence and fatigue or objective sleep measures. Despite this deficiency, a direct correlation between subjective improvement of congestion and sleep has been demonstrated. However, placebo-controlled, double-blinded, large randomized clinical trials that subjectively and objectively assess the outcomes of intranasal corticosteroid use on allergic rhinitis with impaired sleep, productivity, and daytime somnolence are needed.

BIBLIOGRAPHY

Camhi SL, Morgan WJ, Pernisco N, et al. Factors affecting sleep disturbances in children and adolescents. *Sleep Med.* 2000;1:117.

Canova CR, Downs SH, Knoblauch A, et al. Increased prevalence of perennial allergic rhinitis in patients with obstructive sleep apnea. *Respiration.* 2004;71:138.

Craig TJ, Mende C, Hughes K, et al. The effect of topical nasal fluticasone on objective sleep testing and the symptoms of rhinitis, sleep, and daytime somnolence in perennial allergic rhinitis. *Allergy Asthma Proc.* 2003;24:53.

Hughes K, Glass C, Ripchinski M, et al. Efficacy of the topical nasal steroid budesonide on improving sleep and daytime somnolence in patients with perennial allergic rhinitis. *Allergy.* 2003;58:380.

Juniper EF, Rohrbaugh T, Meltzer EO. A questionnaire to measure quality of life in adults with nocturnal allergic rhinoconjunctivitis. *J Allergy Clin Immunol.* 2003;111:484.

Kessler RC, Almeida DM, Berglund P, et al. Pollen and mold exposure impairs the work performance of employees with allergic rhinitis. *Ann Allergy Asthma Immunol.* 2001;87:289.

Kiely JL, Nolan P, McNicholas WT. Intranasal corticosteroid therapy for obstructive sleep apnoea in patients with co-existing rhinitis. *Thorax.* 2004;59:50.

Kremer B, den Hartog HM, Jolles J. Relationship between allergic rhinitis, disturbed cognitive functions and psychological well-being. *Clin Exp Allergy.* 2002;32:1310.

Krouse HJ, Davis JE, Krouse JH. Immune mediators in allergic rhinitis and sleep. *Otolaryngol Head Neck Surg.* 2002;126:607.

Marshall PS, O'Hara C, Steinberg P. Effects of seasonal allergic rhinitis on selected cognitive abilities. *Ann Allergy Asthma Immunol.* 2000;84:403.

McLean HA, Urton AM, Driver HS, et al. Effect of treating severe nasal obstruction on the severity of obstructive sleep apnea. *Eur Respir J.* 2005;25:521.

Mintz M, Garcia J, Diener P, et al. Triamcinolone acetonide aqueous nasal spray improves nocturnal rhinitis-related quality of life in patients treated in a primary care setting: the Quality of Sleep in Allergic Rhinitis study. *Ann Allergy Asthma Immunol.* 2004;92:255.

Stuck BA, Czajkowski J, Hagner A-E, et al. Changes in daytime sleepiness, quality of life, and objective sleep patterns in seasonal allergic rhinitis: a controlled clinical trial. *J Allergy Clin Immunol.* 2004;113:663.

Urschitz M, Guenther A, Eggebrecht E, et al. Snoring, intermittent hypoxia and academic performance in primary school children. *Am J Respir Crit Care Med.* 2003;168:464.

Wilken JA, Berkowitz R, Kane R. Decrements in vigilance and cognitive functioning associated with ragweed-induced allergic rhinitis. *Ann Allergy Asthma Immunol.* 2002;89:372.

Sinusitis

Kevin C. Welch, MD and Andrew N. Goldberg, MD, MSCE, FACS

GENERAL CONSIDERATIONS

Inflammation or infection of the paranasal sinuses is termed *sinusitis*. Because sinusitis as a clinical entity rarely exists without associated rhinitis, the Sinus and Allergy Health Partnership (SAHP) has recommended the use of the term *rhinosinusitis* when referring to this disease entity. Acute and chronic rhinosinusitis affect nearly 20% of the U.S. population annually. The direct and indirect health care expenditures exceed $3.5 to $5.8 billion per year. The impact of rhinosinusitis results in nearly 25 million visits to physicians annually, and for these reasons, it remains a subject of active research in both the medical and pharmaceutical communities.

Classification of Rhinosinusitis

Rhinosinusitis is typically viral or bacterial; however, it can also become manifest as a result of other causes of inflammation such as chemical irritation or radiation. In the clinical setting, virtually all episodes of acute bacterial rhinosinusitis (ABRS) are preceded by viral rhinosinusitis (VRS), or the common cold. Studies consistently show that distinguishing VRS from ABRS is often difficult because the two conditions possess similar symptom profiles and the available imaging modalities have failed to reliably distinguish between the two disease entities (Table 8–1). This results in both the inappropriate treatment of VRS with antibiotics and the potential development of antibiotic resistance among the flora in the nasal cavity and nasopharynx that commonly cause ABRS. However, as the duration of the viral illness increases, the likelihood of a bacterial suprainfection increases. Therefore, the clinical diagnosis of ABRS may be made after 7 to 10 days of persistent VRS symptoms or definitive worsening of symptoms after 5 to 7 days from the onset of the upper respiratory infection. This diagnosis is suggested by the presence of two major symptoms or one major symptom and two minor symptoms in the appropriate time course (Table 8–2).

Bacterial rhinosinusitis is arbitrarily categorized in terms of the duration of symptoms. Acute bacterial rhinosinusitis is diagnosed when signs and symptoms have been present for less than 4 weeks. Subacute bacterial rhinosinusitis is diagnosed when signs and symptoms have been present for 4 to 12 weeks. Chronic rhinosinusitis (CRS) is diagnosed when signs and symptoms have been present for greater than 12 weeks. In addition to the presence of symptoms, imaging is recommended in the diagnosis of CRS.

ANATOMY

The anatomy of the nose and paranasal sinuses is highly variable and often complex. Knowledge of the anatomy and relationships (Figs. 8–1 and 8–2) of the paranasal sinus structures to each other and to other vital organs (orbit, optic nerve, and carotid artery) permits an understanding of the pathophysiology of rhinosinusitis as well as the factors that impede treatment and lead to recurrent disease. Each sinus is lined with mucosa consisting of ciliated pseudostratified columnar epithelium. The cilia propel mucus and debris toward the natural ostium of each sinus in a predictable fashion (Fig. 8–3).

The Septum and Turbinates

The septum anatomically divides the nasal cavity into two halves. It is composed of four bony and cartilaginous elements: the quadrilateral cartilage (anterior), the perpendicular plate of the ethmoid bone (superior and posterior), the vomer bone (inferior and posterior), and the maxillary crest (along the floor of the nasal cavity). It is lined with ciliated pseudostratified columnar epithelium. It is estimated that as many as 80% of septums are deviated in some fashion; however, these deviations are often asymptomatic and infrequently the cause of disease. Significant septal deviations may cause nasal obstruction or compress the middle turbinate, thus obstructing the ostiomeatal complex and preventing sinus outflow.

Table 8–1. Symptoms of viral rhinosinusitis.

Sore throat
Rhinorrhea
Cough
Fever, typically <102 degrees for <3 days
Hoarseness

The turbinates are mucosa-lined structures that arise from the cartilaginous nasal capsule during the 8th week of embryological development. Typically, three turbinates on each side (superior, middle, and inferior turbinates) persist into adulthood. The majority of each turbinate is lined with ciliated pseudostratified columnar epithelium, and olfactory tissue can be found on the middle and superior turbinates. The inferior and middle turbinates contain numerous venous plexuses that under parasympathetic stimulation dilate in a cyclic fashion to alter the patency of the nasal cavity. This natural phenomenon is known as the nasal cycle. Additionally, the mucosa lining these turbinates is particularly responsive to external irritants and allergens that can lead to nasal obstruction and rhinorrhea.

The Ostiomeatal Complex

The confluence of drainage pathways from the maxillary sinus, frontal sinus, and anterior ethmoid sinuses forms the ostiomeatal complex (OMC) (Fig. 8–4). The OMC is not an anatomic structure per se but rather a pathway that when obstructed by inflamed mucosa or a mass may cause subsequent sinus obstruction and ultimately infection. Familiarity with the OMC is particularly important in understanding the pathophysiology of acute and

Table 8–2. Major and minor symptoms of rhinosinusitis.

Major Symptoms	Minor Symptoms
Facial pain or pressure	Headache
Nasal obstruction or blockage	Fever
Nasal discharge	Halitosis
Change in smell	Fatigue
Purulence	Cough
Fever	Otologic symptoms

Adapted from Sinus and Allergy Health Partnership. Antimicrobial Treatment Guidelines for Acute Bacterial Rhinosinusitis. *Otolaryngol Head Neck Surg* 130 (suppl 1):S1, 2004.

chronic rhinosinusitis, and this outflow pathway should be examined in great detail when reviewing computed tomography scans in patients (discussed later). Obstruction of the ostiomeatal complex helps one understand how disease in this region can lead to secondary obstruction of the maxillary and frontal sinuses.

The Paranasal Sinuses

MAXILLARY SINUS

The maxillary sinus represents an expansion of the lateral nasal wall (infundibulum) into the maxillary bone that occurs around the 8th week of gestation. Subsequent pneumatization is biphasic: the first phase in early childhood and the second phase in adolescence. Through most of its expansion, the floor of the maxillary sinus remains at the same level as the floor of the nasal cavity; however, during its final growth, the floor of the maxillary sinus may pneumatize the maxillary alveolar process and rest 5 to 10 mm below the floor of the nasal cavity. The ostium of the maxillary sinus is located on the medial wall of the sinus and is approximately 2 to 3 mm in diameter. An accessory ostium located posterior to the natural ostium is identified in 15% to 20% of cases. The cilia of the maxillary sinus direct mucus and debris through the natural ostium and into the middle meatus.

ETHMOID SINUSES

The ethmoid sinuses develop from a series of lamella and grooves that suspend from the cribriform plate and along the lateral nasal wall around the 8th week of gestation. The first lamella typically forms the agger nasi cell superiorly and the uncinate process inferiorly. The second lamella forms the *bulla ethmoidalis*, an anterior ethmoid cell. The third lamella forms the middle turbinate, the medial boundary of the middle meatus. The remainder of the lamellae forms the posterior ethmoid cells and the superior turbinate. Several other ethmoid cells that may develop are of clinical importance. An infraorbital ethmoid or Haller cell may project into the maxillary sinus near the maxillary sinus ostium, which may impede maxillary sinus outflow. A sphenoethmoid or Onodi cell may pneumatize around the optic nerve, posing a surgical risk.

SPHENOID SINUS

The sphenoid sinus develops in early adolescence as epithelium invaginates into the sphenoid bone where pneumatization occurs. The sphenoid sinus is divided by a septum, which typically divides the sinus asymmetrically. The sphenoid sinus possesses two ostia through which the sinus ventilates and drains mucus. These ostia are 2 to 3 mm in diameter and sit superiorly on the anterior face of the sinus near the base of the skull. The sphenoid sinus is clinically significant in that several critical

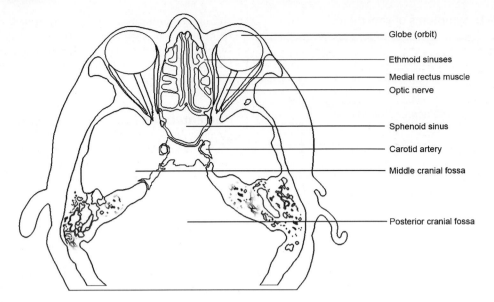

Figure 8–1. Axial anatomy of the nasal cavity and paranasal sinuses. Important anatomic landmarks and relevant sinuses are detailed.

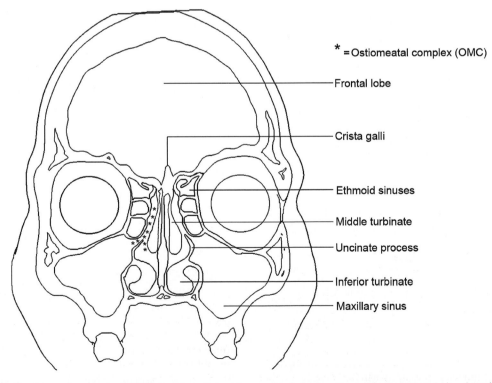

Figure 8–2. Coronal anatomy of the nasal cavity and paranasal sinuses. Important anatomic landmarks and relevant sinuses are detailed along with the ostiomeatal complex (asterisks).

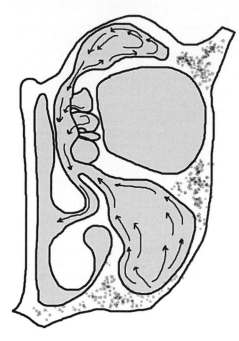

Figure 8–3. The pathway of mucociliary clearance. Cilia beat in a predictable fashion such that mucus and debris are propelled toward the natural ostium of the sinus. Disrupting this flow can lead to stasis or recirculation (if an iatrogenic ostium is created).

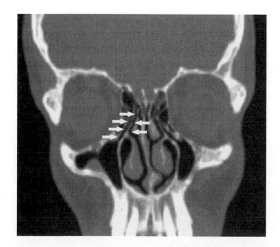

Figure 8–4. A coronal computed tomography image of a patient demonstrating the ostiomeatal complex (arrows defining black space). It should be evident that obstruction of this small region can lead to obstruction in the maxillary or ethmoid sinuses.

structures surround it. The optic nerve usually indents the lateral wall of the sphenoid sinus, and approximately 5% to 7% of patients have no intervening bone between the optic nerve and the sphenoid sinus. The carotid artery also indents the lateral sphenoid sinus wall with 7% of these being dehiscent, that is, with no bone separating the artery and the sphenoid sinus. Posterior and lateral to the sphenoid sinus is the cavernous sinus, a venous plexus structure through which the carotid artery, the oculomotor (CN III) nerve, trochlear (CN IV) nerve, trigeminal (CN V) nerve, and abducens (CN VI) nerve pass. Additionally, the pituitary gland rests superior and posterior to the sinus and can typically be identified as an indentation in the sinus.

FRONTAL SINUS

The frontal sinus represents the superior pneumatization of the frontal bone by anterior ethmoid cells starting around the second year of life. Pneumatization of the frontal bone is occasionally incomplete, with 5% of the population having only a unilateral frontal sinus and 5% of the population having no frontal sinus cells. To complicate matters, ethmoid cells may expand into the frontal sinus causing unique patterns of obstruction. The frontal sinus drains through the frontal recess, which, unlike the other sinuses, is not an ostium or duct but rather a pathway of drainage formed by the walls of specific ethmoid sinuses, chiefly the agger nasi and the *bulla ethmoidalis.*

PATHOPHYSIOLOGY

Acute and chronic rhinosinusitis are different in many respects. The most significant is that ABRS is an exudative process that involves purulence and local neutrophilic infiltration of the sinuses. Chronic rhinosinusitis, however, appears to have multiple etiologies.

ACUTE BACTERIAL RHINOSINUSITIS

The insults that lead to rhinosinusitis have been well characterized. As previously stated, ABRS is usually preceded by viral rhinosinusitis. Whether by local destruction of mucosal epithelium or by upregulation of cytokines and infiltration by host immune cells, viral infections result in inflammation and edema of the nasal and sinus mucosa. Mucosal edema, when in the proper location, can cause ostial obstruction, leading to both stasis of secretions within the sinuses and relative hypoxia. The edema, inflammation, and stasis impair ciliary function, and patients may be susceptible to infection by bacteria colonizing the nasal cavity and nasopharynx. The subsequent bacterial infection leads to more inflammation, edema, and the influx of neutrophils. Therefore, ABRS can be viewed as an exudative and suppurative process.

Chronic Rhinosinusitis

The pathophysiology of chronic rhinosinusitis is more complex and the subject of active research today. The Sinus and Allergy Health Partnership has broadly divided the pathophysiology of CRS into intrinsic and extrinsic factors. In many cases, several overlapping factors may be involved in the pathophysiology of CRS of any given patient.

Intrinsic causes may be subdivided into genetic and acquired causes. The genetic causes include the previously mentioned primary ciliary dyskinesia, cystic fibrosis, or any other ultrastructural abnormality of the cilia. Each sinus is lined with a thin layer of mucosa populated by ciliated pseudostratified columnar epithelium. The cilia beat rhythmically such that the mucous layer (and debris) circulates through the sinus toward the natural ostium. In many instances, such as in the maxillary sinus and sphenoid sinus, this is often against the force of gravity. Ciliary function is easily impaired by changes in temperature, changes in pH, the effects of cigarette smoke, and changes in the consistency of the gel and sol layers of the mucous blanket. Genetic conditions such as primary ciliary dyskinesia or cystic fibrosis can either directly or indirectly impair the ability of the cilia to function effectively. Acquired causes include aspirin sensitivity (i.e., Samter's triad with concomitant asthma and nasal polyposis), hormonal rhinitis, and systemic causes, which are chiefly rheumatologic or autoimmune (e.g., Wegener granulomatosis, sarcoidosis, polyarteritis, and systemic lupus erythematosus). Extrinsic causes are the subject of intense research. This category is subdivided into allergic, bacterial, and fungal.

ALLERGIC

Allergic rhinitis (AR) is discussed extensively elsewhere in this book. Briefly, it is characterized by an abnormal hypersensitivity to extrinsic inhalant allergens that manifest in an IgE-mediated acute-phase response and an eosinophilic delayed-phase response. No causal relationship between AR and CRS has been demonstrated; nevertheless, the association between the two is widely recognized. Studies demonstrate that in the presence of AR, patients with symptoms of CRS demonstrate computed tomography (CT) or endoscopic evidence of CRS approximately 50% of the time. Furthermore, AR is present in 41% to 84% of patients with CRS who need surgery. In patients with CRS, the scoring of severity based on CT exams correlates with the severity of AR in those patients. Moreover, some studies reveal that in patients with concomitant CRS and AR, the benefits of surgery are more lasting when allergic therapy is administered following surgery. In any event, the correlation between AR and CRS is such that concomitant treatment of AR and CRS is appropriate, particularly in the patient who is undergoing surgery.

BACTERIAL

Unlike ABRS, a causal relationship between bacteria and CRS is not as obvious. Determining whether bacterial isolates are infectious causes of CRS or merely contaminants of the paranasal sinuses in patients with CRS, especially those who have undergone surgery, can be difficult. Clear differences exist in ABRS, which is an acute suppurative neutrophilic state, and CRS, which is a TH2 mediated state characterised by circulating lymphocytes, IL-4, and IL-5. This has led to the hypothesis that the presence of bacteria within the paranasal sinuses may incite an inflammatory response. One proposed theory of how this comes about is through bacterial superantigenicity. As opposed to the typical method of antigen presentation to T-cell receptors, superantigens bypass antigen-presenting cells to superstimulate T-cell receptors inappropriately. This leads to activation of large numbers of T cells and the overproduction of cytokines that result in inflammation. Other evidence for the role of bacteria includes the discovery of biofilms in the sinuses of patients with CRS. Biofilms represent the aggregation of bacterial organisms that are protected by a membrane consisting of extracellular matrix. Biofilms are significant in that they provide sufficient shielding of bacteria from antimicrobial agents and may contribute to the survivability of bacteria following antimicrobial administration and the development of resistant organisms.

It is important to recognize that the bacteria in CRS are different from those in ABRS. Their role in the pathogenesis of CRS is unclear and may be only one of several factors required in the development and treatment of CRS.

FUNGAL

Fungal colonization of the nasal cavity is frequently found in healthy volunteers and in patients with CRS. As with bacteria, finding a causal relationship between isolated fungal species and CRS is difficult. Allergic responses to fungal elements have been demonstrated in patients with allergic fungal sinusitis (AFS). These patients have documented IgE-mediated responses to the isolated fungal species, nasal polyposis, CT findings that are characteristic of the disease (heterogeneous opacification of involved sinuses), and a distinct lack of bone invasion. Additionally, non-IgE–mediated responses to fungal species have also been demonstrated in some patients with CRS.

BACTERIOLOGY

The paranasal sinuses are typically sterile environments; however, the nasal cavity and nasopharynx are environments frequently colonized by flora that have been responsible for both acute and chronic rhinosinusitis.

Acute Bacterial Rhinosinusitis

COMMUNITY ACQUIRED

The maxillary sinus has been frequently studied given the relative ease with which an aspiration of contents can be performed in patients who have signs and symptoms consistent with ABRS.

The most common bacterial isolate in community-acquired ABRS in children and in adults is *Streptococcus pneumoniae* (20% to 45% of isolates), an encapsulated gram-positive facultative anaerobe usually occurring in chains or pairs. By age 2, approximately 60% of children are nasopharyngeal carriers of *S. pneumoniae*, and by age 3, almost all children carry this species. These species come in several serotypes, and they are frequently undergoing recombination, which results in a change in serotype or serogroup. The relative hypoxia of an inflamed sinus provides the ideal grounds for replication and growth. Pneumolysin, a soluble 53kDa monomer, is the primary factor in virulent strains of pneumococcus. Pneumolysin binds to cell membrane cholesterol molecules and cross-links them, creating large transmembrane pores that result in cell lysis and death. *S. pneumoniae* resists antibiotic therapy through several mechanisms: efflux of antibiotic molecules, mutations in penicillin-binding proteins, and mutations in the encoding of ribosomal proteins.

Haemophilus influenzae, a gram-negative facultative anaerobe, is isolated in 20% to 35% of cases of ABRS in children and in adults. Nearly half of all children are colonized with *H. influenzae*. With the regular administration of the *H. influenzae* type b vaccine, *H. influenzae* type b strains are found infrequently. However, types a, c, d, e, f, and nontypable (unencapsulated) species are frequently recovered from nasopharyngeal and lateral nasal wall culture swabs. *H. influenzae* also thrive in the hypoxic environment of the inflamed paranasal sinuses. The incidence of resistance to β-lactams in this group is rising with the production of β-lactamase, a family of enzymes that catalyze the hydrolysis of the β-lactam ring that forms the basis of penicillins and cephalosporins. To combat this enzyme, various β-lactamase inhibitors (sulbactam, tazobactam, clavulanic acid) have been manufactured to increase the concentration of the delivered β-lactam. However, strains of *Haemophilus* that are inherently resistant to penicillins through mutations in penicillin-binding proteins are on the rise and effectively nullify the advantage of adding a β-lactamase inhibitor to a penicillin.

The frequency of other species isolated in ABRS varies from study to study and in the age of the patient. In children, the third most common isolate (15% to 20%) is *Moraxella catarrhalis*; however, in adults, this organism is isolated in only about 5% to 7% of cases of ABRS. *M. catarrhalis* is a gram-negative aerobe that, like *H. influenzae*, produces β-lactamases as its primary

defense against antibiotic agents. More than 90% of isolates are known to produce three closely related β-lactamases, making them virtually resistant to penicillins not containing a β-lactamase inhibitor. Cephalosporins still show good activity against this organism, however. Various streptococcal species and anaerobes also occur as pathogens in about equal frequencies (5% to 7%) in cases of pediatric and adult ABRS. Interestingly, approximately 20% to 35% of isolates in the pediatric population may be sterile.

NOSOCOMIAL ACQUIRED

Nosocomial ABRS often occurs in the setting of a prolonged hospital stay or in patients suffering maxillofacial trauma or head trauma, nasotracheal intubation, nasogastric intubation, or patients with burn injuries. These organisms are generally gram-negative organisms: *Pseudomonas aeruginosa*, *Serratia marcescens*, *Klebsiella pneumoniae*, and *Proteus* species. Additionally, *Staphylococcus aureus* is also frequently isolated. These organisms may be responsible for the development of ABRS or they may be the consequence of impaired mucociliary clearance and simply colonizing agents.

Chronic Rhinosinusitis

The role of bacteria in CRS is not clear. Directed cultures of patients with CRS have demonstrated a wide variety of bacterial pathogens that are often quite different from those isolated in ABRS. The two most common isolates are *S. aureus* and coagulase-negative staphylococci. These bacteria are also known for their biofilm production, and *S. aureus* is particularly known for its superantigenicity. Coagulase-negative staphylococci are frequently found in healthy subjects, and their role in infection of other areas of the body is often called into question; therefore, one must ask the question of whether coagulase-negative staphylococci are simply contaminates, infectious causes, or inflammatory "mediators" in CRS. Gram-negative species commonly isolated in CRS include *P. aeruginosa*, *Escherichia coli*, and *Enterobacter* species. Other organisms isolated include viridans streptococci, *Prevotella*, *Peptostreptococcus*, and *Fusobacterium*. Finally, as in ABRS, *S. pneumoniae*, *H. influenzae*, and *M. catarrhalis* are also isolated; however, these three agents are not found as frequently as *S. aureus* and coagulase-negative staphylococci.

Proper identification of the involved bacterial agents in CRS involves a direct culture of the involved sinus. Maxillary puncture is the gold standard for diagnosis; however, this can be done only with the maxillary sinus. Nasal cultures correlate poorly with antral puncture isolates and are not clinically helpful. Endoscopically directed cultures using a culturette or suction trap correlate nicely with antral puncture and are commonly used to determine the bacteriology of sinusitis. Trephination of the frontal sinus can be carried out, although this typically requires a procedure in the operating room and is seldom used outside of the context of urgent treatment of a complicated acute frontal sinusitis. Identification of any offending organisms should begin with Gram stain quantification as well as aerobic and anaerobic culture. Fungal cultures are commonly used in the clinical setting, although the significance of a positive culture for fungus is unclear. Pathologic examination of debris from the sinuses can confirm fungal involvement and suggest speciation, although this method is typically reserved for tissue obtained during surgery for sinusitis. As previously discussed, the overlapping etiologies in CRS lead one to question whether isolated organisms simply represent colonization or are causative of sinus inflammation.

DIAGNOSIS

The symptoms of ABRS and CRS are often nonspecific, and although there are established major and minor criteria for making the diagnosis, they should be made within the context of the duration of symptoms, physical examination findings, adjunctive measures, and, in the case of CRS, imaging.

History and Physical Examination

The diagnosis of ABRS or CRS begins with a thorough history of the illness. As stated before, the duration of illness is important in making the distinction between viral rhinosinusitis and acute bacterial rhinosinusitis. Patients with symptoms (Tables 8–1 and 8–2) persisting beyond 7 to 10 days or symptoms worsening after 5 to 7 days have a history more consistent with acute bacterial rhinosinusitis. When these patients have either two major criteria or one major criterion and two minor criteria in this context, the diagnosis of acute bacterial rhinosinusitis is more likely. The previous or current usage of antibiotics by the patient for the present illness or past illnesses should be noted.

Pattern of illness is important to characterize. Acute bacterial rhinosinusitis or acute exacerbations of CRS are typically preceded by a viral upper respiratory infection. Nasal congestion and obstruction with discolored nasal drainage also accompanies these episodes. Facial pressure, although not headache, is common, and care should be taken to distinguish rhinosinusitis from other causes of headache. Pain in the temporal area, a bandlike sensation around the head, and pain in the occipital area are not generally seen in sinusitis. Pain characterized as constant, cyclical, or occurring daily is also atypical and should prompt additional questions to determine migraine (which can present with throbbing facial pain, congestion, and nasal discharge if in the trigeminal distribution), tension headache, cluster headache, or headaches associated with hormonal changes.

Comorbid illnesses such as allergic rhinitis, asthma, or causes of ciliary dysfunction (e.g., cystic fibrosis or primary ciliary dyskinesia) should be ascertained because they may be misinterpreted as rhinosinusitis or complicate treatment of rhinosinusitis. Additionally, a history of smoking tobacco or inhalation of environmental irritants should also be noted.

The physical examination of the patient should be carried out systematically for all patients. The general appearance of the patient should be assessed to identify patients who appear ill or in distress. The ears should be examined for signs of otitis media (serous or purulent effusions), which can occasionally be seen in children and adults related to upper airway respiratory illnesses or obstruction of the eustachian tube orifices due to mucosal edema or a mass. The eyes should be carefully observed for evidence of lid edema, erythema, chemosis, and eye proptosis and for any restriction of movement, all of which may suggest an orbital complication. Additionally, periorbital "allergic shiners" (venous engorgement of the skin around the eyes) and Denne-Morgan lines (folds beneath the lid) may provide evidence of atopic disease. The external nose should be examined for signs of deviation or trauma as well as for a transverse nasal crease (which occurs as a result of rubbing the nose, "the allergic salute") signifying atopic disease. The nasal cavity should be examined with a speculum and a light source, and it should be carried out prior to and following decongestion. The examination should make note of any septal deviation, the size of the inferior turbinates, the quality of the nasal mucosa (e.g., erythematous, boggy, or atrophic), the quality of any nasal discharge (e.g., clear, mucoid, or purulent), or for the presence of polyps, masses, or any other lesions.

Although transillumination of the sinuses can be performed for the frontal and maxillary sinuses, it is neither sensitive nor specific for maxillary or frontal sinusitis. Transillumination cannot be used to identify disease in the ethmoid sinuses or the sphenoid sinus.

Whenever possible, an endoscope, either flexible or rigid, should be used to examine beyond the anterior nasal cavity. The endoscope provides a superior and detailed view of the relevant anatomic structures in the nasal cavity when compared to visualization with the headlight and speculum. The first inspection with endoscope should involve inspection of the inferior meatus, nasal floor, and nasopharynx. Next, the endoscope should be used to inspect the middle meatus and middle turbinate. Finally, the endoscope should be used to inspect the middle meatus complex. The examiner should make note of any masses, polyps, or exudates and from where they arise.

The oral cavity should be examined for the presence of any abnormality that may be related to rhinosinusitis (maxillary alveolar dental infection or polyp within the posterior oropharynx) or paranasal sinus neoplasm that has invaded the oral cavity. The neck should be examined for signs of lymphadenopathy.

Diagnostic Imaging

A direct coronal CT scan with 1- to 2-mm cuts is considered the most appropriate scan to characterize the radiographic findings in rhinosinusitis. An alternative at some institutions uses fine-cut axial scans 1 mm or less in slice thickness that can be reformatted to display images in the coronal plane. Although CT scanning is not recommended in the routine imaging of ABRS or CRS, patients who are unresponsive to appropriate medical therapy, patients who present a diagnostic dilemma, and patients with a suspected complication of rhinosinusitis should undergo radiographic evaluation with CT scanning.

CT findings in patients with VRS may be indistinguishable from those with ABRS; therefore, these imaging modalities do not aid in the differentiation of the two diseases or change the management of either. This is an important point because patients presenting with complaints of rhinosinusitis can display radiographic abnormalities of the paranasal sinuses within 72 to 96 hours of symptom onset, and the vast majority of the patients will show resolution of their radiographic abnormalities without the use of antibiotics. Clinical history plays a very important role in the timing and interpretation of the CT images. Patients are not generally imaged during an exacerbation of rhinosinusitis because scans will virtually always demonstrate mucosal thickening and are better imaged after resolution to characterize residual disease. However, patients being evaluated for complications of rhinosinusitis should obtain a coronal and axial CT scan with bone and soft tissue windows with intravenous contrast material immediately to aid in evaluation and management.

Magnetic resonance imaging (MRI) should be employed whenever a neoplasm of the sinuses is suspected. Use of MRI for evaluation of intracranial complications can also be helpful.

Plain radiographs are neither sensitive nor specific for rhinosinusitis but may be used to confirm the presence of fluid in the sinuses; however, there is often subjectivity to their interpretation, thus limiting their utility.

Culture

For patients who have failed standard medical therapy, a culture should be obtained. As previously stated, in the setting of community-acquired ABRS in adults, an endoscopic-directed culture of the middle meatus correlates well with cultures obtained through a maxillary "sinus tap" (the gold standard) performed with a needle through the canine fossa. Cultures of the nasal cavity are not recommended. In children, the carriage rates for the organisms responsible for ABRS are much higher than in adults, and endoscopic-directed cultures do not correlate well with maxillary sinus taps. However, consideration to developing maxillary dentition should be given before performing a puncture through the canine fossa and an alterative puncture site in the inferior meatus in the nasal cavity can be used.

Because the organisms are different in nosocomial-acquired ABRS, a maxillary sinus tap or endoscopically directed culture may be beneficial for culture information.

TREATMENT

Medical Therapy

The primary endpoints in the treatment of rhinosinusitis are the eradication of disease, the improvement in symptoms, and the reestablishment of normal paranasal sinus function.

ADJUNCTIVE TOPICAL AND SYSTEMIC THERAPY

Acute VRS is treated with conservative measures: nasal saline irrigation, topical or systemic decongestants, mucolytics, and analgesic medication. Unfortunately, there is no cure for the common cold. It is inappropriate to treat VRS with antibiotics. When VRS has persisted for more than 7 to 10 days or worsens after 5 to 7 days, it is reasonable to presume that suprainfection with bacteria has occurred and ABRS is present. As with VRS, the administration of topical or systemic decongestants and mucolytics is appropriate in ABRS.

Antibiotic Therapy

The selection of the proper antibiotic depends on the patient's history of antibiotic use and the probability of any one or more of the well-established bacterial causes of ABRS to be present. The Sinus and Allergy Health Partnership, in coordination with the Centers for Disease Control and Prevention has established guidelines for the treatment of ABRS. The guidelines are broadly separated based on the severity of the infection and on whether the patient has recently taken antibiotics. These guidelines are based on the most up-to-date susceptibilities of the various bacteria to available antibiotics.

Mild disease For patients with mild ABRS (Table 8–3) who have not taken antibiotics in the past 4 to 6 weeks, an appropriate first-line antimicrobial agent is amoxicillin (1.5 to 4 g/d), amoxicillin/clavulanate (1.75 to 4 g/d), cefpodoxime, cefuroxime, or cefdinir. Patients not improving within 72 hours of administration are presumed to have resistant organisms and should be switched to a fluoroquinolone or a combination of antibiotics. For those that are allergic to penicillin derivatives, trimethoprim/sulfamethoxazole, doxycycline, or a macrolide may be prescribed.

Table 8–3. Antibiotic treatment guidelines for mild acute bacterial rhinosinusitis with no recent antibiotic use.

Starting Therapy	Efficacy	Second Therapy for Medical Failures
Amoxicillin/clavulanate	91%	
Amoxicillin	88%	Flouroquinolone
Cefpodoxime	87%	Amoxicillin/clavulanate
Cefuroxime	85%	Ceftriaxone
Cefdinir	83%	Amoxilcillin/clavulanate or clindamycin and cefixime
Penicillin-Sensitive Patients		
TMP/SMX	83%	
Doxycycline	81%	Fluoroquinolone
Azithromycin, clarithromycin	77%	Rifampin and clindamycin

Adapted from Sinus and Allergy Health Partnership. Antimicrobial treatment guidelines for acute bacterial rhinosinusitis *Otolaryngol Head Neck Surg* 130 (suppl 1):S1, 2004.

Moderate disease or prior antibiotic use Patients who have moderate ABRS or have used antibiotics in the past 4 to 6 weeks (Table 8–4) should be administered a fluoroquinolone, gatifloxacin, levofloxacin, or moxifloxacin, or high-dose amoxicillin/clavulanate (4 g/250 mg). Patients allergic to penicillin and/or cephalosporins should be administered a fluoroquinolone or rifampin/clindamycin. Patients who do not improve within 72 hours should be reevaluated and consideration be given to obtaining a culture either endoscopically or via transantral puncture.

CHRONIC RHINOSINUSITIS

For patients with CRS, the same adjunctive measures (nasal saline irrigations and topical decongestants) should be deployed. Antimicrobial therapy for CRS is controversial. There are no FDA-approved antibiotics for the treatment of CRS, and this is largely because of the issues previously discussed in the pathophysiology of CRS. Several retrospective and prospective studies have shown subjective improvement in patients with CRS who have been treated with 4 to 6 weeks of antibiotics, topical or systemic corticosteroids, and adjunctive measures. These subjective results have been correlated with improvements in CT and endoscopic grading. These studies, however, have been confounded by the coadministration of topical or systemic corticosteroids. Nevertheless, it is reasonable to treat patients with chronic sinusitis with 3 to 6 weeks of antibiotics, topical corticosteroids, a short course of systemic corticosteroids,

Table 8–4. Antibiotic treatment guidelines for mild acute bacterial rhinosinusitis with recent antibiotic use or moderate acute bacterial rhinosinusitis.

Initial Therapy	Efficacy	Second therapy for medical failures
Fluoroquinolone	92%	Re-examine/culture
Amoxicillin/clavulanate	91%	Re-examine/culture
Penicillin-Sensitive		
Flouroquinolone	92%	Re-examine/culture
Clindamycin + rifampin	92%	Re-examine/culture

Adapted from Sinus and Allergy Health Partnership. Antimicrobial Treatment Guidelines for Acute Bacterial Rhinosinusitis *Otolaryngol Head Neck Surg* 130 (suppl 1):S1, 2004.

and a brief period (3 to 5 days) of topical decongestants. Oral corticosteroid dose commonly employs a taper of prednisone from approximately 60 mg to 10 mg over a 2- to 3-week period.

Recently, particular attention has been given to the use of macrolide antibiotics, which have been long known to have an antiinflammatory effect through increased eosinophilic apoptosis and reduction of eosinophilic mediators. Several recent studies have demonstrated that prolonged therapy (2 to 3 months) results in subjective (quality-of-life survey results) and objective (endoscopic grading) improvement as well as decreased circulating IL-8 in patients with CRS treated with macrolide antibiotics versus placebo. This method of therapy has not yet been put into common practice at the time of this writing.

Surgical Therapy

Surgical treatment of ABRS is not frequently needed; however, it may need to be performed in patients who suffer from recurrent acute infection, are refractory to medical management, or develop complications. Functional endoscopic sinus surgery (FESS) is employed as surgical therapy for these patients and in patients who are refractory to medical management with CRS. This procedure is considered functional because it is a mucosal-sparing operation that maintains the physiology of the sinuses by widening the natural ostia of the sinuses, preserving the natural mucociliary clearance. All sinuses may also be surgically drained from either an external, intranasal, or combination of the two approaches when necessary. External approaches to the sinuses are uncommon for routine nonemergent treatment of sinusitis because less invasive endoscopic approaches can virtually always be employed. The frontal sinus and ethmoid sinuses may be drained by making an incision in the skin along the medial and superior aspect of the orbital rim and entering into the sinus with a drill or osteotome. The maxillary sinus may be drained by making an incision in the gingivolabial sulcus (intraorally) and entering the sinus through the anterior maxillary sinus wall (i.e., the canine fossa). Alternately, the maxillary sinus may be entered intranasally, beneath the inferior turbinate by creating a nasoantral window. These procedures are not functional because they disrupt the natural flow of cilia within the affected sinuses and may contribute to stasis and recirculation.

The most common complications related to sinus surgery include bleeding and postoperative scarring or synechiae. For those patients with an intact sense of smell, there is a small risk of postoperative anosmia. Given the proximity of the sinuses to the skull base (Fig. 8–5), the risk of a cerebrospinal fluid leak is present if aggressive dissection of the sinuses is undertaken.

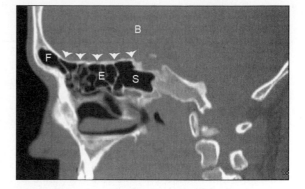

Figure 8–5. Parasagittal anatomy of the frontal (F), ethmoid (E), and sphenoid (S) sinuses in relationship to the skull base (arrowheads) and brain (B).

Other rare complications include injury to the orbit (e.g., globe, extraocular muscles, and hematoma) or injury to the carotid artery and optic nerve.

It is important that patients be informed that surgery is not a cure for CRS, rather an adjunct to the proper—and often indefinite—medical management of chronic rhinosinusitis. Unless anatomic obstruction is the sole cause of rhinosinusitis, it is likely that the underlying pathophysiology (e.g., allergic rhinitis, mucosal hyperreactivity, ciliary dysfunction, etc.) will persist after surgery unless managed with the appropriate medical therapy. Nevertheless, when appropriately employed, medical and surgical therapy can help obtain long-term relief of clinical signs and symptoms of chronic rhinosinusitis. Several studies show that symptomatic improvement can be sustained in 80% to 98% of patients over 8 years, and improvement in objectively measured outcomes such as olfaction, ciliary beat frequency, and olfactory threshold can be accomplished as well.

COMPLICATIONS

Untreated ABRS resolves spontaneously in nearly all cases without evidence of sequelae. However, infectious complications do occur, and these typically result from the direct extension of disease into neighboring structures or hematogenous spread of infection via thrombophlebitis and bacteremia.

Orbital Complications

The orbit is lateral to the ethmoid sinuses and superior to the maxillary sinus. Directly overlying the orbit are supraorbital ethmoid air cells and the frontal sinus. Direct extension of bacteria into the orbit can occur from any of these sinuses. Chandler's classification divides orbital complications into five groups. Group 1 is preseptal cellulitis, which becomes manifest with eyelid edema and erythema. Group 2 is orbital cellulitis, which is marked by proptosis and potentially decreased ocular movement (due to edema) and vision. A group 3 complication arises when a subperiosteal orbital abscess is found. Group 4 complications involve the formation of an orbital abscess. Group 5, the most severe, is cavernous sinus thrombosis, which occurs via direct extension or retrograde movement through a plexus of valveless veins into the cavernous sinus. Cavernous sinus thrombosis is typically evident with proptosis, ophthalmoplegia, and loss of vision. Wide-spectrum antibiotics and a sinusotomy of the responsible sinus are indicated. The use of anticoagulation is controversial. Despite aggressive treatment, mortality is high (approximately 50% to 80%).

Approximately two thirds of orbital complications require surgery. Indications for surgery include abscess formation, progressive loss of visual acuity, or lack of improvement in 48 to 72 hours. Surgery may be carried out with the endoscope; however, external approaches are often employed because nasal mucosa is edematous and friable and the patient is at higher risk for postoperative synechiae in an endoscopic approach.

Intracranial Complications

Intracranial complications usually arise from the frontal sinus and its valveless venous communications with central blood drainage patterns. Frontal bone osteomyelitis may occur with or without a frontal subperiosteal abscess (also known as Pott's puffy tumor). Intracranial extension may lead to meningitis, epidural abscess formation, or a brain abscess. Sagittal sinus thrombosis is particularly worrisome and has a high morbidity and mortality. Consultation with a neurosurgeon is recommended.

FUNGAL RHINOSINUSITIS

Fungal colonization of the nasal cavity and nasopharynx is common in healthy volunteers and patients with CRS. Fungal elements may proliferate to cause local forms of disease within the nasal cavity or paranasal sinuses. When circumstances (allergy or immunocompromised state) permit, the fungal elements may proliferate to cause more significant disease, or fungal rhinosinusitis. Fungal rhinosinusitis occurs in several forms; however, it can be simplified into allergic fungal sinusitis (AFS) and invasive fungal sinusitis.

Allergic Fungal Sinusitis

Allergic fungal sinusitis is documented in a patient with CRS who demonstrates evidence of fungal elements on nasal smears or cultures, documented IgE-mediated allergy to the isolated fungal organism, allergic mucin (dense eosinophilic-rich secretion), nasal polyposis, and a required lack of invasion of paranasal sinus bone. Erosion or expansion of the paranasal sinus bone is frequently found; however, invasion is not present. Typical isolates include *Bipolaris*, *Alternaria*, and *Curvularia* species.

Management of allergic fungal sinusitis is frequently frustrating. However, the mainstays of treatment include débridement of nasal polyps, conservative functional endoscopic sinus surgery, and extirpation of allergic mucin. Postoperative medical management involves topical and systemic corticosteroids and, in some cases, administration of antifungal therapy (e.g., itraconazole). There currently is no consensus, however, regarding the proper dose or length of corticosteroids and the effectiveness of systemic or topical antifungal medications.

Invasive Fungal Sinusitis

Invasive fungal sinusitis comes in acute (fulminant) and chronic forms. As the name implies, the hallmark of invasive fungal sinusitis is invasion of soft tissue and bone. The most common agents causing acute invasive fungal sinusitis include *Aspergillus*, *Rhizopus*, *Mucor*, and *Candida*. Risk factors for invasive forms of fungal sinusitis include diabetes (especially ketoacidosis), immunocompromised states (bone marrow transplantation, chronic immunosuppression), or patients with leukemia.

Fungal elements invade local tissues to cause tissue necrosis, which is manifest as necrotic-appearing or dark insensate tissue within the nasal cavity seen on endoscopy. Manipulated tissue typically does not bleed. Because fungal elements persist in this environment, delivery of systemic antifungal agents is impaired. The cornerstones of therapy include reversal of the underlying medical condition, aggressive surgical débridement of the infected region, and prolonged administration of systemic antifungal agents (typically amphotericin-B or voriconazole). The prognosis for patients with invasive fungal sinusitis is poor, especially when there is intracranial extension or systemic spread. Treatment of rhinocerebral fungal sinusitis involves a multidisciplinary approach and requires aggressive débridement of all infected tissue, control of the underlying medical condition, and prolonged administration of antifungal antibiotics.

EVIDENCE-BASED MEDICINE

The observation that many patients with acute bacterial rhinosinusitis will improve without the administration of antibiotics, coupled with increasing incidence of antibiotic resistance in the community, prompts one to review critically the clinical effectiveness of antibiotics in the treatment of acute bacterial rhinosinusitis and the incidence of adverse outcomes in patients not receiving treatment.

A recent meta-analysis of more than 15,000 patients examining the efficacy of antibiotic treatment in patients with acute bacterial rhinosinusitis or acute exacerbations of chronic rhinosinusitis revealed that the administration of antibiotics reduced the risk of failure to treat completely by 25% to 30% if administered within 7 to 14 days. The spontaneous recovery rate (patients administered placebo) was approximately 65%. Penicillins, especially amoxicillin/clavulanate, were found to be significantly more effective than cephalosporins within the first 25 days of treatment; however, there were no significant differences 25 to 45 days after treatment. Clinical efficacy among other antibiotics (including azithromycin, telithromycin, and gemifloxacin) were comparable.

Results of this meta-analysis agree with published findings of the Sinus and Allergy Health Partnership, the Institute for Clinical Systems Improvement, and the American College of Physicians.

CONCLUSION

Rhinosinusitis is common and has a tremendous impact on society in terms of productivity and health care expenditures. The most common form is VRS, which should be treated conservatively. When ABRS results, the use of antibiotics directed toward the most likely causative agents is typically indicated. Treatment should be modified depending on the efficacy of the primary therapy and whether antibiotics have been used within 4 to 6 weeks of initiating therapy. Chronic rhinosinusitis is a complex syndrome that has no clear etiology at this time. Active research into the pathophysiology may ultimately lead to effective preventative measures and medical therapies for this disease entity. Oral antibiotics, oral and topical corticosteroid therapy, and adjunctive measures appear to improve patient quality of life and reduce disease burden. When surgery is indicated, functional endoscopic sinus surgery can be carried out with significant improvement in quality-of-life measures when appropriate follow-up and medical management is employed after surgery. With this understanding, rhinosinusitis can be effectively managed.

BIBLIOGRAPHY

Benninger MS, Ferguson BJ, Hadley JA, et al. Adult chronic rhinosinusitis: definitions, diagnosis, epidemiology and pathophysiology. *Otolaryngol Head Neck Surg.* 2003; 129(suppl 3):S1.

Bernstein JM, Kansal R. Superantigen hypothesis for the early development of chronic hyperplastic sinusitis with massive nasal polyposis. *Curr Opin Otolaryngol Head Neck Surg.* 2005;13:39.

Casiano RR. Treatment of acute and chronic rhinosinusitis. *Semin Respir Infect.* 2000;15:216.

Chandler JR, Langenbrunner DJ, Stevens ER. The pathogenesis of orbital complications in acute sinusitis. *Laryngoscope.* 1970;80:1414.

Ferguson BJ. Mucormycosis of the nose and paranasal sinuses. *Otolaryngol Clin North Am.* 2000;33:349.

Ferguson BJ, Stolz DB. Demonstration of biofilm in human bacterial chronic rhinosinusitis. *Am J Rhinol.* 2005;19:452.

Gwaltney JM Jr, Phillips CD, Miller RD, et al. Computed tomographic study of the common cold. *N Engl J Med.* 1994;330:25.

Kennedy DW, Senior BA. Endoscopic sinus surgery: a review. *Prim Care.* 1980;25:703.

Kuhn FA. Lateral nasal wall and sinus surgical anatomy: contemporary understanding. In: Johnson JT, et al., eds. *Maintenance Manual for Lifelong Learning.* Dubuque, Iowa: Kendall/Hunt; 2002:203.

Kuhn FA, Swain R Jr. Allergic fungal sinusitis: diagnosis and treatment. *Curr Opin Otolaryngol Head Neck Surg.* 2003;11:1.

Marple BF, Brunton S, Ferguson BJ. Acute bacterial rhinosinusitis: a review of U.S. treatment guidelines. *Otolaryngol Head Neck Surg.* 2006;135:341.

Murr AH, Goldberg AN, Vesper S. Fungal speciation using quantitative polymerase chain reaction (QPCR) in patients with and without chronic rhinosinusitis. *Laryngoscope.* 2006;116:1342.

Pinto JM, Baroody FM. Chronic sinusitis and allergic rhinitis: at the nexus of sinonasal inflammatory disease. *Journal of Otolaryngology.* 2002;31(suppl 1):S10.

Sinus and Allergy Health Partnership. Antimicrobial treatment guidelines for acute bacterial rhinosinusitis 2004. *Otolaryngol Head Neck Surg.* 2004;130(suppl 1):S1.

Vogan JC, Bolger WE, Keyes AS. Endoscopically guided sinonasal cultures: a direct comparison with maxillary sinus aspirate cultures. *Otolaryngol Head Neck Surg.* 2000;122:370.

Allergic Diseases of the Ear

Doris Lin, MD, and Steven W. Cheung, MD

GENERAL CONSIDERATIONS

The ear has multiple targets for allergic diseases (Table 9–1). The external ear may be afflicted with contact dermatitis to earrings or hearing aid molds, eczema, or sensitization to ear drops or fungus. The middle ear may be plagued with persistent effusion secondary to eustachian tube dysfunction or chronic inflammatory response to allergens. The inner ear may be troubled by Ménière's disease and cochlear hydrops, both disorders with possible allergic bases.

ALLERGIC DISEASES OF THE EXTERNAL EAR

Chronic Otitis Externa

The skin of the pinna and external ear may be afflicted in two major ways. Eczema of the auricle or external auditory canal (EAC) may manifest as erythematous, scaling, and pruritic dermatitis. Atopic eczema is the most common type of eczema and closely associated with asthma and allergic rhinitis. The usual treatments are with emollients that maintain skin hydration and topical steroids to reduce inflammation. Another type of eczema seen is seborrheic eczema, which is most commonly seen on the scalp as dandruff but can spread to the face and ears. The condition is thought to be caused by yeast and can be treated with an antifungal cream if necessary. Chronic otitis externa that follows the use of topical antimicrobial drops, particularly those containing neomycin, can actually be a Gell and Coombs Type IV hypersensitivity reaction. Symptoms generally resolve with discontinuation of the offending agent; however, occasionally topical steroid drops may be needed to accelerate recovery.

Contact Sensitivity

Some patients may develop contact sensitivity to certain plastic molds attached to hearing aids. The problem manifests as a localized skin reaction. Boiling the hearing aid mold in water for 30 seconds, substituting a different material for the mold, or plating a thin film of gold onto the mold may reduce symptoms. Along this vein, patients may develop contact sensitivity to nickel and chromium in earrings. Treatment often involves use of earring posts of surgical stainless steel or 14-karat gold or titanium.

Dermatophytid Reaction

The auricle or EAC can be the site of a dermatophytid reaction in a sensitized individual. Usually there is a primary site of fungal infection. The fungus or their allergenic products spread hematogenously to a secondary site, causing an allergic skin eruption. Resolution requires treatment of the primary fungal infection, desensitization with an allergenic extract of the infecting fungus, and control of any secondary bacterial infections. The most common fungus involved is *Trichophyton*, although *Candida* (Oidiomycetes) and *Epidermophyton* have also been described. Common sites for the primary fungal infection include the nails (onychomycoses), skin, and vagina (monilial vaginitis).

ALLERGIC DISEASES OF THE MIDDLE EAR

Otitis media with effusion (OME) can impair hearing significantly, cause profound mucosal changes, delay speech development, and result in permanent middle ear damage. OME is the most common cause of hearing loss in children today and causes a conductive hearing loss with a flat tympanogram (Fig. 9–1). Of particular interest is OME refractory to conventional antibiotic treatment and surgical therapy such as myringotomy, tonsillectomy, adenoidectomy, tympanostomy tube placement, and even radical mastoidectomy. Chronic mucosal inflammation is a major finding in these cases. The role of allergy in these cases is under active investigation and discussed in the following sections.

Table 9–1. Otologic manifestations of allergy.

External Ear

Chronic external otitis
Sensitization to ear drops
Contact sensitivity (hearing aid ear molds, earrings)
Dermatophytid reaction
Eczema

Middle Ear

Eustachian tube dysfunction
Patulous eustachian tube
Otitis media with effusion
Chronic otitis media

Inner Ear

Ménière's disease
Vestibular hydrops
Cochlear hydrops
Dizziness
Tinnitus

Eustachian Tube Dysfunction

Eustachian tube dysfunction (ETD) is a major factor in the development of OME. Upper respiratory infections and allergies contribute to ETD, and in some cases contribute to a patulous Eustachian tube. Patients with patulous Eustachian tube may complain of autophony (abnormal awareness of their own voice), reverberation, or tinnitus resembling the sound of an ocean roar. Provocative intranasal challenges of pollen, house dust mites, and histamine worsen ETD. Allergic rhinitis results in a significantly higher rate of Eustachian tube dysfunction, particularly during childhood, as demonstrated by nasal turbinate changes (Fig. 9–2). Bernstein proposes that Eustachian tube dysfunction in the setting of allergy may be a result of retrograde spread of edema and congestion of nasal mucosa, decreased mucociliary function that permits secretions to cover the ostium and subsequent intraluminal inflammation, or obstruction of the Eustachian tube orifice from hypersecretion by seromucous glands. These symptoms can be alleviated with specific allergy therapy, including immunotherapy and elimination diets depending on the offending agent.

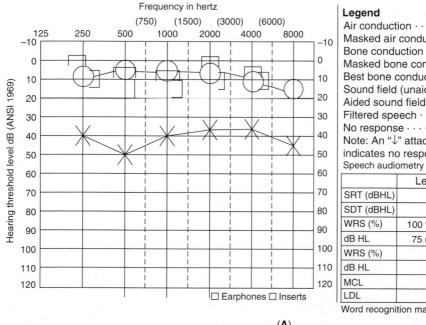

(A)

Figure 9–1. Example of an audiogram (**A**) from a patient with a left otitis media and resultant conductive hearing loss. This patient also has a flattened left tympanogram (**B**) resulting from a tympanic membrane stiffened by fluid in the middle ear. The normal right ear is shown for comparison.

Tympanogram

Right

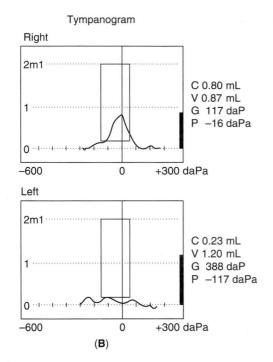

C 0.80 mL
V 0.87 mL
G 117 daP
P −16 daPa

Left

C 0.23 mL
V 1.20 mL
G 388 daP
P −117 daPa

(B)

Figure 9–1. *(Continued)*

Otitis Media with Effusion

OME often results from ETD or can be the result of chronic inflammation or microbial infection. The causative contribution of allergy to OME is unknown, with a broad range of attribution (0% to 95%) reported

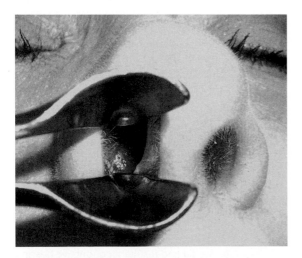

Figure 9–2. An enlarged and boggy right inferior turbinate from a patient with allergic rhinitis.

in the literature. The controversy regarding the role of allergy in OME is reflected in different types of skin and in vitro testing, and heterogeneous types of allergens included in each study. Many would agree that OME caused by allergy is most likely from ETD secondary to an allergic reaction in the proximal Eustachian tube or nasopharynx. However, some studies have demonstrated the presence of histamine and other biologic mediators of inflammation in the middle ear fluid of patients with OME, suggesting that the middle ear is also a primary target of allergic reactions.

An argument against a significant role of allergy in the pathogenesis of OME is that although allergy is typically considered seasonal with regional variation, OME has its highest incidence in the winter, regardless of region. In addition, an IgE-mediated reaction is brief and not typically long enough to cause significant ETD. Also, there is no clear evidence for an intranasal challenge directly producing a middle ear effusion. Although intranasal challenges have resulted in ETD, the duration of dysfunction is insufficient to result in OME. Even complete Eustachian tube obstruction produced by sectioning the tensor veli palatine muscle in an animal model takes 1 to 4 weeks to result in a middle ear effusion. Intranasal provocative challenge persists for only several hours to a few days.

Counter arguments contend that winter is the time of year when dust and mold counts tend to be highest. Intranasal challenges of histamine, pollen, and house dust mites result in ETD, albeit of unclear sufficient duration to cause OME. Epidemiologic studies have shown that patients with OME have an increased prevalence of atopic conditions, such as allergic rhinitis, eczema, and asthma. More than 50% of patients with OME have allergic rhinitis, whereas 21% of patients with allergic rhinitis have OME. One study of 20 patients with OME refractory to medical and surgical management showed that allergy immunotherapy in patients tested with the radioallergosorbent test (RAST) resulted in preservation of hearing and elimination of recurrent infections for 3 years when compared with controls. Although small, this study encourages consideration of allergic factors in patients with refractory OME to conventional treatments.

Food Allergy in Otitis Media with Effusion

Few studies address the role of food antigens in OME. One study of 56 children found food allergies in children with OME (45%) were significantly higher than in children without complaints of food allergy or OME (18%). Another study of 104 children with recurrent otitis media found that 78% had food allergy diagnosed by skin prick or IgE tests and food challenge. They reported that 86% of the children with food allergy who were treated with food elimination had significant amelioration of OME, as documented by clinical examination and tympanometry. Food challenge resulted in recurrence of OME in 94% of the children with food allergies who underwent challenge. A few studies have suggested that cow's milk allergy in infancy, even when treated properly, is associated with significantly higher rates of recurrent OME. A few of these studies address possible mechanisms for this association. These include nasal congestion induced by food allergy, direct middle ear mucosal damage by food immune complexes, and other hypersensitivity response. One study demonstrated elevated serum IgG response, but a lack of IgE response, to foods in otitis-prone children compared with controls. More definitive studies are needed in this area. Nevertheless, current results encourage consideration of a food elimination diet in select patients before surgical intervention.

ALLERGIC DISEASES OF THE INNER EAR

Ménière's Disease

Ménière's disease is characterized by aural fullness, tinnitus, vertigo, and fluctuating sensorineural hearing loss (SNHL). Two related variants are cochlear hydrops (fluctuating SNHL without vertigo) and vestibular hydrops (imbalance without fluctuating SNHL). The etiology of Ménière's disease is unclear and has been attributed to anatomic, infectious, immunologic, and allergic factors. The target organ appears to be the endolymphatic sac. The mainstays of medical therapy have included diuretic therapy (particularly thiazide diuretics), carbonic anhydrase inhibitors, vasodilators, salt reduction (<1.5 g/day) and dietary restrictions. Surgical therapy is reserved for cases refractory to medical management. These include chemical labyrinthectomy (intratympanic aminoglycoside), surgical labyrinthectomy, endolymphatic shunt, and vestibular nerve section.

Both inhalant and food allergies have been linked with symptoms of Ménière's disease and cochlear hydrops. Patients with Ménière's disease have a 40% rate of allergy, as measured by skin or in vitro testing, which is twice as high as that reported for the general population. The success of sedating antihistamines in the treatment of Ménière's disease is usually attributed to vestibular suppressant effects, but allergic reaction suppressant properties may also contribute to clinical improvement. Dietary restrictions on sodium, caffeine, nicotine, alcohol, and foods containing theophylline (e.g., chocolate) improve symptoms in patients with Ménière's disease, although the mechanism has usually been attributed to fluid regulation of the endolymphatic sac. Regardless, immunotherapy and food elimination diets have mitigated both allergic and labyrinthine symptoms in Ménière's disease.

EVIDENCE-BASED MEDICINE

Studies over the last few years have focused on the possible roles of allergy in OME. Allergic rhinitis and nasal/nasopharyngeal inflammation resulting in ETD is associated with increased rates of OME. Allergy-related mediators (IL-4, IL-5, IL-6, regulated on activation, normal T-cell expressed and secreted [RANTES], eosinophil cationic protein [ECP], tryptase, IgE) isolated from middle ear effusions have been shown to be elevated. The role of food allergy in OME and in other allergic diseases of the ear is under active investigation. For OME and Ménière's disease, an allergic basis of disease and treatment should be considered in cases refractory to conventional medical and/or surgical management.

BIBLIOGRAPHY

Derebery MJ, Berliner KI. Allergy and the contemporary otologist. *Otolaryngol Clin N Am.* 2003;36:989.

Mabry RL, Ferguson BJ, Krouse JH. *Allergy, the Otolaryngologist's Approach.* American Academy of Otolaryngic Allergy, Washington, D.C. 2005.

Hurst DS. Association of otitis media with effusion and allergy as demonstrated by intradermal skin testing and eosinophil cationic protein levels in both middle ear effusions and mucosal biopsies. *Laryngoscope.* 1996;106:1128.

Doyle DW. The link between allergic rhinitis and otitis media. *Curr Opin Allergy Clin Immunol.* 2002;2:21.

Lazo-Saenz JG, Galvan-Aguilera AA, Marinez-Ordez VA, et al. Eustachian tube dysfunction in allergic rhinitis. *Otolaryngol Head Neck Surg.* 2005;132:626.

Bernstein JM. Role of allergy in eustachian tube blockage and otitis media with effusion: a review. *Otolaryngol Head Neck Surg.* 1996;114:562.

Bernstein JM. The role of IgE-mediated hypersensitivity in the development of otitis media with effusion: a review. *Otolaryngol Head Neck Surg.* 1993;109:611.

Hurst DS. Allergy management of refractory serous otitis media. *Otolaryngol Head Neck Surg.* 1990;102:664.

Pettigrew MM, Gent JF, Triche EW, et al. Association of early-onset otitis media in infants and exposure to household mold. *Paediatric Perinatal Epidemiol.* 2004;18:441.

Aydogan B, Kiroglu M, Altintas D, et al. The role of food allergy in otitis media with effusion. *Otolaryngol Head Neck Surg.* 2004;130:747.

Nsouli TM, Nsouli SM, Linde RE, et al. The role of allergy in serous otitis media. *Ann Allergy Asthma Immunol.*1994;73:215.

Juntti H, Tikkannen S, Kokkonen J, et al. Cow's milk allergy is associated with recurrent otitis media during childhood. *Acta Otolaryngol.* 1999;119:867.

Derebery MJ: Allergic management of Ménière's disease: an outcome study. *Otolaryngol Head Neck Surg.* 2000;122:174.

Nguyen LHP, Manoukian JJ, Sobol SE, et al. Similar allergic inflammation in the middle ear and the upper airway: Evidence linking otitis media with effusion to the united airways concept. *J Allergy Clin Immunol.* 2004;114:1110.

Cough and Allergic Diseases

10

Eric M. Chen, MD, FACP, FAAAAI, FACAAI

Cough is one of the most common reasons for physician office visits. The majority of cough is self-limiting and often treated symptomatically. In some epidemiologic surveys, however, up to 18% of the population has a persistent cough. If the cough persists for longer than 8 weeks, it is considered a chronic cough. When this occurs, a more comprehensive approach needs to be taken to discern the etiology of the cough. Allergic diseases, also known as atopy, are among the chief causes of cough. Atopy is the sixth leading cause of chronic disease in the United States. Thus, it is important to understand how allergic diseases can cause cough.

DEFINITION AND PHYSIOLOGY

Cough is a protective mechanism to expel offending agents from the respiratory tract. The mechanics of cough can usually be characterized into four phases:

1. Inspiration
2. Compression (expiration against a closed glottis)
3. Expulsion (opening of glottis with expulsive airflow)
4. Recovery (restorative inspiration)

This combination of actions is orchestrated by an extensive neuron network. Involuntary cough is primarily initiated by the vagus afferent nerves. The pharynx is innervated by the glossopharyngeal nerve and a branch of the superior laryngeal nerve. The larynx is innervated by the superior and recurrent laryngeal nerves, which join the vagus nerve. The trachea and bronchi are innervated by three types of nerve fibers called rapid adapting receptor (RAR), slowly adapting stretch receptor (SAR), and C fibers (Table 10–1). RARs are triggered mainly by mechanical stimuli and some inflammatory mediators. SARs are nerve fibers that inhibit inspiration. C fibers are triggered primarily by noxious chemicals and some mechanical irritants.

CAUSES OF COUGH

The causes of cough are numerous and can be multifactorial. The etiology of a cough can be sought out by a careful history, diagnostic tests, and response to treatment. The most common causes of cough are upper airway cough syndrome (UACS), previously known as postnasal drip syndrome (PNDS), asthma, and gastroesophageal reflux disease (GERD).

The American College of Chest Physicians' Evidence-Based Clinical Practice Guidelines concluded from four prospective studies that these three etiologies comprised greater than 92% of patients with cough (who had normal chest radiographs, were nonsmokers and not on angiotensin-converting enzyme inhibitors). Table 10–2 lists the potential causes of cough.

Upper Airway Cough Syndrome (Postnasal Drip Cough)

UACS, or postnasal drip syndrome, is the most common cause of cough. The physical drainage of nasal mucus down the posterior pharynx to the larynx and upper airway induces cough. UACS includes allergic, nonallergic, and infectious rhinitis. Note that the cough may be due to more than one of these etiologies. The strategy is to discern the primary and secondary causes. The history that suggests UACS includes tickling of the throat, hoarseness, throat clearing, and congestion of the throat. This type of postnasal drip cough is often alleviated by drinking or eating. The action of swallowing causes the reflexive closure of the epiglottis. A closed epiglottis shunts the postnasal drip to the esophagus bypassing the posterior pharynx and larynx. This may be the main reason why taking a cough drop and drinking water both help relieve symptoms of cough.

Allergic Rhinitis and Cough

Allergic rhinitis affects as many as 20% to 25% of the population. It is defined as an inflammatory response of the nasal mucosa to airborne antigens. This action is mediated by an IgE antibody. Allergic rhinitis often presents as postnasal drip, nasal congestion, rhinorrhea, and eustachian tube dysfunction. Postnasal drip causes both mechanical and inflammatory mediators to trigger the cough reflex in the larynx and trachea.

Table 10–1. Respiratory innervations.

Location	Innervations
Pharynx	Glossopharyngeal nerve and branch of superior laryngeal nerve
Larynx	Superior and recurrent laryngeal nerves
Trachea and Bronchi	Rapid adapting receptor (RAR) Slowly adapting stretch receptors (SARs) C Fibers

Table 10–2. Causes of cough.

Upper airway cough syndrome (UACS)
  (postnasal drip cough)
   Allergic rhinitis
   Nonallergic rhinitis
    Vasomotor rhinitis
    Nonallergic rhinitis with eosinophilia syndrome
    (NARES)
    Rhinitis medicamentosa
    Gustatory rhinitis
   Infectious rhinitis/sinusitis
   Pertussis
   Mycoplasma
   Chlamydia
Irritant inhalation (e.g., tobacco smoke, noxious fumes)
Angiotensin-converting enzyme inhibitor (ACE-I)
  cough
Asthma
  Cough variant asthma (CVA)
Nonasthmatic eosinophilic bronchitis
Gastroesophageal reflux disease (GERD)
Pulmonary infection
  Bronchitis
  Pneumonia
  Tuberculosis
Chronic obstructive pulmonary disease
  (COPD)/emphysema
Aspiration/foreign body obstruction
Congestive heart failure
Pulmonary embolism
Interstitial lung disease
Bronchiectasis
Cystic fibrosis
Sarcoidosis
Vasculitis
Respiratory tumors
Anatomic abnormality of the larynx/trachea
Psychogenic cough

The history attained from the patient can usually be subdivided into seasonal versus perennial symptoms. Patients who suffer from these symptoms in spring are affected by grass and tree pollen. Symptoms occurring during the fall are typically caused by weed pollen. The perennial symptoms are usually triggered by dust mites, animal proteins, and mold spores. Itching of the nose and eyes is the key symptom that distinguishes allergic rhinitis from other causes. Although sneezing is an associated symptom, it is not unique to allergic rhinitis. Sneezing can be due to infectious, mechanical, or chemical nasal irritation.

Physical examination findings that may help in ascertaining allergic rhinitis include the appearance of posterior pharynx "cobblestoning" and/or observation of mucus draining down the posterior pharynx. Tests such as allergy skin tests and the radioallergosorbent test (RAST) can help establish or rule out allergic causes. However, allergy testing alone without a clinically significant history will lead to an inaccurate diagnosis. Ultimately, the use of a daily intranasal corticosteroid for 2 weeks is the most practical solution for discerning allergic rhinitis from other causes. If symptoms improve, then the likely cause is allergic rhinitis. Asking the patient to assign a percentage of improvement with this therapy is helpful in modifying the treatment plan. If the patient is still symptomatic after using the intranasal corticosteroid, adjunctive therapy with a daily leukotriene receptor antagonist for an additional 2 weeks may be beneficial.

Nonallergic Rhinitis and Cough

A significant etiology of chronic cough that is often overlooked is nonallergic rhinitis with postnasal drip. It encompasses vasomotor rhinitis, nonallergic rhinitis with eosinophilia syndrome (NARES), rhinitis medicamentosa, and gustatory rhinitis. Nonallergic rhinitis is usually perennial, triggered by irritants, and has negative IgE allergy skin tests or RAST.

VASOMOTOR RHINITIS

Vasomotor rhinitis is defined as rhinorrhea, nasal congestion, and postnasal drip cough caused by nasal mucosal autonomic nerve instability or dysfunction. The autonomic nerve instability causes vasodilation and vascular leakage leading to mucosal edema as well as triggering an overproduction of mucus. The stimuli for vasomotor rhinitis usually consist of physical and chemical irritants. These common irritants include odors, smoke, fumes, changes in temperature, and changes in barometric pressure/humidity. A positive correlation between the patient's history and exposure to the irritants is the key to diagnosing this entity. Avoidance of the offending agent, if possible, is the first course of action. However, if this is not possible, medications can serve as a diagnostic tool as well as a treatment option.

If nasal congestion is elicited in the patient's history, the use of azelastine nasal spray two puffs per nostril twice a day for a 2-week trial would be in order. If the nonallergic rhinitis symptom is mostly rhinorrhea, then a 2-week trial of nasal ipratropium bromide, 0.03% or 0.06% one to two puffs per nostril up to four times a day, would reduce mucus production.

NONALLERGIC RHINITIS WITH EOSINOPHILIA SYNDROME

NARES occurs when eosinophils are found in the nasal mucosa. This syndrome has all of the symptoms of vasomotor rhinitis with the addition of itching of the nose and eyes. The IgE allergy skin test or RAST is negative in NARES. A nasal swab for eosinophils is conducted with Hansel's stain to help make the diagnosis. NARES is treated with an intranasal corticosteroid to inhibit the eosinophils and inflammatory mediators.

RHINITIS MEDICAMENTOSA

Rhinitis medicamentosa is defined as paradoxical nasal congestion due to the overuse of topical nasal vasoconstrictors (e.g., oxymetazoline). The long-term use of topical vasoconstrictors (typically alpha agonists) can cause tachyphylaxis or a need for more of the drug to maintain the effect that was initially attained with the medication. Withdrawal of the topical vasoconstrictor causes a rebound vasodilatory effect, which leads to nasal congestion. Associated with this phenomenon is a postnasal drip cough due to overproduction of mucus. The treatment is cessation of the topical nasal vasoconstrictor. It may take up to 2 weeks before the congestion resolves completely.

GUSTATORY RHINITIS

Gustatory rhinitis is rhinorrhea, nasal congestion, and/or postnasal drip caused by the act of eating or drinking. This is a vagal reflex that causes vasodilation of the nasal mucosa and an increase in mucus production. Rhinorrhea is the most common symptom, and ipratropium bromide nasal spray is the drug of choice. Again, if there is a nasal congestion component, azelastine may be helpful.

Infectious Rhinitis and Cough

Infectious postnasal drip cough can occur with viral infection, sinusitis, and/or from a postinfectious cause. Patients who have viral infections experience malaise, clear mucus drainage, nasal congestion, postnasal drip cough, myalgia, and sometimes fevers. Treatment using saline rinses, decongestants and mucolytics usually help resolve symptoms of cough in a couple of weeks. If coughing persists, bacterial sinusitis needs to be considered.

Bacterial sinusitis can be diagnosed with a history of purulent drainage that persists for longer than 10 days and sometimes with symptoms of maxillary tooth pain. Sinus radiographs or computed tomography (CT) scans tend to be the studies of choice. The common bacterias associated with sinusitis are *Streptococcus pneumonia, Haemophilus influenzae,* and *Moraxella catarrhalis* in children. In chronic sinusitis, anaerobic bacteria may play a role. The treatment method should consist of a three-step approach:

1. Decrease nasal mucosa swelling with intranasal corticosteroid with or without a short burst of oral steroids to allow for proper mucus drainage.
2. Loosen up thick mucus with a mucolytic (e.g., guaifenesin).
3. Neutralize the bacteria with the appropriate antibiotic (e.g., amoxicillin or penicillin alternative).

Acute sinusitis requires 2 weeks of treatment; chronic sinusitis requires 4 to 6 weeks of treatment. If a sinus radiograph or CT sinus is positive, and the patient does not respond to antibiotics, fungal sinusitis needs to be considered. Fungal sinusitis requires surgical resection.

Postinfectious cough can comprise 11% to 15% of upper respiratory tract infections. This is the type of cough that lingers for longer than 3 weeks. It usually resolves before the eighth week of symptoms. The two organisms of interest are *Bordetella pertussis* and *Mycoplasma pneumoniae.* Although culturing or antibody titers can be attempted, a trial of an oral macrolide for 2 weeks would be the most practical course of action.

Angiotensin-Converting Enzyme Inhibitor Cough

With the rise of diabetes and hypertension in the general population, the use of angiotensin-converting enzyme inhibitors (ACE-I) has become more prevalent. It can cause a persistent cough in up to 35% of its users. The mechanism is believed to be the inhibition of ACE, which normally degrades bradykinin and substance P. These mediators induce upper airway cough. This class of medications is unusual because the cough can occur much later after the initial use of the medication. The cough may take up to 3 months to resolve after discontinuation of the ACE-I.

Asthma and Cough

Cough is one of many symptoms associated with asthma. However, there tends to be an overdiagnosis of asthma as the cause of chronic cough. The definition of asthma can be elusive. Its most basic definition is hyperresponsive airway disease that is reversible. This hyperresponsive airway is driven most of the time by chronic inflammation of the bronchioles triggered by atopic, physical, or chemical irritation. The chronic inflammatory mediators then cause bronchial smooth muscle constriction and an overproduction of mucus that necessitates clearing the airway with coughing.

Although symptoms of cough, dyspnea, and wheezing may suggest asthma, the need for allergy skin tests/RAST, pulmonary function tests, and response to treatment are important. Spirometry with pre- and post-short-acting bronchodilator agents (e.g., albuterol) showing a forced expiratory volume in 1 second (FEV_1) increase of greater than 12% and 200 mL is a practical approach to showing reversible airway disease. However, if the patient is not actively having bronchospasm, the spirometry may yield a normal result. A better and more definitive test is a methacholine challenge. This test induces airway reactivity if the patient has underlying asthma. Patients are given increasing sequential doses of methacholine, and spirometry is administered after every dilution. A provocative concentration that causes a 20% reduction from the baseline forced expiratory volume in the first second ($PC_{20}FEV_1$) or a decrease in specific conductance of 35% to 45% from the baseline at less than 16 mg/mL of methacholine is considered a positive methacholine challenge.

An adequate trial of asthma medications is the last step to diagnosing asthma, after having considered and treated UACS and other potential causes of cough. An inhaled corticosteroid used on a daily maintenance schedule with or without a long-acting beta agonist is the drug of choice depending on severity. If the patient has a severe cough or shortness of breath, using a trial of prednisone, 40 mg once a day for 7 days, will help control the inflammation more efficiently. Leukotriene receptor antagonists can also be added later, if symptoms persist.

Cough Variant Asthma

Cough variant asthma (CVA) is a subset of asthma that can present as cough alone with a normal physical examination and a normal spirometry. Patients with CVA tend to have a more sensitive cough reflex but less bronchial reactivity when compared to classic asthmatics. A methacholine challenge may assist in confirming bronchial reactivity, but it does not necessarily establish the diagnosis of CVA. The definitive diagnosis depends on resolution of symptoms after being treated with asthma medications.

Nonasthmatic Eosinophilic Bronchitis

Nonasthmatic eosinophilic bronchitis is a steroid responsive chronic cough found in nonsmokers who have sputum eosinophils without variable airflow obstruction. The sputum should contain a nonsquamous cell sputum eosinophil count of greater than 3%. Methacholine challenges in patients with no asthmatic eosinophilic bronchitis usually yield a normal result. It can be associated with occupational exposures as well as allergens. The treatment is avoiding offending agents and using asthma anti-inflammatory medications.

Gastroesophageal Reflux Disease and Cough

Gastroesophageal reflux disease (GERD) frequently causes a persistent cough. It is defined as a retrograde movement of gastric material from the stomach to the esophagus. Common symptoms of GERD include heartburn, regurgitation, sour taste in the back of the mouth, and coughing. In a normal individual, it can occur 50 times a day. Some studies suggest that the patient may not detect symptoms of GERD 75% of the time.

GERD causes cough in two ways. Gastric material (frequently acid) can make its way up the esophagus to the larynx and cause direct irritation. However, this is not always necessary. Acid or other caustic agents (e.g., pancreatic enzymes or bile) can irritate the distal esophagus. This stimulation of the vagal reflexes can cause bronchoconstriction or cough. The diagnostic procedures that may be helpful are 24-hour esophageal pH monitoring and barium esophagography. The 24-hour esophageal pH monitoring is the most sensitive and specific test for measuring acid in the esophagus. However, by itself this test does not establish causation. Barium esophagography helps determine if there is an esophageal lesion from nonacid GERD. Perhaps the most helpful information for diagnosing GERD is a significant resolution of the persistent cough after a 1- to 3-month trial of antireflux treatment. The preferential choice of antireflux treatment is a proton pump inhibitor. This therapy would then be followed by changes in diet and lifestyle modifications to reduce acid production.

SYMPTOMATIC TREATMENT OF COUGH

The goal in treating cough is always to find the etiology. However, symptomatic relief is needed if the source of the cough is unknown or the treatment of the underlying process requires a prolonged course. Usually, the medications are divided into peripheral and central acting agents (Fig. 10–1).

First-generation antihistamines have some local anticholinergic effects in the nasal passages and seem to have some consequence in reducing cough symptoms for upper respiratory tract infections (URIs). Inhaled ipratropium bromide also has peripheral cough suppressing effects for URI and COPD. Interestingly, other anticholinergic inhalers do not seem to have the same effect. In some studies, guaifenesin, an expectorant, decreases symptom of cough in URI and bronchiectasis.

The central acting cough suppressants are believed to act on the brainstem. Dextromethorphan is the most commonly used nonsedating, nonaddicting agent.

Codeine and other opioids have modest effects on chronic bronchitis cough. Some studies suggest codeine is not very effective for URIs.

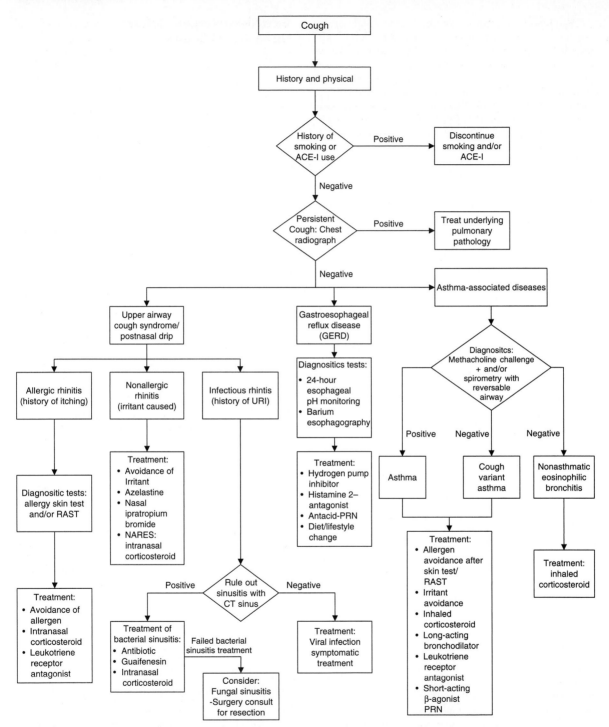

Figure 10–1. Approach to treating the common causes of cough.

CONCLUSION

Cough can be a common presentation for many diseases. Because allergic diseases can affect up to 25% of the general population, atopy should always be a consideration in the differential diagnosis of cough. Allergic diseases play a significant part in UACS (postnasal drip) and asthma, which are the two most common causes of cough. The advent of modern allergy medications has allowed for a powerful way of teasing out the atopic component of cough. It can be used as a diagnostic tool as well as a therapeutic treatment. Having the patient assign a percentage of effectiveness to the different medications can help distinguish between the primary and secondary causes. Thus, integrating therapeutic trials with the history and diagnostic testing can help elucidate the complex etiologies of cough.

EVIDENCE-BASED MEDICINE

Hartl D, Griese M, Nicolai T, et al. Pulmonary chemokines and their receptors differentiate children with asthma and chronic cough. *J Allergy Clin Immunol.* 2005;115:728–736.

This study attempts to use bronchioalveolar lavage fluid (BALF) chemokines and their receptors to distinguish between children with allergic asthmatic cough from children with chronic nonatopic cough. A total of 37 children were sampled: 12 patients with allergic asthmatic cough, 15 patients with idiopathic nonatopic chronic cough, and 10 healthy control patients, ranging from ages 3 to 17. The allergic asthmatic children had a significantly higher level of $CCR4^+CD4^+$ cells (TH2), thymus- and activation-regulated chemokine (TARC), and macrophage-derived chemokine (MDC) as compared to the nonatopic chronic cough children and control. In the nonatopic chronic cough group: $CXCR3^+CD8^+$ cells (TH1) and levels of IFN-gamma-inducible T cell alpha chemoattractant (ITAC) were significantly elevated as compared to the atopic asthmatics as well as the controls. This study helps validate the association of atopy and TH2 chemokines, providing a useful method for distinguishing atopic cough versus nonatopic cough.

Niimi A, Torrego A, Nicholson AG, et al. Nature of airway inflammation and remodeling in chronic cough. *J Allergy Clin Immunol.* 2005;116:565–570.

This study tries to evaluate if there are unique characteristics of inflammation or remodeling as a result of asthmatic cough versus nonasthmatic cough. A group of 62 patients were subdivided into: 33 nonasthmatic chronic cough patients, 14 asthmatic cough patients, and 15 healthy controls. These patients underwent bronchoscopy with biopsies and had capsaicin cough sensitivity assessment. The group with nonasthmatic cough had significant mast cell hyperplasia, increased smooth muscle area, and increased cough sensitivity not seen in the asthmatic cough patients or the control. There was also a positive correlation between the increased cough sensitivity in relation to goblet cell hyperplasia and epithelial shedding. The asthmatic cough group had increased submucosal eosinophils and neutrophils. The results show that airway remodeling was prominent in nonasthmatic as well as asthmatic cough patients. This suggests that the chronic cough itself is the cause of the airway remodeling.

BIBLIOGRAPHY

Bolser DC. Cough suppressant and pharmacologic protussive therapy: ACCP evidence-based clinical practice guidelines. *Chest.* 2006;129(suppl):238S.

Brightling CE, Ward R, Goh KL, et al. Eosinophilic bronchitis is an important cause of chronic cough. *Am J Respir Crit Care Med.* 1999;160:406.

Bronsky EA, Druce H, Findlay SR, et al. A clinical trial of ipratropium bromide nasal spray in patients with perennial nonallergic rhinitis. *J Allergy Clin Immunol.* 1995;95:1117.

Chang AB, Glomb WB. Guidelines for evaluating cough in pediatrics: ACCP evidence-based clinical practice guidelines. *Chest.* 2006;129(suppl):260S.

Chung KF, Widdicombe JG. Cough. In: Mason RJ, ed. *Murray & Nadel's Textbook of Respiratory Medicine.* 4th ed. London: Elsevier; 2005:831.

Fujimura M, Sakamoto S, Kamio Y, et al. Cough receptor sensitivity and bronchial responsiveness in normal and asthmatic subjects. *Eur Respir J.* 1992;5:291.

Hartl D, Griese M, Nicolai T, et al. Pulmonary chemokines and their receptors differentiate children with asthma and chronic cough. *J Allergy Clin Immunol.* 2005;115:728.

Irwin RS, Baumann MH, Bolser DC, et al. Diagnosis and management of cough executive summary: ACCP evidence-based clinical practice guidelines. *Chest.* 2006;129(suppl):1S.

Irwin RS, French CL, Curley FJ, et al. Chronic cough due to gastroesophageal reflux: clinical, diagnostic, and pathogenetic aspects. *Chest.* 1993;104:1511.

Irwin RS, Madison JM. The diagnosis and treatment of cough. *N Engl J Med.* 2000;343:1715.

Israili ZH, Hall WD. Cough and angioneurotic edema associated with angiotensin-converting enzyme inhibitor therapy: a review of the literature and pathophysiology. *Ann Intern Med.* 1992;117:234.

Niimi A, Torrego A, Nicholson AG, et al. Nature of airway inflammation and remodeling in chronic cough. *J Allergy Clin Immunol.* 2005;116:565.

Pratter MR. Overview of common causes of chronic cough: ACCP evidence-based clinical practice guidelines. *Chest.* 2006;129(suppl):59S.

Pratter MR, Brightling CE, Boulet LP, et al. An empiric integrative approach to the management of cough: ACCP evidence-based clinical practice guidelines. *Chest.* 2006;129(suppl):222S.

Urticaria and Angioedema

Bettina Wedi, MD, PhD, and Alexander Kapp, MD, PhD

Urticaria, commonly known as hives, is one of the most common dermatologic conditions seen by allergists. It is characterized by acute or chronic superficial swelling of the skin that is almost invariably associated with itching. Lifetime incidence is higher than 20%. The mechanism is local vasodilation and increase in capillary permeability with plasma leakage and IgE-mediated or nonimmunologic activation of mast cells causing mediator release, predominantly of histamine. The itching can be pricking or burning and is usually worse in the evening or nighttime. Typically the lesions are rubbed and not scratched; therefore, excoriated skin is usually not a consequence of urticaria.

Angioedema is caused by a similar mechanism but is localized deeper in the dermis, subcutaneous, and submucosal tissues. Urticaria and angioedema can occur anywhere on the body. Angioedema most often involves the eyelids, lips, and genitalia but sometimes also the tongue and laryngopharynx, which can be life threatening and causes anxiety (symptoms occur often at nighttime). Systemic symptoms such as fatigue, respiratory, gastrointestinal, and arthralgic symptoms are rare.

Urticaria is not a single disease but a reaction pattern. The clinical pictures are of heterogeneous etiology and therefore subclassified into distinct groups.

CLASSIFICATION OF URTICARIA

The different subtypes within the three main groups of urticaria, spontaneous urticaria (about 80%), physical urticaria (about 10%), and special types of urticaria (<10%), should be clearly defined (see Table 11–1).

Two or rarely more subtypes of urticaria can occur in the same patient, such as chronic urticaria and dermographism or delayed pressure urticaria. In these cases urticaria is more often difficult to treat and is long persisting.

Other diseases such as urticaria vasculitis and urticaria pigmentosa, although associated with the name urticaria for historical reasons, are no longer grouped under the heading urticaria.

SPONTANEOUS URTICARIA

About two thirds of spontaneous urticaria is acute (allergic or nonallergic) and about one third is chronic urticaria (nonallergic).

Acute Urticaria

DEFINITION

Acute urticaria is defined as spontaneous wheal and flare reaction of less than 6 weeks' duration (Fig. 11–1). Most often a single episode lasts for 1 or 2 weeks. Angioedema is associated in more than 50% of cases. Acute urticaria is a common skin disease in medical emergency service. There is no gender preference.

CLINICAL SYMPTOMS

The size, number, and shape of wheals (elevated erythema) vary considerably and can develop anywhere on the body. Sometimes the lesions become annular, arcuate, or polycyclic when confluent. Urticarial wheals are always very itchy but are not scratched, so secondary skin lesions like erosions are rarely seen. General symptoms like fever, arthralgia, headaches, or cardiovascular disturbances may accompany an exacerbation. Involvement of the tongue and pharynx is often associated with hoarseness, difficulty swallowing, and dyspnea.

PATHOGENESIS AND DIAGNOSIS

Most common is *acute nonallergic urticaria,* in which most cases are associated with an acute upper respiratory or genitourinary infection and/or a pseudoallergic reaction (particularly to cyclooxygenase I inhibitors such as aspirin and other nonsteroidal anti-inflammatory drugs [NSAIDs]). In contrast, atopic *acute allergic urticaria* caused by IgE-mediated allergy (e.g., to food allergens, hymenoptera stings, and drugs such as penicillin) can be found more frequently (Table 11–2).

Diagnosis is based on a careful history to identify potential triggering factors (ask for atopic diseases, known allergies, drug intake, signs of infections), and

Table 11–1. Classification of urticaria subtypes.

Urticaria Group	Subtype of Urticaria	Definition
Spontaneous	Acute	Spontaneous wheals <6 wk
	Chronic	Spontaneous wheals >6 wk
Physical	Cold	Cause: cold (air/water/wind)
	Delayed pressure	Cause: vertical pressure (latency of 3–8 h)
	Localized heat	Cause: local heat
	Solar	Cause: ultraviolet and/or visible light
	Dermographic	Cause: mechanical shear forces
	Vibratory	Cause: vibratory forces (pneumatic hammer)
Special type	Aquagenic	Cause: water contact of any temperature
	Cholinergic	Cause: increased body temperature
	Contact	Cause: contact with urticariogenic substance
	Exercise induced	Cause: physical exercise

physical examination (blood pressure, pulse, lung auscultation). If a cause cannot be identified by history, no investigations are needed because of the self-limiting nature of acute urticaria.

MANAGEMENT (PROGNOSIS)

Medical supervision (inpatient care) is recommended in case of dyspnea, hypotension, and generalized severe urticaria. Causal treatment includes stopping of culprit drug intake, removing insect stinger, and prescription of antibiotics in bacterial infections. Symptomatic treatment consists of low-sedating H_1 antihistamines up to fourfold daily (consider potential side effects when increasing the dose!) and, if favored, also local treatment with antipruritic and cooling lotions. In severe cases (associated severe angioedema), often additional administration of glucocorticosteroids, up to 100 to 250 mg intravenous (IV) prednisolone and H_1 antihistamine (IV), are needed, maybe repeatedly. In progressive cases, anaphylactic shock treatment including proper administration of epinephrine is mandatory.

Most cases improve promptly after IV treatment with antihistamines and glucocorticosteroids. However, symptoms may reoccur several hours later (in most patients total symptoms persist less than 2 weeks). Therefore, outpatients should take low-sedating antihistamines in adequate doses (up to fourfold) for 1 to 2 weeks and should be provided with a rescue medication (e.g., drinkable corticosteroid), for severe symptoms. There is no prognostic factor identifying patients at risk for progression to chronic urticaria (less than 1%). Adequate treatment of acute urticaria is able to inhibit progression to chronic urticaria.

Chronic Urticaria

DEFINITION

Urticaria is chronic if it persists for more than 6 weeks with nearly daily whealing episodes. Urticaria with less frequently occurring bouts over a long period is called

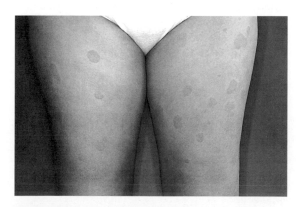

Figure 11–1. Typical wheal and flare reaction in spontaneous urticaria.

Table 11–2. Common causes of acute allergic urticaria and/or angioedema.

Foods (peanuts, shellfish, milk, eggs, tree nuts, soy, latex-associated fruits such as banana, kiwi, avocado, chestnut)
Drugs (β-lactam antibiotics)
Insect venoms, fire ants

episodic and more likely to have an identifiable environmental trigger. Chronic urticaria usually persists on average for 3 to 5 years. In 40% of patients where it lasts more than 6 months; chronic urticaria is still present 10 years later, and in 20%, even after 20 years. Lifelong prevalence is about 0.5% and as far as known does not vary greatly across the world. Chronic urticaria is most common in middle-aged adults, particularly in women, but also occurs in infants and children (Fig. 11–2).

CLINICAL SYMPTOMS

Clinical symptoms are similar to acute urticaria but persist longer than 6 weeks. As in acute urticaria, at least half of the patients suffer from concomitant and sometimes life-threatening angioedema. Approximately 10% to 20% of patients have recurrent angioedema without urticaria. In chronic urticaria, systemic symptoms are possible.

Quality of life is significantly impaired equal to that experienced by patients with severe atopic dermatitis, psoriasis, or triple coronary arterial disease. The main reasons for decreased quality of life are intense pruritus, particularly in the evening and night, and sleep disturbances. Secondary, often psychosocial problems develop.

PATHOGENESIS AND DIAGNOSIS

The diagnosis of chronic urticaria is based on a thorough history considering potential triggering factors, a physical examination including a test for dermographism, laboratory investigations, and, if needed, additional specific procedures. Patient diaries are very helpful to become aware of the fluctuating intensity of the disease.

Every attempt should be made to find an underlying etiology in each patient because the identification and elimination of causal factors represent the best therapeutic approach. IgE-mediated hypersensitivity due to exogenous allergens is generally very rarely the cause of symptoms in chronic urticaria, and there is no increased frequency of atopy. The implication of genuine food allergy is exceptional, in contrast to acute urticaria. Thus routine skin prick tests to inhalant and food allergens are of little value. However, many direct and indirect releasing factors may be involved. Possible mechanisms include autoimmune mechanisms, infectious diseases (viral, bacterial, fungal, parasites), particularly *Helicobacter pylori*–associated gastritis, pseudoallergic mechanisms, and others, such as internal diseases and malignancies. It is often overlooked that several of these mechanisms may be active in a single patient.

About a third of patients show evidence for an autoimmune pathogenesis caused by functional mast cell–stimulating IgG antibodies against the alpha subunit of the high-affinity IgE receptor and more rarely against IgE itself. Indicative is a positive autologous serum skin test (ASST) performed by a specialist, although the clinical relevance is far from clear (ASST can be still positive after resolution of urticaria). At present, there are no commercial sources of direct measurement of these autoantibodies. In addition, about 30% of chronic urticaria cases are also associated with antithyroid antibodies.

Aspirin and NSAIDs (Table 11–3) aggravate symptoms and evoke exacerbations by a non–IgE-mediated pseudoallergic mechanism in a third of patients. Often regular intake of these drugs is not reported. Other mast cell–activating drugs are morphine, codeine, muscle relaxants, polymyxin, and dextran. Rarely, nonallergic hypersensitivity reactions to food additives play a role, but generally they have no role unless proven by a double-blind, placebo-controlled challenge.

Figure 11–3 outlines a reliable diagnostic procedure. With regard to the long duration of the annoying skin disease, a well-directed workup based on a thorough history is indicated. An expert opinion should be sought in severe and unusual cases.

In case of prolonged duration of individual wheals (more than 24 hours) and resolution with purpura and pigmentation, biopsies should be taken to exclude vasculitis by histology and immunofluorescence that may be indicative for systemic disease like lupus erythematosus, which is usually associated with extracutaneous manifestations.

Although very rare, chronic urticaria can be associated with malignant diseases. Moreover, genetic syndromes (e.g., Muckle-Well syndrome, hyper-IgD syndrome,

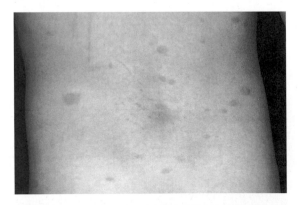

Figure 11–2. Chronic urticaria combined with dermographic urticaria in a child.

Table 11–3. Common NSAIDs triggering urticaria and angioedema.

Acetylsalicylic acid (aspirin)
Ibuprofen
Diclofenac
Naproxen
Metamizole

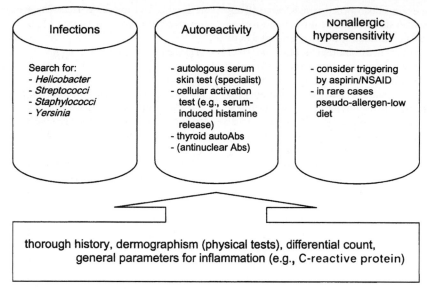

NSAID = nonsteroidal antiinflammatory drug.

Figure 11–3. Recommended diagnostic schedule in chronic urticaria.

chronic infantile neurologic cutaneous and articular syndrome), hematologic (e.g., Schnitzler syndrome), and immune disorders (e.g., systemic lupus erythematosus, hypocomplementemic urticaria vasculitis syndrome) may present with (often nonitching!) urticaria-like skin lesions. Other differentials include scabies; arthropod reactions; urticarial stages of autoimmune bullous skin diseases, such as bullous pemphigoid; and early stages of vasculitis and erythema multiforme.

It has been shown that 20% to 30% of *children* with acute urticaria, of which almost all were associated with acute infections, progressed into chronic urticaria. Accordingly, persistent chronic, often bacterial infections (e.g., with streptococci, staphylococci, but also with *H. pylori*) are common in childhood chronic urticaria. Furthermore, as in adults, positive autologous serum skin tests indicating autoreactivity can be found in a third. In children and young adults, serology for Epstein-Barr virus and cytomegalovirus should be included in the diagnostic workup.

MANAGEMENT (PROGNOSIS)

The goal is to maximize quality of life and ability to work or to attend school and to minimize drug-related side effects such as sedation. Relevant outcomes of treatment trials include pruritus, wheal size, number and frequency, loss of awakening, overall physician and patient assessment, and permanent remission of disease.

Unspecific trigger factors should be avoided, for example, intake of aspirin/other NSAID (in favor of acetaminophen), alcohol, overheating, ACE inhibitors in case of angioedema (often also sartans). Specific and sufficient treatment of identified persistent bacterial and parasitic infections can result in complete remission. In single cases with challenge-proven nonallergic hypersensitivity reactions to food additives, dietary avoidance for 3 to 6 months may be helpful.

Long-acting low-sedating antihistamines are the mainstay of symptomatic treatment and can be given the highest grade of recommendation according to the criteria of evidence-based medicine. They reduce itch and wheal duration and numbers and also increase quality of life. To administer an adequate dose in chronic urticaria, it is common practice to exceed the licensed dose. The current European Guideline recommends an increased dose up to fourfold the normal dose while considering the side effects. Due to the long-term duration of the disease, low-sedating H_1 antihistamines are preferred, particularly when increased dosage is needed. H_1 antihistamines demonstrating high-quality evidence in chronic urticaria treatment include azelastine, cetirizine, desloratadine, ebastine, fexofenadine, levocetirizine, loratadine, and mizolastine (in alphabetical order). Management is better achieved by taking antihistamines daily, not just when the patient is symptomatic.

As general rule, antihistamines are safe, but potential side effects such as impairment of performance, sedation, interaction with CYP450 enzymes, liver, cardiac side effects, and nephrotoxicity should be considered for the respective choice. It is best to avoid all antihistamines in pregnancy, although teratogenic effects have not been proven. Flawless studies investigating alternatives in chronic urticaria are rare. Glucocorticosteroids (30 to 40 mg of prednisone per day) should only be used after a trial of maximal dose of antihistamines. Moreover, replacement of one H_1 antihistamine with another should be tried because of individual differences in responsiveness.

Particularly patients with autoimmune urticaria are frequently treatment resistant. Therapeutic strategies for chronic urticaria resistant to low-sedating H_1 antihistamine monotherapy are problematic and not standardized. The data on treatment alternatives are totally insufficient from an evidence-based viewpoint, and the risk-benefit profile for each alternative (off-label use) should be carefully considered before treatment. This applies especially to immunosuppressive agents. Only in the case of cyclosporine A can a third grade of recommendation for treatment be given for severely affected patients (2.5 to 5 mg/kg/day). Cyclosporin A appears to be effective in a third, in another third urticaria reappears after discontinuation, and a third do not respond.

Chronic urticaria subgroups (i.e., with positive autologous serum skin test and/or intolerance to aspirin/food additives) might benefit from addition of leukotriene antagonists. Chloroquine and dapsone may be worth of further investigation within randomized controlled trials. The choice of a combination of an H_1 antihistamine with a H_2 antihistamine is not justified nowadays. Table 11–4 gives a practical stepwise approach for the treatment.

If chronic urticaria persists for longer than 6 months, prognosis is increasingly bad. After 10 years, more than 40% still suffer from the disease. Regarding chronicity and impairment of daily life and occupational disability,

it is also legitimate to treat the psychological factors involved in chronic urticaria.

PHYSICAL URTICARIA

Physical urticaria is a distinct group that is caused by external physical stimulus and should be clearly differentiated from spontaneous urticaria, although both can coexist. Usually the wheals resolve within 2 hours except in delayed pressure urticaria and delayed dermographic urticaria. Although clinically impressive, to date, neither the pathomechanisms have been clarified nor are sufficient data available to recommend treatment schedules based on an evidence-based view. Prognosis of physical urticaria is worse than chronic urticaria.

Physical urticaria is diagnosed by a thorough history, clinical examination, and provocation procedures using standardized physical tests. These tests are not without risk. Infection as an etiology of physical urticaria has been subject of controversy. Autoreactivity, that is, a positive autologous serum skin test or autoantibodies against IgE receptor/IgE or against thyroid has not been described.

Dermographic Urticaria

DEFINITION AND PATHOGENESIS

Dermographic urticaria (synonyms: factitial urticaria, symptomatic dermographism) develops within a few minutes after mechanical shearing forces and presents with intensely itching wheals. It is possible to write on the skin (Fig. 11–4). In contrast, urticarial dermographism is asymptomatic. Dermographic urticaria is

Table 11–4. Recommended treatment for chronic urticaria with and without angioedema.

Line	
First	Low-sedating H1-receptor antagonists daily (consider up to fourfold dose)
	Adequate treatment of identified triggering factors (e.g., triple therapy for *Helicobacter pylori*, antibiotics for streptococci, or L-thyroxine in case of thyroid autoimmunity)
	Avoid overheating, tight clothing, alcohol, aspirin/NSAID, ACE inhibitors, and angiotensin II receptor blocker
	Reassure patient about the benign nature of the condition and the difficulties in treatment
	Optional topical treatment (2% menthol or 2% polidocanol in aqueous cream or lotion)
Second	Try another low-sedating H1-receptor antagonists (increased dose) *and/or* Add leukotriene antagonist
Third	Consult expert for nonstandard therapies: (hydroxy-)chloroquine, dapsone, oral low-dose corticosteroids, cyclosporine A, doxepin, oxatomide, ketotifen, sulfasalazine, IVIG, plasmapheresis, interferon-γ, methotrexate, cyclophosphamide, colchicine, warfarin, stanozolol, coxibs

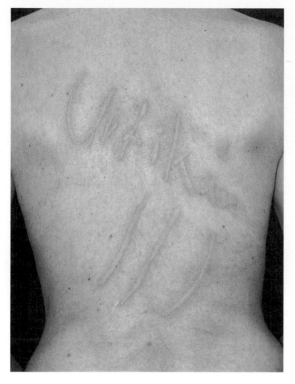

Figure 11–4. Writing on the skin in dermographic urticaria.

the most frequent subtype of physical urticaria with a mean duration of 6.5 years, and it is often combined with spontaneous chronic urticaria. Dermographic urticaria can occur after infections or may be drug induced (e.g., penicillin).

CLINICAL SYMPTOMS AND DIAGNOSIS

Rubbing and touching the skin and also wearing of clothes result in local itchy wheals that again are rubbed (vicious circle). Simply scratching the skin for a length of about 10 cm with a pen produces linear wheals beyond the area of contact. More standardized is the use of a dermographometer (spring-loaded stylus). Thorough history guides further investigations to exclude infections or drugs as causative agents.

MANAGEMENT (PROGNOSIS)

Treatment is similar to chronic urticaria with low-sedating H_1 antihistamines given regularly and at adequate dose (up to fourfold the normal dose). Additional low evidence exists for ketotifen. The patient should be reassured about the benign nature of the disorder. Dermographic urticaria is distressing but not life threatening.

Delayed Pressure Urticaria

DEFINITION AND PATHOGENESIS

Sustained vertical pressure is the eliciting factor of delayed pressure urticaria. Delayed pressure urticaria is more common in middle-aged men and persists for an average of 6 to 9 years, often resulting in disability to work. It may be associated with chronic urticaria.

CLINICAL SYMPTOMS AND DIAGNOSIS

Deep, painful swellings develop 6 to 8 hours after sustained pressure and persist for up to 2 days. Typical localizations are the palms and soles, buttocks, back, and skin under straps and belts. The condition may be accompanied by systemic symptoms of malaise, arthralgia, myalgia, and leukocytosis.

Standardized pressure test consists of applying weight in amount of 0.5 to 1.5 kg/cm^2 for 10 minutes in different areas (back, ventral, and dorsal thigh) (Fig. 11–5). Evaluation of the testing area should be done at least after 30 minutes, 3 hours, 6 hours, and 24 hours. Only definite raised wheals occurring after several hours indicate delayed pressure urticaria. Elicited wheals that persist for more than 24 hours should be biopsied to exclude vasculitis.

MANAGEMENT (PROGNOSIS)

Delayed pressure urticaria responds poorly to antihistamines, even in increased doses. Nevertheless, they represent the mainstay of treatment. Some patients are well controlled by additional low-dose corticosteroids (e.g., 40 to 20 mg prednisone), others by treatment with dapsone (100 to 150 mg/day). Other low-evidence alternatives are methotrexate (15 mg/week), montelukast, ketotifen plus nimesulide, sulfasalazine, or topical clobetasol propionate 0.5% ointment.

Cold Urticaria

DEFINITION AND PATHOGENESIS

Cold bodies or cold water, also cold air and cold food/drinks, can provoke cold urticaria and angioedema within minutes. Mainly young adults are affected with an average duration of 5 years. It may coexist with cholinergic urticaria.

CLINICAL SYMPTOMS AND DIAGNOSIS

Immediate, but rarely delayed reactions occur after cold exposure at the size of localized cooling but may also be generalized following lowering of the body temperature. Infectious diseases such as syphilis, borreliosis, hepatitis, infectious mononucleosis, and HIV infections can induce cold urticaria, but unrecognized bacterial infections are also reported. Cold provocation can be done by applying ice-filled metal cylinders, ice cubes, and/or

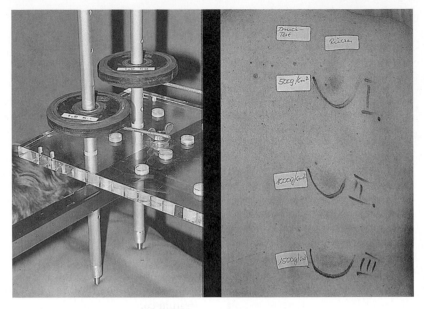

Figure 11–5. Left: Standardized pressure test applying 500 g/cm², 1000 g/cm², and 1500 g/cm² for 10 minutes. Right: Reading after 24 hours revealed wheals of delayed pressure urticaria.

cold water for 1 to 10 minutes (Fig. 11–6). Ideally the threshold temperature is defined. Recently low-voltage Peltier thermoelectric elements have been used to standardize cold provocation. Depending on the history, cold ventilator wind provocation may also be used.

MANAGEMENT (PROGNOSIS)

Identified infectious diseases should be treated adequately. Low-sedating H_1 antihistamines are the first line in

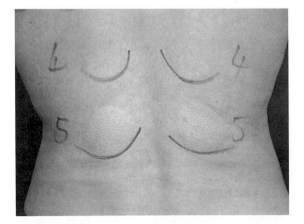

Figure 11–6. Significant swelling of the skin ("peau d'orange") developing 5 minutes after a 5-minute exposure to ice-filled copper cylinders to the back.

treatment. In idiopathic cases, antibiotic treatment (e.g., with oral doxycycline or penicillin, intramuscular, intravenous or orally) is worth trying. Other low-evidence alternatives are cyproheptadine, ketotifen, and montelukast.

Localized Heat Urticaria

DEFINITION AND PATHOGENESIS

Localized heat urticaria is a rare phenomenon that is developed by direct contact with a warm object such as air or water.

CLINICAL SYMPTOMS AND DIAGNOSIS

The eliciting temperature ranges from 38°C to more than 50°C. Ideally the threshold temperature should be defined using a 38°C warm arm bath for 10 minutes (if negative, the temperature may be increased) or to apply a glass tube containing hot water (38°C to 50°C for 1 to 5 minutes). Wheals occur immediately and are often small sized and fleeting.

MANAGEMENT (PROGNOSIS)

Evidence-based treatment is not available. Skin hardening to heat or chloroquine may be tried.

Solar Urticaria

DEFINITION AND PATHOGENESIS

Solar urticaria is rare. It comprises only 4% of all photosensitive skin disorders. Wavelengths ranging from

280 to 760 µm, mostly ultraviolet (UV) light, are the eliciting physical stimulus. Women in their third or forth decade of life are predominantly affected.

CLINICAL SYMPTOMS AND DIAGNOSIS

Within minutes of light exposure, pruritic wheals develop, although constantly exposed areas might be not involved. Provocation is done using specific wavelengths of a monochromator and, for example, a slide projector (visible light) for 10 minutes to determine the minimal urticarial dose (MUD). The lesions usually fade 15 minutes to 3 hours after onset. When forming a differential list, in addition to systemic lupus erythematosus or erythropoietic protoporphyria, more common polymorphous light eruptions should be considered.

MANAGEMENT (PROGNOSIS)

Treatment can be frustrating. Low-sedating H_1 antihistamines are the first line of treatment. Photo hardening of the skin may be effective. Other low-evidence possibilities include plasmapheresis, cyclosporin A, photopheresis, plasma exchange, and IV immunoglobulins or hydroxychloroquine.

Vibratory Urticaria (Angioedema)

DEFINITION AND PATHOGENESIS

Very rarely, strong vibrating forces (e.g., pneumatic hammer) result in vibratory urticaria and/or angioedema.

CLINICAL SYMPTOMS AND DIAGNOSIS

The symptoms are reproduced by a vibrating machine.

MANAGEMENT (PROGNOSIS)

Exposure to vibrating forces is the treatment of choice.

SPECIAL TYPES OF URTICARIA

Cholinergic Urticaria

DEFINITION AND PATHOGENESIS

Cholinergic urticaria is subclassified as a special type of urticaria because it is rather caused by a short increase in body temperature and not by external physical stimuli. The rise in body temperature can be the result of physical exercise, passive warmth (hot bath), or emotional stress. Cholinergic urticaria is common in young adults, lasting for an average of 5 to 6 years. It may coexist with cold urticaria.

CLINICAL SYMPTOMS AND DIAGNOSIS

The wheals are fleeting, typically only of pinhead size, and disappear within several minutes to 1 hour. In severely affected patients, systemic symptoms, such as nausea, headache, and dizziness, may be observed. In exercise-induced urticaria/anaphylaxis, which is the main differential diagnosis, usually the wheals are larger than pinhead size and persist for a long period. For diagnostic purposes, usually cholinergic urticaria is provoked by ergometer exercise or by running in place for 5 to 15 minutes.

MANAGEMENT (PROGNOSIS)

As in other urticaria subtypes, low-sedating H_1 antihistamines (in increased dose) regularly and/or 60 minutes before characteristic triggering situations are the mainstay of treatment. Nevertheless they often fail. It is difficult to achieve exercise tolerance. Ketotifen may be an optional medication to use. Efficient treatment with danazol has been described, but adverse effects have to be considered.

Aquagenic Urticaria

DEFINITION AND PATHOGENESIS

Aquagenic urticaria is very rare. Contact to water of any temperature liberates a water-soluble allergen from the stratum corneum that diffuses into the dermis.

CLINICAL SYMPTOMS AND DIAGNOSIS

After water contact, small-sized wheals occur in the contact area. In contrast, in aquagenic pruritus itch develops without urticaria. Challenge test is performed by application of water compresses at approximate body temperature (37°C) for 30 minutes.

MANAGEMENT (PROGNOSIS)

In most cases, prophylactic treatment with low-sedating H_1 antihistamines is sufficient.

Contact Urticaria

DEFINITION AND PATHOGENESIS

Contact urticaria develops after contact to an urticant that may cause an immunologic (IgE dependent) or nonimmunologic reaction (IgE independent). Examples of allergic contact urticants are food, latex, and animals; these mainly play a role in atopic individuals (particularly in atopic dermatitis), whereas nonallergic contact urticants have a direct effect on blood vessels and include irritants such as balsam of Peru, benzoic acid, and cinnamic aldehyde in cosmetics. Contact to stinging nettles is the most common form of nonallergic contact urticaria.

CLINICAL SYMPTOMS AND DIAGNOSIS

Contact urticaria is characterized by immediate whealing and itching at sites of penetration of substances through the skin or mucous membranes. In immunologic contact urticaria, the reaction may spread beyond the site of contact and progress to generalized urticaria/anaphylaxis. Most reactions occur at work; therefore, details of the patient's employment are essential. If IgE-mediated reactions are suspected, skin prick test and specific IgE measurements are indicated. Other commonly used tests are open application tests with readings at 20, 40, and 60 minutes or chamber tests applied for 15 minutes with similar reading.

MANAGEMENT (PROGNOSIS)

Several episodes of contact urticaria can result in protein contact dermatitis. Therefore, early diagnosis is critical to educate the patient to avoid the contact.

ANGIOEDEMA WITHOUT URTICARIA

Angioedema is defined by sudden, pronounced swelling of the lower dermis and subcutis and is often more painful than itchy. Frequently the mucous membranes are involved, and resolution can take up to 3 days.

CLASSIFICATION OF ANGIOEDEMA WITHOUT URTICARIA

Recurrent angioedema without urticaria must be regarded as a separate entity. To diagnose, hereditary (only 5% of all angioedema without urticaria) and acquired angioedema due to C1 inhibitor (C1 INH) deficiencies (very rare) must be excluded. Angioedema without urticaria and normal C1 INH may be of pharmacologic (ACE inhibitor induced), pseudoallergic (NSAID induced), allergic (IgE mediated), infectious (e.g., *H. pylori* induced), physical (e.g., in cold urticaria), or of an unknown (idiopathic) nature (Table 11–5). ACE-inhibitor angioedema is the most common cause of acute angioedema in accident and emergency hospital departments, and up to 20% may be life threatening.

Non–C1 INH Deficient Angioedema Without Urticaria

DEFINITION AND PATHOGENESIS

Recurrent angioedema without urticaria occur in 10% to 20% of patients who present for urticaria consultation (Fig. 11–7). Particularly angioedema of the tongue and laryngopharynx (sometimes with serious breathing difficulties) can be triggered through a pharmacologic effect by angiotensin-converting enzyme (ACE) inhibitors, angiotensin II receptor blockers (sartans), and particularly to omapatrilat (vasopeptidase inhibitor). These drugs cause decreased bradykinin degradation, resulting in increased bradykinin levels. Angioedema occurs in about 0.6% of patients receiving ACE inhibitor treatment and is more common in African Americans. In most cases this side effect occurs within 3 months of starting the drug, but occurrence after several years is also possible. Angioedema in omapatrilat-treated patients is more frequent (1.2%).

Other drug-related triggers include aspirin (usually a higher dose than 100 mg/day dose) and other NSAIDs. Sometimes persistent bacterial infections, such as those in chronic urticaria, may be associated.

CLINICAL SYMPTOMS AND DIAGNOSIS

Angioedema without urticaria, like angioedema with urticaria, most often involves the eyelids, lips, and genitalia but sometimes also the tongue and laryngopharynx, which can be life threatening and cause anxiety (symptoms occur often at nighttime). ACE inhibitor angioedema may also present with sudden abdominal pain, diarrhea, and vomiting.

A search for a dysfunction or deficiency in the C1 INH is obligatory to exclude hereditary angioedema (HAE).

Table 11–5. Classification of angioedema *without* urticaria.

Angioedema	Subtype	Cause
Non–C1 INH deficient	Pharmacologic	ACE inhibitor induced (class effect)
	Pseudoallergic	NSAID induced (usually with urticaria)
	Allergic	IgE mediated (usually with urticaria)
	Infectious	e.g., associated with *Helicobacter pylori* infection (80% with urticaria)
	Physical	Exposure to vibration, cold, pressure
	Idiopathic	No identifiable cause
C1 INH deficient (e.g., type III)	Hereditary, type I	C1 INH protein deficiency, low C4
	Hereditary, type II	C1 INH dysfunction, low C4
	Hereditary, type III	Normal C1 INH, normal C4, low C1q, exclusively in women
C1 INH deficient	Acquired, type I	Secondary to lymphoma, immune complex–mediated depletion of C1 INH
	Acquired, type II	Autoimmune, autoantibodies against C1 INH

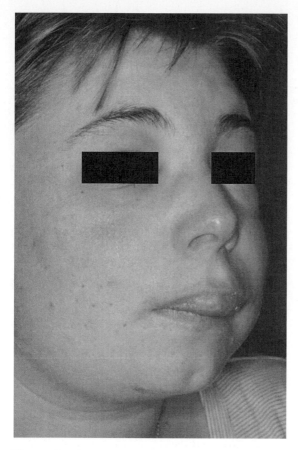

Figure 11–7. Attack of recurrent idiopathic angioedema of the left eye and upper lip.

MANAGEMENT (PROGNOSIS)

In recurrent angioedema, ACE inhibitors, sartans, and NSAIDs should be avoided. Occasionally, angioedema may continue for some weeks or even months after the ACE inhibitor has been withdrawn. Antihistamines are of little value but may attenuate severity or frequency of angioedema. Randomized controlled trials focusing on recurrent non–C1 INH-associated angioedema without urticaria are not available. Treatment is similar to chronic urticaria but often emergency treatment is needed. A dose of 40 to 60 mg of prednisone can be used; if needed, the treatment may be extended by additional 1 or 2 days. For life-threatening episodes, parenteral corticosteroids, adrenaline, or even intubation or tracheotomy may be necessary.

Hereditary Angioedema

DEFINITION AND PATHOGENESIS

HAE is a rare autosomal dominant condition with a prevalence of 1:50,000 in the general population. It is caused by a deficiency (type I, 85%) or dysfunction (type II, 15%) of C1 INH, and there is no sex bias in these classic forms. A third (type III) form occurs exclusively in women with quantitatively and functionally normal C1 INH activity related to estrogens.

CLINICAL SYMPTOMS AND DIAGNOSIS

HAE develops more slowly compared to ordinary angioedema, often beginning with prodromi, and can be associated with colicky abdominal pain. Laryngeal involvement can be life threatening, and treatment with corticosteroids/antihistamines is ineffective. HAE may develop spontaneously or after trauma, particularly with dental maneuvers. Most cases are diagnosed in childhood and have a positive family history. The attacks become worse at puberty and usually decrease in frequency and severity after the age of 50. The main sites involved are the face, hands, arms, legs, genitalia, and buttocks. Glossal, pharyngeal, or laryngeal involvement with sometimes fatal outcome is feared. In one large series, 10% had at least one required intubation or tracheostomy.

Laboratory findings reveal decreased protein levels of C1 INH in 85% of patients (in most cases, 15% to 20% of normal value) and dysfunctional inhibitor in 15% of cases (in most cases, 15% to 20% of normal values). The level of complement C4 is decreased. The C1-esterase deficiency should be detected by both antigenic and functional assays.

MANAGEMENT (PROGNOSIS)

Treatment of HAE is difficult. For acute attacks, C1 INH concentrate or fresh-frozen plasma should be administered. Intubation or tracheotomy may be necessary. Corticosteroids and antihistamines are not helpful; subcutaneous adrenaline may be tried. Prophylactic treatment involves anabolic androgens (danazol and stanozolol) that increase the serum levels of C1 INH and should be prescribed in the lowest effective dosage (hepatotoxicity, liver tumors, hirsutism). In mild HAE, avoidance of provoking factors, ACE inhibitors, estrogens together with C1 INH, or fresh-frozen plasma prophylactically before dental or surgical procedures may be sufficient.

In the near future (launch for 2007), a selective peptidometic bradykinin B2-receptor antagonist (icatibant) may be available for HAE.

Acquired C1 INH Deficiency Angioedema

DEFINITION AND PATHOGENESIS

Clinically this condition is similar to HAE, but the onset occurs in the fifth and six decades of life. Two types are differentiated. In type I, C1 INH depletion may the result of circulating immune complexes secondary to malignancy (e.g., B-cell lymphoma, myeloma). In type II, autoantibodies directed against C1 INH itself are generated.

CLINICAL SYMPTOMS AND DIAGNOSIS

Clinical symptoms are similar to that seen in HAE. Most acquired C1 INH deficiencies are found in the setting of lymphoproliferative disease in older patients with negative family history.

Laboratory assessment should include C1 INH protein level and function and levels of C4 and C1q. The laboratory findings in both types of acquired C1 INH deficient angioedema are similar to that in HAE, except that C1q levels are also decreased.

EVIDENCE-BASED MEDICINE

Zuberbier T, Bindslev-Jensen C, Canonica W et al. EAACI/GALEN/EDF guideline: definition, classification and diagnosis of urticaria. *Allergy.* 2006;61:316.

This European guideline is the outcome of the 2nd International Consensus Meeting on Urticaria and provides the definition and classification of urticaria, taking into account the recent progress in identifying causes, eliciting factors, and pathomechanisms of this disease.

Zuberbier T, Bindslev-Jensen C, Canonica W et al. EAACI/GALEN/EDF guideline: management of urticaria. *Allergy.* 2006;61:321.

This European guideline is the outcome of the 2nd International Consensus Meeting on Urticaria and provides a management approach for different urticaria subtypes, including evidence-based evaluation of published randomized controlled treatment studies.

Wedi B, Kapp A: Chronic urticaria: assessment of current treatment. *Exp Rev Clin Immunol.* 2005;1:459.

This review summarizes in detail available randomized placebo-controlled treatment trials in urticaria. The consensus described the earlier references was based on these data.

Wedi B, Kapp A. Evidence-based therapy of chronic urticaria. *J Dtsch Dermatol Ges.* 2007;5:146.

This concise evidence-based review provides practice-oriented treatment procedures for chronic urticaria.

Wedi B, Raap U, Kapp A: Chronic urticaria and infections. *Curr Opin Allergy Clin Immunol.* 2004;4:387.

This overview emphasizes the role of infections in chronic urticaria.

Federman DG, Kirsner RS, Moriarty JP, et al. The effect of antibiotic therapy for patients infected with *Helicobacter pylori* who have chronic urticaria. *J Am Acad Dermatol.* 2003;49:861–864.

This is a systematic review of existing studies looking at antibiotic therapy targeted at *H. pylori* for the treatment of chronic urticaria. The authors concluded that resolution of urticaria was more likely when antibiotic therapy was successful in eradication of *H. pylori* infection than when patients who were infected did not achieve eradication.

BIBLIOGRAPHY

Bowen T, Cicardi M, Farkas H, et al. Canadian 2003 International Consensus Algorithm for the Diagnosis, Therapy, and Management of Hereditary Angioedema. *J Allergy Clin Immunol.* 2004;114:629.

Bracho FA. Hereditary angioedema. *Curr Opin Hematol.* 2005;12:493.

Federman DG, Kirsner RS, Moriarty JP, et al. The effect of antibiotic therapy for patients infected with *Helicobacter pylori* who have chronic urticaria. *J Am Acad Dermatol.* 2003;49:861.

Grattan CE. Autoimmune urticaria. *Immunol Allergy Clin North Am.* 2004;24:163.

Grattan CEH, Sabroe RA, Greaves MW. Chronic urticaria. *J Am Acad Dermatol.* 2002;46:645.

Kaplan AP. Chronic urticaria and angioedema. *N Engl J Med.* 2002;346:175.

Kaplan AP. Chronic urticaria: pathogenesis and treatment. *J Allergy Clinical Immunol.* 2004;114:465.

Kaplan AP, Greaves MW. Angioedema. *J Am Acad Dermatol.* 2005;53:373.

Kontou-Fili K, Borici-Mazi R, Kapp A, et al. Physical urticaria: classification and diagnostic guidelines. An EAACI position paper. *Allergy.* 1997;52:504.

Wedi B, Raap U, Kapp A. Chronic urticaria and infections. *Curr Opin Allergy Clin Immunol.* 2004;4:387.

Wedi B, Kapp A. Chronic urticaria: assessment of current treatment. *Exp Rev Clin Immunol.* 2005;1:459.

Wedi B, Kapp A. Evidence-based therapy of chronic urticaria. *J Deutsch Dermatol Ges.* 2007;5:146.

Zuberbier T, Bindslev-Jensen C, Canonica W, et al. EAACI/GALEN/EDF guideline: definition, classification and diagnosis of urticaria. *Allergy.* 2006;61:316.

Zuberbier T, Bindslev-Jensen C, Canonica W, et al. EAACI/GALEN/EDF guideline: management of urticaria. *Allergy.* 2006;61:321.

Atopic Dermatitis

12

Satoshi Yoshida, MD, PhD, FACP, FAAAAI, FACAAI

Atopic dermatitis (AD) is a chronic, highly pruritic, inflammatory skin disease frequently seen in patients with a history of respiratory allergy and allergic rhinitis. The prevalence of AD in children has been steadily increasing since 1920s, and it now affects more than 10% of children at some point during their childhood. The term *atopic dermatitis* was first introduced in 1933 in recognition of the close association between AD and respiratory allergy. However, there has been considerable debate over whether AD is primarily an allergen-induced disease or simply an inflammatory skin disorder found in association with respiratory allergy. Recent studies, however, suggest that the mechanisms underlying asthma and AD have greater similarities than differences. Overall, atopy can be defined as a familial hypersensitivity of skin and mucous membranes against environmental substances, associated with increased immunogloblin E (IgE) production and/or altered nonspecific reactivity in different organ systems, for example, skin in the case of AD and lung in the case of asthma. Allergic reactions play a role in some patients but not necessarily in all. In many patients different factors such as a disturbance of skin function, infection, and mental and/or physical stresses are potentially more relevant. Immunologic disturbances are reflected in the elevated IgE production and T-cell dysregulation observed in AD. Nonspecific altered reactivity is reflected in increased releasability of chemical mediator secreting cells and bronchial, nasal, and skin hyperreactivity. Each disease that forms the atopic triad has important immunologic parallels. However, they involve a different regional sphere of immunologic influence; for example, the skin-associated lymphoid tissue in AD as opposed to bronchial-associated lymphoid tissue in asthma.

PATHOGENESIS OF ATOPIC DERMATITIS

The current review examines the cellular and immunologic mechanisms underlying AD as well as the potential role of microbial superantigens in the pathogenesis of AD. An understanding of the relative contributions of allergens, IgE, T cells with skin homing capability,

Langerhans cells, keratinocytes, eosinophils, and mast cells to the inflammatory process in AD may lead to improved treatments for this potentially debilitating disease. The concept that AD has an immunologic basis is supported by the observation that patients with primary T-cell immunodeficiency disorders frequently have elevated serum IgE levels, eosinophilia, and eczematoid skin lesions indistinguishable from AD. Laboratory observations suggest an underlying immunoregulatory abnormality in AD (Table 12–1). IgE play pivotal roles in the pathogenesis of AD (Table 12–2). A number of studies have also demonstrated an increased frequency of allergen-specific T cells producing increased IL-4 and IL-5 but little IFN-γ in the peripheral blood and skin lesions of patients with AD. It should be pointed out, however, that the majority of allergen-specific T-cell clones are TH0-type cells with the potential for development into either TH1 or TH2 cells after they have infiltrated into the skin. The data just described support an important role for TH2 cell development early in the atopic skin process. The ability of TH0 cells to develop into the TH1 or TH2 pathway depends on a number of determinants, including the cytokine milieu in which T-cell development is taking place, the host's genetic background, pharmacologic factors, and the costimulatory signals used during T-cell activation (Table 12–3). There is supportive data for each of these determinants in AD.

IMMUNOHISTOLOGY OF ATOPIC DERMATITIS

The histologic features of AD depend on the acuity of the skin lesion. Uninvolved or clinically normal-appearing skin of patients with AD is histologically abnormal and demonstrates mild hyperkeratosis and a sparse perivascular cellular infiltrate consisting primarily of T lymphocytes. Acute lesions are characterized by marked intercellular edema (spongiosis) of the epidermis and a sparse epidermal infiltrate consisting primarily of T lymphocytes. In the dermis, there is a marked perivenular inflammatory cell infiltrate consisting predominantly

Table 12–1. Peripheral blood findings in atopic dermatitis.

- Increased IgE levels
- Eosinophilia
- Increased basophil spontaneous histamine release
- Decreased CD8 suppressor/cytotoxic number and function
- Increased expression of CD23 on mononuclear cells
- Chronic macrophage activation with increased secretion of GM-CSF, prostaglandin E2, and IL-10
- Expansion of IL-4 and IL-5 secreting TH2-type cells
- Decreased numbers of IFN-γ secreting TH1-type cells
- Increased serum IL-2 receptor levels
- Increased serum eosinophil cationic protein levels
- Increased soluble E-selectin levels
- Increased soluble vascular cell adhesion molecule-1 levels
- Increased soluble intercellular adhesion molecule-1 levels

of T lymphocytes and occasional monocyte macrophages. Essentially all T cells infiltrating into the skin lesion express high levels of cutaneous lymphocyte antigen (CLA), which functions as a skin homing receptor for T lymphocytes. Eosinophils, basophils, and neutrophils are rarely present in the acute lesion. Mast cells, in various stages of degranulation, are present in normal numbers. In chronic lichenified lesions, the epidermis is hyperplastic with elongation of the rete ridges, prominent hyperkeratosis, and minimal spongiosis. There is an increased number of IgE-bearing Langerhans cells in the epidermis, and macrophages dominate the dermal mononuclear cell infiltrate. The number of mast cells are increased in number but are generally fully granulated. Increased numbers of eosinophils are observed in chronic AD skin lesions. Although the role of eosinophils in the pathogenesis of AD is not completely understood, it is thought to contribute to tissue injury in AD through the production of reactive oxygen intermediates and release of cytotoxic granules.

Table 12–2. Multifunctional role for IgE in atopic dermatitis.

- IgE-dependent late-phase skin reaction
- Allergen presentation by IgE-bearing Langerhans cells
- Allergen-induced activation of IgE-bearing macrophages
- IgG/IgM antibodies to IgE
- IgE autoreactivity to human proteins

Table 12–3. Factors contributing to the development of TH2 cells.

- Genetic background (e.g., IL-4 promoter polymorphism)
- Cytokine milieu in which antigen presentation takes place (i.e., IL-4)
- Antigen-presenting cell (e.g., Langerhans cells)
- Nature of antigen (e.g., allergens vs. parasites)
- T/B cell costimulatory signals (i.e., CD28/B7.2) (CD86) interactions
- Pharmacologic factors (i.e., prostaglandin E2, cAMP phosphodiesterase activity)

Cutaneous Infections: Role for Superantigens

Aside from food and inhalant allergens, fungal and bacterial skin infections exacerbate AD. Viral infections include herpes simplex, vaccinia, warts, molluscum contagiosum, and papilloma virus. The most common viral infection is herpes simplex, which tends to spread locally or can become generalized. Superficial fungal infections also appear to occur more frequently in atopic individuals. Recurrence of dermatophyte infections have occasionally been documented to coincide with flaring of AD. Recently there has been considerable interest in *Malassezia furfur,* also known as *Pityrosporum ovale* or *Pityrosporum orbiculare,* as a pathogen in AD. *M. furfur* is lipophilic yeast commonly present in the seborrheic areas of the skin. IgE antibodies against *M. furfur* are commonly found in patients with AD and most frequently in patients with head and neck dermatitis, but rarely outside of AD. The greatest attention has focused on the contribution of *Staphylococcus aureus* colonization and infection to the severity of AD. *S. aureus* is found in more than 90% of AD skin lesions. In contrast, only 5% of normal subjects harbor this organism, and its localization is mainly in the nose and intertriginous areas. The importance of *S. aureus* in AD is supported by the observation that not only patients with impetiginized AD but also patients with AD without superinfection show clinical response to combined treatment with antistaphylococcal antibiotics and topical corticosteroids. Recent studies suggest that one strategy by which *S. aureus* exacerbates or maintains skin inflammation in AD is by secreting a group of toxins known to act as superantigens, which stimulate marked activation of T cells and macrophages (Table 12–4). Several lines of investigation concluded that superantigens may induce an atopic process in the skin. It is therefore of interest that superantigens have recently been demonstrated to induce T-cell expression of the skin-homing receptor through stimulation of IL-12 production. In the case of AD, it has been proposed that staphylococcal superantigens secreted at the skin surface

Table 12–4. Evidence for role of staphylococcal superantigens in atopic dermatitis.

- Majority of *Staphylococcus aureus* isolates secrete superantigens.
- Majority of patients with atopic dermatitis (AD) produce IgE antibodies to superantigens.
- AD severity correlates with presence of IgE antibodies to superantigens.
- Superantigens augment allergen-induced skin inflammation.
- Superantigens induce dermatitis on application to skin by patch testing.
- Chronic eczema develops in patients recovering from toxic shock syndrome.
- Superantigens induce the cutaneous lymphocyte antigen skin-homing receptor on T cells.
- Peripheral blood mononuclear cell from AD, as compared with normal control subjects, have higher proliferative responses to superantigens.
- Superantigens induce corticosteroid resistance.
- Treatment with a combination of antistaphylococcal antibiotics and topical corticosteroids is more effective than using either medication alone.

---

could penetrate inflamed skin and stimulate epidermal macrophages or Langerhans cells to produce IL-1, tumor necrosis factor (TNF), and IL-12. These mechanisms would tend to markedly amplify the initial cutaneous inflammation in AD and perhaps also create conditions favoring staphylococcal skin colonization. Peripheral blood mononuclear cell from children with AD have been reported to have a significantly higher proliferative responses to both *S. aureus* and staphylococcal enterotoxin B, as well as diminished production of IFN-γ in response to *S. aureus* and staphylococcal enterotoxin B. In contrast, peripheral blood mononuclear cell from children with AD were more likely to produce IL-4 in response to *S. aureus*. Impaired IFN-γ production to *S. aureus* in vivo may result in failure to eradicate this organism from the skin. Persistence on the skin could contribute to inflammation by causing continued T-cell activation, release of proinflammatory mediators, and corticosteroid resistance. Furthermore, by eliciting an IgE response, staphylococcal toxins could exacerbate AD by activating mast cells, basophils, or other Fc receptor-bearing cells. Note that other staphylococcal proteins/toxins such as protein A and alpha toxin could also participate in the induction of skin inflammation by releasing TNF-α from epidermal keratinocytes or direct cytotoxic effects on skin keratinocytes.

THE DIAGNOSIS OF ATOPIC DERMATITIS

Atopy is universally recognized as a complex genotypic diathesis that manifests as a syndrome of immunologic aberrations. It would indeed be an oxymoron to make the diagnosis of AD without establishing atopy in the personal or family history and examination. A history of atopy is best obtained by specifically asking for the recognized clinical signs and symptoms of the atopic triad and not by the confusing question "Are you allergic?" In 1980 Hanifin and Rajka published diagnostic criteria for AD that have become universally accepted as the standard for

the diagnosis of that clinical entity. The diagnosis of AD can only be made by the presence of three essential criteria (each of which is included in the Hanifin and Rajka major and minor features of AD): personal or (first-degree) family history of atopy, pruritus, and eczema. Since then, significant progress in our understanding of AD, both on the clinical level and immunopathogenetic level, compels us to consider a reexamination of those original criteria. The discordance is often eloquently supported by the clinical observations of well-reputed "proallergic" investigators and skeptics. However, most of the controversy seems to be the result of one's interpretation of the indistinctive designation *allergy*, which is defined as "an altered state of immune reactivity"; but the term is still, almost exclusively, associated with what most physicians recognize as "immediate" or type I (IgE/mast cell) hypersensitivity instead of the full gamut of immunologic phenomena. As Leung so clearly reports, "an understanding of the immunologic basis of AD is likely to have important clinical implications in our approach to the diagnosis and management of AD" (see Table 12–1). Pruritus must be considered a quintessential feature of AD; pruritus is variable, fluctuating from mild to extremely intense. The itch of AD should be regarded as more than merely the result of a "lowered threshold." That common dermatologic dictum that "AD is an itch that erupts, rather than an eruption that itches" is not accurate. AD is an itch that when scratched erupts. If the atopic patient's itch is not rubbed or scratched, the skin (when provoked) may get red (vasodilate), but no eczema appears until it is traumatized. This can be described as an isomorphic response, or Koebner phenomenon, commonly noted in psoriasis and other skin conditions. An erythema caused by certain histamine-releasing or vasodilatory foods (i.e., alcohol, spices) is a more common trigger of pruritus than the IgE-mediated reaction. Because the former is nonimmunologic, it is dose related and does not depend on prior sensitization. Many patients with AD benefit from avoiding the flushing foods that trigger rosacea (i.e., hot and spicy foods; hot drinks [including hot cider, hot chocolate, coffee, or tea]; soy, and vinegars). The clinical implication of recognizing the many triggers of itch suggests that the pharmacologic mediator causing the pruritus may be different for each trigger. Despite the fact that histamine is the most abundant pruritogenic mediator in our body, its role as the major causation of itch in the patient with atopy remains questionable. Pruritus is the basic bane of atopic individuals. Although immunomodulators may offer symptomatic relief for some patients with AD, the ultimate goal of management for the patient with AD is the identification and avoidance of all the triggers of the pruritus. *Eczema* is a nonspecific term often confounding the clinical and histopathologic description of various unrelated inflammatory diseases. The eczemas include such disparate diseases as allergic contact dermatitis, AD (which may include nummular eczema, dyshidrotic eczema, and eyelid dermatitis), pityriasis rosea, lichen simplex chronicus, and seborrheic dermatitis. These eczemas do not all have clinical and histologic features in common. What is more, the clinical morphologic condition of each entity can undergo evolutionary changes, proceeding through three distinct stages, namely acute, subacute, and chronic. The eczema of AD, we must remember, is the isomorphic response of scratching the itchy, atopic skin; and the clinical morphologic condition (oozy and/or vesicular and/or scaly and/or crusted and/or lichenified) is inherently never stationary and is constantly undergoing an evolutionary process (i.e., acute, subacute, and chronic).

DIFFERENTIAL DIAGNOSIS

We have to rule out some kinds of skin diseases as follows: infant seborrheic eczema, infant xerantic eczema, congenital ichthyosis including sex-linked recessive ichthyosis caused by steroid sulfatase deficiency, bullous congenital ichthyosiform erythroderma, scabies, pediatric dermatomyositis, mycosis fungoides (skin malignant lymphoma), Pautrier microabscess, photo-contact dermatitis, contact dermatitis, chronic actinic dermatitis, and dermatitis due to Cryptomeria (cedar) pollen.

COMPLICATIONS

We have to pay attention to common complications as follows: Kaposi varicelliform, streptococcal impetigo, body trichophytosis, atopic alopecia, systemic lupus erythematodes, syphilis, and thyroid diseases.

THE TREATMENT OF ATOPIC DERMATITIS

American Academy of Dermatology and Joint Council of Allergy, Asthma, and Immunology (American Academy of Allergy, Asthma, and Immunology; AAAAI and American College of Allergy, Asthma, and Immunology; ACAAI) published the guideline of care for AD. The treatment of AD consists of these five pivotal structures:

- Avoidance of allergens (i.e., radioallergosorbent test [RAST] and/or skin test strongly positive allergens should be avoided)
- Skin care (i.e., skin hydration, moisturizers, phototherapy, and others)
- Avoidance of irritants/treatment for pruritus and deterrent to skin scratching (i.e., antihistaminic agents)
- Antiallergic inflammation (i.e., topical corticosteroids, topical calcineurin inhibitors, other antiallergic therapies)
- Exclusion of exacerbation factors (i.e., appropriate skin care, avoid of subclinical infections)

Major impediments to effective management of AD are ambivalence relating to skin care versus allergy as the management priority, uncertainty about bathing and moisturizing, and hesitation about adequate topical corticosteroid therapy. At the initial assessment, an AD evaluation form focuses on history and physical features essential to diagnosis and provides a review of trigger factors and past therapies:

1. Age of onset and clinical course of disease.
2. Personal and family history of atopic conditions.
3. Trigger factors
   a. Infections
   b. Bathing/moisturizing errors
   c. Irritant exposure
   d. Heat/sweating
   e. Emotional stress
   f. Allergic diseases
4. Review of past and current therapy
5. Physical features

During and after this assessment, we highlight with the patient/parent the steps needed for successful prevention, management, and therapy. Patients can quickly be taught increased awareness of (1) signs of infection with staphylococcal and herpes simplex infection along with the need to request antibiotic or antiviral medications; (2) irritating skin care products, clothing (such as wool or rough and occlusive fabrics), hobbies, habits (such as excessive hand washing), and job exposures; (3) the pruritus produced by overheating from excessive ambient temperatures and physical activity and clothing or bedding that are too warm; (4) stressful situations that cause anger and frustration that in turn cause increased pruritus; and (5) allergens that cause real symptoms (in contrast to the often myriad of positive skin tests and RAST reports), whether from foods, airborne sources, or chemicals that have contact with the skin.

Skin Hydration and Moisturizers

Atopic skin shows enhanced transepidermal water loss associated with impaired function of the water permeability barrier. The latter is formed by intercellular lipid lamellae found between the horny cells of stratum corneum. Both epidermal hydration and skin surface lipids were reduced, referring to an abnormality of the hydrolipid film. Hydration of the skin is best accomplished through soaking baths. Bathing might also reduce colonization by S. aureus. To prevent evaporative effects, which are damaging to the skin barrier, patients need to apply medication or moisturizer immediately after bathing or wetting their skin. Use of moisturizers together with hydration may help reestablish and preserve the stratum corneum barrier. Daily moisturizer therapy can also increase high-frequency conductance, a parameter for the hydration state of the skin surface. This allows for ranking the efficacy of moisturizers according to the duration of effects or the magnitude of increase in the hydration level of the stratum corneum. The urea treatment significantly increased skin capacitance, indicating increased skin hydration. The water barrier function, reflected by transepidermal water loss values, improved, whereas skin susceptibility to sodium lauryl sulfate was significantly reduced. Thus certain moisturizers could improve skin barrier function and reduce susceptibility to irritants. Adding a moisturizer to a low-potency topical corticosteroid improves clinical parameters in patients with AD. Moisturizers decrease the need for topical corticosteroids. Ceramide-dominant emollient is added to standard therapy in a group of children with "stubborn-to-recalcitrant" AD. Transepidermal water loss decreased concomitantly, whereas stratum corneum integrity and hydration status improved. In addition, ultrastructure of the stratum corneum revealed extracellular lamellar membranes, which were largely absent in baseline samples. Errors in bathing and moisturizing are the major cause of persistent AD. Physicians and patients have too long been stymied in their therapeutic endeavors by two true but opposing facts about bathing. On one hand, bathing dries the skin: wetting followed by evaporation causes stratum corneum contraction and fissures, impairing the epidermal barrier. On the other hand, bathing hydrates the skin: moisturizer is applied within 3 minutes to retain hydration, keeping the barrier soft and flexible. Until this paradox is explained to the patient, there can be only confusion. Although an infrequent bathing regimen may work for some people, daily bathing is preferred because it cleanses and hydrates and enhances penetration of corticosteroids, and people are more relaxed and comfortable when they bathe. A 20-minute soaking bath is optimal for hydrating the stratum corneum, although even a brief shower helps. The choice of soap may not be very important; but, if patients are concerned, we note that Dove (Lever Brothers, New York, NY) and Olay Sensitive Skin bars (Procter & Gamble, Cincinnati, OH) have reduced irritancy. The important issues are the "3-minute rule" (i.e., application of moisturizer [or topical corticosteroid] within 3 minutes before water evaporates) and the use of a proper nonfragrance moisturizer, either ointment (e.g., petrolatum, Neutrogena Hand Cream [Neutrogena, Los Angeles, CA], Aquaphor [Beiersdorf, Norwalk, CT], Albolene [Menley & James Laboratories, Horsham, PA], and Plastibase [E. R. Squibb Princeton, NJ]) or cream (e.g., Cetaphil [Galderma Laboratories, Fort Worth, TX], Vanicream [Pharmaceutical Specialties, Rochester, NY], Acid Mantle [Doak Dermatologics, Fairfield, NJ], DML [Person & Covey, Glendale, CA], and Aveeno Moisture Cream [Rydelle Laboratories, Racine, WI]). Never use lotions (Table 12–5).

Avoidance of Irritancy

Patients with AD have a lowered threshold of irritant responsiveness and need to avoid irritancy. In addition, patients with AD have an abnormal stratum corneum, even in noninvolved skin, that contributes to diffusional water loss after application of a topical irritant, confirming a functional abnormality. In addition, inflammatory changes, including spongiosis, perivenular mononuclear infiltrate, and activated eosinophils, can be seen, suggesting that nonspecific triggers might contribute to chronic inflammation in AD. Because soaps and detergents are potential irritants, patients are often advised to completely avoid them. However, cleansers might be useful, especially in patients with frequent skin infections. In a double-blinded, placebo-controlled study, use of an antimicrobial soap containing 1.5% triclocarban resulted in reduction in S. aureus colonization and significantly greater clinical improvement. In addition, patients are often counseled

Table 12–5. Optimal bathing and moisturizing for severe dermatitis or during flares.

- Tub bath for severe flaring or for very dry skin; bathe twice daily for 20 minutes (until fingertips wrinkle), using lukewarm water only. Wet compresses if bathing is painful or for nighttime itch control Shower, acceptable when skin is under good control or when flare is mild.
- Avoid washcloths, rubbing, scrubbing, or overuse of soap After bathing, dry off only partially by patting with a towel—do not rub.
- While some water is still on the skin, within 3 minutes and before leaving the bathroom: apply steroid ointment/cream to red itchy areas. Apply moisturizer (not lotions) to other areas.
- Moisturizing should be repeated as often as necessary to keep skin soft throughout the day.

to avoid swimming in chemically treated pools, although such activity can in fact be beneficial to some patients. Patients should be instructed to use a gentle cleanser to remove chlorine or bromine and then apply a moisturizer. Environmental factors that can modulate the effect of irritancy include temperature, humidity, and texture of fabrics. Temperature in home and work environments should be temperate with moderate humidity to minimize sweating. Occlusive clothing should be avoided, and loose-fitting cotton or cotton-blend garments should be substituted to help with overheating. The most important quality of clothing fabrics might be nonabrasiveness and breathability. Texture or roughness, rather than whether a fabric is natural or synthetic, determines tolerability and skin irritancy.

Treatment for Pruritus and Deterrent to Skin Scratching

Appropriate use of antihistaminic agents is variable for the treatment of pruritus and as a deterrent to skin scratching. The second generation of antihistaminic agents, such as cetirizine, loratadine, and fexofenadine, are good to take during the day without their uncomfortable side effects (i.e., drowsiness, malaise, and hydrodipsia). However, they are not effective for the control of strong itching. In such cases, the first generation of antihistaminic agents, such as diphenhydramine, chlorpheniramine, and hydroxyzine, are effective. The strongest drug for the treatment of pruritus and as a deterrent to skin scratching is hydroxyzine. Despite the side effect of drowsiness, the efficacy of controlling pruritus in patients with AD and restraining their skin scratching is indispensable for treatment. Administration of 30 to 50 mg of diphenhydramine hydrochloride (Benadryl, Belix, or Banophen in the United States; Restamine in Japan), three times a day, or 25 to 50 mg of hydroxyzine pamoate (Atarax-P) before sleep for more than moderate AD patients is good to restrain involuntary scratching of the skin. Control of pruritus and a deterrent to skin scratching especially during sleep is so important for patients with AD because unconscious skin scratching could provoke the exacerbation factor of AD. As mentioned earlier, the first generation of antihistaminic agents have a strong effect with strong side effects; the second generation of antihistaminic agents have a mild effect with mild side effects. Olopatadine hydrochloride (Patanol in the United States; Allelock in Japan) fall in the middle rank of antihistaminic agents. Also, topical diphenhydramine ointment (Dermarest in the United States; Restamine in Japan) is very effective for the control of pruritus without major side effects. This ointment is usually used with topical corticosteroids for the treatment of AD. Of course, both drugs can be used together. Some physicians use topical diphenhydramine ointment and topical corticosteroids in the daytime, and they prescribe a 25- to 50-mg capsule of hydroxyzine before sleep for the control of pruritus. Deterrence of skin scratching is critical for the treatment of AD. These different drugs must be prescribed with the understanding that the character of each of them conforms to each skin condition of patients with AD. Generally speaking, so-called antiallergic agents without antihistaminic effect are thought to be *ineffective* for either the control of pruritus or the deterrence of skin scratching.

Avoidance of Allergens

Food allergens play a role in a subset of patients with AD, with milk, egg, peanut, soy, wheat, and fish accounting for approximately 90% of the foods found to exacerbate the condition. Removal of proven food allergens from the patient's diet can lead to significant clinical improvement. Patients should avoid implicated foods completely because even small amounts of the food allergen can contribute to food-specific IgE synthesis. Following the natural history of food-related AD is important because most patients become tolerant to food allergens, even in the face of positive skin test results. Although food challenges have generally been performed to help define clinical allergy, more recently, specific IgE levels to several food allergens by the Pharmacia Immuno-CAP system (Pharmacia, Uppsala, Sweden) have predictive value in terms of clinical relevance. Serial measurements with this assay have proved to be of value in following the natural history of patients' food allergies to help determine when a food could be reintroduced or food challenge performed. The possibility of preventing AD through dietary manipulation has been considered. Restricting the mother's diet starting in the third trimester of pregnancy and during lactation and the child's diet during the first 2 years of life resulted in decreased prevalence of AD in the prophylaxis group compared with a control group at 12 months of age but not at 24 months. Follow-up at 7 years of age showed no difference between the prophylaxis and control groups for AD or respiratory allergy. Breastfeeding did not affect the lifetime prevalence of AD in a large ethnically and socially diverse group of children. In contrast, infants who were breastfeeding exclusively for more than 6 months had a significantly lower prevalence of eczema at 1 year and 3 years compared with infants who were breastfed for less than 1 month or were intermittently breastfeeding. The benefits of breast-feeding infants with AD have been described, although sensitization to allergens in the mother's diet transferred through breast milk is a potential problem for at-risk infants. The degree of sensitization to aeroallergens also is associated with the severity of AD. In addition, patients with dust mite sensitivity likely need to avoid other triggers that could contribute to chronic skin inflammation. The use of polyurethane-coated cotton encasings compared with cotton encasings resulted in clinical benefit even in patients not sensitized to house dust mites, suggesting that impermeable covers could reduce exposure to other allergens as well as irritants or possibly even superantigens. With respect to early dust mite allergen exposure, the authors of a placebo-controlled trial of mite-impermeable covers reported an inverse correlation between dust mite allergen exposure at 3 months of age and development of AD during the first year of life, even after adjusting for potential confounders.

Avoidance of Exacerbation Factors

Patients with severe/persistent AD have been affected by the several exacerbation factors. We have to identify those in each patient with AD; thereafter we must try to remove/avoid each exacerbation factor in each patient to improve clinical condition. Major exacerbation factors are as follows, which are mentioned in order of frequency by our investigation: shampoo or soap, hair treatment, inappropriate topical medicine, subclinical infection (e.g.; chronic tonsillitis, pyorrhea, paranasal sinusitis, urinary tract infection), cosmetics, house dust, ticks, folk remedies, pollens, bathing habits, psychosocial factors, occupation, 4-hydroxybenzoate (paraben), and other preservatives.

Probiotics

Perinatal administration of the probiotic *Lactobacillus rhamnosus* strain GG reduces the incidence of AD in at-risk children beyond infancy. Different studies, which included not only infants but also children up to 13 years of age, showed that treatment with lactobacillus was beneficial in patients with AD and allergies.

Topical Corticosteroids

Since their introduction approximately 50 years ago, topical corticosteroids have been the mainstay of treatment for AD, showing efficacy in both acute and chronic disease. By acting on multiple resident and infiltrating cells, primarily through suppression of inflammatory genes, they are effective in reducing inflammation and pruritus. In addition, topical corticosteroids might have an effect on bacterial colonization in AD, reducing the density of *S. aureus*. Topical corticosteroids are available in extremely high (class 1) to low (class 7) potencies (Table 12–6). Choice of which topical corticosteroid preparation to prescribe depends in large part on the severity and distribution of eczematous lesions. Patients need to be informed about the potency and potential side effects of their prescribed topical corticosteroid. In general, using the least potent corticosteroid that is effective should be the rule. This approach needs to be balanced by the possibility that initiation of therapy with a topical corticosteroid that is too weak might result in persistence or worsening of AD, which in turn can lead to decreased adherence to the treatment regimen. In addition, patients might be prescribed a high-potency corticosteroid with instructions to discontinue it within 7 to 14 days without a plan to step down, resulting in rebound flaring of their AD, similar to what is frequently seen after oral corticosteroids. Therapy-resistant lesions have been treated with potent topical corticosteroids under occlusion, although this approach needs to be used cautiously, primarily for hand or foot eczema, to avoid systemic side effects. Prescribing topical corticosteroids in inadequate amounts can contribute to suboptimally controlled AD, especially in patients with widespread disease, because it takes approximately 30 g of medication to cover the entire body of an average adult. In children, the fingertip unit (FTU), defined as the amount of topical medication extending from the tip to the first joint on the palmar aspect of the index finger, is a measure for applying topical corticosteroids. Approximately 1 FTU is needed to cover the hand or groin, 2 FTUs for the face or foot, 3 FTUs for an arm, 6 FTUs for the leg, and 14 FTUs for the trunk. Topical corticosteroids have typically been applied twice daily, and using them more frequently might increase side effects without significant clinical benefits. Fluticasone propionate cream is safe and effective in children and infants with AD as young as 3 months of age even when applied on the face and over a significant percentage of body surface for up to 1 month. In addition, once-daily treatment is effective for topical fluticasone propionate and mometasone furoate, which might improve adherence with the treatment regimen. In a different approach, a short course of a potent topical steroid applied for 3 days was found to be equal in clinical efficacy to chronic use of a low-potency corticosteroid. Given the concern over side effects associated with chronic use, topical corticosteroids have not been considered appropriate for maintenance therapy, especially on normal-appearing skin in AD. However, several studies with fluticasone propionate in patients as young as 3 months of age have shown that once control is achieved with a once-daily regimen, long-term control can be maintained with twice-weekly therapy. Of note, during the maintenance phase of the study, the corticosteroid preparation was applied to areas that appeared to have healed, which resulted in delayed relapses compared with placebo therapy. Patients with AD might not respond appropriately to topical corticosteroid therapy. Reasons for this might include ongoing exposure to irritants or allergens, *S. aureus* superinfection, inadequate potency of the steroid preparation, or insufficient amount dispensed. Other causes for apparent treatment failure include steroid allergy and possibly corticosteroid insensitivity. However, a much more practical reason for

Table 12–6. Potency chart of topical corticosteroids.

Brand Name	Generic Name
CLASS 1: Superpotent	
Clobex Lotion, 0.05%	Clobetasol propionate
Cormax Cream/ Solution, 0.05%	Clobetasol propionate
Diprolene Gel/ Ointment, 0.05%	Betamethasone dipropionate
Olux Foam, 0.05%	Clobetasol propionate
Psorcon Ointment, 0.05%	Diflorasone diacetate
Temovate Cream/ Ointment/Solution, 0.05%	Clobetasol propionate
Ultravate Cream/ Ointment, 0.05%	Halobetasol propionate
CLASS 2: Potent	
Cyclocort Ointment, 0.1%	Amcinonide
Diprolene Cream AF, 0.05%	Betamethasone dipropionate
Diprosone Ointment, 0.05%	Betamethasone dipropionate
Elocon Ointment, 0.1%	Mometasone furoate
Florone Ointment, 0.05%	Diflorasone diacetate
Halog Ointment/ Cream, 0.1%	Halcinonide
Lidex Cream/Gel/ Ointment, 0.05%	Fluocinonide
Maxiflor Ointment, 0.05%	Diflorasone diacetate
Maxivate Ointment, 0.05%	Betamethasone dipropionate
Psorcon Cream 0.05%	Diflorasone diacetate
Topicort Cream/ Ointment, 0.25%	Desoximetasone
Topicort Gel, 0.05%	Desoximetasone
CLASS 3: Upper Mid-Strength	
Aristocort A Ointment, 0.1%	Triamcinolone acetonide
Cutivate Ointment, 0.005%	Fluticasone propionate
Cyclocort Cream/ Lotion, 0.1%	Amcinonide
Diprosone Cream, 0.05%	Betamethasone dipropionate
Florone Cream, 0.05%	Diflorasone diacetate
Lidex-E Cream, 0.05%	Fluocinonide
Luxiq Foam, 0.12%	Betamethasone valerate
Maxiflor Cream, 0.05%	Diflorasone diacetate
Maxivate Cream/ Lotion, 0.05%	Betamethasone dipropionate

Brand Name	Generic Name
CLASS 3: Upper Mid-Strength (Continued)	
Topicort Cream, 0.05%	Desoximetasone
Valisone Ointment, 0.1%	Betamethasone valerate
CLASS 4: Mid-Strength	
Aristocort Cream, 0.1%	Triamcinolone acetonide
Cordran Ointment, 0.05%	Flurandrenolide
Derma-Smoothe/ FS Oil, 0.01%	Fluocinolone acetonide
Elocon Cream, 0.1%	Mometasone furoate
Kenalog Cream/ Ointment/Spray, 0.1%	Triamcinolone acetonide
Synalar Ointment, 0.025%	Fluocinolone acetonide
Uticort Gel, 0.025%	Betamethasone benzoate
Westcort Ointment, 0.2%	Hydrocortisone valerate
CLASS 5: Lower Mid-Strength	
Cordran Cream/Lotion/ Tape, 0.05%	Flurandrenolide
Cutivate Cream, 0.05%	Fluticasone propionate
Dermatop Cream, 0.1%	Prednicarbate
DesOwen Ointment, 0.05%	Desonide
Diprosone Lotion, 0.05%	Betamethasone dipropionate
Kenalog Lotion, 0.1%	Triamcinolone acetonide
Locoid Cream, 0.1%	Hydrocortisone butyrate
Pandel Cream 0.1%	Hydrocortisone probutate
Synalar Cream, 0.025%	Fluocinolone acetonide
Uticort Cream/ Lotion, 0.025%	Betamethasone benzoate
Valisone Cream/ Ointment, 0.1%	Betamethasone valerate
Westcort Cream, 0.2%	Hydrocortisone valerate
CLASS 6: Mild	
Aclovate Cream/ Ointment, 0.05%	Alclometasone dipropionate
DesOwen Cream, 0.05%	Desonide
Synalar Cream/ Solution, 0.01%	Fluocinolone acetonide
Tridesilon Cream, 0.05%	Desonide
Valisone Lotion, 0.1%	Betamethasone valerate
CLASS 7: Least Potent	
Topicals with hydrocortisone, dexamethasone, methylprednisolone, and prednisolone	

therapeutic failure with topical corticosteroids is nonadherence to the treatment regimen. A significant number of patients or caregivers admit to nonadherence with topical corticosteroids because of fear of adverse effects.

Topical Calcineurin Inhibitors

Topical corticosteroids have been the traditional mainstay of topical drug therapy for AD because of broad immunosuppressant and antiinflammatory effects. However, topical steroids are associated with adverse local effects, such as dermal atrophy, striae, telangiectasia, perioral dermatitis, acneiform eruptions, as well as a risk of systemic effects such as hypothalamic-pituitary-adrenal axis suppression. The development of nonsteroid topical immunosuppressants has been an historic development in therapy of AD. Topical calcineurin inhibitors are an important class of medications that have clinical efficacy in AD, as displayed in a broad set of clinical trials and in extensive clinical use. Topical calcineurin inhibitors were developed after the utility of systemic cyclosporin A, a potent inhibitor of T cells, was noted in the treatment of eczematous dermatitis and psoriasis. Cyclosporin A had been used for prevention of organ transplant rejection after solid organ transplants and as a systemic immunosuppressive for a broad set of conditions. Cyclosporin A is not useful as a topical medication, presumably because of its large molecular size, which impedes its ability to penetrate skin. Its use orally is associated with a risk of serious systemic effects, particularly renal toxicity. Tacrolimus (Protopic) is another potent immunosuppressant used to prevent graft rejection. Tacrolimus, however, is active topically and is effective for treatment of AD. It has been marketed by Asteras (Deerfield, IL) as Protopic ointment (0.03% and 0.1% for children 2 years of age and older and adults, respectively). Pimecrolimus (Elidel) is an ascomycin derivative with potent calcineurin inhibition developed specifically to treat inflammatory skin conditions, the result of a prospective screening of hundreds of compounds. Pimecrolimus is the active agent of Elidel cream 1% (Novartis Pharmaceutical, East Hanover, NJ), a formulation approved by the Food and Drug Administration (FDA) for use in patients 2 years of age or older with mild to moderate AD. Both tacrolimus and pimecrolimus work through inhibition of phosphorylase activity of the calcium-dependent serine/threonine phosphatase calcineurin and the dephosphorylation of the nuclear factor of activated T-cell protein (NF-ATp), a transcription factor necessary for the expression of inflammatory cytokines, including IL-2, IL-4, and IL-5. Also, they might inhibit the transcription and release of other T-cell–derived cytokines, including IL-3, IFN-γ, TNF-α, and GM-CSF, which can contribute to allergic inflammation. The majority of the studies of topical pimecrolimus and tacrolimus

discussed earlier assessed efficacy of these medications as primary monotherapy of AD, with topical or systemic steroids used as "rescue" for disease flares. Clearly, new steroid-free topical agents might offer improved long-term management options for patients with AD. Evolution of topical therapy will likely include combinations of topical antiinflammatory agents including calcineurin inhibitors and topical corticosteroids, although the optimal combination therapy has yet to be defined. With evolving therapeutic options, guidelines for care of AD, perhaps similar to those used for treatment of asthma, might prove useful and are being developed.

TACROLIMUS

Tacrolimus (FK 506) is a macrolide lactone isolated from *Streptomyces tsukubaensis.* Tacrolimus-binding receptors (the major ligand is FKBP12, also known as macrophilin) have been found on a number of cells. Tacrolimus inhibits the activation of a number of key cells involved in AD, including T cells, Langerhans cells, mast cells, and keratinocytes. Tacrolimus 0.03% and 0.1% ointments are safe and effective in the treatment of children (older than 2 years of age) and adults with AD. According to product labeling, less common adverse events (less than 5%) of varicella zoster infections (mostly chickenpox) and vesiculobullous rashes were more common in patients treated with tacrolimus ointment 0.03% compared with vehicle during clinical trials. An average of 2.2 g of tacrolimus was used per day. The outcome measure, a modified eczema and severity index score, showed 61% improvement from baseline after 3 months of treatment and 71% of baseline at 1 year. Pruritus decreased throughout the treatment course, and application site burning diminished within the first few days of tacrolimus use. In other long-term studies, *S. aureus* colonization decreased during long-term therapy with tacrolimus ointment, and cutaneous infection rates decreased with extended use beyond 1 year.

PIMECROLIMUS

Unlike FK 506 and cyclosporin A, the ascomycin derivative pimecrolimus was developed specifically to treat inflammatory skin conditions. Pimecrolimus binds to FKBP/macrophilin and interferes with calcineurin action, apparently with preferential drug distribution to the skin. Topical pimecrolimus appears to be effective topically for AD with little systemic absorption in children and adults with AD. In one study, the systemic availability of topical pimecrolimus was measured in 22 infants age 3 to 23 months, with pimecrolimus 1% cream applied twice daily for 3 weeks to all affected areas including the face and neck. There was a wide range in body surface area involvement, ranging from 10% to 92%. Pimecrolimus blood concentrations were consistently low, with approximately a third of the samples below the assay limit of quantitation (0.1 µg/mL), 71% were below 0.5 µg/mL, and fully 98% of the samples were below 2 µg/mL. Long-term pharmacokinetic studies with repeated application of pimecrolimus did not significantly accumulate in the blood and appeared to have minimal adverse systemic risks. The poor absorption of pimecrolimus and absence of experience with the drug systemically have made it difficult to interpret the low serum levels seen in topical use studies. However, the pharmacokinetics of systemic pimecrolimus given orally have been studied in patients with moderate to severe chronic plaque psoriasis as well as in healthy subjects. In the psoriasis study, patients received pimecrolimus (5 mg every day to 30 mg twice a day) for 4 weeks. Blood concentrations reached steady state after 5 to 10 days, and drug exposure demonstrated linear dose dependency. No serious adverse events or clinically significant changes in physical examination or laboratory safety tests were reported in this study. Multiple clinical studies have demonstrated the efficacy and safety of pimecrolimus 1% cream in AD. A low rate of burning and stinging was seen in pimecrolimus patients, lower, although not significantly, than with vehicle cream. Although not approved by the FDA for use in children younger than 2 years of age, multiple studies of pimecrolimus 1% cream have been performed in this age group, showing excellent tolerance and effectiveness. Long-term therapy with pimecrolimus 1% cream for 6 months and 1 year investigated whether the early treatment of the signs and symptoms of AD with pimecrolimus could influence long-term outcome by preventing disease progression. Patients received twice daily treatments of the study medication at the first signs of AD for up to 12 months. Emollients and moderately potent topical steroids were permitted for maintenance or if study medication was insufficient to treat flares. The primary efficacy was the incidence of flares, and topical corticosteroid intervention was necessary. Both an eczema area and severity index and pruritus scores were used to assess the efficacy of pimecrolimus in AD maintenance.

Historically, combination therapies with different classes of drugs have been used to maximize efficacy while managing the risk of adverse events. Combining a calcineurin inhibitor and corticosteroids should be no different in this regard. Using a topical calcineurin inhibitor as a first-line pharmacologic agent for the treatment of early signs and symptoms of AD, as opposed to treating only more severe exacerbations, necessitates an excellent safety and tolerability profile to ensure practicability and compliance. In this respect, neither skin atrophy nor hypothalamic-pituitary-adrenal axis suppression has been observed with topical calcineurin inhibitors, making them more suitable than topical steroids for frequent or prolonged use, especially on larger body surfaces or on areas especially prone to atrophy with steroid use. Building on the positive experience of combining pimecrolimus with steroids sequentially and concomitantly once daily, an appealing treatment strategy would be to use a topical calcineurin inhibitor twice daily and add a mid-potency steroid such as fluticasone propionate or mometasone once daily. Data from several studies suggest that using pimecrolimus as a first-line pharmacologic agent to treat early signs and symptoms of AD prevents the progression to more severe exacerbations in approximately 50% of the cases, reducing the need for topical steroids. If, despite such early intervention, the addition of a mid-potency steroid is warranted to treat breakthrough flaring of AD, it can be used in short pulses, maximizing the benefit-risk ratio and enhancing patient compliance.

Specialized Therapy

A broad array of therapies are used for AD. Although it is beyond the scope of this chapter to address all of them comprehensively, phototherapy and systemic immunomodulatory agents are briefly discussed here.

PHOTOTHERAPY

Broad-band UV-B, broad-band UV-A, narrow-band UVB (311 nm), UV-A-1 (340 to 400 nm), psoralen plus ultraviolet light of A wavelength (PUVA), and combined UV-A-B phototherapy are useful adjuncts in the treatment of AD. These therapies are well established, although relapse can occur after cessation of treatment. Most patients in a broad set of studies experienced improvement in symptoms as well as reduction in topical corticosteroid use. The photoimmunologic effects of UV-A phototherapy with and without psoralen are presumably mediated through Langerhans cells and eosinophils, whereas UV-B's immunosuppressive effects occur through blocking of antigen-presenting Langerhans cells and altered keratinocyte cytokine production. Photochemotherapy with PUVA might be indicated in patients with severe widespread AD. Studies comparing the different modes of phototherapy are limited. Short-term adverse effects with phototherapy might include erythema, burns, pruritus, and pigmentation. Long-term adverse effects include premature skin aging and cutaneous malignancies. Limited descriptive studies of extracorporeal phototherapy with UV-A and methoxypsoralen have been reported, and this method is not widely used.

SYSTEMIC IMMUNOMODULATORY AGENTS

A broad set of systemic immunomodulatory agents have been used for severe AD refractory to topical therapies. There is documented extensive clinical use and clinical experience with systemic corticosteroids and cyclosporin A. Systemic glucocorticoids such as oral prednisone are highly immunosuppressive but generally avoided in the treatment of chronic AD because of systemic toxicities. Rarely, short courses of oral glucocorticoids might be initiated for acute exacerbations of AD while other treatment measures are being introduced. If used, intensive topical therapy should be initiated during systemic treatment to prevent rebound flaring of AD. Cyclosporin A is a potent immunosuppressive that works by inhibiting calcineurin. Multiple studies have demonstrated that both children and adults with severe AD refractory to conventional treatment can benefit from short-term cyclosporine treatment. Various oral dosing regimens have been recommended; 5 mg/kg has generally been used with success in short-term and long-term (1 year) use, whereas some authorities have advocated body-weight independent daily dosing of adults with 150 mg (low dose) or 300 mg (high dose) daily of a cyclosporine microemulsion. Treatment with cyclosporine has been associated with reduced skin disease and improved quality of life. Discontinuation of treatment, however, generally results in rapid relapse of skin disease. Possible side effects include elevated serum creatinine level, renal impairment, or hypertension. Other systemic therapies include recombinant human IFN-γ, tacrolimus, and intravenous immunoglobulin. Antimetabolites have been used for AD including mycophenolate mofetil, a purine biosynthesis inhibitor used as an immunosuppressant in organ transplantation, methotrexate, and azathioprine. These systemic agents all have significant risks of systemic toxicities, requiring careful monitoring and restricted use. Other systemic medications such as leukotriene receptor antagonists have been suggested as useful, but they have limited peer-reviewed evidence to support routine use. Oral pimecrolimus has been used in clinical trials with some efficacy, although published data are limited. Usefulness of new biologic agents such as infliximab and etanercept in AD is unknown at present.

FUTURE PERSPECTIVE

Corticosteroids, calcineurin inhibitors, UV therapy, and the immunosuppressant macrolides are all therapeutic agents that are likely to be effective in controlling the complex inflammatory cascades of chronic AD. However, future studies are needed to focus on strategies preventing the initial development of AD. Given the central role of TH2 cytokines and chemokines in the development of allergic skin inflammation, strategies directed at reducing TH2 responses and blocking the action of chemokines by antagonists of CCR3 and CCR4 will be important. Further studies are also needed to examine the potential role of IFN-γ, IL-12, and IL-18 in restoring the shift toward a more balanced TH0 response with equal production of TH1 and TH2 cytokines. There is also a strong rationale for examining the effect of therapeutic agents capable of blocking the actions of IL-4 and IL-5. Anti-IL-5 antibody blocks eosinophil infiltration in sensitized animals whether administered before or after allergen challenge. It would be of interest to determine the clinical effects of blocking the action of IL-4 in patients with AD. Elimination of the IgE response may have less importance in patients with continuing TH2-mediated allergic inflammatory responses. Thus the combination of several approaches will be needed to effectively interrupt the complex inflammatory cascades associated with allergic diseases including AD.

EVIDENCE-BASED MEDICINE

Diagnosis

To confirm the diagnosis of AD in a patient with dermatitis, allergist-immunologists are specifically trained to diagnose it. Defining IgE-mediated sensitivity (by means of skin or in vitro testing) is useful in the differential diagnosis.

Joint Task Force on Practice Parameters. Disease management of atopic dermatitis: an updated practice parameter. American Academy of Allergy, Asthma and Immunology, American College of Allergy, Asthma and Immunology. *Ann Allergy Asthma Immunol.* 2004;93(suppl):S1. Evidence grade: IV

Management (Indirect Outcome)

For patients whose AD responds poorly to treatment, allergist-immunologists are specifically trained and experienced in managing atopic dermatitis in both children and adults.

Hoare C, Li Wan Po A, Williams H. Systematic review of treatments for atopic eczema. *Health Technol Assess.* 2000;4:1. Evidence grade: Ia

BIBLIOGRAPHY

Allen R, Chambers S, Kownacki S. *Pimecrolimus.* Oxfordshire, UK: CSF Medical Communications; 2004.

Beltrani VS. The clinical manifestations of atopic dermatitis. In: Leung DYM, ed. *Atopic Dermatitis: from Pathogenesis to Treatment.* Au, 2002.

Hanifin JM, Rajka G. Diagnostic features of atopic dermatitis. *Acta Dermato Venereol Suppl (Stockh).* 1980;92(suppl):44.

Hill LW, Sulzberger MB. *Yearbook of Dermatology and Syphilology.* Chicago: Year Book Medical Publishers; 1933.

Available at: http://www.aad.org/professionals/guidelines/

Available at: http://www.aaaai.org/professionals/resources/rgce/

Kay J, Gawkrodger DJ, Mortimer MJ, et al. The prevalence of childhood atopic eczema in a general population. *J Am Acad Dermatol.* 1994;30:35.

Kieffer M, Bergbrant I-M, Faergemann J. Immune reactions to *Pityrosporum ovale* in adult patients with atopic and seborrheic dermatitis. *J Am Acad Dermatol.* 1990;22:739.

Kolmer HL, Taketomi EA, Hazen KC, et al. Effect of combined antibacterial and antifungal treatment in severe atopic dermatitis. *J Allergy Clin Immunol.* 1996;98:702.

Leung DYM, Eichenfield LF, Boguniewicz M. Atopic dermatitis (atopic eczema). In: Freedberg IM, Eisen AZ, Wolff K, eds. *Fitzpatrick's Dermatology in General Medicine*. 6th ed. New York: McGraw-Hill; 2003:1180.

Leung DYM, Harbeck R, Bina P. Presence of IgE antibodies to staphylococcal exotoxins on the skin of patients with atopic dermatitis: evidence for a new group of allergens. *J Clin Invest*. 1993;92:1374.

Leung DYM. Pathogenesis of atopic dermatitis. *J Allergy Clin Immunol*. 1999; 104(suppl):S99.

Reynolds NJ, Franklin V, Gray JC, et al. Narrow-band ultraviolet B and broad-band ultraviolet A phototherapy in adult atopic eczema: a randomized controlled trial. *Lancet*. 2001;357:2012.

Rosenfeldt V, Benfeldt E, Nielsen SD, et al. Effect of probiotic Lactobacillus strains in children with atopic dermatitis. *J Allergy Clin Immunol*. 2003;111:389.

Ruzicka T, Reitamo S, eds. *Tacrolimus Ointment*. Berlin: Springer; 2004.

Allergic Contact Dermatitis

Bettina Wedi, MD, PhD

DEFINITION, CLASSIFICATION, EPIDEMIOLOGY

Allergic contact dermatitis (ACD), a subtype of contact dermatitis, is a common inflammatory skin condition caused by direct contact with an allergy-causing substance. Over 3000 contact allergens have been identified. ACD affects approximately 1% of the general population, equally as likely in infancy as in adulthood (apparently increasing in children). In affected individuals, ACD has a serious impact on their quality of life. Moreover, in severe, persistent conditions, the disease is sometimes job threatening or life threatening. Occupational contact dermatitis is the second cause of recognized occupational diseases with considerable economic impact. Occupational ACD is most common in hairdressers, printers, machine tool operators, chemical, gas, and petroleum plant operatives, car assemblers, and machine tool setters.

Airborne contact dermatitis is caused by dust, pollen, or volatile substances and is located on air-exposed areas, for example, to the preservative methylchloroisothiazolinone/methylisothiazolinone (MCI/MI) in paintings (Fig. 13–1). Passive exposure via social contacts, termed "consort" or "connubial" dermatitis should also be considered (e.g., ACD of the face in a mother due to benzoyl peroxide acne treatment of her son). Several episodes of contact urticaria (e.g., to meat, vegetables, or spices) may result in protein contact dermatitis (Fig. 13–2). Systemic ACD after systemic intake of the allergen (e.g., orally ingested nickel, balsam of Peru, or spices) is a rare subtype of ACD, although at least systemic ACD to nickel may be underdiagnosed because nickel represents the most common occupational as well as public contact allergen. Baboon syndrome (formerly called mercury exanthema) is a special type of systemic ACD, symmetrically involving the intertriginous areas (buttocks, axillae) and is most common after drug intake. ACD to food is uncommon but more frequent in food handlers. It frequently involves the hands or fingertips (e.g., by diallyl disulphide in garlic) but can also be present around the mouth or on the face (e.g., by urushiol, the allergenic oleoresin of *Toxicodendron* plants, present in mango and cashew nuts). In photoallergic contact dermatitis, additional exposure to ultraviolet light is needed.

ACD can occur at any time, after many years of contact with a substance or after a few exposures. Irritant contact dermatitis (ICD) (common irritants: water, cleaning agents, acids, alkalis, oils, organic solvents) facilitates the development of sensitization and thus often precedes ACD (e.g., cleaners who perform wet work and develop ICD, prompting them to start wearing rubber gloves. They then become allergic to the rubber accelerators in the gloves).

Recognizing Those at Risk

- Atopic dermatitis: The pattern and the frequencies of observed sensitizations do not differ greatly between atopic dermatitis patients and nonatopic individuals (exception: bufexamac). No association exists between atopic dermatitis and reactions to nickel.
- Stasis dermatitis: There is higher risk for developing ACD to materials and agents applied to the areas of stasis dermatitis and leg ulcers (e.g., neomycin).
- Otitis externa: There is higher risk for ACD to topical neomycin and topical corticosteroids.

PATHOGENESIS

Immunology

ACD is caused by specific T lymphocyte–mediated sensitization to low molecular weight substances (haptens). Protein haptenation is one of the key molecular events in skin sensitization. It is a rule without exception that ACD will only develop if molecules are able to penetrate the skin and behave as haptens, that is, bind to cell surfaces in the epidermis or dermis, modify self-skin protein(s), and thus induce immunization. For protein haptenation to occur, a chemical must be electrophilic;

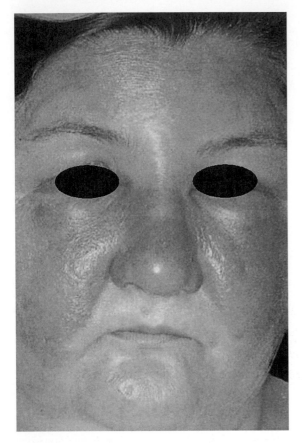

Figure 13–1. Airborne contact dermatitis to the preservatives methylchloroisothiazolinone/methylisothiazolinone (MCI/MI) in paintings.

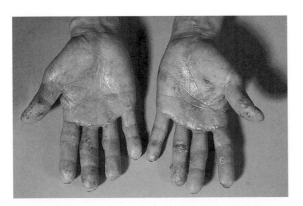

Figure 13–2. Protein contact dermatitis in a baker to wheat flour.

for example, it must have a polarized bond such as halogenated compounds or be a cation such as Ni2+. Importantly, a chemical can also be converted to a protein-reactive species by air oxidation or cutaneous metabolism.

The hapten-carrier complex is processed by Langerhans cells that after migrating to draining lymph nodes present the complex to CD4+ cells. Activated CD4+ cells then secrete cytokines, which induce expression of adhesion molecules and MHC on keratinocytes and endothelial cells, as well as activation of keratinocytes to secrete proinflammatory cytokines. Other T cells and proinflammatory cells then undergo chemotaxis to the site of cytokine secretion.

The initial sensitization typically takes 10 to 14 days from initial exposure to a strong contact allergen such as poison ivy. Once an individual is sensitized to a chemical, ACD develops within hours to several days of exposure. CD4$^+$ CCR10$^+$ memory T cells persist in the dermis after ACD clinically resolves.

It is widely accepted that sensitization is specific. However, very recent data demonstrated that with an increasing strength of a positive reaction to nickel or to fragrance mix, the likelihood of further positive reactions to unrelated contact allergens increased significantly. This recent finding can raise new questions with regard to the concept that sensitization is in any case and throughout an exclusively allergen-specific process.

Histology

Histologically contact dermatitis is characterized by spongiosis (intraepidermal edema) and a mononuclear infiltrate. Thickening of the epidermis (acanthosis) with hyperkeratosis and parakeratosis may be seen in the epidermis and stratum corneum. Some dermatohistopathologists believe they can differentiate allergic from irritant contact dermatitis because ICD may show epidermal necrosis and less intercellular edema, whereas ACD may be associated with the presence of eosinophils.

CLINICAL SYMPTOMS

Acute ACD is characterized clinically by intense pruritus, erythema, vesiculation, and weeping and crusty deposits, whereas in chronic ACD thickened skin and lichenification predominate in addition to erythema and pruritus. Quality of life is impaired similar to patients with psoriasis or hair loss.

Clinical symptoms vary at different areas of the body due to different thicknesses of the skin. For example, erythema and edema predominate in thin skin (eyelids, penis, scrotum), whereas scalp, palms, and soles may exhibit few clinical signs of ACD. Location of the skin or mucosal lesions often points to the offending allergen(s) (Fig. 13–3), for example, nickel in a trouser

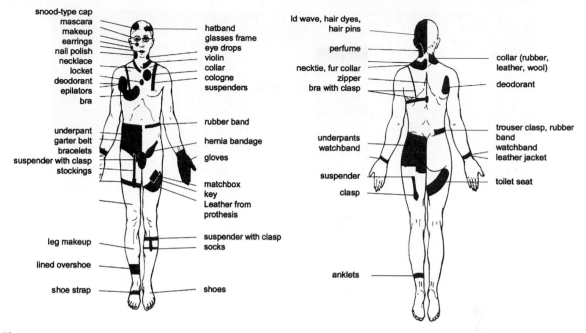

Figure 13–3. Clues to distribution.

button, chromate in leather shoes, metals in dental prosthesis (Fig. 13–4), or chemicals in ophthalmologic preparations causing dermatitis around the eyes. However, sometimes detective work is needed to uncover the allergen(s) (Fig. 13–5).

DIAGNOSIS

Telling ACD apart from ICD can be very difficult because both cannot be easily differentiated by clinical, histologic, or electron microscopic examination. Differences in clinical distribution and morphology are useful guides but dangerous to rely on uncritically (undress the patient completely!). A detailed history is crucial in evaluating individuals with ACD to identify potential causes of ACD. Patients with ACD require a much more detailed history compared to those with most other dermatologic disorders. If occupational ACD is suspected, it should be considered that the material safety data sheets often provide incomplete data and it is frequently necessary to contact the manufacturer.

The demonstration of a type IV immune reaction remains the specific point of difference, which is done by appropriate patch testing that requires three office visits and must be done by a clinician with detailed experience in the procedures and interpretation of results.

In protein contact dermatitis, patch testing and prick testing should be combined to test for type I and type IV immune reaction.

Some substances need additional exposure to sunlight to cause ACD. Thus, if photoallergic contact dermatitis is suspected, additional photopatch testing (irradiation with 10 J/cm^2 ultraviolet A [UVA]) should be performed.

In systemic ACD (usually associated with a strong positive patch test), challenges are recommended (e.g., oral provocation with nickel) (Fig. 13–6).

Patch Test Procedure

Potential causes of ACD and the materials to which individuals are exposed should be patch tested (sensitivity and specificity between 70% and 80%). Approximately 25 chemicals appear to be responsible for as many as half of all cases of ACD. Based on the principles of evidence-based medicine, patch testing is cost effective only if patients are selected on the basis of a clear-cut clinical suspicion of contact allergy and only if patients are tested with chemicals relevant to the problem. Frequent allergens in children and adolescents include nickel (and cobalt), fragrance mix, rubber chemicals, PPD (paraphenylenediamine), and thiomersal (due to presence in vaccines and usually irrelevant). Tables 13–1A and 13–1B present the important contact and occupational contact allergens.

The Finn chamber was designed in the 1970s; this is the standard method for patch testing individuals to chemicals (Fig. 13–7) not found in the thin-layer rapid

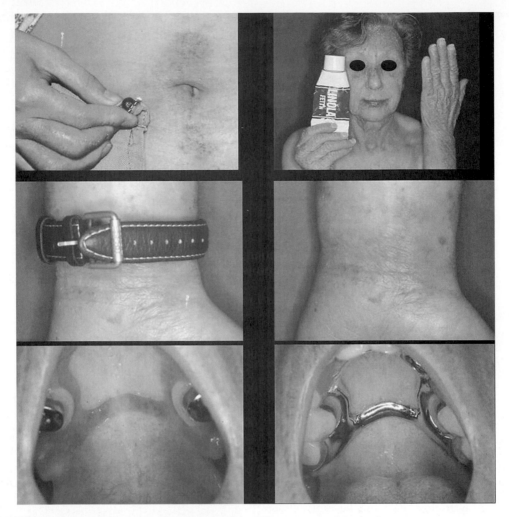

Figure 13–4. Examples of allergic contact dermatitis in different areas of the body.

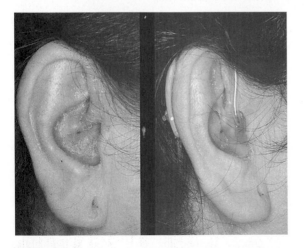

Figure 13–5. Allergic contact dermatitis to acrylics in hearing aid.

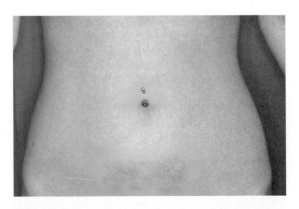

Figure 13–6. Positive double-blind oral provocation test with nickel.

Table 13–1A. Important contact allergens and sources.

- Nickel sulphate (jewelry, zippers, paper clips, coins, keys, metal industry, food)
- Cobalt chloride (inks, varnishes, enamels, fertilizers, feed additives, humidity indicators)
- Chromate (tanned leather, cement)
- Rubber accelerators or antioxidants (gloves, shoes, waistband)
- Cosmetic ingredients, preservatives, fragrances (makeup, perfume, soaps, shampoos, nail products, sunscreens, moisturizers, cleansers, hair dyes)
- Colophony (coniferous tree resin; strings wax, adhesives, mascara)
- Plants, wood (families: Toxidendron, Primulaceae, chrysanthemum, Liliaceae)
- Topical medications (iatrogenic topical treatment: creams, adhesive patches, eye drops, suppositories)

Table 13–1B. Important occupational contact allergens.

- Rubber chemicals in protective gloves
- Epoxy resins in surface coatings or glues
- Hairdressing chemicals
- Chromate, nickel
- Fragrances
- Coconut diethanolamine
- Colophony/rosin (adhesives)
- Acrylates (denture making)
- Preservatives (metalworking fluids, glues)

use epicutaneous (TRUE) test, which became available in the United States in the 1990s. Patch testing must be performed by health care providers trained in the proper technique. Patch test screening series, which pick up approximately 80% of allergens, vary from country to country.

The proper concentration of each chemical should be used. This usually means undiluted substances for leave-on products and dilutions for wash-off products. Hairy areas should be shaved and the areas cleaned with plain water. Occlusion of the patch tests is usually for 48 hours and the reading after removing (according to the labeling), but again at least after 72 hours. Additional reading after 96 hours and sometimes also later (e.g., for corticosteroids, neomycin) may be recommended. A positive patch test shows up as a

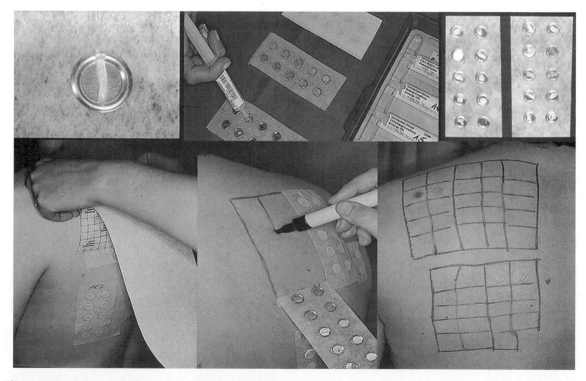

Figure 13–7. Patch test procedure using Finn chambers.

Table 13–2. Interpretation of patch test results according to International Contact Dermatitis Research Group criteria.

–	Negative reaction
(+) or ?	Doubtful reaction (faint homogeneous erythema, no infiltration)
+	Weak positive reaction (erythema, mild infiltration, papules)
++	Strong positive reaction (erythema, infiltration, papules, vesicles)
+++	Extreme positive reaction (coalescing vesicles, bullous reaction)
IR	Irritant reaction (discrete patchy erythema without infiltration)
NT	Not tested

Note: Photopatch tests are graded similarly by just adding the prefix Ph.

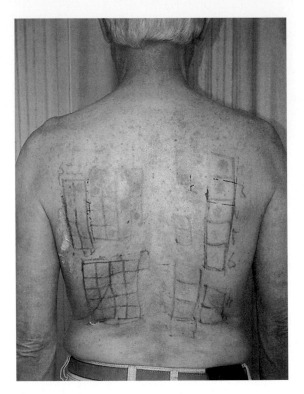

Figure 13–8. Angry back syndrome.

miniature eczema during the following few days. Interpretation should be performed according to standardized International Contact Dermatitis Research Group (ICDRG) criteria (Table 13–2). A "crescendo" or "plateau" reaction is more likely associated with an allergic reaction, whereas a "decrescendo" reaction points to an irritant reaction. The relevance of each reaction should be assessed and recorded as present, past, or unexplained.

The routine patch test was supplemented with a SLS (sodium lauryl sulphate) patch test to identify increased irritability. This allows interpretation of doubtful (erythematous) or even positive (erythematous and infiltrated) patch test reactions to certain allergens, which are at the same time marginal irritants when patch tested. Irritability might also imply increased susceptibility to contact allergy. Another possibility to clarify doubtful cases is a repeated open application test (ROAT).

Repeat Open Application Test

ROAT is most useful when a 1+ reaction to a chemical is found (e.g., in a leave-on product) to determine whether the reaction is significant. The chemical is applied twice a day for a week to the antecubital space of the upper arm, for example. If the individual develops dermatitis following a few days of repeated application of the suspected product, the weak patch test reaction is relevant.

Angry Back or Excited Skin Syndrome

If a large number of positive patch test reactions to unrelated allergens (more than five) occur (Fig. 13–8), retesting the patient sequentially to a small series of these allergens may be necessary to exclude nonspecific false-positive reactions. Angry back is most likely in individuals who have active dermatitis or who have a strong positive patch test reaction, both of which may induce local skin hyperreactivity.

Pitfalls

False-positive reactions occur if irritant allergen concentrations are used or in angry back syndrome. Table 13–3 presents the causes for false-negative reactions. In ACD of the eyelid, tapping of the skin may be needed to get positive patch test reactions. Table 13–4 lists the adverse reactions of patch testing. Contact with allergens via the patch test rarely induces contact allergy, the risk depending on the type and dose of the allergen. Active sensitization is defined as a negative patch test followed by a flare-up of this initial negative test reaction after 10 to 20 days, and then a positive patch test reaction when retested already observed after 2 or 3 days.

The patch test is not capable of predicting the development of ACD and is not recommended in the diagnosis of unspecific symptoms that do not involve the skin. Unnecessary repetition of patch testing should be clearly avoided.

Table 13–3. Causes for false-negative patch test reactions.

- Low allergen concentration
- Topical or systemic concomitant therapy: glucocorticoids, calcineurin inhibitors, immunosuppressives
- Recent ultraviolet radiation
- Immunocompromised patients
- Inappropriate allergen choice
- Testing with cosmetic products
- Variability of individual threshold reactivity
- Improper testing techniques: inappropriate vehicle, poor contact of the allergen to the skin, failure to perform delayed readings (important in elderly patients and in testing of neomycin, corticosteroids, paraphenylenediamine, cobalt)
- Missing cofactors: sweating, disrupted skin, ultraviolet A

In contrast to Europe, in the United States sensitization to urushiol in poison ivy is very common (50% to 80%). An individual who never has been sensitized to poison ivy may develop only a mild dermatitis 2 weeks following the initial exposure but typically develops severe dermatitis within 1 to 2 days of the second and subsequent exposures. The hallmark of the diagnosis of poison ivy is linear skin lesions. Patch testing is not recommended because of the strong sensitization potential. The presence of small amounts of urushiol in mango and cashew nuts should be considered.

MANAGEMENT

Accurate diagnosis of the type of ACD and the eliciting factors are the key to proper management. Strict avoidance of the offending allergen(s) is the treatment of choice. However, detection and avoidance of the allergen is often easier said than done.

Evidence-based medicine data for treatment showed good- and fair-quality evidence for potent or moderately

Table 13–4. Adverse reactions of patch tests.

- Irritation on the back from the presence of the patches
- Hyper- or hypopigmentation
- Excessive reaction
- Persistence of reaction (e.g., to gold chloride)
- Exacerbation of ACD in some cases (pointing to relevance?)
- Risk of sensitization (potent sensitizers: e.g., paraphenylenediamine, plant oleoresins)
- Delayed reactions (after 2–3 wk) point to the development of sensitization

potent topical steroids. Other treatments are not evidence based but commonly used, such as symptomatic treatment with cool compresses with saline. Tanning agents are helpful for acute vesicular dermatitis and emollients, in chronic lichenified dermatitis. Sedating oral antihistamines may help diminish pruritus. Patients should avoid using topical antihistamines, including topical doxepin, because of the apparently high risk of iatrogenic ACD to these agents.

Acute severe ACD (e.g., to poison ivy), often needs to be treated with a 2-week course of systemic corticosteroids. Most adults require an initial dose of 40 to 60 mg. The oral corticosteroid is tapered over a 2-week period, but a complicated tapering regimen probably is not necessary given the short duration of systemic corticosteroids.

Topical calcineurin inhibitors/immunomodulators are approved for atopic dermatitis and may be prescribed for cases of ACD when they offer safety advantages over topical corticosteroids (e.g., avoidance of cutaneous atrophy). Pimecrolimus is a topical treatment often helpful for ACD of the face. Tacrolimus appears to be the most helpful topical immunomodulator for ACD of the hands.

Chronic ACD that is not controlled well by topical corticosteroids may benefit from psoralen plus UVA (PUVA) treatments.

Recent evidence-based medicine data regarding prevention of ACD demonstrated fair-quality evidence for the topical skin protectant and quaternium-18-bentonite to prevent rhus dermatitis and for diethylenetriamine pentaacetic acid to prevent nickel, chrome, and copper dermatitis.

In occupational ACD, barrier creams use should not be overpromoted because they may confer a false sense of security. After-work emollients should be encouraged and made readily available in the workplace.

In proven systemic ACD to food ingredients (e.g., to nickel or balsam of Peru), restricted diets are recommended.

Patch test results, their relevance, and potential cross-reactive allergens should be explained in detail to the patient. An allergy pass and information sheets (e.g., lists of alternatives) should be given (see www.contactderm. org: contact allergen replacement database). Susceptible individuals prone to ICD need career advice.

EVIDENCE-BASED MEDICINE

Bourke J, Coulson I, English J. Guidelines for care of contact dermatitis. *Br J Dermatol.* 2001;145:877.

Guidelines for the management of contact dermatitis on behalf of the British Association of Dermatologists presenting evidence-based guidance for treatment, with identification of the strength of evidence available at the time of preparation of the guidelines, including details of relevant epidemiologic aspects, diagnosis, and investigation.

Uter W, Johansen JD, Orton DI, et al. Clinical update on contact allergy. *Curr Opin Allergy Clin Immunol.* 2005;5:429.

Concise review summarizing recent clinical research findings in contact allergy and addressing new allergens.

Saary J, Qureshi R, Palda V, et al. A systematic review of contact dermatitis treatment and prevention. *J Am Acad Dermatol.* 2005;53:845.

Very recent evidence-based review of contact dermatitis treatment and prevention.

Brancaccio RR, Alvarez MS. Contact allergy to food. *Dermatol Ther.* 2004;17:302.

Comprehensive review of contact allergies to food spices and food additives.

BIBLIOGRAPHY

Andersen KE. Occupational issues of allergic contact dermatitis. *Int Arch Occup Environ Health.* 2003;76:347.

Bourke J, Coulson I, English J. Guidelines for care of contact dermatitis. *Br J Dermatol.* 2001;145:877.

Brancaccio RR, Alvarez MS. Contact allergy to food. *Dermatol Ther.* 2004;17:302.

Brasch J, Schnuch A, Uter W. Strong allergic patch test reactions may indicate a general disposition for contact allergy. *Allergy.* 2006;61:364.

Cohen DE, Heidary N. Treatment of irritant and allergic contact dermatitis. *Dermatol Ther.* 2004;17:334.

Divkovic M, Pease CK, Gerberick GF, et al. Hapten-protein binding: from theory to practical application in the in vitro prediction of skin sensitization. *Contact Dermatitis.* 2005; 53:189.

Hausermann P, Harr T, Bircher AJ. Baboon syndrome resulting from systemic drugs: is there strife between SDRIFE and allergic contact dermatitis syndrome? *Contact Dermatitis.* 2004;51:297.

Heine G, Schnuch A, Uter W, et al. Type-IV sensitization profile of individuals with atopic eczema: results from the Information Network of Departments of Dermatology (IVDK) and the German Contact Dermatitis Research Group (DKG). *Allergy.* 2006;61:611.

Kutting B, Brehler R, Traupe H. Allergic contact dermatitis in children: strategies of prevention and risk management. *Eur J Dermatol.* 2004;14:80.

Li LY, Cruz PD Jr. Allergic contact dermatitis: pathophysiology applied to future therapy. *Dermatol Ther.* 2004;17:219.

Nakada T, Hostynek JJ, Maibach HI. Use tests: ROAT (repeated open application test)/PUT (provocative use test): an overview. *Contact Dermatitis.* 2000;43:1.

Saary J, Qureshi R, Palda V, et al. A systematic review of contact dermatitis treatment and prevention. *J Am Acad Dermatol.* 2005;53:845.

Saint-Mezard P, Rosieres A, Krasteva M, et al. Allergic contact dermatitis. *Eur J Dermatol.* 2004;14:284.

Uter W, Johansen JD, Orton DI, et al. Clinical update on contact allergy. *Curr Opin Allergy Clin Immunol.* 2005;5:429.

Uter W, Schnuch A, Geier J, et al. Epidemiology of contact dermatitis. The information network of departments of dermatology (IVDK) in Germany. *Eur J Dermatol.* 1998;8:36.

Pediatric Asthma

Sixto F. Guiang, MD

The pediatric patient is not a miniature adult, so goes the old teaching. The pediatric patient is a constantly changing patient. There are ever-changing landmarks of growth and development, all of which may be of minor significance in the adult patient but significant in a growing patient. There is also the matter of medical intervention causing alterations in growth and development, altered in the course of treatment as a result of the effect of drugs used to control the patient's asthma or the effect of the disease itself. Then there is the involvement of a third-party caretaker whose cooperation, training, and ability to understand the clinician's instructions may be pivotal in the success or failure of any therapeutic regimen no matter how well intentioned.

There are certain areas of uniqueness in pediatric asthma that makes it worthwhile to allocate a few pages in a discussion of pediatric asthma. First, the highest incidence of the disease occurs in children, and the recently described rise in incidence has occurred in children. Second, a delay in the diagnosis and thus a delay in the initiation of treatment can have far-reaching consequences. Third, permanent changes of remodeling can occur even at an early age. There are also some unique albeit subtle characteristics in pediatric asthma hyperresponsiveness, defined by the drug concentration needed to decrease airway function significantly, a hallmark of asthma in all age groups, which seems heightened in infants and children, although this decreases with further maturation. In fact, a heightened degree of hyperresponsiveness has been described even in normal infants.

A question often asked is about the link between pediatric asthma and adult asthma. What are the characteristics in the pediatric asthmatic that would alert one to monitor even more closely a pediatric asthma patient who is more likely to progress to persistent asthma in adulthood?

Several general observations can be made in this regard: First, severe asthma in early life is associated with significantly higher incidence of allergic rhinitis at 35 years of age. Second, having a history of atopic dermatitis in early life is significantly associated with persistent wheezing at age 29 to 32 years. Third, among children

who wheezed during the first year of life, low lung function is a significant predictor of subsequent wheezing. Stated differently, children with moderate symptoms have moderate symptoms as adults. Children with severe symptoms have severe symptoms as adults. Generally speaking, 75% of persistent wheezers in children can be predicted to have persistent wheezing by 35 years of age. Children who have recurrent episodes of airway obstruction during their early years of life as a consequence of viral respiratory infections, as in respiratory syncytial virus (RSV) infections, but who do not become sensitized to local aeroallergens, are highly likely to remit in their airway symptoms by early adolescence. However, these same patients are highly likely to have recurrences of their asthma symptoms if they should start smoking, even if they have been in remission for an extended period. Those early wheezers who eventually become atopic are at risk for developing persistent asthma. Transient wheezers do not wheeze as adolescents or adults. However, if they become atopic, they are at increased risk of having mild persistent asthma as adults. Persistent asthma in childhood continues to maintain reduced airway function in adults, and if inflammation persists, they may end up having severe asthma in adulthood.

EPIDEMIOLOGY OF PEDIATRIC ASTHMA

About 5 million youngsters younger than 18 years of age in the United States have asthma. This figure includes 825,000 children younger than 5 years. Each year, children with asthma miss 1.4 million school days, three times the school absences of children without asthma. Asthma interferes with school sporting events, school trips, and play activities. For children younger than 15 years, asthma accounts for 3.5 million doctor visits, 658,000 emergency department visits for wheezing, and more than 8.7 million prescriptions.

The cost for asthma care for the average patient with asthma also rises as a result of time lost from work for parents and caregivers. Worldwide, the incidence of asthma has risen, particularly in the pediatric age group.

Because asthma is the leading cause of school absences, time lost over an extended period of time ultimately reflects on the overall performance of the student during his or her formative years and in the end the asthmatic's role and contribution to society as an adult.

ASTHMA IN THE PRESCHOOL-AGE CHILD

By definition, asthma is a "chronic inflammatory disease characterized by recurrent episodes of wheezing, breathlessness, chest tightness, and coughing. Additionally, there is widespread but variable air flow obstruction." Strunk points out in defining asthma in the preschooler that the difficulty with this definition is that a number of other respiratory conditions meet some of these features and yet may not be asthma. Not all that wheezes is asthma, so goes an old teaching. In arriving at a diagnosis in this age group, it has been suggested that one start with a concept that asthma belongs to a group of conditions exhibiting hyperactive airways. (also meaning responding to medications like albuterol). There is no specific test for asthma. Rather, one goes through a series of elimination processes until the diagnosis is arrived at. To this end are three necessary ingredients in the process, namely a chest radiograph, a sweat test to rule out cystic fibrosis, and allergy skin tests to determine sensitization to offending aeroallergens or foods antigens. A barium swallow under fluoroscopy is desirable to rule out structural abnormalities of the mediastinum and/or cardiovascular abnormalities, as in vascular ring, all of which may produce the same symptoms. A sweat test, the second part of a cost-effective assessment, is deemed necessary in spite of the much lower incidence of this disease because both conditions share a number of clinical features. Then of course there is always the possibility of the youngster suffering from both conditions.

With regard to skin testing, the question that always arises both from the clinician's and the parent's perspective is how early does one justify skin testing. Skin testing can be performed at any age when the clinical history, especially the family history, warrants it or when history suggests the possibility of sensitization to an aeroallergen or food allergens. Certainly we are all aware that atopic dermatitis is the first leg of the atopic march and would make skin testing an even more reasonable option. At the minimum, skin test for dust mites, cockroach, and, in inner-city patients, even mouse antigen would be reasonable. The most common food allergens include milk, egg, wheat, peanut, tree nuts, soy, fish, and sesame seed. Pollen allergy appears to herald allergic rhinitis rather than asthma, whereas sensitization to dust mite may antedate asthma. When the history of food allergy suggests a frightening reaction to a particular food, it is good practice to resort to in vitro testing for that suspected food because a skin test by itself can have the potential for a violent systemic reaction. Anaphylaxis from peanut allergy comes under this category. In a typical office setting, a patient is generally brought to the office because of "allergies" manifested by persistent cough interspaced with wheezing, nasal stuffiness, with or without fever. There may be a history of prior spitting up or a "choking spell" after ingestion of a suspected food allergen, unresponsive to repeated courses of antibiotics.

In some cases the diagnosis of asthma had already been arrived at because a sibling has asthma or because there is a strong history of asthma in the family. In this scenario, three conditions immediately come to mind: First, the possibility of asthma; second, the possibility of chronic sinus disease; and third, the possibility of aspiration or a foreign body in the lower respiratory tract. Sinus disease in the preschooler may present itself as a persistent cough. Although wheezing may be reported, cough is more often than not the presenting symptom. Invariably previous caregivers had given a course of antibiotics, and the parents would more often report a transitory response only to end up in a relapse a few days later. This bit of information in the history can be a valuable clue for the presence of sinus infection (a temporary relief of symptoms followed by a relapse or a concomitant sinus disease may be the reason for poorly controlled asthma). Sinus disease is generally poorly responsive to bronchodilator therapy or even steroids and often seen by caregivers as exacerbated by upper respiratory infections (URIs). The presence of nasal polyps at any age in the pediatric population makes a sweat test mandatory. Aspiration may be suggested by a history of a frequent practice of propping the bottle during feedings, a history of choking spells following food, or the unwise practice of offering nuts or popcorn to toddlers less than 4 years of age. Response to medication may be similar to asthma. If one inquires further about stains of vomited material in the beddings, especially after heavy meals (picnics, parties, birthday parties in particular where birthday cakes are often laced with various nuts of various sizes), foreign body in the lower respiratory tract enters the differential diagnosis. A chest fluoroscopy is always an essential part of a workup when foreign body is under consideration because a simple chest radiograph may miss a foreign body, especially if it was very recent episode.

Asthma usually presents exacerbations following viral respiratory illness, exposure to irritants and pollution, or tobacco smoke and will show a dramatic response to steroids, inhaled corticosteroids (ICSs), and bronchodilators. All causes of reactive airway disease need to be considered, including food-induced asthma, bronchopulmonary dysphasia, cystic fibrosis, anatomic abnormalities in the mediastinum (vascular rings), congestive heart failure, bronchiolitis, and pertussis. Just a word about the first episode of bronchiolitis occurring for the first time in any infant: Bronchiolitis is clinically indistinguishable from bronchial asthma. There are laboratory studies designed to identify viral antigens to pinpoint any of the six different viruses that can cause acute bronchiolitis. The clinical picture of pertussis may not be typical because of the attenuation of the disease by previous immunizations, but the presence of leukocytosis with a preponderance of the lymphocytic series may provide the clue.

NATURAL HISTORY OF CHILDHOOD ASTHMA

There are risk factors in the development of asthma. (1) Males have a higher incidence of asthma, but the female sex has a higher deficit in pulmonary function. (2) Atopic status is strongly associated with attacks of wheezing and dyspnea. Children with atopic dermatitis (after all, this is the first lag of the atopic march) or elevation of total serum IgE are strongly associated with the increased prevalence of asthma. (3) A potential genetic component appears likely in the face of the old-time observation that asthma tends to cluster in families. (4) History of viral infections, especially RSV, although other viruses may produce the clinical picture of bronchiolitis; especially those hospitalized for bronchiolitis have reduced pulmonary functions, a feature that appear to be a predictor of bronchial hyper reactivity. (5) Outdoor air pollution: Oxidant pollution such as nitrogen dioxide and ozone may enhance the effects of aeroallergens by increasing airway permeability. (6) Indoor pollution such as increased levels of house dust mite exposure may affect the incidence of asthma and wheezing. (7) Maternal cigarette smoking definitely increases the risk both for the onset or exacerbation of asthma. (8) A recent study investigating genetic polymorphisms among Chinese preschool-age and school-age children found a higher frequency of the "regulated upon activation normal T cell expressed and secreted" (RANTES)-28G allele among children with near-fatal asthma compared with children with mild to moderate asthma.

Will My Child Outgrow the Asthma?

This is a question often asked. Current figures show that 50% of adults who report having had childhood asthma no longer have symptoms. Airway responsiveness in childhood tends to predict airway responsiveness in adulthood.

Children with a parental history of asthma or eczema, who in addition have eosinophilia, allergic rhinitis, and wheezing without colds, have at least a sevenfold increase in risk of active asthma during their school years. The transient wheezers without a history of parental atopy, and who do not have eosinophilia, may be expected to be free of symptoms by the time they enter elementary school.

DIAGNOSIS OF ASTHMA IN THE OLDER CHILD OR ADOLESCENT

The first step in arriving at a diagnosis of asthma, like any other medical condition, is a detailed history. What are the symptoms of concern to the parent or caregiver? When do they occur? Are they repetitive? When they have been in progress for a number of months, it helps to know if a seasonal variation exists. One favorite method in getting an accurate idea of the seasonality of asthma symptoms in any given patient is to refer to the holidays as landmarks (because most parents often do not remember the exact dates of asthma exacerbations). How was the patient on New Year's Day? On Valentines Day? On April Fools Day? On Labor Day? On Memorial Day? On the Fourth of July? On school opening day? After the first frost? On Thanksgiving? Christmas Day? By using these holidays as benchmarks for dates, a more accurate idea of approximate dates of wellness or exacerbations can be obtained. The caregiver's assessment of the severity of the patient's problem can be obtained by asking him or her to give a "grade." Give the child a grade on how well you think the child is with 10 the best and 1 or 2 the poorest or 5 in between. This allows one to gauge the caregiver's ability to judge the patient's wellness state. It is necessary to ask how often the patient has symptoms, how much he or she is restricted in play/or sports activities. How much school does the child miss over a month or all year since the beginning of the school year? It is important to have a list of medications currently used or previously used. One reliable source of this (because often the parents or patient has had so many drugs used he has lost track) is the pharmacist, who usually has a computerized list of drugs used in the preceding 6 or 12 months. It is important to know how many canisters of albuterol have been used the preceding months. Does the patient/caregiver fully understand the difference between the "controller medication" and the "rescue medication"? Have they been given refillable rescue medication or on an as-needed basis (PRN) or as a nonrefillable item? I stress this point because sooner or later the patient or caregiver finds that the rescue inhaler works immediately, and soon the controller medication is neglected and often missed and at times even entirely omitted. The number of visits to the emergency department is important information as is the number of unscheduled visits to the primary care clinician. There are patients who resort to unconventional or alternative caregivers like a chiropractor, herbalist, or acupuncturist. One sure way to alienate a patient is to speak disparagingly about an alternative care provider with whom the patient may have already developed a close relationship. One wants to make certain that the patient is not on any asthmatogenic drugs like β-blockers for migraine prophylaxis or hypertension.

On physical examination, the common stigmas of allergy may already be apparent in an allergic child (as described by Meyers many years ago as the allergic salute: dark circles under the eyes, allergic shiners, Dennie sign, transverse crease at the dorsum of the nose and adenoid fasciae, and the pale nasal mucosa of allergic rhinitis). There may already be a history of several sets of ventilation tubes installed to alleviate middle ear effusion. A tuning fork in the older child may betray the presence of effusion or pneumatic insufflations with a pneumo-otoscope to detect the degree of mobility of the tympanic membranes. One detects pain over the sinus areas (the maxillary sinuses and frontal) by pressure over the areas, which should include a digital palpation of the roof of the mouth (that when exquisitely tender is a common finding in acute or subacute maxillary sinus disease). The search for concomitant sinus disease can be rewarding in making the differential diagnosis in the preschool child and in looking for clues as to why an asthmatic child remains uncontrolled. Tachypnea may or may not be present along with hyperexpansion of the chest. Widespread wheezing may be noted even on tidal breathing and when absent one can often be elicited by having the patient forcefully blow a lighted match or pretend to blow a birthday candle on a cake. Pay close attention to examination of the fingernail beds and toenail beds for cyanosis and early evidence of clubbing, hardly ever seen in asthma but when present may suggest another differential diagnosis.

Objective measurements: A pulmonary function test using standard spirometry is the gold standard in establishing the presence of airway obstruction and demonstrating reversibility after a bronchodilator. It is also a desirable measurement for demonstration of airway obstruction following exercise. This parameter, however, is not adaptable to all ages but may be attempted as early as in patients 4 to 7 years of age. Remember too that giggling, laughing, and crying can be considered the equivalent of exercise in the asthmatic toddler/infant.

ASSESSING SEVERITY OF THE DISEASE BEFORE INITIATION OF THERAPY

Any treatment plan needs to be based on the physician's assessment of the severity of the disease. Table 14–1 shows the classification of asthma severity, from the National Asthma Expert Asthma Expert Panels (NAEP) guidelines.

In children, a recent survey revealed that the majority of pediatric asthma patients have mild persistent or mild intermittent asthma symptoms. An important point to remember is that mild persistent asthma in children should not be considered a benign disease because it can have life-threatening exacerbations. Reliance on symptom severity as a guide to whom to treat is often of limited usefulness. This is clearly pointed out in studies showing poor correlation between symptoms and airway obstruction. Furthermore, in one study forced expiratory volume in 1 second (FEV_1) has been found generally normal in children classified with severe persistent asthma on the basis of symptoms.

A word about exercise-induced asthma (EIA) in children: It is often not formally recognized as a diagnosis in children. EIA is discussed in detail elsewhere in this text, but some points regarding EIA in children are appropriate at this time. Although premedication with short-acting β-adrenergic drugs is effective in the management of most EIA, special consideration should be given to EIA in children. There are studies assessing the effect of ICS use in exercise-induced symptoms in mild asthma demonstrating that ICS when used daily (instead of as needed before exercise) can protect against

Table 14–1. Classification of asthma severity.

	Days with Symptoms	Nights with Symptoms	PEF/FEV$_1$	PEF Variability
Step 4 Severe persistent	Continuous	frequent	<60%	>30%
Step 3 Moderate persistent	Daily	>5/mo	>60–<80%	>30%
Step 2 Mild persistent	2–4/wk	3–4/mo	>80%	20–30%
Step 1 Mild intermittent	<2/wk	<2/mo	>80%	<20%

exercise-induced bronchoconstriction in children with near normal pulmonary function.

Once the severity of asthma is determined, initiation of therapy may be started at the highest dose and as control is achieved, the dose of the ICS selected can then be gradually titrated to the least amount of the drug to achieve control. In some instances, a short pulse of oral corticosteroid (OCS) may be justified to tide over the patient at his or her worse.

GOALS OF TREATMENT

Total control is possible in 40% of cases. It is possible to achieve well-controlled asthma in 80% of patients. To achieve total control or good control, however, requires sustained treatment. When goals are not achieved in spite of maximum dose of ICS, an "add-on drug" (combination therapy) may be in order. Combination therapy may result in lowered doses of ICS. The goals of treatment include (1) prevention of chronic and troublesome symptoms, (2) maintaining normal activity levels, (3) providing optimal pharmacotherapy with minimal adverse effects, and (4) meeting the patients and/or the family's expectations.

Definition of Good Control

From the expert panel guidelines, the definition of well-controlled asthma includes asthma symptoms twice a week or less, use of rescue medication twice a week or less, no nighttime or early morning awakenings, no limitation of activity at school, home, or place of work, and the asthma is well controlled from the assessment of the patient, family, and caregiver.

The addition of newly approved drugs may be a consideration in patients who are already using the maximum doses on ICS or ICS with long-acting β-adrenergic drugs (LABA) or patients requiring OCSs. Coexisting sinus disease or gastroesophageal reflux disease (GERD) should also be ruled out in such cases. When severe symptoms are associated with infiltrates and high levels of serum IgE, bronchopulmonary aspergillosis enters the differential diagnosis. Details on the nature of this complication are discussed elsewhere in this text.

MANAGING BRONCHIAL ASTHMA IN CHILDREN

Managing the child with asthma as outlined in the *Guide for Managing Asthma in Children* covers four components. The first component entails assessment and monitoring.

History is paramount in the assessment of the asthmatic child. One needs to obtain information about nighttime and morning symptoms, school absences, and whether the patient is able to keep up with peers in play or sports. Older children may report "not feeling well" a

good part of the time. In general, information about the youngster's performance in school and whether or not he or she limits participation in sports and play, tailored to what degree the asthma allows the patient to do, are of value in assessing the patient's status.

In the older child capable of performing spirometry, periodic assessment is recommended. Spirometry should be done on the initial visit and after treatment. It will also serve to establish when normal or near normal pulmonary function has been attained. Performing a spirometry every year thereafter assures the clinician that a normal or near normal pulmonary function test (PFT) has been maintained or restored following modifications of any regimen.

Every child, if old enough, or his parent or caregiver should be able to recognize thorough adequacy of symptom control. Based on preconceived perceptions on what is acceptable control, previously agreed on modifications in medication can be added or modified and/or when the clinician should be consulted.

The second component in the management of asthma in children addresses *controlling factors contributing to severity*. For viral URIs, using currently available vaccines like the flu vaccine and reducing exposure to infections is desirable. The preschool nursery is a common conduit for these respiratory infections. Utilization of these facilities should be thoroughly weighed as to its practicality for any individual family and above all affordability, which varies from one family to another.

Tobacco smoke is certainly a completely avoidable irritant, and most parents when told that smoking cessation is really something they are doing not just for themselves but principally for their loved ones invariably are more than willing to make the necessary changes in their lifestyles. Wood stoves are likewise avoidable.

Dust mite antigens are present in every home in the country, and although eliminating this antigen completely is an impossible task, dust control measures significantly contribute to the well-being of the dust mite-sensitive patient. Dust mites dwell where food for them is abundant. Human dander is the source of food for mites, so understandably they are mostly found in pillows, mattresses, and box springs. Of equal importance is the need to lower the humidity in the home to below 50%. Parents need to know that high humidity is conducive to enhanced mite growth. In parts of the country often experiencing freezing weather, it might be a worthwhile effort to have the mattresses, box springs, and pillows taken outdoors overnight because temperatures below freezing significantly reduce the mite population. Often overlooked is the need to use a mattress cover, box spring covers, and pillow covers in beds other than the patient's where the patient shares the room with someone else, usually the parents.

In inner-city dwellings, cockroach antigen and mouse antigens can be an important part of the environmental milieu. Cockroaches thrive best when garbage and food leftovers are left exposed. The use of boric acid traps allows one to avoid using poisons rather than adding another hazard for accidental ingestions. For mold allergens, attentions can be directed to leaky faucets and wet areas. As in dust mite avoidance, reducing humidity to less than 50% can minimize mold exposure.

For patients sensitized to pollens, confinement in air-conditioned rooms is undoubtedly the best barrier to pollen exposure but is not practical. In areas where clothesline drying of laundry is commonly practiced, the moist laundry allowed to dry on a clothesline collects pollens, bringing into the home quantities of pollen where it is recirculated for an indefinite period. The hair collects pollens, so a typical pollen allergic patient may bring in a bagful of pollens to bed. So asking patients to wash their hair at night instead of in the morning can be helpful. In patients with coexisting allergic conjunctivitis, contact lenses are a drawback. Pollen grains can potentially be trapped underneath these lenses, creating an ever-present reservoir of antigens. On the contrary, eyeglasses act as a windshield and thus theoretically block the entry of allergen directly to the eyes.

As you can imagine, all these measures cost money to implement, and perhaps the greatest obstacle to all the above is poverty. And the greatest number of poorly controlled asthma in children is found in poverty-stricken areas.

The third component in managing asthma in children is *pharmacologic therapy*. Attention has been called earlier to the need to assess the severity of the child's asthma before embarking on treatment (Table 14–1).

There are two approaches to the pharmacologic management of asthma in children. The one preferred by most practitioners is an aggressive approach where one attempts to control symptoms as rapidly as possible by using a dose higher than the perceived requirement for any given level of severity. This is usually accomplished by adding short burst of OCS usually prednisone or prednisolone) for a 3- to 10-day period added to the selected ICS. As soon as control is achieved, the dose is then titrated to a level that will maintain control.

The alternative approach is to select a dose level appropriate for the perceived severity of the condition as outlined in Table 14–1, gradually titrating the dose upward until the desired level of control is achieved. Elsewhere in this text are the various preparations currently available for use in children in the United States. The use of inhaled corticosteroids remains the gold standard for the treatment of chronic persistent asthma. In making the selection from the various preparations available, the following considerations are worth mentioning:

1. All currently available ICSs are efficacious.
2. The safety profile of ICS is clearly superior to OCSs.
3. The currently available ICSs are beclomethasone dipropionate, budesonide, flunisolide, fluticasone, triamcinolone, and mometasone.
4. Fluticasone is minimally suppressive even in high doses but is very cortisol suppressive when administered by metered-dose inhaler (MDI).
5. One study determined that a 10% cortisol suppressive effect was produced in these five ways:
   a. 936 μg for flunisolide (47% of highest recommended dose via chlorofluorocarbon [CFC] MDI).
   b. 787 μg of triamcinolone (49% of highest recommended dose via MDI).
   c. 548 μg of beclomethasone dipropionate (65% of highest recommended dose via CFC MDI).
   d. 445 μg (22% of highest recommended dose) of fluticasone dipropionate via dry powder inhaler.
   e. 268 μg of budesonide (17% of highest recommended dose via dry powder inhaler).
   f. 111 μg of flunisolide (6% of highest recommended dose) via a CFC MDI.

These figures suggest that flunisolide delivered via a CFC MDI, fluticasone via dry powder inhaler, and budesonide via dry powder inhaler have a relatively wide margin of safety with regard to cortical suppression if administered with the recommended dosing limits.

Asthma is a condition associated with significant morbidity and mortality. The benefits of ICS in this disease have been well established over the years and the all too familiar side effects should not deter anyone from using these drugs. The adverse effects can be minimized by using the least amount of the drug to bring about the desired result because undesirable side effects tend to increase with increasing doses. There comes a time when further increasing the dose, the desired effects plateau, and further increases produce no further improvement in symptom scores and objective measurements. This would make the ideal time to introduce currently available nonsteroidal drugs to the regimen. This includes the long-acting β-agonists (LABAs), the leukotriene antagonists (LKTRs), and theophylline. When theophylline is added as a steroid-sparing drug, serum levels not to exceed 5 μg/mL would be preferred.

The fourth component in the management of asthma in children is patient education. There are important steps to forming a partnership with the patient and his family and or/care givers. This can be achieved by providing clear and easily understandable written information to all relevant caregivers, including older children, parents, caregivers, child care providers, teachers, coaches, scout leaders, camp counselors, and school and camp nurses.

Written instructions can be given at each visit, allowing ample time for people to study and understand implications of all information. It may be helpful to provide patients and caregivers with access to the Internet various website addresses like those of the American Academy of Allergy, Asthma and Immunology or the American College of Allergy, Asthma and Immunology, or similar organization sites where appropriate printed information is available.

Even medically trained individuals can absorb only so much information during any given time, so it is always good practice to offer information a little bit at a time as a short discussion at each subsequent visit. Provide information in a way that is easily understood and accepted, respecting cultural differences among patients at all times. Note: This responsibility can easily be delegated to trained personnel in the clinicians' offices given the proper training.

The fourth component in the management of asthma in children is patient education. The asthmatic patient should learn more and more about asthma like the diabetic patient learns more and more about diabetes. The patient must learn nature of the drugs being taken and the reasons for their use. Such patients should be made familiar with the modes of delivery of each inhaled drug. When patients fully understand the reasons for any advice given, they are more likely to be receptive to their doctors' recommendations.

PEAK FLOW MONITORING

It is not very unusual to find quite a disconnect between the patient's perception of what is adequate control and what is poorly controlled asthma. Even with the input of the parents or caregivers, there is often a mistaken perception of what is desirable or optimum control. This is one of the situations when peak flow monitoring might be of value. It is also desirable where there is a history of severe exacerbations of moderate to severe bronchial asthma.

The patient's "personal best" is obtained at a time when the child "feels good" and does not have any symptoms. Personal best is the highest peak expiratory flow (PEF) number the patient can achieve over a 2- to 3-week period. A course of OCS may be necessary to optimize asthma control and establish as a result a "personal best."

When determining a personal best, always use the same peak flow meter. Record the PEF twice a day for 2 weeks and from the data obtained, select a number that represents the patient's personal best.

The Peak Flow Zone System illustrated in Figure 14–1 allows the clinician to issue instructions to the patient, parent, or caregiver on what therapeutic steps to take in any given clinical situation.

Some clinicians find this system undesirable as in instances where the parties concerned feel they are already overburdened with what would appear to the patient or his parents "too many things to do over and

above administering medications" and could theoretically reduce even more patient compliance.

IMMUNOTHERAPY AS A TREATMENT OPTION

Immunotherapy (IMT) as a treatment option dates back to the early 1900s. Most clinicians prefer to wait until a patient is at least 5 years old before immunotherapy is given serious consideration. This stems primarily from the overall "fear of shots" in all age groups. However, when there is a distinct cause-and-effect relationship between an antigen identified either in vitro or in vivo, and when undesirable side effects have been experienced with conventional therapy, immunotherapy certainly is a viable option.

A family strongly opposed to getting rid of a cat is one instance. Cat antigen immunotherapy has been demonstrated to be efficacious. A number of studies have also repeatedly shown similar effects with dust mite immunotherapy. In some instances, IMT has allowed clinicians to successfully eliminate the need for maintenance controller medication. In others, clinicians have been able to reduce the doses of controller medication used. There are data to suggest that immunotherapy in dust mite (DM) sensitized patients appear to prevent the development of new sensitivities. Lesser established is the role of pollen immunotherapy in bronchial asthma. IMT for allergic rhinoconjunctivitis has had a favorable effect on bronchial asthma. In the final analysis, the decision is dictated by the families' expressed desires. The mechanism underlying amelioration of symptoms following IMT has been established and is described elsewhere in this text.

WHEN DOES REFERRAL TO AN ASTHMA SPECIALIST BECOME DESIRABLE?

1. When the asthma is severe by definition. The following defines severe asthma:
   a. Treatment with continuous or near continuous OCS (more than 50% of the year).
   b. Requirement of high-dose ICS to achieve control of mild to moderate persistent asthma. The preceding is in association with two of the minor criteria listed next.
2. When the goals of treatment are not being met after 3 to 6 months of treatment; earlier if the child appears unresponsive to treatment.
3. When signs and symptoms are atypical or there are problems in the differential diagnosis.
4. When there are other comorbid conditions (sinusitis, allergic rhinoconjunctivitis).

Cutpoints for Peak Expiratory Flow (PEF) Monitorng

- PEF ≤ 80% of the child's personal best before a short-acting bronchodilator indicates a need for additional medication.
- PEF ≤ 50% of the child's personal best indicates a severe asthma exacerbation.

Cutpoints should be tailored to the child's needs and PEF patterns. The emphasis is not on a specific PEF value but, rather, on changes from one reading to the next.

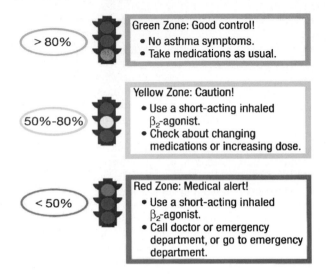

The Peak Flow Zone System

% Personal Best

> 80%

Green Zone: Good control!
- No asthma symptoms.
- Take medications as usual.

50%-80%

Yellow Zone: Caution!
- Use a short-acting inhaled β_2-agonist.
- Check about changing medications or increasing dose.

< 50%

Red Zone: Medical alert!
- Use a short-acting inhaled β_2-agonist.
- Call doctor or emergency department, or go to emergency department.

Asthma changes over time. Patient monitoring and follow-up are important.

Janie Doe: PEF personal best = 280 L/min

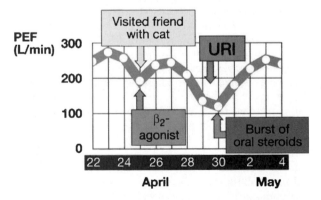

Figure 14–1. The Peak Flow Zone System. (Used by permission of the American Academy of Allergy, Asthma and Immunology. Pediatric asthma: promoting best practice, guide for managing asthma in children. 1999-2004.)

5. When additional diagnostic testing is deemed necessary (pulmonary function tests [PFTs], skin testing, immunodeficiency workup).
6. When immunotherapy as part of the contemplated treatment is an option.
7. When the child is younger than 3 years of age and has severe persistent asthma.

EVIDENCE-BASED MEDICINE

Can my child have a pet? This is a question that is asked of us quite often. What should we tell allergic families about pets? For many years we told our patients not to have any pets because if the child is not allergic to one now, with continued exposure, he or she eventually will be. Recent developments would suggest we may need to rethink this concept.

Evidence has shown in recent years that exposure to a farming environment confers protection against atopy and, as a result, allergic diseases (rhinitis, eczema, and asthma). This protection is not confined to any single antigen but rather sensitization to any allergen.

Martinez and his group at the University of Arizona at Tucson studied a population of 1246 newborns and followed them prospectively to 13 years of age. The aim of the study was to investigate whether pet exposure in early life decreases the subsequent risk of frequent wheezing and/or allergic sensitization. The main outcome measures were as follows: time to first report of frequent wheezing (more than three episodes in the past year), skin prick test reactivity at 6 years and 11 years of age, and total serum IgE at 9 months, 6 years, and 11 years of age. They found that children living in households with more than one indoor dog were less likely to develop frequent wheezing than those not having indoor dogs. This inverse association was confined to children without parental asthma. The lack of relation between exposure to dogs and the development of asthma in children with parental history of asthma could be interpreted as the fact that asthmatic parents make every effort to avoid exposure or may already know they cannot tolerate such exposures. Neither cat nor dog exposure in early life was associated with skin prick test reactivity or elevated total serum IgE at any age. In three published studies, this protection was limited to children with a genetic predisposition to atopy.

Marks, writing in the same issue of the *Journal of Allergy and Clinical Immunology* makes the following observations regarding Martinez's findings: "there are three separate phenomena attributed by this publication to animal exposure in early life:

1. An increased risk of sensitization to cat allergen has been observed during the first 3 years of life in children who are exposed to this allergen in infancy.
2. A reduced prevalence of sensitization to specific pet allergens has been observed in later childhood and adulthood in genetically predisposed individuals who were exposed to the relevant allergen source in early life. This is believed to be immunologic phenomena, which might be explained by the development of specific IgG4 antibody as part of the modified TH2 responses described by Platte-Mills. Custovic et al have suggested that the difference in effect between early and late childhood might reflect the maturation of the immune response from initial sensitization to later tolerance.
3. A reduced tendency to develop sensitization to all allergens has been observed. This has been noted

mainly in relation to farm animals, but it has also been attributed to dog ownership in childhood. The presence of siblings at home and child care attendance has a similar effect. The protection does not seem to be limited to those with a genetic predisposition. This nonspecific protective effect is probably not attributable to a direct immunologic mechanism. The hygiene hypothesis has been invoked to explain this observation."

Are we then ready to recommend acquisition of pets to forestall the development of sensitization? Maybe not so fast because it is still sound advice to tell people who have a pet allergy and existing asthma to avoid having pets. For instance, we know that the onset of specific sensitization is related to the level of environmental exposure to that antigen. How practical is it to expose a nonsensitized infant purposely to pets to abort the development of cat- or dog-induced atopy? As a practical matter, for most families with an atopic background, someone in the family, either one or both parents, may already be allergic to a cat so that obtaining a cat to prevent sensitization of the infant is no longer an option for that family.

BIBLIOGRAPHY

Apter AJ, Szefler SJ. Advances in adult asthma and pediatric asthma. *J Allergy Clin Immunol*. 2004;113:407.

Apter AJ, Szefler SJ. Advances in adult and pediatric asthma. *J Allergy Clin Immunol*. 2006;117:512.

Bisgaard JH, Szefler SJ. Understanding mild persistent asthma in children: the next frontier. *J Allergy Clin Immunol*. 2005;115:708.

Covar RA, Cool C, Szefler SJ. Progression of asthma in childhood. *J Allergy Clin Immunol*. 2005;115:700.

Limb SL, Brown KC, Wood RA, et al. Irreversible lung function deficits in young adults with a history of childhood asthma. *J Allergy Clin Immunol*. 2005;116:1213.

Marks GB. What should we tell allergic families about pets? *J Allergy Clin Immunol*. 2002;108:500.

Martinez FD. Links between pediatric and adult asthma. *J Allergy Clin Immunol*. 2001;107:449s.

Pediatric asthma, promoting best practice, guide for managing asthma in children. American Academy of Allergy, Asthma, and Immunology; 2004.

Remes ST, Rodriguez JA, Holberg C, et al. Dog exposure in infancy decreases risk of frequent wheeze but not atopy. *J Allergy Clin Immunol*. 2002;108:509.

Szefler SJ, Spahn JD. Advances in pediatric and adult asthma. *J Allergy Clin Immunol*. 2005;115:470.

Szefler SJK. Advances in childhood asthma: hygiene hypothesis, natural history of asthma and management. *J Allergy Clin Immunol*. 2003;111:785s.

Wentzel S, Szefler SJ. Managing severe asthma. *J Allergy Clin Immunol*. 2006;117:508.

Adult Asthma

15

Eric C. Chenworth, DO and Daniel E. Maddox, MD

The adult population presents a different set of challenges than seen in the pediatric asthma patient. Special considerations in adult asthma patients include numerous potential medical comorbidities and complex differential diagnoses.

The concept of asthma as a disorder involving airway inflammation is now well established. Although there is heterogeneity in its presentation, the asthma phenotype is well defined and can usually be diagnosed without excessive difficulty. The goal of appropriate diagnosis and treatment, of course, is to normalize and maintain the quality of life for patients with asthma, including social and occupational considerations. In spite of the current understanding of various pathophysiologic perturbations, asthma remains a considerable cause of morbidity and, in some instances, even mortality.

The primary goals of this chapter are to address basic diagnostic considerations (including differential diagnosis), classification of severity, and treatment of the adult asthmatic patient. A brief discussion regarding asthma pathogenesis is also included, although a detailed review of asthma pathogenesis is beyond the scope of this chapter.

DEFINITION

Asthma is a disorder of chronic airway inflammation associated with episodic and at least partially reversible airflow obstruction. Asthma is more a clinical rather than a laboratory diagnosis, which is discussed in greater detail later. It is essential to exclude other potential disease processes that may mimic asthma, thus reinforcing the importance of exploring potential alternative diagnoses.

EPIDEMIOLOGY

An estimated 15 million people in the United States suffer from asthma. Roughly two thirds of these are adults. The prevalence of asthma is increasing in many industrialized nations. According to U.S. Department of Health and Human Service data, the prevalence increased significantly in all groups measured between 1980 and 1994 (Fig. 15–1). In addition to an increase in asthma prevalence, the overall age-adjusted asthma mortality rate appears to be increasing as well. The increase in asthma death rates appears to be higher for blacks than whites. Socioeconomic factors may also play a significant role in asthma-related morbidity and mortality. Similar trends seem to occur throughout most industrialized nations. The overall cost of asthma in the United States has been estimated at approximately $11.3 billion annually.

PATHOGENESIS

The pathogenesis of asthma is incompletely understood. Considering the variable clinical manifestations and inheritance patterns, it is likely that asthma is more of a syndrome rather than a discrete disease entity with a single structural or genetic cause. That said, the clinical features among asthmatic patients seem to be similar enough to develop some useful generalizations regarding asthma pathogenesis.

Historically, the focus of thought regarding asthma pathogenesis was on airflow obstruction secondary to bronchoconstriction. Although this is clearly a component of asthma and an element of asthma diagnosis, the emphasis has now shifted to the inflammatory nature of the illness. Now, the bronchoconstriction or airway hyperresponsiveness (AHR) is often viewed as a marker of underlying inflammation.

Many different cell types have been implicated in asthma pathogenesis. These include eosinophils, lymphocytes, dendritic cells, smooth muscle, epithelial cells, and endothelial cells. In severe asthma or with certain comorbidities, neutrophils may also play a significant role.

For example, asthmatic patients tend to develop an eosinophilic infiltration in their airways. Additionally, the recruitment of T helper 2 (TH2) cells seems to play a significant role in the initiation and maintenance of airway inflammation. Variations in T-cell responsiveness to corticosteroids may correlate with clinical steroid-resistant asthma. Dendritic cells also appear to play a central role in the development of the asthma phenotype,

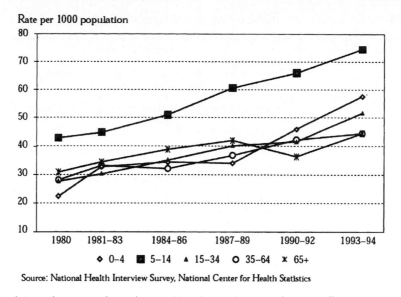

Rate per 1000 population

◆ 0–4 ■ 5–14 ▲ 15–34 ○ 35–64 ✕ 65+

Source: National Health Interview Survey, National Center for Health Statistics

Figure 15–1. Trends in asthma prevalence by age. Note increasing prevalence in all age groups, although less marked in adults. NIH NHLBI Data Fact Sheet: Asthma Statistics. Available at: http://www.nhlbi.nih.gov/health/prof/lung/asthma/asthstat.pdf.

particularly in extrinsic asthma. This is not surprising, considering the role of the dendritic cell in providing a link between innate and adaptive immunity. These cells (dendritic cells) appear to aid in directing the type of adaptive immune response (TH1 vs. TH2). In asthma a TH2 response is favored.

Analysis of mRNA transcripts in bronchial T-cell infiltrates shows submucosal lymphocyte expression of the cytokines that are usually secreted by TH2-type T cells (IL-4, IL-5, IL-13, and granulocyte-macrophage colony-stimulating factor [GM-CSF]). Additional mediators of inflammation, such as histamine, leukotrienes, neuropeptides, and platelet activation factor, are released by local mast cells and eosinophils. These factors in turn may initiate proinflammatory cascades in the extracellular milieu leading to the formation of vasoactive species such as kallikrein. The release of these inflammatory mediators results in changes favoring both smooth-muscle contraction and proliferation, resulting in bronchoconstriction, airway narrowing, and airway glandular hypersecretion. Although a complex array of cytokines, inflammatory mediators, second messengers, and transcription factors have a significant role in the development and pathogenesis of asthma, much work is still required to understand the global process. Ultimately, chronic airway inflammation may lead to irreversible airway narrowing ("remodeling") in a subset of patients.

Also of interest is the question of whether immunoglobulin E (IgE) plays a direct role in asthma. In addition to the role of allergen-specific IgE in allergic asthma, there appears to be a correlation between total IgE level and asthma, even in patients without evidence of allergic sensitivity.

ASTHMA DIAGNOSIS

As with any illness, an accurate diagnosis is necessary to allow for appropriate treatment. The cornerstone of asthma diagnosis is patient history, supplemented with a limited number of diagnostic studies. It is helpful to remember the working definition of asthma as a disorder of chronic airway inflammation with associated intermittent episodes of symptomatic airflow obstruction that is at least partially reversible. These intermittent episodes of airflow obstruction may be manifested by coughing, a sensation of breathlessness, and chest tightness. Symptoms tend to be worse at night and/or associated with specific triggers, such as exercise.

A careful history is necessary not only to look for clues to possible asthma but more importantly to exclude other diseases that may be causing or contributing to the patient's symptoms. It is essential to ask questions pertaining to potential coronary artery disease, thromboembolic disease (especially pulmonary embolism), gastroesophageal reflux, infectious diseases, malignant processes, and other potential pulmonary diseases (Table 15–1).

It is surprisingly common to find multiple systemic and pulmonary processes leading to respiratory symptoms, particularly in older patients. One should always be mindful of overall activity level and conditioning,

Table 15–1. Considerations in the differential diagnosis of asthmatic adults.

System	Selected Diseases
Cardiovascular	Coronary artery disease, heart failure, valvulopathy, pulmonary hypertension, pulmonary embolism
Infectious	Pneumonia, particularly atypical organisms, acute bronchitis
Neoplastic	Lung cancer, carcinoid
Other pulmonary disease	Chronic obstructive pulmonary disease, ABPA, idiopathic pulmonary fibrosis, bronchiectasis, pulmonary eosinophilia, cystic fibrosis, pulmonary manifestations of connective tissue diseases, hypersensitivity pneumonitis, sarcoidosis, asbestosis
Gastroesophageal	Gastroesophageal reflux disease
Hematologic	Anemia, systemic mastocytosis
General	Deconditioning, obesity
Psychiatric	Anxiety, vocal cord dysfunction

It is important to remember that although many of these disease processes may mimic asthma, they (or their treatments) may also coexist with and contribute to the severity of asthma.

tobacco use, and drugs of abuse. A complete occupational history is essential. Potential comorbidities also need to be considered, such as chronic obstructive pulmonary disease (COPD), vocal cord dysfunction, heart disease, anemia, connective tissue disease, risk factors for infectious diseases, and potential malignancies. Although the differential is quite extensive, it is usually possible to focus on important historical elements.

A detailed physical examination, focused by historical information, is essential. This should include careful cardiac and pulmonary auscultation. Wheezing in asthma is typically expiratory and musical. However, wheezing is not always present. When asthma is well controlled or the patient is not suffering an acute exacerbation, wheezing generally is not heard. Never forget, however, that if an asthma exacerbation becomes severe enough to critically limit airflow (either directly or because of patient fatigue), wheezing may resolve. This can be an ominous sign and suggests impending respiratory collapse. The quality of airflow is also important. Many diseases, including asthma and COPD, may result in diminished airflow noted on auscultation. The presence of stridor suggests an upper airway process. Inspiratory Velcro-type crackles may represent an interstitial process such as idiopathic pulmonary fibrosis. Expiratory crackles often represent an alveolar process such as infectious infiltrate or pulmonary edema. The neck should be examined for evidence of jugular venous distension, which suggests a volume overload state that is commonly seen in various cardiac diseases and renal failure. Extremities should also be examined closely for signs of clubbing, cyanosis, and edema. The presence of clubbing suggests an alternative pulmonary process other

than asthma, such as idiopathic pulmonary fibrosis or cystic fibrosis. Clubbing is not a characteristic of asthma, even when asthma is severe. Dependent edema is another sign of cardiac, renal, or other processes resulting in a volume overload state. The ears, nose, throat (ENT) components of the physical examination are also important, with particular attention to possible rhinitis, sinusitis, nasal polyposis, and postnasal drip. It is important not to overlook vital signs (including weight because asthma may be more severe in obese patients).

Diagnostic Studies

In addition to the history and physical examination, a limited set of diagnostic studies may be useful in supporting a clinical diagnosis of asthma. These include pulmonary function testing, measurement of sputum eosinophils, exhaled nitric oxide, allergy skin testing, chest radiograph, and complete blood count. Other diagnostic studies may be suggested by elements of the patient's history and physical examination. A thorough discussion of all of these modalities is beyond the scope of this chapter.

PULMONARY FUNCTION TESTING

Pulmonary function testing is essential at the time of initial diagnostic evaluation and of cardinal importance in guiding the ongoing management of the patient. Ideally, the initial assessment of pulmonary function should include plethysmographic determination of total lung capacity as well as diffusing capacity. These parameters provide the earliest abnormalities definable in asthma—specifically, elevations in residual volume and diffusing capacity are reflective of air trapping. These changes often antedate any significant abnormalities in the spirometric flow-volume curve and can thus illuminate further the decision-making process surrounding the transition from as-needed medication to regular daily administration in patients with mild asthma. Once a thorough assessment of lung function has been made for the asthmatic patient, simple spirometry may suffice for continuing follow-up of the patient's response to therapy. Many asthmatics subconsciously decrease their level of activity or avoid exercise completely as their asthma worsens; this tendency underscores the unreliability of symptoms reporting alone and highlights the importance of periodic reassessment of pulmonary function with spirometry.

Spirometry Spirometry should generally include baseline and postbronchodilator expiratory flow-volume loops. Although the flow-volume curve may be normal in many asthmatics not suffering from an acute exacerbation, asthmatics often have a "scooped" or scalloped appearance to the descending limb of the expiratory flow-volume curve typical of obstructive lung disease. The FEV_1-to-FVC ratio (the ratio of forced expiratory volume in 1 second, FEV_1, to the forced vital capacity, FVC) is generally below 0.7 in a patient with significant airflow obstruction at the time of testing. The degree of obstruction can then be further characterized by the FEV_1. However, it is important to remember that airflow obstruction (at least in the absence of severe remodeling) is variable; thus many mild asthmatics have a normal baseline spirometry. Of significant importance in asthma is demonstration of bronchodilator responsiveness, which is defined as an increase in FEV_1 of at least 200 mL and 12%. Forced expiratory flow (FEF_{25-75}) may also be reduced, suggesting small airways obstruction (Fig. 15–2).

Methacholine challenge In patients with a normal baseline spirometry whose primary presenting symptom is cough and whose history suggests bronchial hyperreactivity, a methacholine challenge may offer additional insight into the level of activity of the lower airway inflammatory process. However, methacholine challenge is neither sensitive nor specific for asthma. For example, a positive response, although expected in asthma, may simply reflect the occurrence of a respiratory viral infection or other inflammatory process within the 6 weeks preceding the test. Similarly, a negative response does not entirely rule out the diagnosis of asthma. Methacholine challenge may be most useful in providing additional insight into the care of patients with persistent cough, if a positive test remains persistently positive (Fig. 15–3).

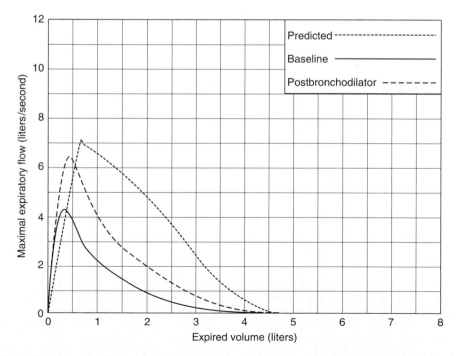

Figure 15–2. Positive bronchodilator response in an asthmatic patient. Notice the shift in the flow-volume curve upward and to the right. A significant bronchodilator response is generally considered to require an FEV_1 of 200 mL and 12%.

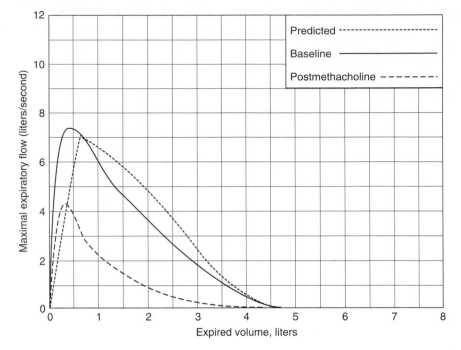

Figure 15–3. Positive methacholine challenge. Notice the impressive decrease in airflow following administration of low-dose methacholine. For a methacholine challenge to be positive, the FEV_1 must decrease by at least 20%.

EXHALED NITRIC OXIDE

Exhaled nitric oxide (eNO) is gaining increasing acceptance as a marker of airway inflammation in asthma. However, accurate interpretation is plagued by many problems. The ambient nitric oxide (NO) level significantly impacts measurement. Results are often poorly reproducible between different pulmonary function laboratories. Additionally, there is a lack of consensus on values that define normal. Methodologic challenges are presented by the fact that NO is evolved from the nasal and sinus airways in much higher concentrations than are normally present in the lower airways, necessitating special procedures to avoid cross-contamination of sampling. Note that eNO may be elevated in other inflammatory airway diseases, including bronchiectasis, chronic bronchitis, and eosinophilic bronchitis. Thus eNO measurement itself is *not* diagnostic of asthma. However, eNO may be helpful in monitoring an individual's response to therapy because this marker is expected to decrease with successful therapy. Proponents have suggested that eNO might help predict which individuals with mild persistent asthma would respond better to an inhaled steroid versus a leukotriene antagonist, although data are presently too preliminary to make such a recommendation.

CHEST RADIOGRAPHY

Although the majority of patients with asthma have normal chest films, too many competing diagnostic possibilities will be missed if chest radiography is overlooked in the initial evaluation. Important findings include hyperinflation, airway wall changes, alveolar and interstitial processes, nodules, masses, and adenopathy. Abnormalities of the cardiac silhouette and cardiothoracic ratio require further evaluation. Acute processes, such as pneumonia, may be present and can lead to a more difficult course in ill asthmatic patients presenting with a flare of respiratory symptoms. When asthma is in flare, atelectasis is a very frequent finding. This may often lead to a radiographic diagnosis of pneumonia, which is erroneous. The best means of distinguishing atelectasis from true pneumonia is by serial imaging. An area of atelectasis will usually have radiographically resolved by the third day of therapy, whereas a true pneumonic infiltrate will require 2 full weeks or longer for complete resolution.

SPUTUM EOSINOPHILS

Sputum eosinophils are another marker of airway inflammation in asthma. However, these may also be elevated in chronic rhinosinusitis and eosinophilic bronchitis. It is usually necessary to induce sputum to provide an appropriate sample with the exception of some patients presenting with an asthma flare. Although simple Wright's staining of sputum smears may be helpful when eosinophils predominate, a more reliable assessment is provided by processing sputum samples to yield homogeneous fluids that permit comprehensive counting of all cellular elements in the sputum. This provides an accurate expression of eosinophils reported as a percentage of total sputum leukocytes. Although helpful as an adjunctive measure of control of airway inflammation in asthma, measurement of sputum eosinophils is insufficient alone to diagnose asthma or initiate therapy.

ALLERGY TESTING

Evaluation for allergic sensitivity is often of significant benefit to patients with asthma and should be considered an essential component of a thorough diagnostic evaluation. Relying on clinical history may help guide a decision about testing for seasonal allergens, but there are no reliable historical features that identify patients with dust mite or indoor mold sensitivity. Allergy testing must be done to recognize such patients accurately. Although not a diagnostic test for asthma per se, the information provided may greatly assist in management. Allergy testing should primarily evaluate sensitivity to aeroallergens. This can include perennial allergens such as house dust mite, animal danders (as directed by history), molds, and cockroach. Assessment of seasonal allergens such as tree, grass, and weed pollens is also helpful but can be guided by the patient's history. Determination of total serum IgE can be beneficial, particularly in patients with severe persistent asthma and evidence of aeroallergen sensitivity because the level may impact therapeutic options.

ASTHMA MANAGEMENT

Classification of Severity

Because initial decision making surrounding asthma therapy is today closely tied to asthma severity, some scheme for stratifying new patients is useful. In the 1997 National Asthma Education and Prevention Program (NAEPP) Guidelines for the Diagnosis and Management of Asthma, asthma severity was stratified on the basis of whether symptoms were intermittent or persistent. Persistent asthma was then further stratified as mild, moderate, or severe based on severity and frequency of symptoms. This classification has been helpful in identifying appropriate initial therapeutic interventions for asthma patients (Table 15–2). It is critical to understand that all asthmatics can have severe exacerbations; these may be life threatening. This is independent of the classification of asthma severity.

Asthma control should be reevaluated regularly, the frequency of which should be determined by the patient's overall severity. Whenever possible, medications, particularly oral or inhaled steroids, should be titrated downward to minimize potential side effects. The stepping up and down of asthma therapy is discussed in more detail later. New NAEPP guidelines will be published in the near future. These will place greater and more detailed emphasis on the stepwise approach to asthma management.

Management

As previously mentioned, asthma management should be tailored according to a patient's needs and asthma

Table 15–2. Classification of asthma severity.

Severity	Symptoms (Daytime)	PEF or FEV$_1$ (%)	Daily Medications
Severe persistent (step 4)	Continual daily symptoms Frequent nocturnal symptoms	≤ 60	• High-dose inhaled corticosteroids + long-acting β$_2$-agonists • Systemic corticosteroids if needed; however, goal of therapy is to maintain control with inhaled corticosteroids and β$_2$-agonists
Moderate persistent (step 3)	Daytime symptoms daily Nocturnal symptoms >1 night/wk	>60–80	• Low/medium-dose inhaled corticosteroids and long-acting β$_2$-agonists • May use leukotriene modifier or theophylline as adjunctive medications
Mild persistent (step 2)	> 2 d/wk but <1x/d >2 nights/mo but <1 night/wk	≥80	• Low-dose inhaled corticosteroids • Alternatively, may use leukotriene modifier, cromolyn, or nedocromil
Mild intermittent (step 1)	≤2 d/wk ≤2 nights/wk	≥80	• No daily medications

FEV$_1$, forced expiratory volume at 1 second; PEF, peak expiratory flow.
Modified from Stepwise approach for managing asthma, Appendix A-1, NAEPP Expert panel report: Guidelines for the diagnosis and management of asthma; update on selected topics 2002. Available at: http://www.nhlbi.nih.gov/guidelines/asthma/asthmafullrpt.pdf.

severity. The guidelines should be followed whenever possible. Asthmatics of all severities should have ready access to inhaled short-acting β-agonists. Additionally, a plan should be in place for monitoring of asthma control and treatment of exacerbations. Many clinicians approach this with an "asthma action plan," governed both by asthma symptoms and serial home peak-flow measurements. Sample asthma action plans are included in the National Institutes of Health NAEPP practice guidelines (available online at http://www.nhlbi.nih.gov/guidelines/asthma/asthmafullrpt.pdf or from the American Lung Association, http://www.lungusa.org). Although commonly recommended, there is insufficient evidence to state that asthma action plans are effective for all patients. Studies suggest that those patients who present for unscheduled office visits or emergency department care of asthma on a recurring basis benefit most from the creation of asthma action plans. Therefore, this approach should be carefully tailored to each situation.

Education is critical in achieving appropriate asthma control. Patients should be instructed on appropriate use of inhaler devices, including spacer use where relevant. Oral hygiene following the use of inhaled steroids is encouraged for prevention of thrush. Perhaps the most critical educational point that patients must learn early, and be frequently reminded about, is the difference between daily or "controller" medications and rescue medications. Daily (controller) medications include corticosteroids (generally inhaled), leukotriene modifiers, and less commonly cromolyn and theophylline. These may be used in conjunction with long-acting β-agonists (LABAs), particularly in moderate or severe asthma. Short-acting β-agonists, such as albuterol, should generally be used as rescue medications for prompt relief of symptom exacerbation and as premedication prior to exercise.

Some patients with refractory asthma and demonstration of positive skin tests or elevated specific IgE to aeroallergens may respond to treatment with the anti-IgE monoclonal antibody omalizumab. Dosing is based on body weight and pretreatment total serum IgE level (consult the manufacturer's recommendations). It is generally reserved for severe asthma, largely because of cost and convenience factors. Once given, it is no longer possible to follow the patient's IgE levels as a reflection of the activity of their disease. A subset of asthma patients may respond favorably to inhaled quaternary amine anticholinergic medications such as ipratropium bromide. Although this class of medications alone is not considered sufficient as therapy in asthmatic patients, it may be a useful adjunct in some patients. There is limited experimental evidence in animal models that this class of medications may potentially limit airway remodeling, thus potentially expanding the future role of these drugs in asthma. However, at present there is not enough evidence to make such a recommendation.

Allergy vaccine immunotherapy is beneficial in asthmatics with known aeroallergen sensitivities, resulting in improvement both in nonspecific bronchial hyperreactivity and in reductions in responsiveness to specific aeroallergens. There is also evidence that this may result in decreased symptoms and medication use. However, immunotherapy should not be started in patients with unstable asthma. Yearly influenzae vaccine may be important in decreasing infection-related asthma exacerbations and has been shown to be safe in this population.

Exercise-Induced Asthma

This topic is covered thoroughly in Chapter 16. Suffice it to say here that virtually all asthmatics can be provoked to symptoms, given a sufficiently strenuous task in cool, dry air environments. Patients whose asthma symptoms occur only in circumstances of exercise should not be considered as having a separate disorder—they simply have asthma that is mild enough to require a potent provoking stimulus to manifest symptoms. Patients who engage in a regular exercise program that predictably provokes asthma symptoms usually benefit from premedicating themselves before exercise. This is helpful not only in preventing symptoms but allows the patient to exercise more comfortably, thus encouraging a higher activity level and healthier lifestyle.

Asthma Exacerbations

Severe asthma exacerbations may occur in patients of any asthma severity or perceived level of control. To ameliorate exacerbations, which may occur in spite of the health care provider's best efforts, an asthma action plan may be helpful, allowing interventions to be initiated prior to the development of severe or even life-threatening symptoms.

Exacerbations may be caused by common respiratory infections, especially viruses (such as rhinovirus) and atypical bacteria, especially *Clamydophila pneumoniae* (formerly known as *Chlamydia pneumoniae*) or *Mycoplasma pneumoniae*. Other factors such as environmental allergens (perennial and seasonal) and occupational exposures are also common causes of exacerbation. Complicating conditions such as allergic bronchopulmonary aspergillosis (mycosis) or other comorbid diseases (as previously described) should be considered as well.

Evaluation of an exacerbation should include a focused history and physical examination including vital signs. Capillary oxygen saturation, spirometry (or peak expiratory flow [PEF] whenever spirometry is not available), and chest radiographs are also important in the evaluation of asthma exacerbations. In patients with a severe exacerbation, an arterial blood gas may be considered. Further evaluation should be guided by the patient's history and findings. Patients should always be asked whether they feel the same as they usually do when their asthma flares. Diagnosis of pulmonary embolism is almost always delayed in patients with asthma unless the alert physician elicits a comment such as "This doesn't quite feel the same as my usual asthma flare."

Initial therapy should be aimed at maintaining adequate ventilatory mechanics and tissue oxygenation. Inhaled β-agonists are necessary early on; however, patient response to bronchodilators must be closely monitored because some patients present in an advanced state of tachyphylaxis to β-agonists. Oxygen supplementation should usually be provided to the tight asthmatic with the goal of maintaining capillary oxygen saturation of at least 90%.

For moderate exacerbations (PEF, 51% to 80% of personal best), it may be necessary to increase inhaled steroids or initiate systemic steroids. For severe exacerbation (PEF, 50% or less of personal best), systemic steroids and immediate emergency medical attention are necessary. If patients with severe exacerbations fail to achieve an adequate response after the first hour of intervention, hospital admission is necessary. Patients with moderate exacerbations with inadequate response to therapy may also be considered for emergent medical evaluation and hospital admission if necessary.

A short course of oral prednisone, in divided daily doses in the range of 40 mg per day for a period of 5 to 10 days, is sufficient for most exacerbations, but duration should be tailored to fit the clinical scenario. Experience with the individual patient's history is generally required to establish whether a taper is necessary (to prevent a rebound exacerbation of the asthma) after a short course of oral steroid therapy.

Patients whose asthma relentlessly worsens and who present in a tight hyperinflated state of breathlessness with little or no favorable response to β-agonist bronchodilators are said to be in *status asthmaticus.* This is a true medical emergency. Such patients should be managed in a hospital emergency department and/or intensive care unit. Simultaneous pursuit of emergent studies and therapy is needed. The evaluation should include arterial blood gases, chest radiography, and visualization of the laryngeal airway. Generalized fatigue, normal to elevated $PaCO_2$, and mental status changes are generally considered indications for endotracheal intubation and initiation of mechanical ventilation. Aggressive use of β-agonists may trigger a significant, albeit transient, hypokalemia, necessitating electrocardiographic monitoring. The addition of inhaled anticholinergic medications (ipratropium bromide) may provide additional benefit when combined with inhaled β-agonists.

Maintaining Asthma Control

As with other chronic health problems, regular follow-up and assessment of control is crucial to manage asthma appropriately. Asthma control issues should be addressed at every office visit. Additionally, follow-up visits should be scheduled at regular intervals, with the frequency determined by asthma severity. These should occur at least once per year for all asthmatics.

Because asthma symptoms do not always correlate with asthma severity, more objective parameters, such as spirometry, are necessary to ascertain the current degree of control. Questions addressing degree of control should generally include the frequency of asthma symptoms, rescue bronchodilator use, nighttime or early morning symptoms, limitations on work, school, or exercise, home PEF measurements, and patient/family member assessment of overall control and comfort (Table 15–3). Validated questionnaires such as the Asthma Control Test (ACT) may be helpful.

Discussions of medication use should not be limited to the frequency of rescue bronchodilator use alone. It is important to ask whether a patient has previously required oral steroids (particularly within the past year), hospitalization, or intubation. Many patients are poorly compliant with controller therapies, particularly inhaled corticosteroids. This may be due to side effects, such as thrush or dysphonia, or other factors, such as inconvenience or medication cost. Alternatively, poor compliance with controller therapies may suggest inadequate asthma education. The patient's inhaler and peak-flow techniques should be regularly reviewed.

The asthma checkup visit should include periodic spirometry. This should be done at least yearly, particularly in patients on regular daily controller therapies and may be done more frequently if necessary. Other measurements such as eNO and sputum eosinophils may provide additional helpful information, although no consensus regarding the indication and timing of such testing has yet emerged.

If the patient's asthma is well controlled, then therapy may either remain unchanged or attempts to step down may occur. For example, a patient on high-dose

Table 15–3. Characteristics of well-controlled asthma.

- Asthma symptoms ≤2x/wk
- Rescue bronchodilator use ≤2x/wk
- No nighttime or early morning awakening
- No limitations on exercise, work, or school
- Patient and provider both describe asthma as well controlled
- Normal or personal best (after aggressive therapy) PEF or FEV_1

Reprinted with permission from Li JT, Oppenheimer LB, Berstein IL, et al. Attaining optimal asthma control: a practice parameter. *J Allergy Clin Immunol.* 2005;116:S3.

inhaled corticosteroids whose asthma has remained well controlled may warrant a change to intermediate dose inhaled corticosteroids. But if a patient's asthma symptoms are not well controlled, and if the patient is appropriately compliant with the current prescribed regimen, then stepping up the level of therapy may be necessary. Recent studies suggest that the dose-response curve of inhaled corticosteroids in asthma is quite shallow. Therefore, addition of a long-acting β-agonist (LABA) or leukotriene blockade may provide more advantage than doubling the dose of inhaled corticosteroids. If a LABA is added, a period of close monitoring is indicated in case the patient should have the Arg/Arg genotype for the β-receptor and as a result suffer worsening of asthma control with regular β-agonist use. Asthma patients should not receive LABA without concomitant inhaled corticosteroid administration.

In many instances, lack of control is due to poor compliance with the prescribed regimen. Again, in these situations, it is necessary to discover the reasons leading to poor compliance and provide further education.

SPECIAL CONSIDERATIONS IN THE MANAGEMENT OF ADULT ASTHMA

Pregnancy and Asthma

This topic, covered in detail in Chapter 18, is an area of significant importance in the management of asthmatic adults. Suffice it to say here that poorly controlled asthma during pregnancy increases the rate of both maternal and fetal complications. Thus, although there is always potential risk associated with any medical intervention during pregnancy, appropriate medical management of asthma prior to and during pregnancy is considered essential.

Heart Disease and Asthma

Aside from providing additional triggers for dyspnea, heart disease complicates asthma management largely as a result of opposing goals in pharmacologic management. β-Antagonists (β-blockers) are a component of standard care for most patients with heart disease, including coronary artery disease (CAD) and heart failure. Unfortunately, even medications that are considered to be β_1 selective do exhibit some β_2 antagonism. This commonly results in exacerbation of asthma and complicates management. The additional physiologic stress due to asthma may also exacerbate the comorbid cardiac condition. Patients with moderate or severe asthma should not be treated with β-blockers. When this class of medications is necessary in mild asthmatics, the lowest possible dose should be used, and the patient must be closely monitored, preferably with before and after spirometry. If the β-blocker can be shown to eliminate a favorable

β-agonist response, or decrease the baseline flow-volume curve in the well asthmatic, then the β-blocker may prove catastrophic if the patient were to have an asthma flare. In the setting of β-blocker–induced asthma, the administration of glucagon and carefully titrated epinephrine may be necessary. Quaternary amine inhaled anticholinergics such as ipratropium bromide may also be helpful in the treatment of β-blocker–associated bronchospasm, although first priority should be to avoid an exacerbation. Mild asthmatics who must be treated with β-adrenergic blockade for cardiac conditions should have access to inhaled anticholinergic medications. Even without concurrent β-blocker administration, it is always necessary to consider both the asthma and any comorbid cardiac diseases as potential causes in any increase in respiratory complaints.

Chronic Obstructive Pulmonary Disease and Asthma

Long-term asthma may result in airway remodeling with resulting irreversible obstruction similar to COPD. Furthermore, many asthmatics, particularly elderly asthmatics with a history of tobacco use, develop a significant component of COPD. Evaluation of such patients is more complex. Complete pulmonary function testing with plethysmographically derived lung volumes and measurements of diffusing capacity, along with chest radiography and in some cases high-resolution chest computed tomography (for quantification of emphysematous changes), are needed in evaluation of this group of patients. It is important to remember that the optimal treatment of COPD is generally regarded as distinct from that of asthma; thus treatment decisions may become more complex. Collection of additional data, such as a sputum cellular profile and blood eosinophil enumeration, may help determine which disease pattern more closely describes the patient. Treatment should be tailored accordingly. This may be a subclass of patients that derive additional benefit from the addition of inhaled long-acting quaternary amine inhaled anticholinergic medications such as tiotropium.

EVIDENCE-BASED MEDICINE

Although an exhaustive discussion of evidence-based care of the adult asthmatic is beyond the scope of this chapter, a brief discussion of some particularly salient issues is provided here. Foremost among these is the present concern regarding salmeterol use in asthmatics. The SMART (Salmeterol Multicenter Asthma Research Trial) study attempted to assess the long-term safety and efficacy of salmeterol in asthmatic patients. This was a randomized, double-blind, placebo-controlled, observational study carried out over a period of 28 weeks in physician-diagnosed asthmatics older than 12 years. The study and control groups received "usual asthma care" along with a metered-dose inhaler containing either salmeterol or placebo. Methodologic problems plagued this study, making it difficult to form solid evidence-based conclusions from this data. For example, follow-up did not assess compliance with or use of inhaled corticosteroids or even compliance with the study drug. There was no overall significant difference in terms of the primary study end point (which was respiratory-related death), although subgroup analysis did suggest an increase in respiratory-related deaths or life-threatening experiences in African American patients when compared with the placebo group. This group of patients, however, had lower prestudy inhaled corticosteroid use, reduced PEF, and more frequent emergency department visits. A more recent meta-analysis was also less than ideal because of such problems; thus the conclusions that warn against LABA use are difficult to accept fully. At present, it appears that LABAs should only be used in patients compliant with inhaled corticosteroid use, and pulmonary function tests should be closely monitored following LABA institution. Differences may possibly be due to β_2-receptor polymorphisms.

In a similar vein, an exciting area of progress in asthma research has been the demonstration that patients with an Arg/Arg phenotype of the β_2-receptor may have an adverse response to regular daily long-term exposure β-agonists. Thus withdrawal or avoidance of β-agonist use in these patients would be the preferred course. The substitution of inhaled anticholinergics may result in particularly significant clinical improvement in this group of patients.

Prevention or reduction of asthmatic airway remodeling remains a challenging area of research. Ideally the mechanisms behind this process will be further clarified in ways that lead to improved therapeutics. There have been some encouraging advances in animal models that await demonstration of practical relevance in humans.

BIBLIOGRAPHY

Glezen W.P., Asthma, influenzae, and vaccination. *J Allergy Clin Immunol.* 2006;118:1199–2006.

Israel E, Chinchilli VM, Ford JG, et al. Use of regularly scheduled albuterol treatment in asthma: genotype-stratified, randomized, placebo-controlled cross-over trial. *Lancet.* 2004;364:1505.

Kanazawa H. Anticholinergic agents in asthma: chronic bronchodilator therapy, relief of acute severe asthma, reduction of chronic viral inflammation and prevention of airway remodeling. *Curr Opin Pulm Med.* 2006;12:60.

Li JT, Oppenheimer LB, Berstein IL, et al. Attaining optimal asthma control: a practice parameter. *J Allergy Clin Immunol.* 2005;116:S3.

NAEPP Expert panel report: Guidelines for the diagnosis and management of asthma, update on selected topics 2002. Available at: http://www.nhlbi.nih.gov/guidelines/asthma/asthmafullrpt.pdf.

Nathan, R.A., Sorkness, C.A., Kosinki M. Development of the Asthma Control Test: a survey for assessing asthma control. *J Allergy Clin Immunol.* 2004;113:59–65.

Nelson HS, Weiss ST, Bleecker ER, et al. The salmeterol multicenter asthma research trial: a comparison of usual pharmacotherapy for asthma or usual pharmacotherapy plus salmeterol. *Chest.* 2006;129:15.

Salpeter SR, Buckley NS, Ormiston TM, et al. Meta-analysis: effect of long-acting β-agonists on severe asthma exacerbations and asthma-related deaths. *Ann Intern Med.* 2006;144:904.

Exercise-Induced Asthma

Laura H. Fisher, MD and Timothy J. Craig, DO

Exercise-induced asthma (EIA), sometimes referred to as exercise-induced bronchospasm (EIB), is extremely common. Prevalence varies, depending on location, investigational criteria, and specific population studied, with increased incidence in developed countries, urban locations, and those in high-performance athletics. The prevalence of EIA in the general population is likely between 6% and 20%. Up to 90% of asthmatics suffer from EIA. This increase in EIA parallels the overall increase in asthma over the past several decades. EIA is also frequently underdiagnosed. In a study of Australian children, 19.5% experienced a fall in forced expiratory volume in 1 second (FEV_1) greater than 15% with exercise. Only 60% of those who had this decline in FEV_1 were known asthmatics. EIA can significantly impair social function and exercise in children. At times, half of children with asthma were unable to compete secondary to symptoms, especially those who participated in outdoor-running sports. Furthermore, asthma inhibited life activities in a third of students over a random 2-week period in Australia. EIB is also a concern in high-performance athletes. Although the incidence of asthma in the general population is 4% to 7%, a much higher proportion of competitive athletes have been diagnosed with asthma, up to 55%, depending on the study.

EIA is second only to viral infections as a cause of acute airway obstruction. Often, EIA is the first presentation of asthma in an individual. Several factors may increase the risk of EIA. Atopy, as measured by positive skin tests, correlates with EIA incidence. Up to 40% of patients with allergic rhinitis have EIA. Genetics may play a part because relatives of asthmatics, who do not have asthma themselves, often have an obstructive pattern on pulmonary function testing with exertion. The increase in obesity and a parallel overall reduction in physical activity and conditioning may be associated with some of the increased incidence of EIB.

The terms *EIA* and *EIB*, although not identical, are often used interchangeably in much of the literature. Some have avoided the term *EIA* in favor of *EIB*, to avoid the mistaken impression that exercise causes asthma. Rather, exercise leads to bronchospasm in susceptible individuals, who may or may not have asthma. In this light, all patients with EIA have EIB, but the reverse is not true. This is especially true of athletes, who demonstrate airway bronchial hyperactivity that may be a consequence of extreme performance conditions and hyperventilation. Perhaps the term *hyperpnea-induced airway irritability* would be the most accurate if ungainly description. Debate is still ongoing regarding the definition among experts in the field.

CLINICAL CHARACTERISTICS

EIA may present with traditional symptoms such as coughing, wheezing, or chest tightness during or within 5 to 10 minutes after exercise. However, the clinician should be aware of atypical presentations such as fatigue, chest pain, persistent postexercise cough, headache, or stomachache (Table 16–1). Cough may be triggered by either neural stimuli or secondary to increased mucus presence. The differential diagnosis of EIA includes intra- and extrathoracic causes of tracheal narrowing, metabolic disorders, and deconditioning (Table 16–2). Vocal cord dysfunction must be considered and may be more common under those undergoing highly stressful athletic performances. Patients with vocal cord dysfunction may have more difficulty on inspiration, rather than on expiration, and they may also demonstrate trouble with phonation during the event and/or inspiratory stridor. Direct visualization of the vocal cords at this time may aide in diagnosis, as may an attenuated or sawtoothed pattern on the inspiratory flow portion of the spirometric flow-volume loop. Cardiac disease and other causes of pulmonary disease should be ruled out, including arterial septal defects, idiopathic arterial hypoxemia of exercise, and arrhythmias. Measurement of response or lack of response to therapies for EIA may assist with the diagnosis. Physicians should be cautious of overdiagnosis of EIA, especially in regard to deconditioning. In Vancouver schoolchildren with refractory EIA, laboratory testing

Table 16–1. Symptoms of exercise-induced asthma.

Typical	Atypical
Coughing	Fatigue
Wheezing	Headache
Chest tightness	Chest pain
Dyspnea/Air hunger	Stomachache

confirmed EIA in only 15% of children. The others had deconditioning, habit cough, and vocal cord dysfunction as well as other miscellaneous causes. Physical examination is important to rule out other etiologies as well as comorbid conditions, such as rhinosinusitis, although the physical and pulmonary examination in most patients with EIA will be normal. Similarly, baseline spirometry done in the office is often normal in patients with EIA, especially in highly conditioned athletes. As with many chronic diseases, a complete and accurate history and physical examination will aid in accurate diagnosis.

DIAGNOSIS

In a study of 166 student athletes, nearly a third who had risk factors for EIA on a simple questionnaire had a 15% drop in their FEV_1 with testing, confirming the

Table 16–2. Differential diagnosis of exercise-induced asthma.

Respiratory	Intra- and extrathoracic tracheal disorders causing tracheal narrowing, uncontrolled asthma, viral or bacterial respiratory infection, emphysema
Cardiac	Coronary artery disease, arrhythmia/tachycardia, congenital defect, idiopathic arterial hypoxemia of exercise, valvular heart disease/congestive heart failure
Neuro/Muscular	Deconditioning, metabolic disorders, neuromuscular disorders
Psychogenic	Vocal cord dysfunction, malingering for secondary gain
Gastrointestinal	Gastroesophageal reflux disease

diagnosis. However, diagnosis based on symptoms alone is often unreliable because different patients have different subjective symptoms that may or may not correlate with objective measures of EIB. A response to therapy, such as with a β-agonist, may more strongly suggest the diagnosis of EIB, with improvement as airway smooth-muscle narrowing is reversed with the bronchodilating β-agonist. Challenge tests may help confirm EIA if history is suspicious to demonstrate effectiveness of acute or chronic therapeutics, to screen athletes in high-risk sports, and to prove need for medication in high-performance Olympic athletes. An exercise challenge test, sport specific if possible, may be the most reliable method of diagnosing EIA. Exercise challenge tests are contraindicated in those with severe airflow limitation and other unstable medical conditions (Table 16–3). A screening baseline electrocardiogram should be considered in those older than 60 years. Patients should be advised to arrive at the test dressed to exercise, after eating only a light meal, and they should not have exercised within 4 hours of the exercise challenge test. This latter requirement is secondary to a refractory period in which a patient may be "protected" from EIB symptoms.

The refractory period may persist up to 4 hours following exercise and raises the risk of false-negative test results. During testing, the patient's FEV_1 is measured at baseline and then at frequent intervals after exercise. Peak flows, although giving less reproducible and reliable results, may also be measured pre- and postexercise. Pulmonary function testing should be done while the patient is in a seated position. Tests are performed at 5, 10, 15, 20, and 30 minutes after exercise, and, some suggest, even at 1 and 3 minutes postexercise. Two to three tests are performed at each time interval, with variability of an accurate test of less than 0.2 L between the two top tests. The diagnosis of EIA is suggested by a reproducible decline of 15% in FEV_1 or peak flow following exercise.

Table 16–3. Contraindications to exercise challenge test.

Respiratory	Low FEV_1 <50–60% predicted; technical inability to perform spirometry
Cardiovascular	Myocardial infarction or stroke within 3 mo; unstable angina; malignant arrhythmia; uncontrolled blood pressure>200/100; aortic aneurysm
Orthopedic	Inability to perform specified exercise

FEV_1, forced expiratory volume in 1 second.

Some researchers use values of a fall of 10%, which suggests an abnormal response, and others a value of 20% from baseline, but 15% is the standard for most field studies. Nonasthmatics usually experience, at most, less than a 5% decline. The response of the normal individual to exercise should be an increase in FEV_1. If the FEV_1 declines with exercise, the FEV_1 should be measured by pulmonary function testing for two readings following the nadir, or to recovery within 5% of the baseline FEV_1. If pulmonary function has returned to the baseline level, the test may be terminated at the 20-minute interval. Obstruction may be reversed with a bronchodilator as needed or when recovery is less than 10%.

Exercise challenge may be performed via cycle ergometer, treadmill, free-running, or step testing. Bronchoconstriction may be easier to provoke with treadmill exercise due to a faster increase in minute ventilation. Cycling is easier than treadmill testing, especially for those with lower extremity weakness or arthritis, and it will identify most patients with EIB, even though treadmill exercise testing produces more rapid bronchoconstriction. Treadmill testing also has proven efficacy in measuring the effectiveness of medications. Of course, field testing of the athlete in his or her chosen event would be most specific although not always practical. To achieve adequate exercise level for testing, patients should reach 80% to 90% of their maximum predicted heart rate (220 minus age), or 30 to 40 mL/kg oxygen consumption. It is important for the patient to reach target heart rate quickly to prevent development of the refractory period. Inspiration of dry, cold air and use of a nose clip to force mouth breathing is more likely to produce EIB sooner. The goal is 8 minutes of exercise, 6 minutes near the desired target rate. If a patient is unable to exercise for whatever reason, stationary hyperventilation may be an adequate alternative. This is usually performed with the patient breathing air with a fixed concentration of carbon dioxide to prevent hypocapnia from hyperventilation. The goal is to achieve 60% to 70% maximal voluntary ventilation. Eucapnic voluntary hyperventilation is sensitive and may be equal or superior to cold air exercise challenge in the identification of airway hyperresponsiveness in elite cold-weather athletes. The eucapnic hyperventilation testing has a limited role because it is expensive, and difficult to perform, and equipment is rarely available. Free-range running may also be a useful measure to diagnose EIA, especially in children in whom formalized testing is more difficult. Arguments have been made for and against this modality.

Exercise and hyperventilation testing are forms of indirect stimuli on the airways because they lead to mediator release with subsequent mediators acting on airway receptors. Methacholine, a form of direct challenge, involves the cholinergic system by binding to airway muscarine 3 (M3) receptors. Methacholine testing can also be used to measure airway responsiveness and is likely to be abnormal in patients with EIB. Methacholine challenge is sensitive but not specific, with most examiners considering significant a PC20 of 8 mg/mL. PC20 is the concentration of methacholine causing a fall in FEV_1 of 20% or greater. Given its high sensitivity, a methacholine challenge test is more useful to exclude asthma with a higher negative versus positive predictive value. The pretest probability of a person having asthma should also be considered in the equation. The American Thoracic Society (ATS) has useful predictive curves illustrating pre- and posttest probability based on PC20 values. Increased bronchial hyperresponsiveness is seen in other disorders such as chronic obstructive pulmonary disease (COPD), congestive heart failure, cystic fibrosis, and even allergic rhinitis. Methacholine testing is not recommended if the patient's FEV_1 is less than 70% predicted, if the patient is unable to perform spirometry, if a patient is pregnant or nursing, or if the patient has other unstable medical conditions. The ATS guidelines include medications that should be avoided prior to testing to prevent false-negative results (Fig. 16–1). β-Blocking agents should be held 48 hours, short-acting bronchodilators 8 hours, long-acting bronchodilators 48 hours, theophylline 24 hours, and sustained-release theophylline 48 hours prior to exercise challenge. Ipratropium should be held 24 hours, cromolyn 8 hours, nedocromil 48 hours, antihistamines 3 days, and leukotriene modifiers 24 hours. Guidelines for tiotropium are not available, but a 5-day hold is probably needed. It may not be necessary to hold inhaled corticosteroids, depending on the information sought from the test. Patients should avoid caffeinated drinks or chocolate on the day of the study. When investigating the possibility of EIA to explain symptoms, baseline asthma should be maximally controlled to avoid skewed results. Patients should not exercise for at least 4 hours prior to testing to avoid inducing a refractory period and therefore a false-negative test.

Another direct challenge is a histamine challenge. Histamine, which binds to airway H1 receptors, may miss a significant number of patients with EIA, as demonstrated by the 30% to 45% of patients who have evidence of EIA in the field but no response to histamine challenge. Histamine is also known to produce false-positive results when testing for EIB. Besides direct challenge, patients with bronchial hyperreactivity with exercise often have increased response to other stimuli, such as adenosine monophosphate (AMP), mannitol, or hypertonic saline. Some have suggested that mannitol inhalation testing may be ideal for diagnosis of EIA. It has correlated well when compared to eucapnic hyperventilation in a study of EIA in summer athletes, remaining sensitive for diagnosis, but is less expensive and easier to perform than hyperventilation testing.

Exhaled nitric oxide (eNO) testing may not be as useful in the diagnosis of EIA. Scollo et al showed that

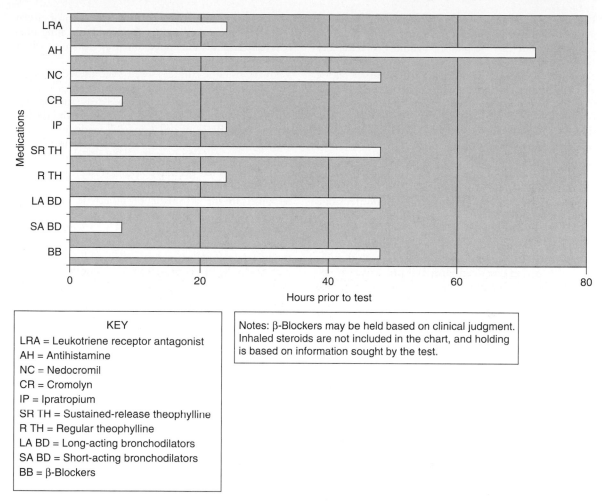

Figure 16–1. Recommended medication holding times prior to exercise challenge test.

KEY
LRA = Leukotriene receptor antagonist
AH = Antihistamine
NC = Nedocromil
CR = Cromolyn
IP = Ipratropium
SR TH = Sustained-release theophylline
R TH = Regular theophylline
LA BD = Long-acting bronchodilators
SA BD = Short-acting bronchodilators
BB = β-Blockers

Notes: β-Blockers may be held based on clinical judgment. Inhaled steroids are not included in the chart, and holding is based on information sought by the test.

eNO levels do not change significantly during symptom induction exercise challenge in children with asthma. Baseline eNO values did correlate with the degree of postexercise bronchoconstriction, however, suggesting eNO may predict hyperresponsiveness to exercise. Other investigators have shown that eNO does change following exercise and that the change correlates with FEV_1. More study is needed, and the majority of these investigative methods are likely more useful in laboratories that are skilled in their use, rather than in general practice.

PATHOPHYSIOLOGY

Within the first few minutes of exercise, bronchodilation secondary to endogenous catecholamine release occurs as a reflexive response, even in some asthmatic patients. This lasts through exercise and even up to 20 minutes postexercise in some patients. Airway obstruction in those with EIB usually peaks 5 to 10 minutes after aerobic exercise with recovery after 30 to 60 minutes. The clinician should be aware that some patients present with shortness of breath during, instead of after, exercise. Unlike asthma exacerbations secondary to other etiologies, the occurrence of a late reaction following pure EIA in the absence of allergen challenge is unusual, but it has been reported in rare instances. In contrast to conventional teaching, Boulet et al and Chhabra et al showed a late response in 30% and 50% of EIA patients, respectively, following exercise. Unfortunately, there were no predictors as to who was at risk for this phenomenon. Following resolution of an acute attack of EIB, many patients experience a refractory period with repeated exertion. During this period, which usually lasts less than 4 hours, resumption of activity results in less bronchoconstriction. Several theories exist, but the mechanism behind this refractory period remains unknown. It has been hypothesized that the refractory period is secondary to the earlier release and depletion of available preformed mediators during the first event. The refractory period may also be secondary to protection from natural catecholamines produced in response to stress on the airway, or it may be due to release of inhibitory mediators as a result of the initial airway insult. Prostaglandins (PGs) may play a role in the refractory period because indomethacin, a PG inhibitor, also leads to protection. Conversely, histamine tachyphylaxis is abolished by indomethacin, implicating an inhibitory role for PGs in the refractory period. Tachyphylaxis can also be prevented with the cyclooxygenase inhibitor flurbiprofen, lending further support to this theory. It is important to note that the refractory period described for EIB is protective for further exercise only. It is not protective for allergen-triggered events.

During exercise, minute ventilation increases to meet expanding oxygen requirements, resulting in the cooling and drying of inhaled air by various mechanisms. As minute ventilation increases, and athletes switch from breathing through the nose to breathing through the mouth, air is not optimally humidified and heated before reaching the lower airway. The severity of EIB is directly proportional to the water content of inspired air, cool air having a more detrimental effect than warm air. Mucociliary clearance is also decreased by hyperpnea of dry air but not warm, humid air. In fact, humidification of inspired air may prevent EIB.

Two theories have been described to explain the pathophysiology of EIB. They are not mutually exclusive and may or may not be the same as the pathology involved in chronic asthma. The first was described in 1986 and is often referred to in the literature as the thermal hypothesis. According to this theory, airway cooling is less of a problem than the rapid rewarming of the airways that follows exercise. Rapid rewarming leads to reactive hyperemia and airway wall edema that contributes to airway narrowing and bronchoconstriction with mediator release. By preventing airway rewarming, the obstructive bronchial response is abrogated. If athletes avoid rewarming by breathing cold air instead of warm air during their recovery period postexercise, FEV_1 decline was reduced from 25% to less than 10%. This thermal theory has been debated. For instance, EIB occurs with hot, dry air as well. Furthermore, technical problems exist in methods used to measure water loss in cold temperatures.

The second theory, dubbed the osmotic hypothesis, states that neither cooling nor rewarming is necessary. The osmotic theory espouses water loss in the airway following hyperpnea as the pathologic cause. This leads to increased cell osmolarity and dehydration of airway cells. In support of the osmotic hypothesis, lung mast cells have been demonstrated to release histamine with a transient osmotic stimulus. Mucus increases in airways following osmotic stimuli as well. As cells dehydrate, an increase in intracellular calcium and inositol triphosphate triggers intracellular mediator release such as mast cell degranulation, with release of histamine and the formation and release of inflammatory mediators such as cysteinyl leukotrienes. In normal individuals, an increase in bronchial blood flow secondary to increased cell osmolarity has been hypothesized to rehydrate cells and clear inflammatory mediators as a protective response. In the asthmatic or otherwise predisposed individual, local inflammation contributes to microvascular leakage and airway edema. Those with EIB may have an exaggerated response to airway dehydration in the presence of inflammatory cells, resulting in airway narrowing with contraction of smooth muscle, increased mucus production, and airway wall edema. Epithelial cells desquamate, and there is leukocyte infiltration and increased vascular leakage. Inflammation in predisposed individuals may further alter cell volume regulation and amplify this process.

Regardless of the pathway that leads to their release, the downstream mediators are powerful inducers of bronchoconstriction and airway narrowing. There are likely multiple stimuli for EIB because combination therapy is often required for effective treatment, with a regimen including agents acting on different mediator pathways. The cysteinyl leukotrienes are direct stimuli of the Cys-LT1 receptor and include LTC4, LTD4, and LTE4. These leukotrienes, produced in mast cells and eosinophils, facilitate bronchoconstriction, increase mucus secretion, and increase vascular permeability. LTC4, LTD4, and LTE4 are all increased following exercise. In fact, increased LTE4 can be measured in the urine following exercise, although its level does not necessarily correlate with the degree of vasoconstriction. Leukotrienes are more potent inducers of EIB than is histamine and include potent vasoconstriction among their downstream events. This may explain the current inferiority of histamine-based diagnostic testing for EIB.

Prostaglandins play a role in the pathophysiology of EIB as well. PGD2 and PGF2a also act as direct stimuli for bronchoprovocation. However, PGE_2 is a protective PG and bronchodilator that is the normal physiologic response to increased osmolarity and hyperpnea in the airway. In the presence of inflammation, cells may not produce the protective PGE_2, leading to increased potentiation of airway damage. Prostaglandin E1 also reduces airway hyperresponsiveness. Histamine and IL-8, a potent chemoattractor for neutrophils, are also increased following EIB. There is likewise an increase in CD25-expressing T cells and CD23-expressing B cells, favoring a TH2 pathway. Chemotactic factors recruit other inflammatory cells to the area, propagating inflammation. Increased sputum and serum eosinophil counts have been documented in some cases of EIB, although not all studies have supported this. Higher eosinophil counts and levels of eosinophilic cationic protein may show active asthma. Neuropeptides may also play a role in EIB and are affected by osmolarity shifts.

TREATMENT

With proper treatment, EIA and EIB should not limit physical activity. A management plan for EIB includes pharmacologic and nonpharmacologic treatments (Fig. 16–2). If possible, athletes should schedule exercise to avoid the coolest time of the day, or the highest pollen time for those with coexistent allergies. Patients should warm up and cool down following exercise for 10 to 15 minutes. Warm-up exercises may increase bronchial blood flow, which may be crucial in clearance of inflammatory mediators from the pulmonary circulation. Furthermore, breathing through the nose rather than the mouth facilitates the warming and humidification of cool, dry air, minimizing the forces contributing to EIB. By covering the face during sports in cold environments, inhaled air is warmed and EIA is lessened. If symptoms limiting physical activity develop, activity may be restarted cautiously when symptoms clear. A refractory period as described earlier has been noted in many athletes following EIB, and this period may be protective for several hours. In fact, a 10-minute warm-up may decrease EIB during active sports participation by taking advantage of this refractory period. Short sprints may be an effective warm-up. By improving overall aerobic fitness, athletes decrease their minute ventilation required for the same amount of work, limiting airway drying and EIB. By this method, regular exercise may help reduce persistent disease. There are some data that exercise training improves symptoms of EIA, by up to 25% improvement in one study. Therefore, exercise should be encouraged and not limited in those with EIB.

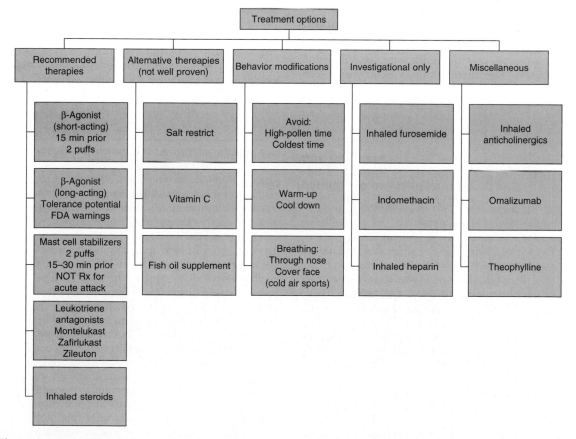

Figure 16–2. Treatment of exercise-induced asthma.

As alternative medicine becomes more popular, some patients may inquire about other, nonmedicinal treatment modalities, such as diet. There are some preliminary, although not conclusive, data that suggest dietary salt restriction may improve EIA. Vitamin C may provide variable protection from EIB but should not replace standard pharmacotherapy. Fish oil supplementation may also be beneficial in asthmatic subjects with EIB. Laser acupuncture, quite a controversial therapy, offered no protection against EIB in pediatric and adolescent patients. Other alternative therapies that may have some merit include hydration, other antioxidants, and magnesium.

β-Agonists inhibit EIA as well as bronchospasm secondary to hyperosmolar stimuli. First-line treatment usually includes 2 to 4 puffs of a short-acting inhaled bronchodilator 15 minutes before exercise. The effects of short-acting bronchodilators prior to exercise may last up to 4 hours. However, in children, only a third were protected at 2 hours and less than half of the children were still protected at 4 hours. Response to bronchodilators may increase with age. Options for inhaled short-acting bronchodilator treatment include albuterol, metaproterenol, or pirbuterol.

Long-acting bronchodilators may also provide protection from EIA symptoms. The Food and Drug Administration (FDA) has issued warnings regarding long-acting bronchodilators and increased morbidity and mortality in some individuals. These warnings should be disclosed to patients. However, there is a long record of study of these medications for EIA. One author reviewed 32 studies of long-acting β-agonists in children, 9 of which referred to the effects of these medications on EIA. Formoterol decreases symptoms of EIA after a single dose and with regular use. Formoterol has a faster onset of action than salmeterol and may be given 15 minutes prior to exercise, whereas salmeterol requires earlier administration at least 60 to 90 minutes before anticipated activity. These long-acting bronchodilators provide protection for a longer duration of time, up to 12 hours after administration, and may be better options for activities or play that may last longer than a few hours. However, the regular use of long-acting bronchodilators should be discouraged as solo therapy if used regularly. A tolerance to and loss of protection with bronchodilators has been demonstrated following long-term use. With twice-daily dosing, salmeterol has a lack of protection from EIB at 9 hours. This tachyphylaxis has been shown for both formoterol and salmeterol, the two long-acting β-agonists currently available for use in the United States. Other side effects of β-agonists commonly include tremor and increased heart rate, which could adversely affect performance in some athletes.

Mast cell stabilizers may also be used prophylactically, decreasing EIA symptoms significantly. Two puffs prior to exercise of either nedocromil sodium or cromolyn sodium provided significant and comparable protection

from EIA and were superior to placebo. A meta-analysis by the Cochrane Database regarding mast-cell stabilizing agents in the prevention of EIB involved 518 participants in 24 trials in 13 countries. All medications evaluated were effective to a varying degree. Patients on mast cell stabilizers had a 7.1% decline in FEV_1 versus a 13.8% decline with anticholinergic agents, but neither were as effective as β-adrenergic agonists. A subsequent study demonstrated no significant change between salbutamol plus nedocromil versus salbutamol alone. In a study of children, the 2-mg dose of sodium cromoglycate is just as effective as the 10-mg dose. Four or more puffs are recommended for the higher performance athlete. Mast cell stabilizers are not effective for aborting symptoms of acute EIB and are useful as prophylactic agents only. The mechanism of action of sodium cromoglycate and nedocromil sodium may include action on ion channels involved in cell volume regulation as well as inhibiting mediator release. They are approved for use by the U.S. and International Olympic Committees (see later). These medications have a very favorable and minimal side-effect profile. Disodium cromoglycate is most commonly associated with postinhalation cough. Nedocromil has an unpleasant taste. In the Cochrane meta-analysis, only 3% of patients on mast cell stabilizers experienced side effects versus 11% on β-adrenergic agonists.

Leukotriene antagonists such as montelukast and zafirlukast, or the 5-lipoxygenase inhibitor zileuton, also have proven efficacy in the treatment of EIB, especially when used regularly. Urinary leukotrienes, which are increased following exercise in those with EIB, decline with montelukast treatment. Similarly to salmeterol, montelukast and zafirlukast provide protection from EIB within 1 hour of ingestion. Montelukast and zafirlukast have a longer half-life than bronchodilators and provide protection from EIB up to at least 12 hours, with efficacy proven to 20 and 24 hours in some investigations. Zileuton provided protection only up to 4 hours. In a comparison of montelukast and salmeterol, although initial efficacy in reduction of EIB was similar with both medications, at 8 weeks, montelukast was superior to salmeterol, probably as a result of loss of protection with the bronchodilator after extended use. Tolerance does not develop to montelukast. Montelukast may be an ideal treatment for children with symptoms of EIB with play, given its long duration of action along with a minimal side-effect profile. Compliance is also improved with montelukast versus inhaled cromolyn.

Other effective treatments for EIB include medications such as inhaled corticosteroids. Inhaled corticosteroids decrease asthma exacerbations, including exacerbations secondary to exercise. For example, budesonide, at a dose of 100 to 400 μg per day, provided 80% protection from EIB symptoms. Corticosteroids decrease mast cells and eosinophils and improve integrity of the epithelial cell airway lining. Corticosteroids may also help in the reversal of vasoconstriction and may have properties that counteract airway edema. Inhaled corticosteroids may not decrease EIB in a dose-related manner, but they do show a dose-related response as measured by methacholine sensitivity. When used regularly, an inhaled steroid demonstrated better protection from EIA versus montelukast. Uncontrolled asthma may be an underlying cause if EIB fails to improve with the treatments just mentioned. According to the ATS guidelines for asthma management, inhaled corticosteroids are first-line therapy for persistent asthma. This includes patients with FEV_1 less than 80% predicted or those with daytime symptoms greater than twice per week or nighttime symptoms greater than twice per month. Patients with persistent symptoms should be treated with daily inhaled corticosteroids. Inhaled corticosteroids are not effective as acute or prophylactic therapy. More concerning, some researchers have found evidence of airway remodeling, secondary to chronic obstruction, not only in those with EIA but also in those who participate competitively and chronically in cold air environments. The development of chronic inflammatory changes in the airway may argue for a role of daily inhaled corticosteroids even in those with EIA symptoms only. In low to moderate doses, no significant adverse effect on bone mineral density or final growth in children has been demonstrated.

Multiple other medications have been used in patients with EIB. Inhaled anticholinergic agents, such as inhaled ipratropium or tiotropium, may be effective. Tiotropium at this time is FDA approved only for use in COPD. Oral β-agonists and methylxanthines are not very effective in the treatment of EIB. However, oral theophylline, used more frequently in the past, did show a degree of protection from EIB correlating with serum concentration of theophylline, albeit not as much as with cromolyn. Currently, more efficacious, faster acting, and safer medications are in existence. Other agents with only minimal, if any, efficacy include antihistamines, calcium channel blockers, and α-agonists. Further data are needed on the effects of omalizumab, an anti-IgE therapy, on EIA. Experimental therapies such as inhaled furosemide, indomethacin, and heparin have also been described in the treatment of EIB but require further study. Furosemide inhibits NAK2CL transport and may inhibit EIA by a mechanism similar to cromolyn. Inhaled indomethacin may inhibit local PG synthesis and/or ion transport, protecting against EIA. Inhaled heparin may inhibit mast cell release. These latter treatments should only be used as a research tool at this time.

SPECIAL CONSIDERATIONS

Many famous sports figures, such as Pittsburgh Steeler Jerome Bettis and track and field athlete Jackie Joyner-Kersee, have succeeded in competitive sports despite having asthma. Elite athletes compose a special group at risk for EIB. A high prevalence of bronchial hyperreactivity

to methacholine of almost 50% has been demonstrated in elite athletes. The majority of these athletes had no personal or family history of asthma prior to this testing. However, some may argue that pathologic findings in this population are the result of the extreme conditions under which these athletes compete, rather than a true form of asthma. Patients who undergo repetitive exercise often have evidence of chronic airway inflammation. In animal models, acute mucosal injury occurs in the airways with dry air inspiration. The changes described in detail earlier, especially in response to airway dehydration with hyperpnea, occur in normal individuals without symptoms of EIB. Airway narrowing may even be a defense mechanism in these individuals. Repetitive exercise itself may be responsible for EIB and related symptoms in elite athletes through IL-8, a potent neutrophil chemoattractant. Increased numbers of neutrophils have been found after heavy exercise but not moderate exercise in athletes. In addition to neutrophils, lymphoid aggregates may play a role in the increase in EIB in elite athletes. In cross-country skiers, 65% had increased lymphoid aggregates following bronchial biopsy versus 25% of controls. Adenosine, another mediator in the asthma cascade, also increases in patients with asthma following exercise.

Environmental factors, including pollutants, may especially have physical effects on the airways of high-performance athletes secondary to the degree to which these athletes are exposed under strain, rather than being secondary to an underlying asthmatic component in these individuals. A full 76% of elite swimmers show signs of repetitive injury to the airway epithelium with remodeling, a process that may be secondary to the effects of chlorine at concentrations higher than those approved by the World Health Organization. Simply sitting in a hot tub caused reduction in the amount of methacholine needed to cause a significant decline in FEV_1 in asthmatics versus control individuals, hypothesized to be secondary to the effects of humidified chemicals on the airway. Similarly, ice skaters are exposed to increased levels of nitrogen oxides, chemicals that may have a detrimental physical effect on the airway. As elite athletes show pathologic changes in their airways consistent with chronic inflammation, regular treatment with inhaled corticosteroids could be considered in this group. However, elite athletes may not respond to traditional medications that usually improve symptoms in asthmatics. Short-acting β-adrenergic agonists are not as effective in elite speed skaters, and cross-country skiers did not have significant improvement with treatment with inhaled corticosteroids despite evidence of airway inflammation.

Regardless of etiology, the extraneous circumstances of elite athletes often require their physicians to be aware of special risks and treatment requirements. The sports associated most often with EIB are cold air sports and/or those requiring the highest minute ventilation

Table 16–4. Sports and risk for exercise-induced asthma.

High-Risk Sport	Lower Risk Sport
Cross-country skiing	Baseball
Figure skating	Swimming
Ice hockey	Football (American)
Distance running	
Basketball	

(Table 16–4). Cross-country skiers, for example, are especially exposed to cold, dry air that may induce EIB by the mechanisms previously described in predisposed individuals. Fifty-five percent of elite Swedish cross-country skiers had EIB by history or testing. Up to 35% of elite figure skaters had a significant postexercise drop in their FEV_1, as do competitive ice hockey players. Conversely, with the exception of the suspected effects of chlorine and chemical exposure as described earlier, athletes who swim are breathing in warm, humidified air that may abrogate some of the effects of hyperventilation and airway cooling and dehydration. Summer sports are associated with less EIA, 16% in the 1996 Summer Olympic Games, a significant decrease compared to the Winter Olympic Games. Sports with vigorous exercise, such as basketball and soccer, are more likely to raise minute ventilation and induce EIB than sports such as baseball. However, as alluded to earlier, even sports previously considered preferable for those with EIB may induce symptoms. Seasonal outdoor activities are also more likely to expose athletes to high pollen counts, which could worsen bronchospasm in susceptible atopic individuals.

Olympics

The incidence of EIB in Olympic athletes is on the rise. As early as 1984, the U.S. Olympic Committee discovered through a screening program that 67 of 597 athletes had asthma or EIB. Each subsequent set of Olympic Games, winter and summer, has seen a rise in the diagnosis of EIB in athletes. Between 1984 and 1996, the percentage of athletes requesting International Olympic Committee (IOC) approval for use of an inhaled β-agonist doubled. In the 2000 summer games, 5.5% of participants notified the IOC of their inhaled β-agonist use for the treatment of EIA. This represented an increase from 3.6% during the Atlanta games. The prevalence of EIA in winter Olympic athletes is much higher, as expected:

17% in 1998 and higher at each subsequent Winter Olympics Games.

This rise has become an important issue in regard to antidoping policies, and certain medications are restricted by the IOC. Since 1976, inhaled bronchodilator usage has been permitted with an accompanying physician's letter. As of 2001, clinical laboratory evidence was required at least a week prior to competition to obtain permission for inhaled bronchodilator use. For the first time, at the Salt Lake City 2002 Olympic Games, athletes with asthma were required to prove their diagnosis with spirometry and medical record documentation. Although inhaled bronchodilators are not likely to enhance performance or offer an additional advantage to asthmatics over nonasthmatic competitors, oral bronchodilators may do so. For this reason, oral β-agonists have been banned. Inhaled formoterol, albuterol, salmeterol, terbutaline, and related medications are restricted. Oral, rectal, intravenous, and intramuscular steroids are prohibited. The National Collegiate Athletic Association (NCAA) permits athletes to use all inhaled, but not oral, β-agonists. Up-to-date guidelines for patients participating in high-performance sports can be obtained from the respective websites of the International Olympic Committee, the U.S. Olympic Committee, the National Collegiate Athletic Association, and the International Skating Union.

Hiking

High-altitude sports also require special consideration for those with EIB. At higher altitudes, the air is cooler and drier, and hikers are at risk for hypoxia. However, Boner et al. documented improved function in asthmatics at higher altitude, hypothesizing that it may be secondary to decreased pollen and dust mite allergen concentrations as well as less pollution at these altitudes. Hypoxia may lead to natural adrenal steroid production that may protect the airway.

SCUBA

Scuba divers are at particular theoretical risk for EIB, which may be life threatening during dives. Because there are nearly 9 million sport divers in the United States alone, this is an important consideration for physicians. Approximately 7% of scuba divers have asthma, similar to the incidence of asthma in the general population. These asthmatic divers may risk higher chance of decompression-related illness and arterial gas embolism by the following mechanism. According to Boyle's law, there is an inverse relationship between the pressure and the volume of a gas. As ascent occurs and pressure decreases, the gas expands, increasing its volume. These effects are more pronounced closer to the surface, so diving in shallow water is not protective.

Furthermore, scuba divers breath cold, dry air that may exacerbate EIA by mechanisms described earlier in this chapter. This, along with possible inhalation of aerosolized hypertonic saline from faulty regulators, aeroallergens introduced when tanks are filled, as well as increased exertional work of breathing, may lead to bronchospasm. With bronchospasm, trapped air may lead to barotraumas with pneumothorax, pneumomediastinum, and sinus and ear barotrauma, a particular problem for those with EIA and nasal congestion, which often go hand in hand. The Thoracic Society of Australia and New Zealand recommends that at-risk divers undergo pulmonary function testing with a cold, dry air inhalation challenge. For those with a positive challenge test, diving may not be recommended. A history of recent active asthma within the past 5 years may also be a contraindication (see section on evidence-based medicine for more information).

SCUBA DIVING AND EIA: EVIDENCE-BASED MEDICINE

Diving with asthma is at least theoretically a risky endeavor because of the mechanisms described earlier in this chapter. Many physicians do not endorse diving for their asthmatic patients. However, many asthmatic patients will continue to dive, whether secondary to improper education regarding the risks or in spite of it. Although a significant amount of research still needs to be done in this area to provide evidence-based recommendations to divers, some recent work in the field merits review.

Hagberg and Ornhagen published a retrospective cohort study in *Undersea & Hyperbaric Medicine* in 2003. They sent a validated questionnaire to dive masters and dive instructors in Sweden to investigate possible risk factors for decompression sickness. Asthma was not a risk factor for decompression sickness symptoms in this cohort. Detractions include the fact that there was a predominance of male versus female divers included in this study, and the study was from an isolated location/population. Although this data may suggest a trend toward safety for the diving asthmatic, further research is warranted.

Cirillo et al. published a report in *Medicine and Science of Sports & Exercise* in 2003 comparing atopic nonasthmatics and healthy subjects. They evaluated pulmonary function tests and the skin-prick test for environmental antigens and then performed methacholine challenge before, immediately after, and 24 hours after a dive. The asymptomatic atopic subjects had a significant decline in the methacholine dose required to cause a 20% fall in FEV_1. Although the number evaluated in this study was only 30 subjects, this does suggest a higher risk in atopic

patients for airway hyperresponsiveness with dives, even if they lack the diagnosis of asthma.

Tetzlaff and Muth distributed questionnaires to scuba divers in Germany, Austria, and Switzerland and published their results in the *International Journal of Sports Medicine* in 2005. Of the divers, 8.7% indicated current asthma and two thirds had regular dyspnea. Only 42.4% were on regular medications. Of 17,386 dives, there were no cases of serious diving injuries in this group. This study demonstrated that asthmatics are definitely diving, and their risk may be no different than those without asthma.

The British Thoracic Society Fitness to Dive Group, a subgroup of the British Society Standards of Care Committee, performed a literature search of major scientific databases as well as a review of major diving-related websites. They published recommendations based on the evidence they reviewed in *Thorax* in 2003. In regard to asthma and scuba diving, they made several recommendations. Those asthmatics with symptoms worsened by exercise, cold, or emotion were advised not to dive. They further stated that asthmatics may be permitted to dive if they are free of asthma symptoms, and have "normal" pulmonary function testing, as defined by an FEV_1 more than 80% or FVC-to-FEV_1 ratio more than 70%, and a negative exercise test with fall in FEV_1 less than 15%. Patients with asthma should monitor peak flows twice per day and refrain from diving with active asthma requiring rescue medication 48 hours prior to a scheduled dive, with PEF drop more than 10% from baseline or with diurnal variation greater than 20%. All these literature-based recommendations were only category C recommendations, suggesting a need for further study.

As in most aspects related to EIA, there is need for further research to provide evidence-based guidelines to minimize patient morbidity and mortality while allowing symptomatic individuals to live normal and full lives.

CONCLUSION

EIB is very common in the general population as well as in elite athletes. Exercise should be encouraged rather than limited because with proper diagnosis and treatment, EIB should not limit performance. Part of the responsibility of the physician caring for patients with EIB includes education of the public. In several studies, despite the high prevalence of EIA in children, teachers did not demonstrate knowledge of the condition or its management. As the subject of EIA/EIB expands, look for further guidelines to aid in the diagnosis and management of the ever-growing percentage of the population with this condition.

BIBLIOGRAPHY

Anderson S, Seale JP, Ferris L, et al. An evaluation of pharmacotherapy for exercise-induced asthma. *J Allergy Clin Immunol.* 1979;64(6 pt2):612.

Anderson SD, Daviskas E. The mechanism of exercise-induced asthma is . . . *J Allergy Clin Immunol.* 2000;106(3):453.

Anderson SD, Holzer K. Exercise-induced asthma: is it the right diagnosis in elite athletes? *J Allergy Clin Immunol.* 2000;106(3):419.

Bisgaard H. Long-acting B2 agonists in management of childhood asthma: a critical review of the literature. *Pediatr Pulmonol.* 2000;29:221.

Boner AL, Niero E, Antolini L, DeStafano G. Biphasic (early and late) asthmatic responses to exercise in children with severe asthma, resident at high altitude. *Eur J Pediatr.* 1985 Jul;144(2):164–6.

Boulet LP, Legris C, Turcotte H, Herbert J. Prevalence and characteristics of late asthmatic responses to exercise. *J Allergy Clin Immunol.* 1987 Nov;80(5):655–62.

Chhabra SK, Ojha UC. Late asthmatic response in exercise-induced asthma. *Ann Allergy Asthma Immunol.* 1998 Apr;80(4):323–7.

Cirillo I, Vizzaccaro A, Crimi E. Airway reactivity and diving in healthy and atopic subjects. *Med Sci Sports Exerc.* 2003;35; 1493–8.

Davies MJ, Fisher LH, Chegini S, et al. Asthma and the diver. *Clin Rev Allergy Immunol.* 2005;29:1.

de Benedictis FM, Tuteri G, Pazzelli P, et al. Combination drug therapy for the prevention of exercise-induced bronchoconstriction in children. *Ann Allergy Asthma Immunol.* 1998; 80(4):352.

Godrey S, Konig P. Inhibition of exercise-induced asthma by different pharmacological pathways. *Thorax.* 1976;31:137.

Guidelines for methacholine and exercise-challenge testing—1999. *Am J Respir Crit Care Med.* 2000;161:309.

Hagberg M, Ornhagen H. Incidence and risk factors for symptoms of decompression sickness among male and female dive masters and instructors–a retrospective cohort study. *Undersea Hyperb Med.* 2003;30(2):93–102.

Langdeau J, Turcotte H, Bowie DM, et al. Airway hyperresponsiveness in elite athletes. *Amer J Respir Crit Care Med.* 2000; 161:1479.

McFadden ER, Gilbert IA. Exercise-induced asthma. *N Engl J Med.* 1994;330:1362.

McFadden ER, Lenner KAM, Strohl KP. Postexertional airway rewarming and thermally induced asthma. *J Clin Invest.* 1986; 78:18.

O'Byrne PM. Leukotrienes in the pathogenesis of asthma. *Chest.* 2006;111:27.

Scollo M, Zanconato S, Ongaro R, Zaramella C, Zacchello F, Baraldi E. Exhaled nitric oxide and exercised-induced bronchospasm in asthmatic children. *Am J Respir Crit Care Med.* 2000;161:1047–50.

Tan RA, Spector SL. Exercise-induced asthma: diagnosis and management. *Ann Allergy Asthma Immunol.* 2002;89(3):226.

Tetzlaff K, Muth CM. Demographics and respiratory illness prevalence of sport scuba divers. *Int J Sports Med.* 2005 Sep;26(7):607–10.

Occupational Asthma

Jonathan A. Bernstein, MD

DEFINITION

Occupational asthma (OA) has been defined as "a disease characterized by variable airflow limitation and/or hyperresponsiveness and/or inflammation due to causes and conditions attributable to a particular occupational environment and not to stimuli encountered outside the workplace." Two types of OA need to be distinguished based on the presence of a latency period (includes most high molecular weight agents and some low molecular weight agents) or absence of a latency period (includes irritant-induced asthma, also known as reactive airways dysfunction syndrome). High molecular weight (HMW) agents refer to plant or animal proteins larger than 1000 kD, such as natural rubber latex, enzymes, or laboratory animal allergens. Low molecular weight (LMW) agents refer to chemicals smaller than 1000 kd that usually require conjugation with endogenous proteins to form a complete hapten capable of eliciting an immunogenic response. Examples include isocyanates, acid anhydrides, and metallic salts. It is important to emphasize that preexisting asthma does not preclude a diagnosis of OA. The term *work-exacerbated asthma* has been recommended for patients with this presentation.

HISTORICAL PERSPECTIVE: INCIDENCE AND PREVALENCE

The first reference to asthma in workers was cited by Hippocrates (460–370 BC) in reference to metal workers, tailors, horsemen, farmhands, and fisherman. Throughout history, physicians have increasingly recognized the relationship between asthma and a variety of occupations.

The incidence of OA is difficult to estimate because there are significant differences among countries, ranging from 10 to 114 per million per year. These differences are largely due to methodological differences in calculating incidence and the types of occupations and employment opportunities in each country. The Sentinal Event Notification System for Occupational Risks (SENSOR) was developed in several U.S. states in the 1980s to encourage reporting of OA cases by physicians and to put them in contact with public health agencies responsible for investigating high-risk workplaces. This program was successful at increasing awareness among physicians about OA; however, as with other notification systems, underreporting was a problem. Other countries have developed voluntary reporting registries to identify an ongoing incidence and prevalence of OA with varying degrees of success. Asthma cases being evaluated for work-related medicolegal benefits have been another source for estimating the incidence of OA.

Overall, it has been estimated that 5% to 15% of all new diagnoses of asthma are occupationally related. More than 250 agents in the workplace have now been associated with causing OA. Cross-sectional studies have provided much of the prevalence data available for many of these agents known to cause OA. The prevalence of OA varies between occupations. For example, studies have found the prevalence of OA among laboratory animal workers is approximately 20%, whereas western red cedar asthma occurs in approximately 5% of workers. The prevalence of OA has been estimated to occur in 7% to 9% of bakers for baker's asthma, 5% to 10% of isocyanate-exposed workers, 20% to 50% of platinum-exposed workers, and up to 60% of enzyme-exposed workers.

The prevalence for OA within a specific occupation depends on many factors, including environmental conditions within the plant, exposure levels, and the number of exposed workers. For example, at first glance, it might appear that isocyanate-exposed workers have a lower prevalence of OA compared to platinum-exposed workers. However, the absolute number of workers exposed to isocyanates (more than 100,000) each year results in a greater absolute number of workers who develop isocyanate-induced OA compared to platinum-exposed workers.

Unfortunately, cross-sectional studies can underestimate the prevalence of OA due to the "healthy worker effect." This phenomenon occurs as the result of symptomatic workers leaving the workplace because of illness, which results in a misleading healthier workforce. Therefore, to obtain more accurate prevalence statistics and information about the causes, risk factors, and natural course of OA, surveillance programs have been established in developed countries, including the United Kingdom, United States, and Finland. The SWORD (Surveillance of Work-Related and Occupational Respiratory Disease) program established in the United Kingdom involves voluntary reporting of occupational illnesses from a variety of industries by pulmonologists and occupational medicine physicians. This program has already yielded useful prevalence data due to the excellent response rate from participating physicians. Thus far, SWORD has identified OA as the most frequently reported occupational respiratory illness and isocyanates as the most common specific cause of OA. As mentioned, the SENSOR program established in the United States has not been as successful in obtaining useful epidemiologic data due to a poor response rate from participating physicians. This is in contrast to Finland's program, which has already compiled enough data to estimate the country's yearly incidence of OA and hypersensitivity pneumonitis.

PATHOGENESIS

Our understanding of asthma has been greatly enhanced with the advent of bronchoscopy, bronchoalveolar lavage, and bronchial biopsies. The pathogenic features of OA are similar to what has been observed in non-OA patients. In general, lung biopsies of patients with OA demonstrate increased numbers of inflammatory cells with a predominance of eosinophils and lymphocytes, increased intercellular spaces between epithelial cells, and thickening of the reticular basement membrane due to deposition of collagen (types I, III, and V). Interestingly, the degree of reticular basement membrane thickening has been demonstrated to differ among different forms of OA. For example, workers with reactive airways dysfunction syndrome (RADS) have thickening that can reach 30 to 40 μm compared to 6 to 15 μm in workers with diisocyanate asthma and 3 to 8 μm in normal subjects. Airway inflammation associated with OA involves similar bioactive mediators and proinflammatory cytokines identified in non-OA. Certain causes of work-related lower respiratory symptoms have been reported to manifest as eosinophilic bronchitis, characterized as a chronic cough with sputum eosinophilia in the absence of bronchial airway hyperresponsiveness. For example, natural rubber latex, mushroom spores, acrylates, and epoxy resins present as eosinophilic bronchitis. Occupational asthma manifesting as neutrophilic inflammation is less common but has been reported with some LMW agents. For non-OA

the presence of neutrophils is believed to be a marker of severity, but their role in different causes of OA is still unclear.

Patients with OA can exhibit the inflammatory phases of asthma similar to non-OA. However, some forms of OA are more commonly associated with either the early airway response (EAR), the late airway response (LAR), or a dual airway response (DAR). For example, whereas an EAR may be more characteristic of HMW agents, an LAR or DAR may be more commonly seen in workers with isocyanates-induced OA. Therefore it is important for the clinician to be familiar with these different disease presentations to avoid missing a diagnosis of OA because symptoms by history begin after leaving the workplace.

MECHANISMS OF OCCUPATIONAL ASTHMA

In general, many HMW and LMW agents known to cause OA involve TH2 proinflammatory cytokines characteristic of IgE-mediated allergic asthma. For example, enzymes commonly used in the detergent manufacturing industry are proteins that have been well documented to cause OA through IgE-mediated mechanism. Acid anhydrides are examples of LMW agents known to cause IgE-mediated OA. However, some LMW chemicals (plicatic acid and diisocyanates) cause OA in nonatopic workers through non-IgE–mediated mechanisms. The mechanism(s) by which these agents cause OA is unknown. The mechanism(s) for irritant-induced asthma, or RADS, also remains elusive. It is believed chronic inflammatory changes occur in these workers as the result of toxic injury to bronchial epithelial cells leading to loss of epithelial-derived relaxing factors combined with neurogenic inflammation and release of bioactive mediators and proinflammatory cytokines by nonspecific activation of mast cells. Ongoing research using a variety of animal models is trying to elucidate further the role of innate and adaptive immune responses in causing a variety of non-IgE–mediated forms of OA.

GENETICS OF OCCUPATIONAL ASTHMA

Several studies have now reported potential and important genetic associations in workers who develop OA. For example, workers with acid anhydride OA express the class II HLA molecule DQB1*501, but this same molecule may be protective against developing OA from isocyanates or plicatic acid. Furthermore, the HLA-DRB1*07 phenotype was more commonly expressed in laboratory animal handlers sensitized to rat lipocalin allergens. More recently, certain glutathione-S transferase polymorphisms, important for protecting cells from reactive oxygen species, might protect workers exposed to isocyanates from developing OA and may also play a protective role against developing non-OA from ozone and diesel exhaust particulate exposures. Finally, N-acetyltransferase genotypes may also be important in OA because recent studies have found that individuals with a slow acetylator genotype had a 7.8-fold risk of developing toluene-diisocyanate (TDI) asthma. A variety of other candidate gene polymorphisms found to be associated with non-OA phenotypes have also been investigated to a lesser extent in OA, such as IL-4Rα S478P and IL-4–589.

DIAGNOSIS OF OCCUPATIONAL ASTHMA

History

Table 17–1 summarizes the criteria for defining OA proposed by the American College of Chest Physicians. The diagnosis of OA requires a detailed and comprehensive history (Table 17–2). An inadequate history can often delay the diagnosis of OA for months or years. To prevent omission of important historical data, administration of a physician-directed history in conjunction with a structured questionnaire is recommended. The occupational history should elicit comprehensive demographic data about the worker, present and past employment history, the nature, duration, and temporal pattern of symptoms, and finally any potential risk factors for OA. It is essential that the physician be familiar with most of the known causative HMW and LMW agents of OA and methodologies used for diagnosis (Table 17–3).

Although questionnaires are essential, they have limitations. Occupational questionnaires are sensitive but not specific and therefore cannot be used to make a diagnosis of OA without confirmatory objective testing. The poor correlation between a history of OA and OA confirmed by specific challenge testing emphasizes the limitations of the medical history. Although several itemized questionnaires have been used to obtain an occupational history by different investigators, there is as yet no standardized instrument available for this purpose. However, several groups of experienced investigators have developed questionnaires, which have been validated by repeated use in cross-sectional or longitudinal studies.

The basic components of a structured occupational questionnaire include an employment history and medical history. The employment history should ascertain information regarding the individual's work process, including all jobs that could be related to specific exposures, work processes in adjacent areas, work-shift hours, and previous jobs where the worker may have been exposed to similar or identical agents. The medical history should determine any relationship of symptoms experienced before, during, or after work to a specific exposure in the workplace; duration of symptoms after leaving the workplace; improvement of symptoms on weekends or vacations; associated upper respiratory and dermatologic symptoms; systemic symptoms such as fever, chills, or temperature; smoking history; preexisting allergy/asthma history; and previous chemical spill exposure.

Table 17–1. Criteria for Defining Occupational Asthma Proposed by the American College of Chest Physicians.

A. Diagnosis of asthma
B. Onset of symptoms after entering the workplace
C. Association between symptoms of asthma and work
D. One or more of the following criteria:
    1. Workplace exposure to an agent or process known to give rise to occupational asthma
    2. Significant work-related changes in FEV_1 or peak expiratory flow rate
    3. Significant work-related changes in nonspecific airway responsiveness
    4. Positive response to specific inhalation challenge tests with an agent to which the patient is exposed at work
    5. Onset of asthma with a clear association with a symptomatic exposure to an irritant agent in the workplace (RADS)
Requirements
    Occupational asthma:
    Surveillance case definition: A + B + C + D1 or D2 or D3 or D4 or D5
    Medical case definition: A + B + C + D2 or D3 or D4 or D5
    Likely occupational asthma: A + B + C + D1
    Work-aggravated asthma: A + C (i.e., the subject was symptomatic or required medication before and had an increase in symptoms or medication requirement after entering a new occupational exposure setting)

FEV_1, forced expiratory volume in 1 second; RADS, reactive airways dysfunction syndrome.

Table 17–2. Key Elements of the Occupational History in the Evaluation of Occupational Asthma.

I. Demographic Information
   A. Identification and address.
   B. Personal data including sex, race, and age.
   C. Educational background with quantitation of the number of school years completed.

II. Employment History
   A. Current department and job description including dates begun, interrupted, and ended.
   B. List all other work processes and substances used in the employee's work environment. A schematic diagram of the workplace is helpful to identify indirect exposure to substances emanating from adjacent work stations.
   C. List prior jobs at current workplace with description of job, duration, and identification of material used.
   D. Work history describing employment preceding current workplace. Job descriptions and exposure history must be included.

III. Symptoms
   A. Categories
      1. Chest tightness, wheezing, cough, and shortness of breath.
      2. Nasal rhinorrhea, sneezing, lacrimation, and ocular itching.
      3. Systemic symptoms such as fever, arthralgias, and myalgias.
   B. Duration should be quantitated.
   C. Duration of employment at current job prior to onset of symptoms.
   D. Identify temporal pattern of symptoms in relationship to work.
      1. Immediate onset beginning at work with resolution soon after coming home.
      2. Delayed onset beginning 4–12 h after starting work or after coming home.
      3. Immediate onset followed by recovery with symptoms recurring 4–12 h after initial exposure to suspect agent at work.
   E. Improvement away from work.

IV. Identify Potential Risk Factors
   A. Obtain a smoking history along with current smoking status and quantitate number of pack-years.
   B. Asthmatic symptoms preceding current work exposure.
   C. Atopic status
      1. Identify consistent history of seasonal nasal or ocular symptoms.
      2. Family history of atopic disease.
      3. Confirmation by epicutaneous testing to a panel of common aeroallergens.
   D. History of accidental exposures to substances such as heated fumes or chemical spills.

The classic presentation of a worker with OA often consists of symptoms that begin at work and resolve or improve either shortly after leaving the workplace at night, during weekends, or while on vacation. However, a worker with OA may not improve away from the workplace because of chronic airway inflammation as a result of persistent workplace exposure to an agent for months or years after the initial onset of symptoms. In addition, patients with RADS typically do not improve away from work. Therefore, the diagnosis of OA should not be overlooked because of the apparent lack of correlation of symptoms to workplace exposure.

Material safety data sheets (MSDSs) are an essential part of the occupational history. They provide valuable information regarding generic chemical names and specific constituents of raw materials being used in the workplace. They also provide standard information about threshold limit values (TLV) and permissible exposure levels (PEL) of potentially toxic and/or sensitizing

agents. When available, assistance from industrial hygienists or safety officers familiar with the workplace and the worker's exposure history should be sought. On occasion, these documents have proprietary agents not specifically listed that may cause OA. Therefore, it may be necessary for the clinician to call the company to obtain this additional exposure information.

Differential Diagnosis

A diagnosis of OA can be incorrectly made in individuals with preexisting asthma or allergic asthma due to nonworkplace allergens. In these cases, symptoms are aggravated by exposure to irritants, physical factors (e.g., cold air), or common indoor allergens (e.g., dust mites) in the workplace. However, it should be emphasized that preexisting asthma does not preclude the development of OA. In these cases, workers may be experiencing work-exacerbated asthma or asthma due to a new

Table 17–3. Etiologic Agents of Occupational Asthma and Reported Immunologic Tests.

Agent	In vivo	In vitro
Azodicarbonamide	Prick tests with 0.1%, 1%, and 5% azodicarbonamide	Not done
Baby's breath	Intradermal titration testing	RAST/histamine release
Bacillus subtilis enzymes	Prick tests with 0.05, 0.5, 5, and 10 mg/mL	RAST/radial immunodiffusion
Buckwheat flour	Prick test with 10 mg/mL	Reverse enzyme immunoassay/ histamine release
Carmine dye	Skin test with *Coccus cactus*	RAST to dyes
Castor bean	Prick test with 1:100 extract	Not done
Chloramine-T, halazone	Scratch test at 10^{-5} dilution	Not done
Chromate	Prick test at 10, 5, 1, and 0.1 mg/mL $Cr_2(SO_4)_3$	RAST to HSA-chromium sulfate
Cobalt	Patch tests	RAST to HSA-cobalt sulfate
Coffee bean	Intradermal titration to coffee bean extract	RAST to coffee bean extract
Diazonium tetrafluoroborate (DTFB)	Not done	RAST to HSA-DTFB
Dimethylethanolamine	Prick tests to dimethylethanolamine undiluted at 1:10, 1:100, and 1:1000	Not done
Douglas fir tussock moth	Cutaneous tests with 1:25 extract	Histamine release
Dyes, textiles	Prick or scratch tests to dyes at 10 mg/mL in 50% glycerine	HSA-dye
Egg proteins	Prick tests with 1:10 w/v egg white, egg yolk, whole egg; prick tests to 10 mg/mL egg white fractions	RAST to egg proteins
Ethylenediamine	Intracutaneous test to 1:100 ethylenediamine	Not done
Furan binder	Not done	RAST to catalyst, sand, and furfuryl alcohol
Garlic	Prick test titrations beginning at 10^{-5} garlic extract	PTRIA for IgE against garlic extract
Grain dust, grain dust mite	Prick and intracutaneous tests with grain dust and grain mite	Not done
Grain weevil	Skin test to weevil extract	Not done
Gum acacia	Skin tests with gum arabic	Not done
Guar gum	Prick tests with 1 mg/mL guar gum	RAST with guar gum
Hexamethylene-diisocyanate (HDI)	Prick tests to HSA-HDI	ELISA to HSA-HDI
Hexahydrophthalic anhydride (HHPA)	Not done	RAST to HSA-HHPA
Hog trypsin	Skin test to trypsin	Histamine release

(Continued)

Table 17–3. Etiologic Agents of Occupational Asthma and Reported Immunologic Tests. (Continued)

Agent	In vivo	In vitro
Laboratory animals	Skin tests with serum and urine extracts from animals	ELISA
Latex	Prick test using low ammonia latex solution	Not done
Locusts	Prick tests with locust extract at 0.1, 1, and 10 mg/mL	ELISA
Mealworm	Prick test titration beginning at 1:20 w/v *Tenibrio molitor* (TM extract)	RAST to TM extract
Diphenol methane diisocyanate (MDI)	Prick test with 5 mg/mL HSA-MDI; intradermal test with 1 µg/mL and 10 µg/mL	ELISA to HSA-MDI
Mushroom	Prick test with mushroom extract	Not done
Nickel	Prick tests with $NiSO_4$ at 100, 10, 5, 1, and 0.1 mg/mL	RAST to $HSA-NiSO_4$
Papain	Skin test with papain at 1.25 to 20 mg/mL	RAST to papain
Pancreatic extract	Prick tests with 1:100 and 1:1000 extracts	Not done
Penicillin	Prick tests to ampicillin at 10^{-3} to 10^{-2} mol/L, benzyl penicilloyl polylysine at 10^{-6} mol/L, and minor determinants at 10^{-2} mol/L	Not done
Penicillamine	Prick tests with penicillamine; major and minor penicillin determinants at 0.01, 0.1, and 1 mg/mL	Not done
Phthalic anhydride (PA) and tetrachlorophthalic anhydride (TCPA)	Prick and intradermal tests to HSA-PA and HSA-TCPA	ELISA; PTRIA to HSA-PA only
Platinum	Prick tests with complex platinum salts from 10^{-3} to 10^{-11} g/mL	RAST to $(NH_4)_2PtCl_2$, RAST to HSA-platinum and histamine release
Poultry mites	Skin tests with 1:10 w/v northern fowl mite (NFM)	RAST to NFM
Protease bromelain	Prick test with bromelain at 10 mg/mL	RAST to bromelain
Redwood	Prick test to redwood sawdust extract	Not done
Spiramycin	Prick tests with 10 and 100 mg/mL spiramycin	Not done
Tobacco	Skin tests with green tobacco extract 10 mg/mL	RAST with green tobacco extract
Toluene diisocyanate (TDI)	Prick test to 5 mg/mL HSA-TDI	RAST and ELISA to HSA-TDI, histamine release
Trimellitic anhydride (TMA)	Prick tests to 3.4 mg/mL HSA-TMA and TMA in acetone	PTRIA with HSA-TMA
Western red cedar (WRC)	Prick tests with 25 mg/mL WRC extract; intracutaneous testing with 2.5 mg/mL WRC	Not done
Wheat flour	Prick tests with 10% w/v extract	RAST to wheat flour and wheat flour components

ELISA, enzyme-linked immunoabsorbent assay; HSA, human serum albumin; PTRIA, polystyrene-tube radioimmunoassay; RAST, radioallergosorbent assay test; w/v, weight (of solute) per volume (of solution).

workplace allergen or chemical exposure. At times, OA must also be distinguished from other diseases, such as chronic obstructive lung disease, pneumoconiosis, bronchiolitis obliterans, and endotoxin-induced asthma-like syndromes such as grain fever or byssinosis. These disorders are differentiated from OA by history, chest radiograph, chest computerized tomography (CT) scan, lung volumes with diffusion capacity, and, if necessary, open lung biopsy. Chest radiographs and diffusing capacity of lung for carbon monoxide (DLCO) are usually normal in workers with OA.

Immunologic Assessment

Immunologic mechanisms have been confirmed for many causes of OA. Therefore, it is important to investigate whether specific immune responses to suspected agents with allergenic potential are involved. Although identification of an immunologic response to a specific agent helps phenotype different forms of OA, it is usually not diagnostic. Such a response may only reflect exposure and/or the immunogenic nature of the inciting agent. Cutaneous sensitization to an offending agent indicates a high risk for OA but lacks the specificity needed to diagnose OA. Several types of immune responses are associated with HMW and LMW agents that cause OA. Type I IgE-mediated immune responses have been identified for the majority of HMW proteins derived from a variety of plant and animal sources known to cause OA. IgE-mediated immune responses have also been identified as the underlying mechanism for several LMW chemical agents, such as acid anhydrides and platinum salts. Although type II cytotoxic, type III immune-complex, and Type IV cell-mediated immune responses have been linked to certain causes of OA, measures of specific IgE are usually the simplest and most readily available tests for diagnosing OA.

HMW antigens are considered complete allergens because they do not require structural modification to elicit a specific immune response. In vivo skin testing and in vitro immunoassays have been used to identify sensitized individuals to these specific allergens. HMW allergens include proteins from animal dander, insect scales, food products, and enzymes used in the food manufacturing and pharmaceutical industries. LMW chemical agents require structural modification to act as complete antigens. Traditionally, these reactive chemicals are coupled to a carrier molecule such as an autologous human protein (e.g., human serum albumin, or HSA). The chemical hapten-protein conjugate forms new antigenic determinants, which are capable of inducing an IgE-mediated response.

The test reagents used in the diagnosis of OA must be characterized and standardized. Standardization of an allergen extract requires identification of the allergen source, the extraction procedure, and its biochemical composition. The allergen source should be fresh and free of contaminants. The extraction process should record characteristics such as temperature, the medium used for extraction, the extraction time period, and the filtration methods utilized. Proper characterization should include total protein content, molecular weight range of proteins, isoelectric points of each protein, and identification of immunologic and allergenic components. The latter can be determined by a variety of techniques, such as the radioallergosorbent test (RAST) or enzyme-linked immunoabsorbent assay (ELISA), Western blotting, leukocyte histamine release assays, and endpoint skin test titration techniques.

LMW chemicals can be conjugated to a carrier protein and used as an antigen for use in immunodiagnostic tests. Platinum chloride salts and sulfonechloramide represent two examples where LMW agents have been directly used as skin test reagents without prior conjugation to proteins. The most common protein carrier used is HSA. Successful hapten-protein conjugation depends on the buffers used, the amount of protein and chemicals used, and the duration and temperature of the reaction. To determine the degree of chemical linkage to protein, the ratio of chemical ligand to protein carrier (mols/mole) must be established. This analysis is essential because antigenicity and allergenicity of the final conjugate may vary with ligand density. The method of analysis depends on the chemical structure of the compound. For example, spectrophotometric analysis is used to assess aromatic compounds, and free amino analysis is used for chemicals that bind to carrier amines. Gas chromatography and mass spectroscopy are the preferred methods for analysis of aliphatic chemical-protein antigens. The ideal range of ligand binding should fall between 10 and 20 molecules of chemical per molecule of protein. Over- or underconjugation of ligand to protein binding can result in poor test antigens. The methods described for biochemical composition of HMW complete proteins can also be used for analysis of hapten-protein conjugates.

Clinical immunologic assessment of workers suspected for OA should include in vivo and in vitro tests when they are available. The prick skin test is the most commonly used in vivo test to assess IgE-mediated hypersensitivity responses to occupational protein allergens. The prick test concentration usually ranges between 0.1 and 10 mg/mL.

In vitro tests can detect specific IgG and IgE antibody responses to a suspected causative occupational agent. RAST requires binding of the specific allergen to a solid phase material, which is then incubated with the subject's serum and radiolabeled anti-human IgE. The number of radioisotopic counts bound is directly proportional to the amount of serum-specific IgE. The RAST test has been largely supplanted by ELISA because the latter does not require use of radioisotopes. This assay differs from the RAST in that the allergen is bound to a plastic well with high binding avidity and then incubated with the subject's serum and anti-human IgE conjugated to alkaline phosphatase. This results in a colormetric change, which is measured by spectrophotometry. The optical density is proportional to the amount of specific IgE in the subject's serum.

For natural protein allergens such as enzymes, ELISA-specific IgE assays are specific assays but tend to be less sensitive than skin prick testing. False-positive reactions can occur in the presence of high serum total IgE levels due to nonspecific binding, and false negatives can occur as the result of binding of a specific isotypic antibody other than IgE.

ELISA assays are also used to measure specific IgG antibodies. The significance of elevated specific IgG antibodies to a workplace allergen is less clear. Some evidence suggests it could represent a biologic marker of exposure to chemicals such as methylene diphenyl diisocyanate (MDI). Specific IgG antibodies to TMA-HSA–conjugated antigens have been found in both trimellitic anhydride–exposed workers with hemolytic anemia and pulmonary hemorrhage as well as in workers with late systemic symptoms, suggesting that such antibodies may have a mechanistic role in cytotoxic or immune complex–mediated responses.

The proper interpretation of an immunologic test used in the diagnosis of OA requires validation against an accepted benchmark, such as the specific bronchoprovocation test (SBPT). Furthermore, proper standardization of an immunoassay always requires the use of well-established positive and negative control sera.

More recently, investigators have developed an in vitro assay for measuring production of monocyte chemoattractant protein-1 (MCP-1) by mononuclear cells cocultured with diisocyanate-HSA antigens. This assay was demonstrated to have a 91% specificity in specific inhalational challenge–confirmed diisocyanate OA. Unfortunately, this assay is not as practical as other immunoassays because it requires immediate processing of fresh peripheral blood mononuclear cells.

Other in vitro assays, such as lymphocyte proliferation and leukocyte histamine release, have been used primarily as research tools in the investigation of workers with OA. Table 17–2 lists several HMW and LMW agents known to induce OA in workers and the reported immunologic tests that have been performed as part of their assessment. It should be emphasized that skin test responses and in vitro specific antibody responses may decline within months or years after removal from exposure from the causative agent, which may limit their clinical utility in the evaluation of workers remotely exposed to an incriminated agent.

Physiologic Assessment

Many approaches have been used in measuring lung function in workers suspected of OA. Ideally, lung function should be monitored in the workplace during a known exposure to a suspected causative agent. However, this may present logistical problems when conditions in the workplace are not suitable for pulmonary function testing. Personnel experienced in proper performance of pulmonary function testing often are not readily available to conduct serial testing of lung function or employers are not cooperative.

Spirometry should include the forced expiratory volume in 1 second (FEV_1), forced vital capacity (FVC), and the maximum mid-expiratory flow rate (FEF_{25-75}). Assessment of cross-shift lung function (i.e., pre- and postshift FEV_1) has been used to correlate asthma symptoms to workplace exposure, but this approach lacks sensitivity for confirming OA. Multiple assessments of PEFR at work (four to five times per day) often capture enough data to diagnose or exclude OA. Furthermore, cross-shift changes in a worker's lung function have been found to be directly proportional to their level of exposure to the sensitizing agent.

Serial measurements of PEFR, when performed properly, correlate moderately well with results of specific bronchoprovocation testing used in the diagnosis of OA. Serial PEFR measurements should be interpreted with caution due to patient noncompliance or the potential for falsification of measurements. Using computerized peak-flow meters that record effort associated with each measurement, reproducibility, and the exact time of the reading may circumvent these problems.

Although not diagnostic, nonspecific bronchial hyperresponsiveness (NSBH) testing with agonists such as methacholine or histamine are essential for confirming the presence or absence of airway hyperresponsiveness, a central feature of asthma. Subjects with a positive methacholine test and evidence of specific IgE to a HMW are more likely to exhibit a positive SBPT to that agent. Negative tests of NSBH are most useful in excluding a current diagnosis of OA in a currently symptomatic exposed worker.

The SBPT is considered the gold standard for diagnosis of OA. This test should only be administered in specially equipped centers under the supervision of physicians experienced in conducting this procedure. Specific provocation testing is very time consuming and expensive to perform and therefore not readily available. However, if performed properly, the SBPT can be performed with minimal risk. Several airway response patterns may be elicited that are characteristic for workers presenting with OA. An isolated EAR is characterized by the immediate onset of asthma symptoms after exposure to an agent that is more commonly associated with IgE-mediated OA. An isolated LAR, which occurs until 4 to 12 hours after exposure to the challenge agent, is more characteristic of nonimmunologic OA induced by LMW chemical agents. Finally, workers with OA may exhibit a DAR characterized by an EAR followed

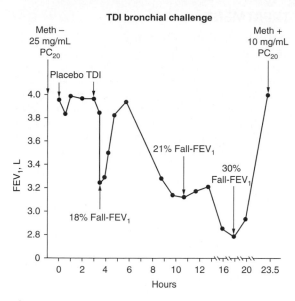

TDI bronchial challenge

Figure 17–1. A dual-asthmatic response in a polyurethane foam worker after bronchoprovocation to toluene diisocyanate (TDI). The early asthmatic response is followed by spontaneous recovery and then a late asthmatic response. The concentration of methacholine required to reduce the forced expiratory volume in 1 second (FEV_1) by 20% (PC_{20}) fell from a baseline of 25 mg/mL to 10 mg/mL, the day after the TDI challenge.

by recovery period and then a LAR. Figure 17–1 is an example of a DAR in a worker diagnosed with diisocyanate-OA by a SBPT. Multiple physiologic patterns have been observed in OA caused by chemicals. For example, workers with diisocyanate-induced OA present 30% to 50% of the time with DARs, 40% of the time with an isolated LAR, and less than 10% of the time with an isolated EAR.

Asthma occurring in the workplace in the absence of a latency period is characteristic of RADS, also referred to as irritant-induced OA. RADS typically occurs after one or more repetitive large inhalational exposure to a toxic chemical agent such as ammonia gas, acidic fumes, smoke, or spray paints. RADS must be differentiated from the irritant symptoms that occur in patients with preexisting asthma. Irritant symptoms disappear promptly after cessation of exposure and are not associated with prolonged bronchoconstriction or bronchial hyperresponsiveness characteristic of RADS. Workers with RADS typically do not manifest airway response patterns seen with OA induced by HMW and LMW agents. Being familiar with the different airway responses associated with various agents known to cause OA can greatly facilitate the correct diagnosis of OA.

Clinical Assessment of Occupational Asthma

The first step for assessing a suspected case of OA is to obtain a careful physician-administered history. As mentioned, an occupational questionnaire is useful in capturing the necessary clinical and exposure information and to help validate information obtained by the physician-administered history. Workers with OA may present with dyspnea, chest tightness, wheezing, and/or cough in or out of the workplace. Upper airway symptoms such as rhinorrhea, nasal congestion, or ocular pruritus preceding the onset of asthmatic symptoms are especially characteristic of IgE-mediated sensitization to HMW agents. Symptoms may begin after immediately starting a work shift (within 1 to 2 hours) or several hours after starting work. Review of MSDSs is often very helpful for identifying agents known to cause OA.

If the history is positive for OA, a test of NSBH (i.e., methacholine or histamine provocation) should be performed at work or within 2 hours after the work shift. Results of this test are usually reported as PC_{20} measurements (provocative concentration of methacholine or histamine causing a 20% decrease in FEV_1). A negative methacholine test (PC_{20} more than 10 mg/mL) would exclude airway hyperresponsiveness (AHR) and is a good negative predictor for asthma. A positive methacholine test indicates the presence of AHR suggestive of asthma but is nonspecific and does not confirm a diagnosis of OA. In this case, assessment of lung function performed at and away from the workplace to demonstrate AHR around the suspected agent is very useful for supporting a diagnosis of OA. When possible, a workplace challenge, which consists of supervised measurements of lung function (i.e., FEV_1) in the actual work site before and during work shifts for at least 1 week of work exposure, should be conducted. Improvement of symptoms and lung function after removal from the workplace with subsequent deterioration after reintroduction into the workplace further supports a diagnosis of OA, except in the case of RADS. If a workplace challenge cannot be performed, PEFR monitoring should be conducted over 2 to 3 weeks at work. The worker should measure and record his or her PEFR every 3 hours while awake or at least four times a day. Work exposure, symptoms, and medication usage should be recorded in a diary during this time. Diurnal variability of greater than 20% at work as compared to normal variability at home is consistent with OA. Visual analysis of weekly plots of PEFR measurements by a blinded physician is the most reliable method of analysis. A consistent pattern of declining PEFRs at work and improvement away from work is strong evidence supporting a diagnosis of OA. PEFR measurements should be interpreted with caution because workers who are seeking compensation could potentially falsify their readings.

The gold standard for the diagnosis of OA is the SBPT. If a specific substance in the workplace is suspected of causing OA and the workplace challenge is equivocal, a SBPT may be necessary. The PC_{20} ascertained by methacholine or histamine testing may be helpful for estimating the initial dose of an occupational agent prior to the specific inhalation challenge test. Because these tests are very time consuming and potentially risky, they should only be performed by experienced individuals. An SBPT should not be performed in workers with severe cardiac or pulmonary disease (FEV_1 less than 60%). Specific inhalation challenge tests have also been used to document causation of OA by new substances in index cases and for medical/legal purposes in proving or excluding a worker's eligibility for workers' compensation. Although specific challenge tests confirm a diagnosis of OA if positive, negative tests do not always exclude the diagnosis in workers who have been removed from the workplace for a period of time during which bronchial AHR to the suspected agent may have resolved. It is therefore important to perform a SBPT either before or shortly after removing the worker from his or her workplace exposure. Another potential problem with specific inhalation challenge testing is poor standardization of methods used among different centers. Furthermore, it may not be possible to reproduce workplace exposure conditions in the laboratory because a number of technical factors, such as temperature, atmospheric pressure, and concentration, must be controlled to assure consistent exposures to chemical agents (i.e., toluene-diisocyanate). In Canada, regional centers have adapted standardized methodologies for performing inhalational challenges that obviate this problem.

In addition to lung function assessment, it is important to identify whether the worker is atopic by skin testing with common aeroallergens and other appropriate allergens, especially when HMW substances are suspected of causing OA. These workers can often be skin-tested using the actual agent they are exposed to, such as flour, coffee beans, castor beans, and egg enzymes (Table 17–3). In vitro assays to measure specific IgE to these proteins can also be performed but are less specific than in vivo skin testing. As previously mentioned, the presence of either a positive prick skin test or serum-specific IgE only indicates IgE-mediated sensitization has occurred and does not prove a clinical diagnosis of OA.

Immunologic testing by RAST or ELISA methods using serum from workers exposed to LMW reactive chemicals is also useful for supporting IgE-mediated sensitization when present. IgG antibodies may represent markers of exposure to a particular chemical antigen. In vivo skin testing to LMW chemical agents has been less reliable for confirming IgE-mediated sensitization. Other in vitro techniques, such as leukocyte histamine release, leukocyte inhibitory factor, and MCP-1, have thus far been reserved for research purposes only.

TREATMENT

Once the diagnosis of OA has been confirmed, the treatment of choice should be to remove the worker from further exposure. Studies evaluating the clinical course of workers after removal from the workplace have found that persistence of their asthma correlated with the duration of exposure and symptoms prior to diagnosis. Individuals with OA caused by diisocyanates or western red cedar wood dust had a better prognosis if they were diagnosed early, relatively well-preserved lung function, and a less AHR. In contrast, symptomatic workers who remained in the workplace for longer periods of time experienced greater deterioration of their lung function, leading to chronic persistent asthma that required increased medication use even after being removed from further exposure. Use of respirators in the work environment generally does not reduce exposure or prevent clinical deterioration. Some studies have suggested that certain types of respirators such as airstream helmets may offer adequate protection for the worker from the offending agent; however, they are generally not considered adequate substitutes for absolute avoidance measures. Pharmacologic treatment of acute or chronic OA is similar to nonoccupational asthma, which involves inhaled corticosteroids, with or without selective long-acting β_2-agonists and leukotriene-modifying agents, theophylline, cromolyn, or nedocromil sodium. Medications can be used in various combinations depending on the severity of the worker's symptoms. Immunotherapy may play a role in the treatment of some forms of OA caused by HMW protein allergens such as laboratory animal proteins.

PREVENTION AND IMMUNOSURVEILLANCE

The primary categories of prevention include reducing exposure to known occupational inciting agents, identifying susceptible workers and removing them from exposure, administering workplace controls to reduce the number of workers exposed or the duration of their exposure, providing personal protective equipment in the workplace, and education of at-risk atopic individuals about avoidance of occupations where the likelihood for developing OA would be increased (e.g., laboratory handlers). Effective prevention of OA requires the cooperation between management and workers in the implementation of good industrial measures aimed at preventing exposure to agents known to cause OA. Every attempt should be made to minimize a worker's exposure to potentially problematic agent(s) through the institution of strict handling procedures. Workers should be continually educated about the importance of adhering to those procedures to avoid inadvertent exposures such as chemical spills. Prescreening of already hired workers for atopy should be considered before assigning employees to jobs where they would have inhalational exposure to sensitizing proteins (e.g., latex, laboratory animals, and enzyme proteins). Comprehensive immunosurveillance programs for detecting and monitoring workers at increased risk for exposure to known inducers of OA need to be implemented in industries that commonly use agents known to cause OA. Industries that have implemented such comprehensive immunosurveillance programs have been successful in reducing the incidence of asthma in the workplace.

EVIDENCE-BASED MEDICINE

Bernstein IL, Bernstein DI, Chan Yeung M, et al. Definition and classification of asthma in the workplace. In: Bernstein IL, Chan-Yeung M, Malo J-L, et al., eds. *Asthma in the Workplace*. 3rd ed. New York: Taylor and Francis; 2006:1.

Asthma in the Workplace is a comprehensive authoritative book on all aspects of OA. This book is an excellent resource for anyone interested in learning more about occupational lung diseases. The book goes into detail regarding pathophysiology, genetics, epidemiology, disease mechanisms, specific causes of OA, clinical diagnosis, treatment, prevention, and surveillance. It is considered the most up-to-date resource on this topic.

Jones MG, Floyd A, Nouri-Aria KT, et al. Is occupational asthma to diisocyanates a non-IgE mediated disease? *J Allergy Clin Immunol*. 2006;117:663.

Diisocyanate OA is the most common cause of OA in the United States. The mechanism for this cause of OA remains elusive, but some studies have demonstrated that specific IgE may be involved and a subset of affected workers. In this study, bronchial biopsies were obtained from workers with positive and negative SBPT to diisocyanates to compare immunohistochemistry changes and the presence of proinflammatory cytokines in these individuals. They found an absence of IL-4 mRNA positive cells but an increased number of IL-5, CD25+, and CD4+ cells in workers with a positive isocyanate challenge, indicating that diisocyanate-induced asthma is likely a non-IgE–mediated disease.

Bernstein DI, Cartier A, Cote J, et al. Diisocyanate antigen-stimulated monocyte chemoattractant protein-1 synthesis has greater test efficiency than specific antibodies for identification of diisocyanate asthma. *Am J Respir Crit Care Med*. 2002;166:445.

Diagnosis of diisocyanate-induced asthma remains problematic and requires a standardized algorithmic approach. Development of diagnostic tests that have increased sensitivity and specificity would improve our ability to diagnose this disease correctly. Monocyte chemoattractant protein-1 (MCP-1) was demonstrated to have a greater sensitivity and specificity than antibody assays in correctly identifying diisocyanate OA.

Bernstein JA. Material safety data sheets: are they reliable in identifying human hazards? *J Allergy Clin Immunol*. 2002;110:35.

MSDSs are an integral part of evaluating workers suspected of having OA. Unfortunately, these documents frequently have limitations that may thwart the clinician's ability to make a correct diagnosis of this disease. Health care personnel should understand how to interpret information provided by MSDSs and recognize that they often contain incomplete information.

BIBLIOGRAPHY

Newman-Taylor AJ, Yucesoy B. Genetics and occupational asthma. In: Bernstein IL, Chan-Yeung M, Malo J-L, et al., eds. *Asthma in the Workplace*. 3rd ed. New York: Taylor and Francis; 2006:87.

Bernstein DI, Cartier A, Cote J, et al. Diisocyanate antigen-stimulated monocyte chemoattractant protein-1 synthesis has greater test efficiency than specific antibodies for identification of diisocyanate asthma. *Am J Respir Crit Care Med*. 2002;166:445.

Bernstein DI, Korbee L, Stauder T, et al. The low prevalence of occupational asthma and antibody-dependent sensitization to diphenylmethane diisocyanate in a plant engineered for minimal exposure to diisocyanates. *J Allergy Clin Immunol*. 1993;92:387.

Bernstein JA, Bernstein IL: Occupationally induced asthma. In: Kaplan AP, ed. *Allergy*. 2nd ed. Philadelphia: WB Saunders; 1997:511.

Bernstein JA: Material safety data sheets: are they reliable in identifying human hazards? *J Allergy Clin Immunol*. 2002;110:35.

Brooks SM, Weiss MA, Bernstein IL: Reactive airways dysfunction syndrome (RADS). Persistent asthma syndrome after high level irritant exposures. *Chest*. 1985;88:376.

Gautrin D, Boulet LP, Boutet M, et al. Is reactive airways dysfunction syndrome a variant of occupational asthma? *J Allergy Clin Immunol*. 1994;93:12.

Bernstein IL, Bernstein, DI, Chan Yeung M, et al. Definition and classification of asthma in the workplace. In: Bernstein IL, Chan-Yeung M, Malo J-L, et al., eds. *Asthma in the Workplace*. 3rd ed. New York: Taylor and Francis; 2006:1.

Bernstein JA, Sarlo K. Enzymes. In: Bernstein IL, Chan-Yeung M, Malo J-L, et al., eds. *Asthma in the Workplace*. 3rd ed. New York: Taylor and Francis; 2006:377.

Jones MG, Floyd A, Nouri-Aria KT, et al. Is occupational asthma to diisocyanates a non-IgE mediated disease? *J Allergy Clin Immunol*. 2006;117:663.

Maestrelli P, Fabbri LM, Mapp CE. Pathophysiology. In: Bernstein IL, Chan-Yeung M, Malo J-L, et al., eds. *Asthma in the Workplace*. 3rd ed. New York: Taylor and Francis; 2006:109.

Becklake MR, Malo J-L, Chan-Yeung M. Epidemiologic approaches in occupational asthma. In: Bernstein IL, Chan-Yeung M, Malo J-L, et al., eds. *Asthma in the Workplace*. 3rd ed. New York: Taylor and Francis; 2006:37.

Park H, Jung K, Kim H, et al. Neutrophil activation following TDI bronchial challenges to airway secretion from subjects with TDI-induced asthma. *Clin Exp Allergy*. 1999;2:1395.

Quirce S. Eosinophilic bronchitis in the workplace. *Curr Opin Allergy Clin Immunol*. 2004;4:87.

Stenton SC. Determinants of whether occupational agents cause early, late, or dual asthmatic response. *Occup Med*. 2000;15:431.

Asthma and Pregnancy

18

Peg Strub, MD

Asthma is one of the most common chronic diseases and affects up to 7% of pregnancies. The recently validated "one-third rule" states that in pregnancies with asthma, a third of the patients will improve, a third will get worse, and a third will stay the same.

Asthma in two thirds of pregnant women will either worsen or show no improvement; the importance of treating all persistent asthmatics with inhaled corticosteroids must be emphasized. One large study showed that in women using inhaled corticosteroids prior to pregnancy, the number of emergency department visits for asthma remained unchanged, and the rate of physician visits for asthma actually decreased after pregnancy.

Despite worsening or unchanged asthma in two thirds of the patients, pregnant women in general report a decrease in asthma symptoms throughout the pregnancy, particularly in the last 4 weeks of pregnancy. This perceived improvement may be explained by hormonal changes or other factors and may lead to difficulties with medication adherence.

ADVERSE PREGNANCY OUTCOMES FOR PATIENTS WITH ASTHMA

Studies have shown that pregnant women with asthma are at increased risk for pregnancy-induced hypertension, preeclampsia, eclampsia, vaginal bleeding, perinatal mortalities, premature birth, low birth weights, and neonatal sepsis. For pregnancies complicated by moderate to severe asthma, studies report an increased incidence of Cesarean section deliveries. Pregnancies with poorly controlled asthma are at risk for intrauterine growth retardation (IUGR).

PHYSIOLOGY

During pregnancy, many physiologic changes occur in the mother. Understanding these changes is important not only for the care of the pregnant patient with asthma but also for the fetus.

Maternal Respiratory Physiology

In early pregnancy, 60% to 70% of women feel dyspneic due to hyperventilation. The mechanism of the hyperventilation is progesterone mediated with a resultant increase in tidal volume. As pregnancy progresses, an up to 50% increase in minute volume occurs with a corresponding increase in oxygen consumption and carbon dioxide production. The increase in carbon dioxide production is partially blunted by an increase in renal excretion of bicarbonate (explaining the polyuria of early pregnancy), resulting in a mild compensatory respiratory alkalosis. During pregnancy, arterial blood gases (ABGs) typically have pH levels at 7.42 to 7.46, P_{CO_2} levels at 26 to 30 mm Hg, and P_{O_2} levels at 99 to 106 mm Hg.

The increased size and pressure of the uterus limits diaphragmatic excursion, lowering residual volume and functional residual capacity. Compensation occurs by increased mobility and flaring of the ribs, as well as by a progesterone-mediated relaxation of bronchial smooth muscle. The net result is that pulmonary function test results remain unchanged for forced expiratory volume in 1 second (FEV_1), forced vital capacity (FVC), the forced expiratory volume in 1 second to forced vital capacity ratio (FEV_1 to FVC), and peak expiratory flow rate (PEFR) (Table 18–1).

Maternal Cardiovascular Physiology

Although central venous pressure remains unchanged, there is a 40% increase in maternal cardiac volume and cardiac output with a marked increase in left ventricular mass, compliance, and end-diastolic volume. Total blood volume increases by 40%, but plasma volume increases more than red cell mass resulting in anemia of pregnancy or physiologic hemodilution (Table 18–2).

Maternal Gastroesophageal Reflux

Gastroesophageal reflux during pregnancy is a common complaint and may exacerbate asthma. The increase in

Table 18–1. Maternal respiratory physiology.

- 60–70% of patients have dyspnea of early pregnancy due to hyperventilation.
- Progesterone-related tidal volume increase.
- Minute ventilation increases up to 50% with increased O_2 consumption and CO_2 production.
- Compensatory respiratory alkalosis (pH 7.42–7.46, P_{CO_2} 26–30, and P_{O_2} 99–106).
- Increased size and pressure of uterus limits diaphragmatic excursion.
- Increased mobility and flaring of ribs.
- Progesterone may relax bronchial smooth muscle.
- Pulmonary function tests remain essentially unchanged.

Table 18–3. Fetal physiology.

- Fetus functions by aerobic metabolism
- Mechanisms allowing fetus to thrive
  - Increase in hemoglobin content
  - Increase in oxygen affinity of fetal hemoglobin
  - Preferential blood flow to vital organs
  - High cardiac output
  - Leftward shift of oxygen dissociation curve
- Acid–base balance important
- Increase in maternal P_{CO_2} may result in fetal acidosis, even with adequate oxygenation

gastroesophageal reflux may be due to progesterone-mediated relaxation of smooth muscle of the esophagus with a resultant increase in intraabdominal pressure (Table 18–2).

Fetal Physiology

The fetus functions by aerobic metabolism, even though the P_{O_2} level of the fetus is one fourth of the P_{O_2} level of the mother. Mechanisms allowing the fetus to thrive include an increase in hemoglobin content and the oxygen affinity of fetal hemoglobin, preferential blood flow to vital organs, high cardiac output, and leftward shift of the oxygen dissociation curve.

A low maternal P_{O_2} is important to normal fetal acid-base balance. An increase in maternal P_{O_2} may affect this balance and result in fetal acidosis, even with adequate oxygenation (Table 18–3).

ASTHMA TREATMENT DURING PREGNANCY

The treatment goal for the pregnant asthma patient is to provide optimal therapy to maintain control of asthma for maternal health and quality of life as well as for

Table 18–2. Maternal cardiovascular physiology.

- Central venous pressure remains unchanged
- 40% increase in maternal cardiac volume
- 40% increase in cardiac output
- Increase in left ventricular mass, compliance, and end-diastolic volume
- Plasma volume increases more than red cell mass: anemia of pregnancy

normal fetal maturation, as per the National Asthma Education Prevention Program (NAEPP). Asthma control is defined as follows:

- Minimal or no chronic symptoms day or night
- Minimal or no exacerbations
- No limitations on activities
- Maintenance of normal or near-normal pulmonary function
- Minimal use of short-acting inhaled β_2-antagonist
- Minimal or no adverse effects from medications. Always consult latest NAEPP guidelines.

Assessment of Asthma

Pregnant women with asthma should have a thorough assessment of their asthma control. Patients should be asked about their frequency of symptoms (particularly at night), how often symptoms interfere with normal activities, and the usage of short-acting β_2-agonists for symptom relief (not for exercise-induced bronchospasm prevention). Validated questionnaires such as the ATAQ, ACQ and the ACT are particularly helpful in classifying the level of asthma control.

In addition, a complete assessment of asthma must include objective measurements. All patients should have pulmonary function testing at their initial evaluation to determine disease severity. Patients should be given a peak flow meter to monitor asthma variability. At subsequent office visits, repeat pulmonary function testing is preferable, but at a minimum, assessment of peak expiratory flow rates (PEFRs) should be checked.

Assessment of the Fetus

All pregnant women should be advised to be attentive to fetal activity. Serial ultrasound evaluations beginning at 32-week gestation may be considered for women with moderate to severe asthma and women with poorly controlled asthma. In addition, after a severe exacerbation, an ultrasound evaluation may be reassuring.

Table 18–4. Guide to asthma severity.

Category	# Symptoms/day	#Symptoms/night	FEV$_1$ or PEFR	PEFR Variability
Intermittent asthma	$\leq$2 d/wk	$\leq$2 nights/mo	$\geq$80%	$\leq$20%
Mild persistent	>2/wk<daily	>2 nights/mo	$\geq$80%	>20–30%
Moderate persistent	Daily	>1 night/wk	>60–<80%	>30%
Severe persistent	Continual	Frequent	$\leq$60%	>30%

Reassurance

Patients need to be reassured about the safety of asthma medications and advised that the risks of treatment are much less than the risks of untreated asthma. Concern about side effects in the fetus may interfere with medication adherence and lead to undertreatment of asthma.

Education

All pregnant women with asthma should receive asthma education emphasizing the important benefits of treatment and its impact on the fetus. Written and verbal instructions should be given on the proper use of medications, spacers, and peak-flow meters. Patients should be taught how to monitor inhaler usage to avoid running out of medication.

Smoking

Any patient who is smoking should be advised to quit and be referred to a smoking cessation program. Besides adversely affecting asthma, smoking has deleterious affects on the mother and the fetus.

Triggers

An assessment of common triggers with instructions on avoidance and control should be part of all patient evaluations. Patients should be educated on ways to minimize exposure to dust mites, cockroaches, pets, pollens, irritants, and odors. Studies reporting that high levels of either total serum immunoglobulin E (IgE) or cockroach-specific IgE are associated with worsening asthma underscore the importance of such environmental controls. Patients with exposure to secondary smoke, including wood-burning stoves and fireplaces, should also be counseled on the importance of avoidance (Table 18–5).

Viral infections are the most common triggers causing severe exacerbations. Influenza vaccines and frequent handwashing are recommended, particularly during the so-called flu season. In nonpregnant patients, increased body weight and high-panic-fear state can worsen asthma and complicate treatment. Although studies are conflicting in pregnancy, increased body weight and high-panic-fear state should still be considered potential triggers.

Treatment Plans

Together with the patient, providers should develop medication regimens that are effective and easy to follow. Providers need to be aware that pregnant patients with asthma may have difficulty following complicated treatment regimens.

All patients should receive a written self-management plan. The plan should emphasize home management of exacerbations, including instructions on when to start oral steroids and when and where to call for help. Ideally, these plans should be based on both symptoms and peak-flow meter.

In addition, it is important to include the obstetrical provider from the beginning. The obstetrical provider will be assessing the patient more regularly, and their involvement in the asthma care team is critical, particularly in reassuring the patient on the safety of the medications.

Medications

Inhaled Short-Acting β$_2$-Agonists

Inhaled short-acting β$_2$-agonists are one of the mainstays of therapy and should be administered only as needed. The preferred medication is albuterol, based on more published data on safety.

Inhaled Long-Acting β$_2$-Agonists

Inhaled long-acting β$_2$-agonists have a profile similar to the inhaled short-acting β$_2$-agonists with the exception that these drugs are retained longer in the lungs. The preferred medication is salmeterol (Serevent), due to the longer availability of the drug in the United States (Table 18–6).

There has been a recent controversy about inhaled long-acting β$_2$-agonists paradoxically increasing the

Table 18–5. Summary of control measures for environmental factors that can make asthma worse.[†]

Allergens
Reduce or eliminate exposure to the allergen(s) the patient is sensitive to, including:

- Animal dander: Remove animal from house, or, at the minimum, keep animal out of patient's bedroom and seal or cover with a filter the air ducts that lead to the bedroom.
- House dust mites:
  - Essential: Encase mattress in an allergen-impermeable cover; encase pillow in an allergen-impermeable cover or wash it weekly; wash sheets and blankets on the patient's bed in hot water weekly (water temperature of >130°F is necessary for killing mites).
  - Desirable: Reduce indoor humidity to less than 50%; remove carpets from the bedroom; avoid sleeping or lying on upholstered furniture; remove carpets that are laid on concrete.
- Cockroaches: Use poison bait or traps to control. Do not leave food or garbage exposed.
- Pollens (from trees, grass, or weeds) and outdoor molds: To avoid exposure, adults should stay indoors, especially during the afternoon, with the windows closed during the season in which they have problems with outdoor allergens.
- Indoor mold: Fix all leaks and eliminate water sources associated with mold growth; clean moldy surfaces. Consider reducing indoor humidity to less than 50%.

Tobacco Smoke
Advise patients and others in the home who smoke to stop smoking or to smoke outside the home. Discuss ways to reduce exposure to other sources of tobacco smoke, such as from child care providers and the workplace.

Indoor/Outdoor Pollutants and Irritants
Discuss ways to reduce exposures to the following:

- Wood-burning stoves or fireplaces
- Unvented stoves or heaters
- Other irritants (e.g., perfumes, cleaning agents, sprays)

[†]Adapted from EPR-2 1997.
[†]From the National Heart, Lung, and Blood Institute: National Asthma Education and Prevention Program Asthma and Pregnancy Working Group. NAEPP expert panel report. Managing asthma during pregnancy: recommendations for pharmacologic treatment-2004 update. *J Allergy Clin Immunol.* 2005;115(1):36.

risks of hospitalization and death in asthmatics. It would be prudent to use inhaled long-acting β_2-agonists only as add-on therapy to medium- or high-dose inhaled corticosteroids, if asthma remains poorly controlled.

INHALED CORTICOSTEROIDS

Inhaled corticosteroids are the cornerstone of therapy for the pregnant woman with persistent asthma. Multiple studies have emphasized the decrease in asthma exacerbations and the improvement in FEV$_1$ with the use of inhaled corticosteroids. Even studies in large birth registries have failed to relate the use of inhaled corticosteroids to any unfavorable perinatal outcome, including increased incidence of congenital malformations. The preferred medication is budesonide (Pulmicort), based on more recently published data (Table 18–7).

ORAL CORTICOSTEROIDS

Studies have shown that oral corticosteroid use has been associated with a decrease in birth weight of approximately 200 g, although without an increased incidence

of small for gestational age (SGA) infants. In addition, there is an association with an increased incidence of isolated cleft lip (without cleft palate) especially when taken during the first trimester (0.3% vs. 0.1% in the general population). The preferred drugs are prednisone and prednisolone because they have limited placental transfer. Oral corticosteroids are used in the treatment of poorly controlled severe persistent asthma or for the treatment of asthma exacerbations. On occasion, a short course of oral corticosteroids may be necessary to gain control of asthma (Table 18–6).

CROMOLYN SODIUM

Cromolyn sodium is safe for pregnancy. It is considered an alternative but not a preferred option for mild persistent asthma (Table 18–6).

THEOPHYLLINE

Theophylline is safe for pregnancy in the usual therapeutic serum level range of 5 to 12 μg/mL. However, theophylline has many side effects and drug-drug interactions. Studies have shown that women treated

Table 18-6. Usual dosages for long-term-control medications during pregnancy and lactation.*†

Medication	Dosage form	Adult Dose
Inhaled Corticosteroids (See Estimated Comparative Daily Dosages for Inhaled Corticosteroids [Table 18-7].)		
Systemic Corticosteroids (Applies to all three corticosteroids.)		
Methylprednisolone	2-, 4-, 8-, 16-, 32-mg tablets	7.5–60 mg daily in a single dose in AM or qod as needed for control
Prednisolone	5-mg tablets, 5 mg/5 mL, 15 mg/5 mL	Short-course "burst" to achieve control: 40–60 mg/d as single dose or two divided doses for 3–10 d
Prednisone	1-, 2.5-, 5-, 10-, 20-, 50-mg tablets 5 mg/mL, 5 mg/5 mL	
Long-Acting Inhaled β₂-Agonists (Note: Should not be used for symptom relief or for exacerbations. Use with inhaled corticosteroids.)		
Salmeterol	DPI 50 µg/blister	1 blister q12h
Formoterol	DPI 12 µg/single-use capsule	1 capsule q12h
Combined Medication		
Fluticasone/ Salmeterol	DPI 100, 250, or 500 µg/50 µg, HFA 45, 115 or 230 µg/21µg	1 inhalation bid; dose depends on severity of asthma. 2 puffs bid; dose depends on severity of asthma
Budesonide/ Formoterol	HFA MDI 80 mg or 160 mcg/4.5 mcg puff	2 inhalations bid; dose depends on severity of asthma
Cromolyn		
Cromolyn	MDI 800 µ/puff Nebulizer 20 mg/ampule	2–4 puffs tid–qid 1 ampule tid–qid
Leukotriene Receptor Antagonists		
Montelukast	10-mg tablet	10 mg qhs
Zafirlukast	20-mg tablet	40 mg daily (20-mg tablet bid)
Methylxanthines (Serum monitoring is important [serum concentration of 5–12 µg/mL at steady state].)		
Theophylline	Liquids, sustained-release tablets, and capsules	Starting dose, 10 mg/kg/d up to 300 mg max; usual max 800 mg/d

DPI, dry powder inhaler; MDI, metered-dose inhaler.
*Adapted from EPR, update 2002.
†Modified from National Heart, Lung, and Blood Institute: National Asthma Education and Prevention Program Asthma and Pregnancy Working Group. NAEPP expert panel report. Managing asthma during pregnancy: recommendations for pharmaco-logic treatment-2004 update. *J Allergy Clin Immunol.* 2005;115(1):36.
Notes: • The most important determinant of appropriate dosing is the clinician's judgment of the patient's response to therapy.
  • Some doses may be outside package labeling, especially in the high-dose range.

with theophylline have a high rate of discontinuance of the drug, and there is an increase in the proportion of women with FEV$_1$ less than 80% of predicted. Oral theophylline is an alternative but not a preferred option for mild, moderate, or severe persistent asthma (Table 18–6).

LEUKOTRIENE RECEPTOR ANTAGONISTS

There are limited studies on leukotriene receptor antagonists available for review, but they appear to be safe in pregnancy. Consequently, leukotriene receptor antagonists would be an alternative but not preferred option for the treatment of mild or moderate persistent asthma (Table 18–6).

IPRATROPIUM

Although there are reassuring animal studies for ipratropium (Atrovent, Atrovent HFA), it should only be used in the treatment of severe asthma exacerbations. In the emergency department, usage is indicated only when the FEV$_1$ is less than 50% or there is impending respiratory arrest.

Table 18–7. Estimated comparative daily dosages for inhaled corticosteroid.

Drug	Low Daily Dose Adult	Medium Daily Dose Adult	High Daily Dose Adult
Beclomethasone HFA 40 or 80 μg/puff	80–240 μg	>240–480 μg	>480 μg
Budesonide DPI 90 or 180 μg/inhalation	180–540 μg	>540–1080 μg	>1080 μg
Flunisolide 250 μg/puff	500–1000 μg	1000–2000 μg	>2000 μg
Fluticasone MDI: 44, 110, or 220 μg/puff DPI: 50, 100, or 250 μg/inhalation	88–264 μg 100–300 μg	264–440 μg 300–500 μg	>440 μg >500 μg
Triamcinolone acetonide 75 μg/puff	300–750 μg	750–1500 μg	>1500 μg
Mometasone DPI 220 μg/inhalation	220 μg	440 μg	>440 μg

Note: Mometasone was added to the table. It only recently became FDA approved. DPI, dry powder inhaler; MDI, metered-dose inhaler.
Source: NHLBI of the NIH and the HHS. Modified from the NAEPP Guidelines.

Treatment Guidelines

The NAEPP has proposed a pharmacologic treatment approach for pregnant women with asthma based on stepwise asthma care (Fig. 18–1). This approach follows established guidelines for intermittent asthma and mild, moderate, and severe persistent asthma. It recommends controller medications for all levels of persistent asthma. Doses of medications used in pregnancy and lactation are included in Table 18–6. These guidelines may be modified to fit the needs of individual patients (Table 18–8).

INTERMITTENT ASTHMA

Patients with intermittent asthma should be treated with inhaled short-acting β_2-agonists, preferably albuterol, as needed. However, it is important to note that even patients with intermittent asthma can experience life-threatening exacerbations and should have treatment plans for exacerbations that include oral corticosteroids (Table 18–8).

MILD PERSISTENT ASTHMA

Patients with mild persistent asthma should be treated with low-dose inhaled corticosteroids, preferably budesonide (Pulmicort), with inhaled short-acting β_2-agonists, preferably albuterol, used as needed.

Alternative but less-preferable treatments include cromolyn, leukotriene receptor antagonists, and sustained-release theophylline (Table 18–8).

MODERATE PERSISTENT ASTHMA

Patients with moderate persistent asthma should be treated with medium-dose inhaled corticosteroids, preferably budesonide (Pulmicort). If control is difficult or cannot be achieved, inhaled corticosteroids can be supplemented with an inhaled long-acting β_2-agonist, preferably salmeterol (Serevent). Inhaled short-acting β_2-agonists, preferably albuterol, should be added as needed. Alternative, but-less preferable treatments include either low-dose or medium-dose inhaled corticosteroids with the addition of sustained-release theophylline or leukotriene receptor antagonist therapy (Table 18–8).

SEVERE PERSISTENT ASTHMA

For patients with severe persistent asthma, the treatment of choice is high-dose inhaled corticosteroid therapy, preferably budesonide (Pulmicort), and an inhaled long-acting β_2-agonist, preferably salmeterol (Serevent). Inhaled short-acting β_2-agonists, preferably albuterol, should be added as needed. Alternative but less-preferable treatment would be high-dose inhaled corticosteroids with sustained-release theophylline. If

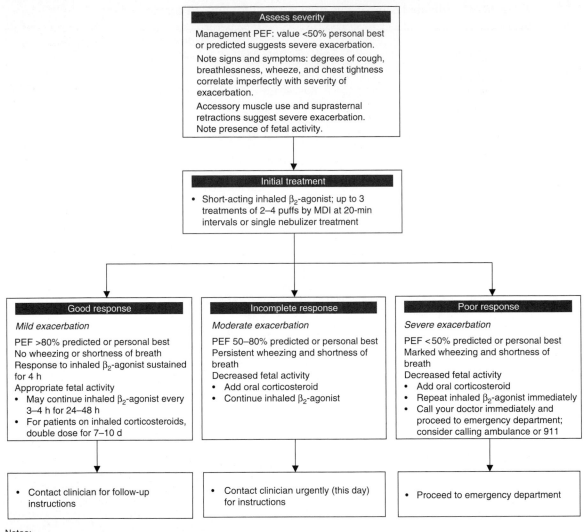

Figure 18–1. Management of asthma exacerbations: home treatment.

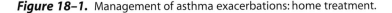

control cannot be achieved with these drugs, oral corticosteroids should be added, as needed, to maintain control (Table 18–8).

ASSIGNMENT OF SEVERITY STEP

All patients should be assigned to the highest step, in which any single feature occurs. For example, nighttime symptoms twice a week will increase the severity assignment to moderate persistent asthma, even if all other symptoms and objective measures are in the mild persistent asthma category (Table 18–8).

OVERUSE OF ALBUTEROL

Patients need to be specifically asked about their use of albuterol or other inhaled short-acting bronchodilators. Overuse of albuterol indicates inadequate asthma control and the need to increase the asthma severity assignment to a higher level. Pharmacy records, if available, can be invaluable in analyzing refill patterns and determining if patients are refilling their inhaled short-acting β_2-agonists too frequently.

The extent of albuterol overuse can be easily estimated by multiplying the number of canisters used by

Table 18–8. Stepwise approach for managing asthma during pregnancy and lactation: treatment.

Classify Severity: Clinical Features Before Treatment or Adequate Control		Medications Required to Maintain Long-Term Control
Symptoms/Day / *Symptoms/Night*	*PFEF or FEV$_1$* / *PEF Variability*	*Daily Medications*
Step 4 **Severe** **Persistent**	Continual / Frequent — $\leq$60% / >30%	• Preferred treatment: • High-dose inhaled corticosteroid AND • Long-acting inhaled β$_2$-agonist AND, if needed, • Corticosteroid tablets or syrup long term (2 mg/kg/d, generally not to exceed 60 mg per day). (Make repeat attempts to reduce systemic corticosteroid and maintain control with high-dose inhaled corticosteroid.) • Alternative treatment: • High-dose inhaled corticosteroid AND • Sustained-release theophylline to serum concentration of 5–12 μg/mL.
Step 3 **Moderate** **Persistent**	Daily / >1 night/wk — >60%–<80% / >30%	• Preferred treatment: • Medium-dose inhaled corticosteroid If needed (particularly in patients with recurring severe exacerbations): • Medium-dose inhaled corticosteroid and long-acting inhaled β$_2$-agonist. • Alternative treatment: • Low-dose inhaled corticosteroid and either theophylline or leukotriene receptor antagonist. If needed: • Medium-dose inhaled corticosteroid and either theophylline or leukotriene receptor antagonist.
Step 2 **Mild** **Persistent**	>2 d/wk but <daily / >2 nights/mo — $\geq$80% / >20–30%	• Preferred treatment: • Low-dose inhaled corticosteroid • Alternative treatment (listed alphabetically): cromolyn, leukotriene receptor antagonist, OR sustained-release theophylline to serum concentration of 5–12 μg/mL.
Step 1 **Mild** **Intermittent**	$\leq$2 d/wk / $\leq$2 nights/mo — $\geq$80% / <20%	• No daily medication needed. • Severe exacerbations may occur, separated by long periods of normal lung function and no symptoms. A course of systemic corticosteroid is recommended.

Modified from National Heart, Lung, and Blood Institute: National Asthma Education and Prevention Program Asthma and Pregnancy Working Group. NAEPP expert panel report. Managing asthma during pregnancy: recommendations for pharmacologic treatment-2004 update. *J Allergy Clin Immunol.* 2005;115(1):36.

200 (puffs per canister) and dividing the result by the number of days between refills. Even the use of one canister, every 2 months, indicates an average of more than 3 puffs of albuterol per day, suggesting suboptimal control that should be evaluated (Table 18–8).

Patients often experience worsening of asthma symptoms during exercise. These patients may require albuterol use prior to exercise. In some cases, alteration of medication regimens may be required to allow for exercise.

GAINING CONTROL OF ASTHMA

Most asthma specialists start a patient at a higher dose of medication to gain control quickly and even consider a short course of oral steroids. Once control is gained, the dosage should be lowered to the minimal medication needed to maintain good control. Reassessment should occur frequently to determine if control can be maintained at a lower dose of medications (Table 18–8).

SPECIALTY CARE

The NAEPP Guidelines recommends that pregnant women with asthma be referred to an asthma specialist if there is difficulty controlling their asthma. The guidelines specifically advise that patients with severe persistent asthma or those requiring step 4 treatment be referred to an asthma clinic or to a specialist. Patients with moderate persistent asthma or who require step 3 treatment may also be considered for referral (Table 18–8).

EXACERBATIONS

During the course of their pregnancy, studies show that 20% of asthma patients have exacerbations severe enough to seek urgent medical care. Approximately 6% require hospital admissions. Severe exacerbations such as those requiring hospital admission, urgent physician visits, or systemic corticosteroids are significantly more likely to occur with severe asthma.

Exacerbations are most common in the late second trimester to early third trimester. The most common reasons for exacerbations are viral infections and non-compliance of inhaled corticosteroid treatment. The importance of regular usage of inhaled corticosteroids for persistent asthma cannot be overemphasized. Studies show that for patients using inhaled corticosteroids before pregnancy, the rate of asthma-related physician visits decreased and the number of emergency department visits was unchanged after pregnancy.

MANAGEMENT OF EXACERBATIONS

The management of the pregnant woman having an asthma exacerbation is set forth in the NAEPP Guidelines (Figs. 18–1 and 18–2). Treatment depends on the severity of the exacerbation with nebulized albuterol and oral steroids used as the primary treatment, particularly at

home. For pregnant women with severe exacerbations in the emergency department, nebulized ipratropium can be added to the nebulized albuterol. Table 18–9 lists the doses of medications for acute exacerbations.

The usual P_{CO_2} in pregnancy is in the range of 26 to 30 mm Hg. For pregnant women presenting with a severe acute asthma exacerbation, a P_{CO_2} of 40 signifies impending respiratory arrest.

Mechanical Ventilation

Fortunately, it is rare for a pregnant woman to require intubation and mechanical ventilation. If needed, intubation should be oral instead of nasal due to airway narrowing. Preoxygenation with 100% oxygen prior to intubation is important to avoid a precipitous drop in oxygen that may occur after even a short period of apnea. Studies show that it is important to maintain cricoid pressure before and after intubation to avoid aspiration and gastric insufflation.

Studies show that patients should be ventilated with respiratory rates of 8 to 12 breaths per minute, tidal volumes of 6 to 8 ml/kg, and high-inspiratory flow rates of 100 to 120 per minute. Hyperventilation should be avoided because a respiratory alkalosis may decrease uterine blood flow and impair oxygenation of the fetus. In addition, it is important to avoid volutrauma and barotrauma.

CONCLUSION

Optimal asthma control during pregnancy is very important for both the mother and the fetus. To achieve this goal, thorough assessments and evaluations are critical, including monitoring with pulmonary function testing and peak-flow meters. Avoidance and control of common triggers needs to be addressed with an emphasis on smoking cessation. Effective treatment must include asthma education and reassurance that treatment is much safer for the fetus than maternal asthma exacerbations and symptoms. The obstetrical provider should be involved as part of the asthma care management team from the start of the pregnancy.

EVIDENCE-BASED MEDICINE

National Heart, Lung, and Blood Institute. National Asthma Education and Prevention Program Asthma and Pregnancy Working Group. NAEPP expert panel report. Managing asthma during pregnancy: recommendations for pharmacologic treatment-2004 update. *J Allergy Clin Immunol.* 2005; 115(1):36.

This paper is a systemic evidence-based review of pharmacologic treatment of pregnancy. Tables from this working paper are highlighted in the chapter. This is a very thorough, well-presented paper.

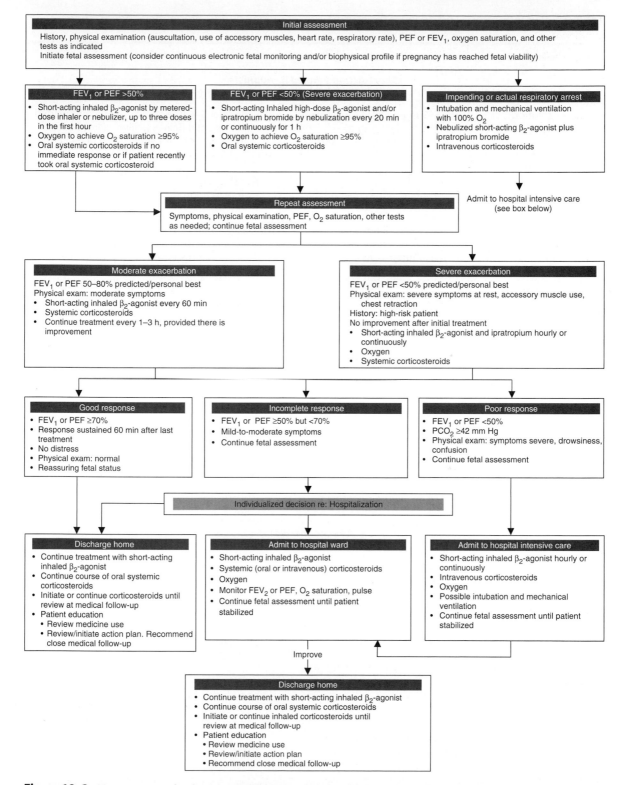

Figure 18–2. Management of asthma exacerbations: emergency department and hospital-based care (NAEPP Report).

Table 18–9. Medications and dosages for asthma exacerbations during pregnancy and lactation.

Medications	Adult Dosages	Comments
Short-Acting Inhaled β₂-Agonists		
Albuterol		
Nebulizer solution (5 mg/mL, 2.5 mg/3 mL, 1.25 mg/3 mL, 0.63 mg/3 mL)	2.5–5 mg q20min for 3 doses, then 2.5–10 mg q1–4h PRN, or 10–15 mg/h continuously	Only selective β₂-agonists are recommended. For optimal delivery, dilute aerosols to minimum of 3 mL at gas flow of 6–8 L/min.
HFA (90 µg/puff)	4–8 puffs q20min up to 4 h, then q1–4h as needed	As effective as nebulized therapy if patient is able to coordinate.
Bitolterol		
Nebulizer solution (2 mg/mL)	See albuterol dose	Has not been studied in severe asthma exacerbations. Do not mix with other drugs.
MDI (370 µg/puff)	See albuterol dose	Has not been studied in severe asthma exacerbations.
Levalbuterol (R-albuterol)		
Nebulizer solution (0.63 mg/3 mL, 1.25 mg/3 mL)	1.25–2.5 mg q20min for three doses, then 1.25–5 mg q1–4h as needed, or 5–7.5 mg/h continuously	0.63 mg of levalbuterol is equivalent to 1.25 mg of racemic albuterol for both efficacy and side effects.
HFA 45 µg/puff	See albuterol dose	
Pirbuterol		
MDI (200 µg/puff)	See albuterol dose	Has not been studied in severe asthma exacerbations.
Systemic (Injected) β₂-Agonists		
Epinephrine		
1:1000 (1 mg/mL)	0.3–0.5 mg q20min for three doses sq	No proven advantage of systemic therapy over aerosol.
Terbutaline (1 mg/mL)	0.25 mg q20min for three doses sq	No proven advantage of systemic therapy over aerosol.
Anticholinergics		
Ipratropium bromide		
Nebulizer solution (0.25 mg/mL)	0.5 mg q30min for three doses, then every 2–4 h as needed	May mix in same nebulizer with albuterol. Should not be used as first-line therapy; should be added to β₂-agonist therapy.
HFA (17 µg/puff)	4–8 puffs as needed	
Ipratropium with albuterol		
Nebulizer solution (each 3-mL vial contains 0.5 mg ipratropium bromide and 2.5 mg albuterol)	3 mL q30min for three doses, then every 2–4 h as needed.	Contains EDTA to prevent discoloration. This additive does not induce bronchospasms.

(Continued)

Table 18–9. Medications and dosages for asthma exacerbations during pregnancy and lactation. (Continued)

Medications	Adult Dosages	Comments
Ipratropium with albuterol		
MDI (each puff contains 18 μg ipratropium bromide and 90 μg albuterol)	4–8 puffs as needed	
Systemic Corticosteroids (Dosages and comments apply to all three corticosteroids)		
Prednisone **Methylprednisolone** **Prednisolone**	40–80 mg/d in 1 or 2 divided doses until PEF reaches 70% of predicted or personal best	For outpatient "burst," use 40–60 mg in 1 or 2 divided doses for 5–10 days in adults

MDI, metered-dose inhaler; PEF, peak expiratory flow; PRN, as needed.
SOURCE: Modified from the NAEPP Report. Child doses taken off table.

Hanania NA, Belfort MA. Acute asthma in pregnancy. *Crit Care Med.* 2005;33(10 suppl):S319.

This article is a review of acute asthma in pregnancy. Physiology during pregnancy and management of the pregnant woman with severe, acute exacerbations are highlighted.

Salpeter SR, Buckly NS, Ormiston TM, et al. Meta-analysis: effect of long-acting β-agonists on severe asthma exacerbations and asthma-related deaths. *Ann Intern Med.* 2006;114:904.

Although no specific reference to pregnancy is made, this paper is a meta-analysis of long-acting inhaled β_2-agonists on severe asthma exacerbations and asthma-related deaths. The article specifically looks at randomized, placebo-controlled trials and the risks of hospitalizations, life-threatening asthma, and asthma-related deaths.

BIBLIOGRAPHY

Bakhireva LN, Jones KL, Schatz M, et al. Asthma medication use in pregnancy and fetal growth. *J Allergy Clin Immunol.* 2005;116(3):503.

Dombrowski MP, Schatz M, Wise R, et al. Asthma during pregnancy. *Am Coll Obstet Gynecol.* 2004;103(1):5.

Haggerty CL, Ness RB, Kelsey S, et al. The impact of estrogen and progesterone on asthma. *Ann Allergy Asthma Immunol.* 2003;90(3):284.

Hanania NA, Belfort MA. Acute asthma in pregnancy. *Crit Care Med.* 2005;33(10 suppl):S319.

Jones KL, Johnson DL, Van Maarseveen ND, et al. Salmeterol use and pregnancy outcome: A prospective multi-center study. *J Allergy Clin Immunol.* 2002;109(1 suppl):S156.

Kircher S, Schatz M, Long L. Variables affecting asthma course during pregnancy. *Ann Allergy Asthma Immunol.* 2002;89:463.

Kwon HL, Belanger K, Bracken MB. Effect of pregnancy and stage of pregnancy on asthma severity: a systematic review. *Am J Obstet Gynecol.* 2004;190(5):1201.

Murphy VE, Clifton VL, Gibson PG. Asthma exacerbations during pregnancy: incidence and association with adverse pregnancy outcomes. *Thorax.* 2006;61(2):169.

Namazy J, Schatz M, Long L, et al. Use of inhaled steroids by pregnant asthmatic women does not reduce intrauterine growth. *J Allergy Clin Immunol.* 2004;113(3):427.

National Asthma Education and Prevention Program. Full report of the expert panel: guidelines for the diagnosis and management of asthma (EPR-3). Draft. January, 2007.

National Heart, Lung, and Blood Institute: National Asthma Education and Prevention Program Asthma and Pregnancy Working Group. NAEPP expert panel report. Managing asthma during pregnancy: recommendations for pharmacologic treatment-2004 update. *J Allergy Clin Immunol.* 2005;115(1):36.

Schatz M: Breathing for two: now we can all breathe a little easier. *J Allergy Clin Immunol.* 2005;115(1):31.

Schatz M, Dombrowski MP, Wise R., et al. The relationship of asthma medication use to perinatal outcomes. *J Allergy Clin Immunol.* 2004;113(6):1040.

Schatz M, Hoffman CP, Zeiger RS, et al. Asthma and allergic diseases during pregnancy. In: Adkinson NF, Yunginger JW, Busse WW, et al., eds. *Allergy: Principles and Practice.* 6th ed. Philadelphia: Mosby; 2003:1303.

Schatz M, Leibman C: Inhaled corticosteroid use and outcomes in pregnancy. *Ann Allergy Asthma Immunol.* 2005;95(3):234.

Salpeter SR, Buckly NS, Ormiston TM, et al. Meta-analysis: effect of long-acting β-agonists on severe asthma exacerbations and asthma-related deaths. *Ann Intern Med.* 2006;114:904.

van Runnard Heimel PJ, Franx A, Schobben AF, et al. Corticosteroids, pregnancy, and HELLP syndrome: a review. *Obstet Gynecol Surv.* 2005;60(1):57.

Pseudo-asthma: When Cough, Wheezing, and Dyspnea Are Not Asthma

19

Miles Weinberger, MD and Mutasim Abu-Hasan, MD

WHAT IS ASTHMA?

Asthma is a disease characterized by hyperresponsiveness of the airways to various stimuli resulting in airway obstruction that is reversible either spontaneously or as a result of treatment. The airway obstruction is from variable components of bronchial smooth-muscle spasm and inflammation that results in edema of the respiratory mucosa and secretions (Fig. 19–1). The clinical pattern can vary from those who get symptoms of asthma only episodically, commonly from viral respiratory infections, to those with chronic asthma resulting in daily or near daily symptoms. In the young child who gets very frequent viral respiratory infections, the distinction can sometimes be difficult. However, the distinction is important because of the different treatment strategies.

WHEN ISN'T IT ASTHMA?

Asthma is diagnosed clinically and suspected when there is cough, wheezing, or dyspnea. However, the same symptoms may be from other causes. The distinguishing characteristic of asthma from other causes of these symptoms is the response to bronchodilator or corticosteroids when the patient is symptomatic. For patients old enough to perform a pulmonary function test, substantial improvement of airway obstruction from an aerosol bronchodilator or a short course of a reasonably high dose of systemic corticosteroid supports the diagnosis of asthma, whereas the failure to completely relieve symptoms and substantially improve lung function argues against asthma as the etiology (Table 19–1). This will be apparent in the subsequent description of clinical problems initially misdiagnosed as asthma that we have indicated as pseudoasthma syndromes.

COUGH THAT IS NOT ASTHMA

Other Inflammatory Airway Diseases

Asthma is the most common chronic or recurrent inflammatory airway disease and a major cause of cough in children. Although there are causes of cough that are unlikely to be confused with asthma, there are several that characteristically are confused with asthma and result in overdiagnosis of asthma with consequent inappropriate treatment. Acute viral bronchitis, colloquially called a chest cold, is a common cause of a generally self-limited cough. Pertussis causes a more prolonged period of cough. It was known in the past as the 100-day cough. Characteristically spasmodic and associated with posttussive gagging or emesis, diagnosis is important to prevent spread to contacts. Pertussis should be suspected for any cough persisting for more than 2 weeks. Diagnosis is most readily made by polymerase chain reaction (PCR) from a properly collected nasal swab (Fig. 19–2). Acute cough beyond infant and toddler years with no prior history is rarely asthma. It is more likely that chronic longstanding cough will be confused with asthma.

Two common diagnoses for cough that need not be considered are postnasal drip and gastroesophageal reflux.

Cystic Fibrosis

Cystic fibrosis is the second most common inflammatory airway disease, occurring in about 1 in 2500 live births in white populations of northern European descent with variable lesser incidence in other ethnic groups and races. Although the mechanisms of airway inflammation are different in these two diseases, both cause airway obstruction, cough, wheezing, and dyspnea. The classical clinical presentation of malabsorption is not always present, and the severity and progression of

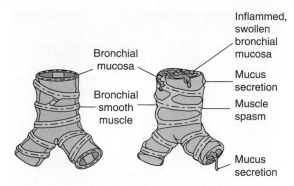

Figure 19–1. Artist's rendition of the two components of airway obstruction in asthma: bronchospasm and inflammation with mucosal edema and mucus secretions.

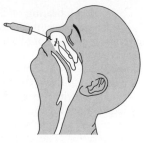

Figure 19–2. Pertussis should be considered for any child with a prolonged period of cough in the absence of a prior history. A flexible wire with a cotton tip is inserted in a nares and left in the posterior nasopharynx for 30 seconds before being withdrawn, appropriately saved as instructed by the laboratory, and sent for polymerase chain reaction (PCR) detection of pertussis. This is far more sensitive than culture. When performed early in the course of pertussis infection, appropriate preventative measures can be provided to all contacts and thereby minimize the spread.

the airway disease is highly variable. Some degree of bronchodilator response may even be present.

Cystic fibrosis should be suspected when symptoms and signs of airway inflammatory disease persist despite a short course of a systemic corticosteroid. The diagnosis of cystic fibrosis is most reliably made by performing a sweat chloride measurement using the classical quantitative pilocarpine iontophoresis method. Most of the various screening methods utilizing assessment by the

Table 19–1. Suggested doses of systemic corticosteroid to use as a diagnostic test for asthma when cough, wheezing, or dyspnea persists.

Complete relief of signs and symptoms with these doses within an absolute maximum of a 10-day period (usually less) is supportive of the diagnosis of asthma, whereas failure to relieve symptoms and normalize physiology warrants pursing alternative diagnoses. These doses are empirical, based on our clinical experience as sufficiently high to provide a definitive answer regarding the steroid responsiveness of the airway inflammation.

Age of Patient	Dosage as Prednisone or Prednisolone
Infant <6 mo	10 mg bid
Infant 6–12 mo	15 mg bid
1–3 y	20 mg bid
3–13 y	30 mg bid
>13 y	40 mg bid

bid, twice daily.

conductivity of sweat are unreliable, having both false-positive and false-negative results. For the test to be valid, duplicate collections of at least 75 mg are required for the filter paper discs or gauze pads with 15 μL being sufficient with the Macroduct collection coil. Measurement of 60 mEq/L chloride with substantial agreement in both samples is generally diagnostic of cystic fibrosis. Measurements of less than 40 mEq/L is generally reassuring that cystic fibrosis is not the cause of the patient's airway inflammatory disease. Levels of 40 to 60 mEq/L should be considered sufficiently suspicious that genetic analysis should be performed for the presence of two mutations of the cystic fibrosis transmembrane regulator, of which there are now more than 1500. Some of the less common mutations are associated with a milder course of the pulmonary disease, and a few are not associated with elevated sweat chlorides. Although rare, constituting less than 1% of patients with cystic fibrosis, awareness of these exceptional cases permits specific treatment rather than fruitless use of antiasthmatic medications that only frustrate the patient and the physician.

PRIMARY CILIARY DYSKINESIA

Primary ciliary dyskinesia is rare and consequently may not be adequately considered when a persistent cough is present. It includes a variety of abnormalities in airway ciliary function that results in absence of normal mucociliary clearance, an important innate host-defense mechanism for the lungs. A continuous movement of the mucous layer of the respiratory mucosa is normally maintained by the rhythmic beating of ciliated respiratory epithelial cells. The absence of the coordinated ciliary movement results in pooling of mucus in the airway with low-grade chronic infection. Cough and slowly progressing bronchiectasis results from this defect. Half will have situs inversus totalis, which is then known as Kartagener syndrome. As with cystic fibrosis, primary ciliary dyskinesia does not respond to usual antiasthmatic medications, and delayed diagnosis results in permanently damaged airways. The diagnosis should be highly suspect in the presence of situs inversus totalis, but the definitive diagnosis can be difficult in the absence of that anatomic abnormality. The classical means of diagnosing has been examination of ciliary structure by electron microscopy. However, this is fraught with errors in interpretation. Examination of coordinated ciliary movement from a nasal or tracheal epithelial sample by light or phase contrast microscopy is probably a more practical means of evaluation.

CHRONIC PURULENT (BACTERIAL) BRONCHITIS

Chronic purulent (bacterial) bronchitis is an entity not well appreciated and only infrequently described. Although chronic bacterial bronchitis is certainly a characteristic of cystic fibrosis, there are young children with no identifiable abnormalities in immunity or other underlying disease who have prolonged periods of cough with neutrophilia and bacteria in their lower airways demonstrable by bronchoalveolar lavage. Some, but not all, have bronchomalacia that may be contributing both to cough and to retaining secretions in the lower airway, which predisposes the child to secondary infection (Fig. 19–3). The bacteriology identified are most commonly the same ones commonly associated with otitis media, *Haemophilus influenzae, Moraxella catarrhalis,* and *Streptococcus pneumoniae.* Although responsive to appropriate antibiotics, some require repeated courses or even maintenance prophylactic antibiotics for an extended period. Resolution with age is common in the absence of an underlying innate or acquired host-defense disorder. Diagnosis requires flexible bronchoscopy and bronchoalveolar lavage with cell count and differential of lavage fluid for evidence of significant neutrophilia and quantitative culture of the fluid.

Tracheomalacia and Bronchomalacia

Inadequate rigidity of the tracheal or mainstem bronchial cartilage results in tracheal collapse, which causes cough by two mechanisms (Fig. 19–4). When secretions are present in the airway, the airway collapse causes pooling of secretions distally. The secretions then act as a continued stimulus for cough. Additionally, collapse of the trachea or mainstem bronchi during increased intrathoracic pressure as in vigorous exhalation

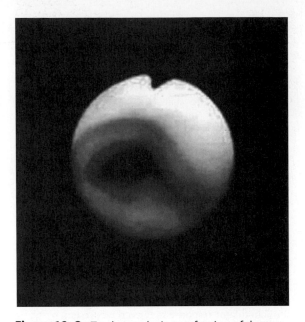

Figure 19–3. Tracheomalacia, a softening of the tracheal rings that are to provide a degree of rigidity to the airway, occurs from either a defect in the cartilage itself or from external compression by the great vessels. The innominate artery (also known as the brachiocephalic trunk) crosses over the lower third of the trachea where a pulsating bulge can often be seen on bronchoscopy. This is a common location for tracheomalacia, as in this picture. Persistent cough occurs when the repeated contact of the anterior and posterior walls of the trachea causes a focus of irritation with a consequent harsh barking cough characteristic of a tracheal cough. Cough may also occur because of inefficient clearing of secretions that results from the collapse of the airway when intrathoracic pressure is increased during coughing.

or coughing can cause the anterior and posterior walls to come into contact, resulting in an irritable focus that stimulates the cough reflex. Although tracheomalacia and bronchomalacia can be troublesome in the infant, some cases do not cause problems until later in childhood. In unusually severe cases of intractable cough from tracheomalacia, surgical aortopexy is needed. This involves placing a suture through the adventitial lining of the aortic arch and the periosteum of the sternum to pull the arch forward. Because the anterior tracheal wall is connected to the aortic arch with fascial tissue, it essentially pulls the anterior wall of the trachea forward, thereby maintaining a more normal tracheal lumen.

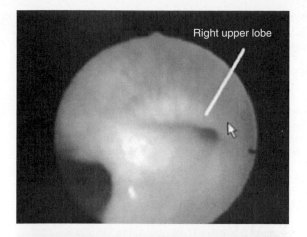

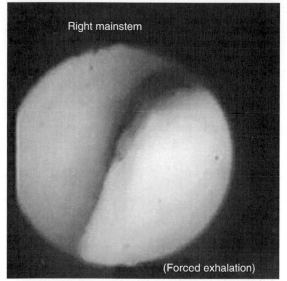

Figure 19–4. Bronchomalacia of the right upper lobe (top) and of the right mainstem (bottom). Depending on the degree of obstruction caused by the malacia, either cough or expiratory monophonic wheezing may be heard. Obstruction occurs on expiration with positive intrathoracic pressure during expiration while negative intrathoracic pressure during inspiration opens the airway. Complete airway obstruction during expiration can result in lobar emphysema from persistent hyperinflation of the lobe distal to the malacia. Decreased clearing of secretions distal to the malacia may result in purulent bacterial bronchitis.

Habit Cough Syndrome

Habit cough syndrome is a troublesome disorder commonly treated as asthma that often causes a great deal of morbidity and ineffective treatment and yet is readily rapidly curable with a simple behavioral technique. The classical presentation of the habit cough syndrome is that of a harsh barking repetitive cough occurring several times per minute for hours on end. It is extremely irritating to those in the presence of the cougher. Characteristic of the habit cough syndrome is the complete absence of cough once the patient is asleep. A variation of the habit cough is habitual throat clearing. As with the classical habit cough, the softer throat clearing occurs up to several times a minute and is completely absent once asleep. Both of these are frequently subjected to multiple diagnostic tests and therapy with anti-asthmatic medications.

This syndrome is sometimes misinterpreted as a tic. However, the so-called cough-tic syndrome involves more vocalization characteristic of Tourette syndrome and does not resemble the true cough or simple throat clearing of the habit cough or habit throat clearing syndrome. In considering treatment and discussing the issue with the family, it is important not to refer to this as a psychogenic cough because that is likely to adversely affect the relationship with the therapist, who will subsequently need the patient rapport to utilize suggestion therapy effectively. Moreover, there is no evidence in all but the rare case of other psychosomatic or psychological problems in these children and adolescents. Testing performed on our patients identified no tendency toward somatization but some tendency to score high, but not pathologically so, on an obsessive-compulsive scale. Perhaps related to this personality characteristic is our observation that most of these patients are academically high achievers.

If not treated with appropriate behavioral intervention, symptoms can continue for months and even years as was demonstrated in a follow-up of diagnoses of habit cough syndrome made at the Mayo Clinic. Treatment with suggestion therapy can provide a sustained cure by the use of various modes of suggestion therapy. We have used a technique that results in complete cessation of symptoms within 15 minutes (Table 19–2).

Other Rare Causes of Chronic Cough

We have seen some particularly unusual causes of chronic cough that were misdiagnosed as asthma. Although unlikely to be frequently encountered, awareness of these entities can encourage further investigation when the pattern of symptoms and response to treatment is not consistent with asthma (Figs. 19–5 and 19–6).

In contrast, postnasal drip is often diagnosed as a cause of cough, whereas the cough is actually more likely to be a manifestation of lower airway inflammation from asthma with the postnasal mucus visualized simply a manifestation of accompanying upper airway inflammation. Similarly, the presence of gastroesophageal reflux is more likely to be a result of coughing rather than a cause.

Table 19–2. Major elements of the suggestion therapy session for the habit cough syndrome.

- Expressing confidence, communicated verbally and behaviorally, that the therapist will be able to show the patient how to stop the cough.
- Explaining the cough as a vicious cycle of an initial irritant, now gone, that sets up a pattern of coughing that caused irritation and further symptoms.
- Encouraging the suppression of cough to break the cycle. The therapist closely observes for the initiation of the muscular movement preceding coughing and immediately exhorts the patient to hold the cough back, emphasizing that each second the cough is delayed makes further inhibition of cough easier.
- An alternative behavior to coughing is offered in the form of inhaling a generated mist or sipping body-temperature water with encouragement to inhale the mist or sip the water every time the patient begins to feel the urge to cough.
- Repeating expressions of confidence that the patient is developing the ability to resist the urge to cough.
- When some ability to suppress cough is observed (usually after about 10 min), asking in a rhetorical manner if the patient is beginning to feel that he or she can resist the urge to cough (e.g., "You're beginning to feel that you can resist the urge to cough, aren't you?").
- Discontinuing the session when the patient can repeatedly answer positively to the question, "Do you feel that you can now resist the urge to cough on your own?" This question is only asked after the patient has gone 5 min without coughing.

WHEEZING THAT IS NOT ASTHMA

In considering wheezing, it is important to consider that patients, parents, and even physicians at times refer to various respiratory sounds as "wheezing" that are not, in fact, wheezing. Wheezing is defined as a continuous musical expiratory sound due to intrathoracic airway obstruction. However, parents may describe inspiratory rattling or stridor as wheezing, and there are many reports of inspiratory sounds from upper airway obstruction being called wheezing by medical personnel.

Partial Airway Obstruction

A cause of true wheezing, partial obstruction of a bronchus can result in wheezing that is commonly misdiagnosed and treated as asthma. A *retained foreign body* in a bronchus is one cause. This needs to be distinguished from a *mucus plug* associated with asthma that

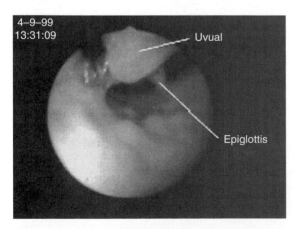

Figure 19–5. The uvula making contact with the epiglottis caused a troublesome cough in this 4-year-old boy treated unsuccessfully for asthma who was able to relate that he coughed because he felt something in the back of his throat. Uvulectomy cured his cough.

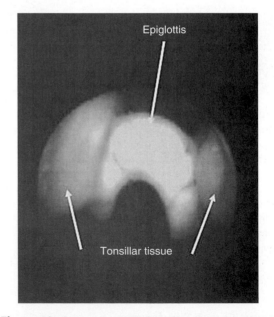

Figure 19–6. Tonsils (the lateral masses in the image) impinging on the epiglottis in a 3-year-old girl caused chronic cough initially treated unsuccessfully for asthma. Tonsillectomy cured her cough.

can also obstruct a bronchus. Another is *bronchomalacia* (Fig. 19–4). Most commonly associated with wheezing in infants, this is associated with little respiratory distress. In contrast to a mucus plug from asthma or other airway inflammatory disease, these causes of partial airway obstruction cause unilateral wheezing that is persistent, whereas the localized wheezing from a mucus plug varies from time to time.

When bronchomalacia occurs in an infant who also experiences recurrent viral respiratory infection–induced asthma, which occurs in 15% to 20% of infants and toddlers to some degree, the persistent wheezing following the initial clearing of symptoms can result in frustrating attempts to clear the wheezing pharmacologically. However, once confirmed to be bronchomalacia by direct observation during flexible bronchoscopy with conscious sedation, no further treatment is indicated. It is important to consider that both tracheomalacia and bronchomalacia can be missed during rigid bronchoscopy where general anesthesia and positive pressure ventilation keep the airway open. That eliminates the increase in intrathoracic pressure from normal ventilator effort that will collapse an airway that is poorly supported because of defective cartilaginous rings.

The natural course of this is resolution with age, apparently as the airway increases in size. It is not known how many eventually become associated with cough as described earlier, but this is probably not an inevitable outcome.

Vocal Cord Dysfunction Syndrome

Vocal cord dysfunction syndrome is a functional disorder of the vocal cords most commonly seen in adolescents. It is commonly misdiagnosed as asthma based on an inappropriate description of "wheezing." The respiratory noise, however, is actually a high-pitched inspiratory stridor due to paradoxical adduction of the vocal cords during inspiration. A variation of the vocal cord dysfunction syndrome manifests itself as abnormal continuous inspiratory and expiratory noise. This latter variation of the vocal cord dysfunction syndrome is characterized by spasmodic closure of the vocal cords with adduction persisting during both inspiration and expiration. Spirometry with a maximal inspiratory effort can readily distinguish the upper airway obstruction of vocal cord dysfunction from the lower airway obstruction of asthma (Fig. 19–7).

Two phenotypes of vocal cord dysfunction syndrome have been described. One type occurs spontaneously with the patient experiencing dyspnea and inspiratory stridor (often described as "wheezing") at various and often unpredictable times. Whether this is a panic or anxiety-induced reaction is speculative. It nonetheless is alarming for those experiencing this and for those observing the reaction. Urgent visits to an emergency department are common, and those who have the spasmodic closure of the vocal cords are more likely than those with just paradoxical movement to experience multiple emergency 911 calls because of the alarming appearance of their respiratory distress. The other phenotype are those that occur only with exercise. This is commonly seen in adolescent athletes during competitive aerobic activities. Typically transient and relieved spontaneously with a period of rest, this phenotype of vocal cord dysfunction syndrome is troublesome predominantly because it interferes with their athletic activities. Although most patients with vocal cord dysfunction syndrome manifest only one of these two patterns, some exhibit both.

The treatment for the spontaneously occurring phenotype of vocal cord dysfunction syndrome is instruction by a speech pathologist familiar with this disorder who can instruct techniques to take control of the vocal cords voluntarily. This is generally effective. Such techniques, however, are not practical for those with exercise-induced vocal cord dysfunction because the techniques would require stopping the activity that was inducing the problem, which results in spontaneous resolution of symptoms anyway. We have found that an anticholinergic aerosol (Atrovent Oral Inhaler) when used prior to exercise prevents the vocal cord dysfunction in these patients, and this observation is consistent with evidence that a vagal reflux is involved in this pattern. For both patterns of vocal cord dysfunction syndrome, the long-term outlook for resolution or accommodation appears favorable.

DYSPNEA THAT IS NOT ASTHMA

Hyperventilation

Attacks of hyperventilation can be confused with asthma, both in those who have asthma and those who do not. Patients who have both asthma and experience hyperventilation attacks cannot readily distinguish the sensation of dyspnea associated with hyperventilation from that associated with their asthma. Spirometry at the time the patient is symptomatic can help distinguish the perception of dyspnea associated with a hyperventilation attack from asthma. A blood gas demonstrating low pCO_2 and high pH without evidence of airway obstruction at the time of symptoms provides supportive evidence for hyperventilation.

Exertional Dyspnea

Dyspnea on exertion in children and adolescents is frequently part of the clinical course of asthma. However, asthma is rarely the diagnosis when there is dyspnea on exertion with no respiratory symptoms other than during exercise. In a study of 142 children and adolescents

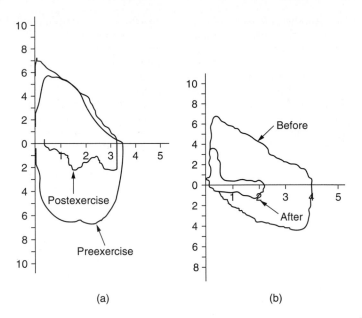

(a)   (b)

Figure 19–7. Flow-volume loops obtained before and when symptomatic in two patterns of vocal cord dysfunction syndrome. On the left is the preexercise flow-volume loop with the midinspiratory and midexpiratory flows about equal and the postexercise loop exhibiting the typical flattening of the inspiratory portion of the flow-volume loop in a 15-year-old girl with exercise-induced inspiratory stridor (that had been described as "wheezing" by the patient's primary care physician). This indicates reversible upper airway obstruction typical of paradoxical vocal cord movement, which was then confirmed by visualizing adduction of the vocal cords on inspiration with flexible laryngoscopy. The flow-volume loops on the right are from a 15-year-old girl with repeated episodes of sudden-onset severe dyspnea who had spontaneous onset of severe dyspnea during our evaluation. Flexible laryngoscopy demonstrated the vocal cords and false vocal cords to be severely adducted, leaving only about a 2-mm opening for air movement. This results in impressive dyspnea from the resulting upper airway obstruction.

with exercise-induced dyspnea referred to us, 100 had been diagnosed and treated as asthma without clinical response. When treadmill exercise was performed with full cardiopulmonary monitoring on 117 of the 142 (Fig. 19–8), exercise-induced bronchospasm was rare despite having reproduced the patient's exercise-induced dyspnea. The most common cause of exercise-induced dyspnea in these patients was physiologic limitation in patients with a wide range of cardiovascular conditioning. Their perception of dyspnea results from the respiratory drive that occurs as a result of the lactic acidosis produced during anaerobic metabolism when exercise exceeds what is commonly called the aerobic threshold. The lowered pH from the metabolic acidosis stimulates the attempt to compensate by increasing respiratory drive to an extent that exceeds the patient's maximal respiratory effort. The result is the perception of dyspnea. Other abnormalities documented included vocal cord dysfunction, restrictive physiology associated with minor chest wall abnormalities, exercise-induced laryngomalacia (Fig. 19–9), and exercise-induced supraventricular tachycardia (Fig. 19–10).

Making the correct diagnosis enables the cessation of ineffective asthma pharmacotherapy and appropriate corrective action. For those with physiologic dyspnea, counseling regarding cardiovascular conditioning and appropriate training can be of considerable value.

CONCLUSION

Although asthma is a common cause of various respiratory symptoms, all that coughs, wheezes, and causes shortness of breath or dyspnea is not asthma. Knowledge of the natural history of asthma and close observation of the response to therapy should quickly lead to an index of suspicion that diagnoses other than asthma need to be considered when there are characteristics that are atypical for asthma. Appropriate diagnostic tests, including spirometry when symptomatic, flexible bronchoscopy with conscious sedation rather than general anesthesia, bronchoalveolar lavage, and treadmill exercise testing with full cardiopulmonary monitoring, can generally result in the appropriate diagnosis and more specific treatment.

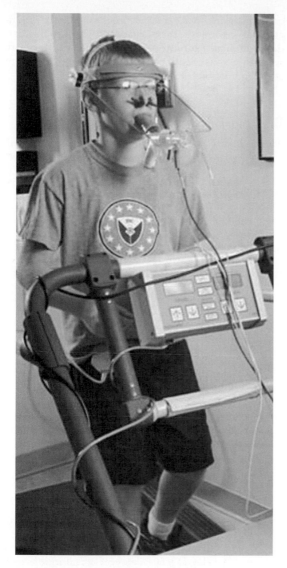

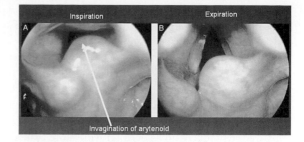

Figure 19–9. Example of exercise-induced laryngomalacia. On the left is the invagination of the right arytenoid partially obstructing the airway on inspiration with clearing of the airway on expiration (right). The result of the obstruction to inspiratory flow is dyspnea and noise on inspiration that can be misdiagnosed as "wheezing." Only with laryngoscopy can this be distinguished from vocal cord dysfunction because both will give the same flattening of the inspiratory portion of the flow-volume loop during exercise. (Reproduced, with permission, from Arora et al. *An unusual case of laryngomalacia presenting as asthma refractory to therapy. Ann Allergy Asthma Immunol.* 2005;95:607.)

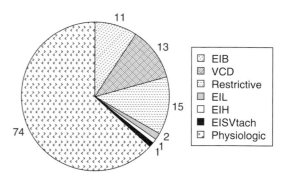

Figure 19–10. Diagnoses among 117 children and adolescents who underwent treadmill exercise testing with progressive incline and duration until symptoms were reproduced during full cardiopulmonary monitoring. Most had been previously diagnosed and treated for asthma, exercise-induced bronchospasm (EIB) was present in only 11. Vocal cord dysfunction (VCD) was associated with the reproduced dyspnea on exertion in 13, 15 had evidence of chest wall restriction (restrictive) associated with minor degrees of pectus deformities and scoliosis, 2 had exercise-induced laryngomalacia (EIL), 1 had exercise-induced hyperventilation (EIH), 1 had exercise-induced supraventricular tachycardia (EISVtach), while the majority, 74, had physiologic dyspnea (physiologic), about one third of whom were highly motivated, well-conditioned athletes, and one third had below-average cardiovascular conditioning.

Figure 19–8. Exercise test with cardiopulmonary monitoring. Continuous measurement is provided for inspiratory and expiratory flow, oxygen utilization, carbon dioxide production, electrocardiogram, and pulse oximetry during progressive treadmill exercise until the patient's symptoms are reproduced. A blood gas is routinely obtained at the completion of the test.

EVIDENCE-BASED MEDICINE

Abu-Hasan M, Tannous B, Weinberger M. Exercise-induced dyspnea in children and adolescents: if not asthma then what? *Ann Allergy Asthma Immunol.* 2005;94:366.

Background: Exercise-induced dyspnea (EID) is commonly attributed to asthma in otherwise healthy children.

This study reports outcome of EID evaluated when other symptoms and signs of asthma were absent or if there was no response to previous use of an inhaled β_2-agonist.

Methods: Physiologic measures included pre- and postexercise spirometry in 142 children and adolescents with the addition of O_2 uptake, CO_2 production, continuous oximetry, and ECG monitoring in 117. Exercise-induced asthma (EIA) was diagnosed if symptoms were reproduced in association with more than a 15% decrease in FEV_1 from baseline. Endoscopy was performed if stridor and/or decreased maximal inspiratory flow were present. Criteria were established for restrictive abnormalities, physical conditioning, exercise-induced hyperventilation, and normal physiologic limitation.

Results: EID, present for a mean duration of 30 months, had been previously attributed to asthma by the referring physician in 98. Symptoms were reproduced during exercise testing in 117. Only 11 had EIA; 74 demonstrated only normal physiologic exercise limitation at the time symptoms were reproduced. Other diagnoses associated with reproduced EID included restrictive abnormalities in 15, vocal cord dysfunction in 13, laryngomalacia in 2, primary hyperventilation in 1, and supraventricular tachycardia in 1.

Conclusion: EIA is not the etiology of EID in most children and adolescents who have no other clinical manifestations of asthma, and it is frequently inappropriately diagnosed in these patients. Exercise testing that reproduces symptoms while monitoring cardiac and respiratory physiology is indicated to identify the various causes of EID when other symptoms or signs of asthma are absent.

Comment: This study illustrates the problem of overdiagnosing asthma in school-age children who experience dyspnea on exertion to varying degrees from various physiologic causes. This is particularly apparent in preadolescents and adolescents when their drive to participate in athletic activities exceeds their level of conditioning. For these children, further cardiovascular conditioning and appropriate aerobic training is indicated. Physiologic abnormalities were identified in other children in this study. Few had evidence for exercise-induced asthma in these children who had no other history of symptoms consistent with asthma. Treadmill exercise testing at a rate and progressive incline sufficient to reproduce their symptoms during full cardiopulmonary monitoring with breath-by-breath analysis permits identification of the physiology present at the time of symptoms.

BIBLIOGRAPHY

Abu-Hasan M, Tannous B, Weinberger M. Exercise-induced dyspnea in children and adolescents: if not asthma then what? *Ann Allergy Asthma Immunol.* 2005;94:366.

Doshi D, Weinberger M. Long-term outcome of vocal cord dysfunction. *Ann Allergy Asthma Immunol.* 2006;96;794.

Hammo AH, Weinberger M. Exercise induced hyperventilation: a pseudoasthma syndrome. *Ann Allergy Asthma Immunol.* 1999;82:574.

Kemp A. Does post-nasal drip cause cough in childhood? *Paediatr Resp Rev.* 2006;7:31.

Leigh MW. Primary ciliary dyskinesia. In: Chernick V, Boat TF, Wilmott RW, et al., eds. *Kendig's Disorders of the Respiratory Tract in Children.* 7th ed. Philadelphia: Saunders Elsevier; 2006:902.

Lokshin B, Lindgren S, Weinberger M, et al. Outcome of habit cough in children treated with a brief session of suggestion therapy. *Ann Allergy.* 1991;67:579.

Lokshin B, Weinberger M. The habit cough syndrome: a review. *Am J Asthma Allergy Peds.* 1993;7:11.

Morice AH. Post-nasal drip syndrome—a symptom to be sniffed at? *Pulm Pharmacol Ther.* 2004;17:343.

Najada A, Weinberger M. Unusual cause of chronic cough in a four-year-old cured by uvulectomy. *Pediatr Pulmonol.* 2002;34;144.

Selvadurai H. Investigation and management of suppurative cough in pre-school children. *Pediatr Respir Rev.* 2006;7:15.

Thomson F, Masters IB, Chang AB. Persistent cough in children and the overuse of medications. *J Paediatr Child Health.* 2002;38:578.

Weinberger M, Abu-Hasan M. Asthma in the pre-school child. In: Chernick V, Boat TF, Wilmott RW, et al., eds. *Kendig's Disorders of the Respiratory Tract in Children.* 7th ed. Philadelphia: Saunders Elsevier; 2006:795.

Weinberger M. Proceedings from the consensus conference on treatment of viral respiratory infection-induced asthma in young children. *J Pediatr.* 2003;142(suppl 2):S1.

Weinberger M. Gastroesophageal reflux is not a significant cause of lung disease in children. *Pediat Pulmonol.* 2004;26(suppl):194.

Wood RE. Localized tracheomalacia or bronchomalacia in children with intractable cough. *J Pediatr.* 1990;116:404.

Hypersensitivity Pneumonitis

Joshua Gibbs, DO and Timothy J. Craig, DO

Hypersensitivity pneumonitis (HP), or extrinsic allergic alveolitis, is an uncommon syndrome that involves the interaction between the immune system and inhaled low molecular weight chemicals, biologic dusts, and medications that manifests as pulmonary disease. Although the antigens can be derived from many different sources, they are approximately 1 μm in diameter, are able to reach the distal airways, and cause similar clinical manifestations. Unlike other allergic diseases, the immune mechanisms do not involve immunoglobulin E (IgE) or a T helper cell type 2 (TH2) response. Inhalation of environmental antigens induces a complex T helper cell type 1 (TH1) response and causes interstitial and alveolar pathology. HP is considered a chronic disease with acute exacerbations. Host deposition of fibrotic tissue ensues in an attempt to repair the damage along with the consequence of progressive pulmonary dysfunction.

The most critical aspect of the treatment strategy is to first recognize the presence of HP and then to remove the subject from exposure to the offending antigen. The identification of the offending agent can pose a significant challenge to clinicians; however, if there is identification of the environment where exposure has taken place, remediation can be performed, which is usually successful in removing the antigen, thus preventing further exposures. Treatment with systemic corticosteroids can reduce symptoms, but corticosteroids will not delay progression of the underlying disease process. This treatment modality should not replace environmental control measures.

HP was initially considered an occupational lung disease because workplace antigens were implicated in causing diseases such as farmer's lung, bagassosis, and mushroom pickers' disease. This dogma has shifted toward HP being a primary home-related disease process. Exposure to common antigens found in or around the home environment has increasingly been implicated in the disease process.

EPIDEMIOLOGY

It is difficult to assess the incidence and prevalence of HP because presentation can vary widely. HP can mimic other histopathologic patterns, such as bronchiolitis obliterans with organizing pneumonia (BOOP), acute eosinophilic pneumonia, usual interstitial pneumonitis/idiopathic pulmonary fibrosis (UIP/IPF), and nonspecific interstitial pneumonitis (NSIP). Many exposed asymptomatic individuals have serum precipitins or elevated T cells in bronchoalveolar lavage (BAL) fluid. These findings represent exposure as opposed to disease in this population. An individual's ability to become sensitized to an antigen depends on factors such as antigenic potential of the inhaled particle, host susceptibility, and the ability of the antigen to disperse in the air.

Prevalence

Most epidemiologic data relates to occupational causes that vary depending on location and industry. The reported prevalence of farmer's lung, the classic example of HP, ranges from 1.6% to 7%. The farmer's lung antigen, *Thermophilic actinomycetes*, is associated with disease predominantly in wet climates. Antigens able to induce HP are derived from microorganisms, animals, plants, organic and inorganic chemicals (Table 20–1). Most of these antigens are derived from organisms that are ubiquitous in the natural environment. Sensitization typically occurs via the aerosol route. Bird handlers have a prevalence of HP that ranges from 20 to 20,000 affected individuals per 100,000 at-risk persons. This population appears to have an increased risk of the disease as compared to farmers because their exposure to the avian antigen is on a more routine basis and is less affected by season and geographic location.

Incidence

The incidence of HP varies and depends on multiple factors. Factors such as the country in question, climates, seasonal changes, cultural differences, and workplace environments all contribute to the variability of indoor mold exposure. Finland in particular seems to demonstrate significant variability based on season. Most cases of farmer's lung occur during April when the indoor feeding season for cattle is ending.

Table 20–1. Antigens in hypersensitivity pneumonitis.

Antigen	Disease	Source
Bacteria: *Thermophilic Actinomycetes*		
Bacillus subtilis	Enzyme/detergent worker's lung Familial hypersensitivity pneumonitis (HP)	Enzyme dust, contaminated house dust
Bacillus cereus *Klebsiella oxytoca*	Humidifier's lung	Ultrasonic cool mist humidifiers
Cephalosporium acremonium	Floor finisher's lung	Moldy wood floors
Mycobacterium avium complex	Hot tub lung	Detergent/cleaning agents Hot tub
Pseudomonas fluorescens *Acinetobacter calcoaceticus* *Mycobacterium chelonae*	Machine operator's lung	Contaminated metalworking fluids
Thermoactinomyces candidus *Thermoactinomyces viridis*	Mushroom picker's lung	Mushroom compost
Thermoactinomyces sacchari	Ventilation pneumonitis	Humidifier, air conditioner
Thermoactinomyces vulgaris	Residential composter's lung	Moldy residential compost
T. vulgaris	Bagassosis	Moldy sugarcane
Faeni rectivirgula	Farmer's lung Potato riddler's lung	Moldy hay, grain, compost, silage Moldy hay around potatoes
Fungi		
Aspergillus spp.	Malt worker's lung Stipatosis Compost lung Tobacco worker's disease	Moldy malt dust Moldy esparto grass Compost Moldy tobacco Contaminated oxygen water humidifier Contaminated soy sauce
Alternaria spp.	Woodworker's lung	Moldy wood dust
Rhizopus and Mucor spp.	Wood trimmer's disease	Moldy wood trimmings
Botrytis cinerea	Wine grower's lung	Moldy grapes
Aureobasidium pullulans	Air-conditioner lung	Moldy water in HVAC systems
Cladosporium spp.	Sauna taker's lung	Contaminated sauna water
Cephalosporium spp.	*Cephalosporium* HP	Contaminated basement (sewage)
Penicillium frequentans	*Suberosis*	Moldy cork dust
Penicillium caseii *Penicillium roqueforti*	Cheese worker's/washer's lung	Cheese mold
Penicillium brevicompactum *Fusarium* spp.	Farmer's lung	Moldy hay

(Continued)

Table 20–1. Antigens in hypersensitivity pneumonitis. (Continued)

Antigen	Disease	Source
Fungi		
Absidia corymbifera *Wallemia sebi*	Farmer's lung in eastern France	Moldy cowshed fodder
Penicillium expansum *Penicillium cyclopium* *Penicillium chrysogenum*	Farmer's lung in eastern France	Moldy wood dust
Penicillium camembertii *Penicillium nalgiovense* *Penicillium chrysogenum*	Salami worker's lung	Salami seasoning
Penicillium and *Monocillium* spp.	Peat moss processor's lung Woodman's disease	Moldy peat moss Moldy oak and maple trees
Pleurotus ostreatus and *Hypsizigus marmoreus* basidiospores	Mushroom worker's lung	Indoor mushroom cultivation
Trichosporum cutaneum *Trichosporon ovoides* *Cryptococcus albidus*	Summer-type/summer house HP	Japanese house dust
Cryptostroma corticale	Maple bark stripper's disease	Wet maple bark
Rhodotorula rubra		Moldy cellar/bathroom walls
Pullularia spp. *Graphium* spp. *Alternaria* spp.	Sequoiosis	Moldy redwood dust
Pezizia domiciliana	El Niño lung	Moldy home from flooding
Lycoperdon puffballs	Lycoperdonosis	Puff ball spores
Candida spp.	Saxophonist's lung	Moldy reed
Epicoccum nigrum	Basement shower HP	Moldy basement shower
Fusarium napiform		Moldy home
Saccharomonospora viridis	Thatched roof disease	Dried grasses and leaves
Streptomyces albus	*Streptomyces albus* HP	Contaminated fertilizer
Animal Protein		
Avian proteins	Bird fancier/breeder/handler's lung, pigeon breeder's disease	Pigeon (pets and wild), duck, chicken, turkey, lovebird, dove, parrot, parakeet, Canada goose, owl
Bovine and porcine proteins	Pituitary snuff user's lung	Heterologous pituitary snuff

(Continued)

Table 20–1. Antigens in hypersensitivity pneumonitis. (Continued)

Antigen	Disease	Source
Animal Protein		
Cat hair, animal pelts	Furrier's lung	Cat hair and fur dust
Rodent urinary proteins	Laboratory worker's lung Gerbil keeper's lung	Laboratory rat or gerbil urine
Oyster/mollusk shell protein	Oyster shell lung	Shell dust
Insect Protein		
Sitophila granarius	Wheat weevil disease Miller disease	Infested wheat flour
Silkworm larvae	Sericulturist's lung disease	Cocoon fluff
Amoebae		
Naegleria gruberi *Acanthamoeba castellani*	Ventilation pneumonitis	Contaminated ventilation system
Chemicals		
Toluene diisocyanate (TDI)	Paint refinisher's disease Bathtub refinisher's lung	Varnishes, lacquer, foundry, casting, polyurethane foam
Diphenylmethane diisocyanate (MDI)	Chemical worker's lung	Urethane paint catalyst
Phthalic anhydride	Epoxy resin worker's lung	Resin, adhesive, foam
Trimellitic anhydride	Plastic worker's lung	Plastics industry
Pyrethrum	Pyrethrum lung	Insecticide
Medications or Drugs		
Fluoxetine, mesalamine, intravesicular BCG, intranasal heroin, β-blockers, nitrofurantoin, HMG-CoA reductase inhibitors, sulfasalazine, minocycline, chlorambucil, procarbazine, cyclosporine, gold, clozapine, amiodarone	Drug-induced HP	Medications
Plant		
Soybean hull		Veterinary feed
Tobacco leaves	Tobacco grower's lung	Tobacco dust
Coffee and tea dust	Coffee/Tea worker's lung	Coffee bean dust or tea leaves
Abreva wood Pine saw dust	Woodworker's lung	Wood dust/sawdust

BCG, Bacille Calmette-Guérin (vaccine); HVAC, heating, ventilating, and air conditioning.
Fink, J.N., Zacharisen, M.C. (2003). Hypersensitivity Pneumonitis. In Adkinson: Middleton's Allergy: Principles and Practice, 6th ed. Vol. 2 (pp. 1374–1375). Philadelphia, PA: Mosby.

The incidence is lowest in October when outdoor feeding for cattle is more common. There is also a positive correlation between the incidence of HP and the average daily rainfall during the preceding haymaking season.

Cigarette smoking is associated with a decreased risk of developing HP. Smoking seems to decrease the risk of developing farmer's lung, pigeon breeder's disease, HP associated with contaminated air conditioners, and Japanese summer-type HP caused by *Trichosporon cutaneum*. Once the disease process has begun, smoking does not mitigate disease severity or slow progression. Smoking may also predispose to a more chronic form of HP.

IMMUNOPATHOGENESIS

Overview

Proliferation of CD8[+] cytotoxic lymphocytes and significantly elevated IgG antibody are central to the pathogenesis of HP. The IgG is likely derived from plasma cells stimulated from CD4[+] T_H1 lymphocytes. Once inhaled antigen is deposited in the lower airway, macrophages ingest the antigen and initiate the inflammatory cascade. Interestingly, only 1% of patients exposed to the implicated antigens progress to manifest the disease. The majority of people exposed to the antigenic particles develop an IgG response. This alone is not sufficient to cause disease when not accompanied by a cytotoxic delayed hypersensitivity CD8[+] response. The factors that determine whether a person will develop the clinical manifestations of HP are not fully delineated. Increased production of macrophage-derived tumor necrosis factor alpha (TNF-α) and expression of the TNF A2 allele, which is associated with increased production of TNF-α, were found with increased frequency in patients with HP. These patients had farmer's lung and had an increased production of TNF-α after hay challenge, but asymptomatic controls with positive antibodies did not have this exaggerated response. Recently, investigators have found that glucocorticoid-induced TNF receptor (GITR) expressed on natural killer T cells (NKT) can increase cytokine production by NKT cells in vitro. They have also demonstrated that this effect can protect against the development of HP in vivo.

There have been no clear correlations between specific major histocompatibility class (MHC) I loci and HP or any specific genetic predisposition for the development of HP. Despite this, pigeon fanciers with HP have a higher frequency of HLA-DRB1*1305, HLA-DRQB1*0501, and TNF-α(308) promoter. Patients with farmer's lung also have a higher incidence of HLA B8. Those with Japanese summer-type HP have a higher frequency of HLA-DQw3.

Acute Phase of Hypersensitivity Pneumonitis

The acute phase of HP is initiated when the inhaled antigen binds specific IgG antibody. Immune complex formation ensues and C5 is elaborated. C5 serves to activate macrophages. Once macrophages are activated, they secrete various chemokines, such as IL-8, macrophage inflammatory protein α1 (MIP-1α), and regulated on activation, normal T-cell expressed and secreted (RANTES). Other cytokines are also elaborated. These molecules initially attract leukocytes, which in this case are predominantly neutrophils, not eosinophils as seen in other forms of pulmonary disease. Circulating T lymphocytes and monocytes are attracted later in the immune response. MIP-α1 contributes to the differentiation of T_H0 cells to T_H1 cells and acts as a chemotactic molecule for macrophages and lymphocytes. Mouse models of HP show that IFN-γ, which is usually produced by activated CD4[+] T_H1 lymphocytes, is required for the activation of macrophages. This activation leads to the formation of granulomas. Other cytokines, such as IL-1 and TNF-α, derived from activated macrophages, act as pyrogens and cause fever. They also cause the acute-phase response seen in HP. Macrophages also elaborate IL-6 and IL-12. IL-12 contributes to the differentiation of B cells into plasma cells and the development of CD8[+] cells into cytotoxic T lymphocytes. IL-12 additionally contributes to the differentiation of T_H0 to T_H1 cells, amplifying the reaction. Human subjects with HP have T lymphocytes in BAL fluid with increased IL-12 receptor.

The adhesion molecule CD80/86, or B-7, is increased on activated macrophages. Activated T cells have increased CD28, which is the ligand for B-7. CD28 and B-7 function as critical costimulatory molecules for antigen presentation and for B-cell activation by CD4[+] T-helper cells. Mouse models of HP show that antagonism of these ligands inhibits inflammation necessary to induce HP. Endothelial adhesion molecules such as E- and P-selectin and ICAM-1 play a crucial role in the migration of inflammatory cells into target tissues. Inhibition of these molecules blocks the recruitment of lymphocytes into pulmonary tissue. BAL fluid in most cases of HP demonstrates higher numbers of CD8[+] cells compared to CD4[+] cells. Higher numbers of CD4[+] cells, however, do predominate early in the immunologic response.

Subacute Phase of Hypersensitivity Pneumonitis

The subacute phase of HP is characterized by granuloma formation. Macrophages that are attracted to lung tissue eventually develop into epithelioid cells and multinucleated giant cells. Lymphoid follicles containing plasma cells form in proximity to the granuloma. This phase of inflammation is also represented by proliferation of CD4⁺ T$_H$1 lymphocytes, which contain the CD40 ligand on their surface. This ligand is critical for the activation of B cells and their subsequent development into plasma cells that produce antibody. Much of the antibody production in HP occurs locally in lung tissue primarily due to this immune response.

Chronic Phase of Hypersensitivity Pneumonitis

The extracellular matrix surrounding the granuloma contains myofibroblasts, which deposit collagen and the proteoglycan versican. The activated macrophages secrete high amounts of TGF-β, a potent inducer of fibrosis and angiogenesis. These pathologic changes are the hallmark of the chronic phase of inflammation. Expression of Fas ligand and CD40 ligand also promote fibrosis. Increased numbers of mast cells are present in the BAL fluid of mouse and human models of HP. They are also found in high numbers in the interstitial tissue in HP. Mast cells can also be found in the BAL fluid of other interstitial lung diseases. The mast cells in BAL fluid in HP have characteristics of the connective tissue type rather than the mucosal type. Mast cells of the connective tissue type may play more of a role in diseases characterized by fibrosis as opposed to diseases such as asthma. Mast cells elaborate inflammatory cytokines that promote fibrosis and recruitment of monocytes and lymphocytes. Neutrophils may play a role in the development of fibrosis in HP. Recently, evidence indicates that alveolar macrophages in patients with pulmonary fibrosis and HP secrete high levels of CCL18, which is a potent inducer of fibroblast collagen deposition. These are possible mechanisms of why fibrosis develops in patients with chronic HP.

CLINICAL PRESENTATION

The presentation of HP can be acute, subacute, or chronic. These various stages can overlap clinically (Fig. 20–1), and individuals can present with a combination of these forms. This presentation is usually determined by level of antigenic exposure. Patients can present with different forms of HP despite being in the same setting where the exposure took place. Why some patients stay healthy, some develop just acute HP, others develop progressive fibrosis, and still others asthma from the same exposure is presently unknown.

Acute Presentation

Signs and Symptoms

The incorrect diagnosis of infectious pneumonia is often made during the acute presentation of HP.

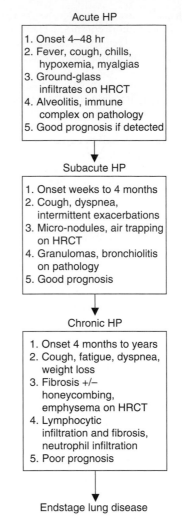

Figure 20-1. Clinical presentation of hypersensitivity pneumonitis (HP).

Symptoms typically consist of fever, cough, dyspnea, chest pain, myalgias, and fatigue. Other symptoms include loss of appetite, weight loss, and wheezing. Symptoms of the acute form are usually abrupt and occur within 4 to 6 hours after exposure to the agent. When the subject is exposed to very large amounts of antigen, the acute presentation can be within only a few hours of exposure. Symptoms typically resolve within 12 hours but may take up to several days after the subject is removed from the offending agent. Physical examination demonstrates rales, but wheezes can be present. Resolution of symptoms with hospitalization often delays the diagnosis because the patient is removed from the source of antigen. Markers of inflammation, such as erythrocyte sedimentation rate, C-reactive protein, and white blood cell count, may be elevated in this form. Neutrophilic leukocytosis usually predominates in acute HP. Elevated inflammatory markers may precede signs and symptoms by several days and may also persist for several days after symptom resolution.

Radiography and Pulmonary Function Testing

Radiographic and spirometric evaluation during the acute form of HP have notable findings. Chest radiograph can demonstrate bilateral interstitial infiltrates in up to 90% of patients, and hilar lymphadenopathy is present about 50% of the time. Spirometry shows a decreased forced vital capacity (FVC) and forced expiratory volume in 1 second (FEV_1). The ratio of FEV_1 to FVC is usually preserved, and total lung volumes (TLC), along with diffusing capacity (D_{LCO}), are decreased. Radiographic abnormalities in acute HP usually resolve along with symptoms within 12 hours to several days after removal from exposure.

Subacute Presentation

SIGNS AND SYMPTOMS

The subacute form is more difficult to diagnose because the associated signs and symptoms mimic many other respiratory disease states. Symptoms begin with coughing, fever, and malaise that resemble bronchitis. The cough can become severe and productive. Wheezes, rales, and rhonchi may be present on examination as the disease severity fluctuates. Low-grade fever may also be present, but this is not a consistent finding in the subacute stage of the disease. Other symptoms, such as arthralgias, myalgias, and fatigue, may be significant, leading one to falsely suspect a rheumatologic disease.

Radiography and Pulmonary Function Testing

Pulmonary function tests in the subacute form reveals a mixed obstructive-restrictive defect that may reverse with bronchodilators. Glucocorticoids often reverse the pulmonary function abnormalities as well. These findings often lead to the misdiagnosis of asthma. Interestingly, approximately 50% of patients have a positive methacholine bronchial challenge, making the distinction with asthma even more difficult. Unlike patients with asthma, patients with HP do not achieve control of their pulmonary symptoms with bronchodilators and inhaled corticosteroids. They require courses of systemic glucocorticoids to control their symptoms.

Chest radiographs may be normal or slightly abnormal in the subacute form. Computed tomography (CT) may be the preferred imaging study to identify any pulmonary abnormalities. Inflammatory markers may be elevated as in the acute form of HP. These markers may be particularly useful when monitoring avoidance-challenge procedures.

Chronic Presentation

SIGNS AND SYMPTOMS

In the chronic form of HP, patients often present to medical attention late in the course of the disease. Patients may be identified by routine chest radiography with minimal or no symptoms. The most common symptom is dyspnea with exertion and a nonproductive cough. Other complaints include weight loss, loss of appetite, and malaise. These nonspecific symptoms may be present for years before medical attention is sought. Lung exam often reveals crackles. Unlike the other stages of HP, wheezes, rales, and rhonchi are unlikely to be found on lung auscultation. Digital clubbing is uncommon in the other two forms of HP but may be present in the chronic form and indicates severe disease.

RADIOGRAPHY AND PULMONARY FUNCTION TESTING

Unlike the other forms of HP, inflammatory markers may be normal. Chest radiography often shows significant pulmonary fibrosis but may be normal. Pulmonary function test (PFT) demonstrates a restrictive pattern where the D_{LCO} will be reduced. CT will have changes consistent with HP or nonspecific endstage *honeycombing,* a term used to describe severe fibrosis.

DIAGNOSIS

HP is frequently misdiagnosed or unrecognized because of its similarity to other interstitial lung diseases and its low incidence in the population. In some instances, respiratory symptoms dominate the clinical picture, whereas in other cases, systemic symptoms predominate. Respiratory symptoms may be intermittent and correlate with exposure to the implicated agent. In other cases, respiratory symptoms may be chronic. The disease process may not be HP, despite identification of a potential exposure. There are other immunologically mediated diseases that mimic HP. An occupational or environmental etiology for respiratory disease must be considered in the differential diagnosis when evaluating patients. The clinician should search for potential antigens when HP is suspected and work to identify a relationship between the timing of exposure and symptoms.

There is no single diagnostic test specific for HP (Table 20–2). The diagnosis is often entertained based on history, physical examination, and environmental and occupational exposure. Radiographic infiltrates that

Table 20–2. Studies used to evaluate HP.

Evaluation	Findings
Laboratory investigation	IgG antibody specific for antigen (Precipitin) Inflammatory markers: leukocytosis, hypergammaglobulinemia, elevated C-reactive protein, elevated erythrocyte sedimentation rate
Arterial blood gas	Possible hypoxemia
Chest radiography	Pulmonary infiltrates, fibrosis, nodules depending on stage of disease, level of antigen exposure, duration of exposure
Computerized tomograph scan	Ground-glass opacities, air trapping, fibrosis
Pulmonary function	Restrictive defect, hypoxemia, impaired D_{LCO}, obstructive defect
Bronchoalveolar lavage fluid analysis	Initially neutrophilic predominance, followed by lymphocyte predominance ($CD8^+$)
Lung biopsy	Lymphocytic infiltration, granulomas, fibrosis

are intermittent in presentation should raise suspicion of HP. Physical examination may reveal crackles and occasionally wheezing on lung auscultation. These findings are nonspecific for HP but may be helpful if present with a compatible history.

Laboratory Findings

Laboratory testing is not particularly revealing in evaluating for the presence of HP. Inflammatory markers such as erythrocyte sedimentation rate and leukocyte count may be elevated. This elevation is most common in acute HP. Serum total IgG is elevated, but IgE and eosinophil count are usually normal. Rheumatoid factor may also be positive, especially with chronic HP secondary to the lung fibrosis.

Serum specific precipitating antibodies are found in many patients with HP. As many as 40% to 50% of asymptomatic individuals exposed to the same antigens have serum IgG antibodies. Positive serum precipitins indicate past exposure to the implicated antigen in sufficient amount to induce a humoral immunologic response but not always the disease. Thus serum precipitins are sensitive but not specific in diagnosing HP. Serum precipitin testing offered by commercial laboratories in general is only helpful in the evaluation of farmer's lung or bird fancier's disease. If exposure to the antigen is related to the home or work environment, this test most likely has little value. If precipitin testing is performed on suspected antigens from the environment where exposure has taken place, the diagnostic yield may be greatly increased. Idiopathic interstitial lung disease (ILD) is one situation when a positive precipitin test is particularly useful. If this is identified in an

individual with ILD, the clinician should search for the implicated antigen and the environment where exposure has taken place. Precipitins can remain positive for months or years after the last known exposure. If antibodies are no longer detectable by gel diffusion, the patient may still respond to specific antigen challenges.

Keep in mind that allergen skin testing to identify allergen-specific IgE antibodies is not indicated in the workup of HP because it is not an IgE-mediated disease. Skin tests are nonspecific and not useful in the evaluation of suspected HP. Cell-mediated hypersensitivity to the suspected antigen may be more reliable in distinguishing patients with HP from asymptomatic individuals who are exposed to the antigen because a cell-mediated immune response is postulated to be integral in the disease pathogenesis.

Radiographic Evaluation

Chest radiography and high-resolution computed tomography (HRCT) of the chest can assist in the evaluation of HP. HRCT is considered more sensitive than chest radiography in supporting the diagnosis of HP and more capable of defining interstitial pathology. The findings on imaging vary according to the stage of HP. Acute HP typically demonstrates bilateral micronodular infiltrates or patchy ground-glass opacities on HRCT. Imaging may also show decreased attenuation and mosaic perfusion due to air trapping from bronchiolitis. These findings correlate on histopathology to peribronchiolar perilymphatic infiltration and active interstitial inflammation, respectively. In subacute HP, linear shadows and small nodules give a reticulonodular appearance on chest radiographs. Chronic HP demonstrates radiographic findings consistent with interstitial fibrosis or honeycombing. The distribution of fibrosis is in the upper and mid-lung zones. This is in contrast to idiopathic pulmonary fibrosis where the fibrosis is in the lower lung zones. Advancing chronic disease causes bronchiectasis, volume loss, and honeycombing. Pleural disease and lymphadenopathy are rare in HP.

Pulmonary Function Testing

Pulmonary function testing typically demonstrates a restrictive defect with abnormal diffusion capacity. Therefore, measuring the FVC and the diffusion capacity (D_{LCO}) are the most useful parameters in pulmonary function testing. FVC reflects static lung volume and D_{LCO} is a measure of gas exchange. The FVC may be normal in early HP, but this value usually becomes progressively reduced as the disease process advances. The FVC can also be used to monitor the effects of glucocorticoids or removal from the environment where the exposure took place. Environmental challenges with the putative antigen can also be monitored with FVC.

The D_{LCO} is a more sensitive indicator of disease presence compared to FVC when measured early in the disease course. Because D_{LCO} measures gas exchange, it is also is a better predictor of oxygen desaturation with exercise. Serial measurements of D_{LCO} can also be used to monitor intervention strategies. Pulse oximetry with exertion can be used in the office as an initial screen for oxygen desaturation with exercise. The finding of oxygen desaturation, particularly during exercise, may be an indicator of insidious interstitial involvement. Arterial blood gas measurement does not seem to have any additional benefit over pulse oximetry.

Because many other interstitial lung diseases produce a similar pattern on spirometry, these findings are not specific for HP. Chronic HP may show an obstructive defect with a reduced FEV_1 to FVC ratio as previously mentioned; however, most cases are restrictive. Severe cases of HP may show significant hypoxemia. A mixed restrictive or obstructive pattern can also be found in HP, confusing the diagnosis with asthma or chronic obstructive pulmonary disease.

Bronchoscopy

Clinical signs and symptoms that are consistent with HP in conjunction with relevant environmental exposure may be sufficient to establish the diagnosis of HP. If uncertainty persists, additional evaluation may be pursued. Bronchoscopy with transbronchial biopsy along with BAL may be performed. Transbronchial biopsy specimens may help differentiate HP from entities such as sarcoidosis, alveolar hemorrhage, and lymphangitic carcinoma, which have their own characteristic findings that differ from HP. To increase the diagnostic yield of biopsy specimens, multiple biopsies should be performed on areas of lung that demonstrate radiographic involvement.

Histologic Analysis

The classic triad of HP on histopathologic analysis is bronchiolitis or bronchiolitis obliterans, patchy NSIP, and scattered nonnecrotizing granulomas. Despite the classic triad on histologic specimens, not all patients with HP demonstrate granulomas and bronchiolitis obliterans. The most common findings on histologic analysis found in farmer's lung as determined by Reyes et al are listed in Table 20–3. One group of investigators found that the only consistent pathologic finding in HP was patchy peribronchiolar pneumonitis with an interstitial infiltrate of predominantly lymphocytes and/or plasma cells. Interstitial infiltrates in HP are predominantly lymphocytes, macrophages, mast cells, and plasma cells. An important distinction between HP and rheumatologic conditions is the absence of vasculitis and necrotizing granulomas.

Neutrophilic inflammation and emphysema may be present if exposure is to a significant degree. Acute HP is characterized by neutrophils that infiltrate the alveoli and respiratory bronchioles. This can manifest as diffuse

Table 20–3. Pathologic findings in hypersensitivity pneumonitis.

Pathologic Findings	% of Cases
Patchy interstitial pneumonitis	100%
Unresolved pneumonia with organizing intraalveolar fibrinous exudates	65%
Patchy interstitial fibrosis of varying severity	65%
Bronchiolitis obliterans	50%
Granulomas with Langhans-type giant cells	70%
Birefringent foreign body material of uncertain nature	60%
Pleural fibrosis	28%
Intraalveolar edema	52%
Variable-size collections of intraalveolar foam cells	65%

Adapted from Reyes CN, Wenzel FJ, Lawton BR, et al. The pulmonary pathology of farmer's lung disease. *Chest.* 1982; 81:142.

alveolar damage. There have been multiple reports of neutrophil and eosinophil presence in lung tissue specimens in patients with HP; therefore, even though lymphocytes are generally found more commonly in this disease, the presence of neutrophils and eosinophils should not exclude HP as a diagnostic possibility. It is important to remember that the presence of the previously described pathologic findings is determined by the stage and duration of the disease as well as the quality of the biopsy.

If the natural course of HP continues without intervention, fibrosis becomes the predominant finding and may resemble other fibrotic pulmonary diseases such as UIP. As compared to UIP, more upper lung field involvement typically occurs in HP. In 1987 Dunhill reported that findings in chronic HP were the same as other endstage lung diseases and that the fibrosis in chronic HP was indistinguishable from the fibrosis manifested by other causes.

Analysis of BAL fluid can assist in the diagnosis of HP. Microbial stains and cultures can be performed on BAL fluid to diagnose infections that can mimic HP. Malignancies can also be diagnosed in some cases as well. In HP, BAL fluid typically reveals a predominant $CD8^+$ lymphocytosis in HP as opposed to the BAL fluid in sarcoidosis, which is characterized by $CD4^+$ lymphocytosis. This is determined by the ratio of $CD8^+$ to $CD4^+$ lymphocytes on the BAL cell differential. This finding depends on the timing of antigen exposure because neutrophils are the predominant cell type present after acute antigen exposure and as HP becomes chronic, the ratio of $CD4^+$ lymphocytes to $CD8^+$ lymphocytes increases. A marked elevation in the $CD8^+$ T cells may indicate a protective effect on the progression to pulmonary fibrosis. Conversely, an elevated $CD4^+$ T cell count may have a predictive role on progression to the fibrotic phase of HP. Unlike diagnosing fungal infections and organic dust toxic syndrome (ODTS), the detection of antigen in BAL specimens has a limited role in the diagnostic workup of HP.

Video-Assisted Thorascopic Surgery

When biopsy samples from transbronchial biopsy and BAL fluid analysis are not sufficient to aid in the diagnosis of HP, video-assisted thorascopic surgery (VATS) can be performed. VATS can provide larger specimens that are required for diagnosing certain entities clinically similar to HP such as vasculitic processes. Patients who have an FVC less than 40% or require supplemental oxygen may not be appropriate candidates for this procedure because of its inherent morbidity. Compared to open lung biopsy, VATS requires less analgesia, has less blood loss, and requires a shorter postoperative stay. Specimens obtained from open lung biopsy and VATS have the same sample adequacy and diagnostic accuracy;

therefore, VATS has become the preferred modality when larger specimens are required.

Environmental History

The environmental history is an important aspect of the investigation when HP is suspected. In the past, HP was viewed as an entity that resulted from a large exposure to an antigen found primarily in the agricultural, industrial, or hobbyist surroundings. Because practices in the workplace have been remedied by the addition of protective equipment, antigen exposure in the occupational setting has substantially diminished. Altering storage of hay has been very effective at decreasing HP in farmers.

The home is an integral part of the environmental investigation when HP is suspected. The investigator should clue in to areas of excessive moisture within the home environment when mold exposure is suspected. Seemingly irrelevant aspects of the home investigation should be considered, such as plumbing irregularities, humidifiers, hot tubs, bird antigens, saunas, animal exposures, forced air-heating and air-cooling system abnormalities, and roof leaks. These represent some reservoirs in the home that can provide enough antigen exposure to cause HP. It is also important to ascertain the daily routine of the inhabitants of a home. Factors such as indoor plants, thermostat settings, cooking habits, and size of the family all play a role in the overall humidity within a home, which may lead to mold overgrowth. If the thermostat is set to a high temperature but fans are used to circulate the air, the air may not be effectively dehumidified. As a result, microenvironments within the home can form where humidity concentrates, such as behind furniture, inside closets, and under beds. These areas of high humidity can lead to overgrowth of antigen that may be difficult to detect. The office or work environment should also be evaluated for these same conditions that can lead to antigen exposure.

Environmental Sampling

Environmental sampling of water, dust, soil, and air that is performed at suspected antigen exposure locations may be helpful. Most areas of antigen exposure are readily detected by inspection that is directed by environmental history under the guidance of the physician. A "musty" odor on initial encounter with the environment in question can serve as a helpful tool. This smell indicates that high levels of mold and/or bacteria are present in the environment. Visual inspection is also employed to ascertain the specific areas of contamination. A clue to significant environmental exposure is the presence of water damage, leaking roofs, or plumbing malfunctions. Again, areas of moisture in the home should be sought because these areas tend to harbor antigen that can cause HP.

Obtaining cultures of contaminated areas in the environment in question can assist in the investigation. The swab technique of areas that have visible mold has no value in quantifying exposure. But the gravity culture technique, if performed on the indoor environment by employing agar plates, can determine a reference level of antigen. This method can also be used to determine the effectiveness of environmental remediation. Unfortunately, even if technically satisfactory samples are obtained, the results may be difficult to interpret and correlate to the clinical presentation. Reliability of air sampling devices and the lack of standardization of this technique make this method of measuring microbes in the environment less useful in the investigation.

Challenge Methods

Direct antigen inhalation, environmental exposure, and in vitro stimulation of lymphocytes are some of the various challenge methods used to help in the diagnosis of HP. Each of these methods has their own advantages and disadvantages.

IN VITRO CHALLENGE

In vitro challenges have been used on blood lymphocytes and lymphocytes derived from BAL fluid. In vitro challenges, much like precipitin testing, do not discriminate between individuals who have been exposed to the antigen and those who are manifesting the clinical disease of HP. This method has been used successfully in diagnosing sensitivity to pigeon antigens in pigeon breeders with positive precipitin testing.

DIRECT ANTIGEN INHALATION

Direct antigen inhalation can be used to identify the causal antigen in all three stages of the disease. Because antigen concentrations are arbitrarily chosen, this procedure may deliver a potentially dangerous dose of antigen to a susceptible subject. It is imperative that patients be prick test negative to the antigen as well, so a potentially lethal asthmatic response can be avoided. Provocative inhalational testing is usually not required for the diagnosis of HP, and if they are to be performed, they should be done in an appropriate setting where correct management can be obtained. To avoid poor outcomes, inhalational challenge is best reserved to be performed by those experienced with the technique.

PFT values that are considered the eligibility cutoff for antigen inhalation is an FVC or D_{LCO} below 50%. Patients should ideally be asymptomatic and off corticosteroids when performing an antigen challenge procedure. Pulmonary function testing may be helpful if performed before and after exposure. Parameters measured before and after challenge include temperature, spirometry, auscultation, and leukocyte count. These values are typically measured every hour after antigen

challenge up to 8 hours. Chest radiographs are also obtained before and after the challenge is performed. Antigen challenge can also be used in chronic HP to differentiate this entity from other forms of ILD.

ENVIRONMENTAL AVOIDANCE CHALLENGE

Environmental avoidance challenge is another method to help detect the presence of HP. The disadvantage of this method is that the implicated antigen cannot be accurately determined. There is also no consensus on the duration of avoidance required to observe a beneficial effect on clinical, laboratory, and pulmonary function parameters. A typical environmental challenge would begin by inducing remission of the disease with a course of corticosteroids followed by restriction to the home environment. Parameters such as chest radiograph, C-reactive protein, sedimentation rate, pulmonary function tests, and white blood cell count are monitored. When symptoms return, the patient is moved to an environment that is known to be free of antigen. Remediation of the home environment is then undertaken. The patient returns home and is followed for a period to see if remediation of the home environment was successful.

Diagnostic Criteria

Diagnostic criteria for HP have been proposed by the American Academy of Allergy Asthma and Immunology. According to these diagnostic guidelines (Table 20–4), if four of the major criteria and two of the minor criteria are fulfilled, then the diagnosis of HP is made. Importantly, other disease processes with similar presentations must be excluded.

TREATMENT
Avoidance of Antigen

The primary objective in the treatment of HP is early identification of the disease and, most importantly, avoidance of the putative agents. Identifying the specific antigen is a challenging endeavor and may not be feasible. Equipment to protect the subject from exposure such as laminar flow high-efficiency particle arrest-filtered helmets may be used. Electrostatic dust filters installed in the air-conditioning system can be effective in lowering mold antigen but may not provide adequate protection. High-efficiency particulate air (HEPA) filters when used in isolation are considered insufficient to remove antigen.

Environmental Remediation

Remediation of the environment is the next step in antigen avoidance. General contractors or the owner of the home are typically sufficient to perform a successful

Table 20–4. Major criteria for diagnosis.

Major Criteria

-----

1. History of compatible symptoms with hypersensitivity pneumonitis (HP) that develop or worsen within hours if exposed to antigen.
2. Historical confirmation of exposure to the offending agent, investigation of the environment, serum precipitin testing, and/or bronchoalveolar lavage fluid antibody.
3. Changes on chest radiography or high-resolution computerized tomography of the chest that is compatible with HP.
4. If bronchoalveolar lavage is performed, the presence of fluid lymphocytosis.
5. If lung biopsy is performed, compatible histologic findings with HP.
6. Reproduction of symptoms and laboratory abnormalities after exposure to the suspected environment or by controlled challenge.

Minor Criteria

-----

1. Basilar crackles on lung examination.
2. Decreased diffusion capacity of pulmonary function testing.
3. Arterial hypoxemia at rest or with exercise.

Note: Four major and two minor criteria are required for diagnosis.

remediation. Once remediation has been implemented, the patient must be monitored for disease progression. Care must be taken to prevent progression to chronic HP or fibrosis by chronic low-level antigen exposure that is subclinical.

Corticosteroids

Corticosteroids may be used to treat acute and subacute HP but should not be substituted for avoidance measures. An appropriate time course and dose would be 2 to 4 weeks of prednisone, 0.5 mg/kg/day. Subacute HP may mandate higher doses of prednisone for a longer duration. The effect of corticosteroids on slowing the progression of the subacute and chronic forms of HP has not been clearly defined.

PROGNOSIS

Early recognition of HP and removal from the offending agent seem to be the most important factors in terms of prognosis. The prognosis is favorable if HP is detected early. Once the person is removed from the offending agent, improvement is typically observed within 1 to 6 months. If identified in the acute stage, the patient may demonstrate restrictive lung disease with reduced diffusion capacity that continues to improve over the course of several weeks. The granuloma and bronchiolitis that occurs in the subacute phase may take longer to resolve even if corticosteroids are implemented. Some patients with farmer's lung may continue to have disease progression and a decline in

lung function despite removal from antigen exposure. Predictors of progressive decline in lung function in farmers include recurrent acute episodes of HP, exposure to areas of swine confinement, bacterial endotoxin exposure, allergy to mites/organic dust, and fungal infections. There also appears to be an increased risk of developing emphysema in farmers with farmer's lung. Chronic fibrotic HP is a slowly progressive disease that is irreversible and can lead to respiratory failure, right heart failure, and death.

EVIDENCE-BASED MEDICINE

Despite the progress in diagnosing and treating HP, there is still a need to determine better diagnostic criteria. Recognition of the disease is a challenge, and clinicians must think of HP in the differential diagnosis of interstitial lung disease. A recent study demonstrated that genetic expression profiles can help differentiate between HP, idiopathic pulmonary fibrosis, and nonspecific interstitial pneumonitis. HP gene signatures were associated with T-cell activation, inflammation, and immune responses. This is in contrast to gene expression in IPF where the genes were associated with remodeling, epithelial cell, and myofibroblasts. This technology may be helpful in identifying patients with HP who present with interstitial lung disease.

There has not been much new information in regard to treating HP, and the major modality of therapy remains antigen identification and avoidance with remediation of the environment of exposure if necessary. Corticosteroids can be helpful but should not supplant avoidance of the putative antigen. There is some evidence that pentoxifylline induces a dose-dependent suppression of TNF-α and IL-10 secretion from alveolar macrophages in patients with HP. Dexamethasone, however, only suppressed the elaboration of TNF-α. These results indicate that there may be some therapeutic potential for pentoxifylline in treating HP.

Further highlighting the importance of early recognition of the disease, preventing fibrosis in patients with HP can impact survival. In a cohort of patients with subacute and chronic HP, it was determined that the presence of fibrosis was related to a 5-year mortality of 27% and a median survival of 12.8 years.

CONCLUSION

In summary, HP remains a diagnostic challenge for the clinician. The pathophysiology involves interaction with an inhaled antigen that is of animal, plant, microbial, organic material, or inorganic material origin. In susceptible individuals, the antigen induces an immune response dominated by a T_H1 cytokine profile including INF-γ and TNF-α. Some MHC class I loci have been identified that predispose the individual to develop HP if the correct exposure takes place. Once the inflammatory process begins, IgG specific for the antigen is elaborated and can be measured serologically. Aside from lymphocytes that tend to be CD8[+] in the case of HP, neutrophils and macrophages are also recruited to the site of inflammation and contribute to the pathogenesis of HP. Granuloma formation occurs as a consequence of inflammation. Ultimately, fibrosis can occur and the disease becomes relatively indistinguishable from other forms of ILD. Clinical manifestations can be protean and include fever, myalgias, cough, dyspnea, and rales on examination. HP is further classified into three stages: acute, subacute and chronic HP. Each stage has its typical clinical findings, and associated radiographic abnormalities including ground-glass opacities, nodules, and fibrosis. Serum precipitins can be measured to assist in diagnosis but may be positive in exposed individuals without clinical symptoms. Obtaining PFTs and bronchoscopy with BAL analysis may be helpful, as well as VATS for tissue diagnosis. Treatment is directed toward identifying the antigen in the environment and using techniques such as direct antigen inhalation or environmental avoidance challenge to verify the diagnosis.

Remediation of the exposure environment may be necessary. Oral corticosteroids can be used to treat symptoms but should not replace removal from exposure to the antigen.

BIBLIOGRAPHY

Camarena A, Juarez A, Mejia M, et al. Major histocompatibility complex and tumour necrosis factor-alpha polymorphisms in pigeon breeder's disease. *Am J Respir Crit Care Med.* 2001;163:1528.

Denis M. Proinflammatory cytokines in hypersensitivity pneumonitis. *Am J Respir Crit Care Med.* 1995;151:164.

Fink JN, Schlueter DP, Sosman AJ, et al. Clinical survey of pigeon breeders. *Chest.* 1972;62:277.

Emanuel DA, Wenzel FJ, Bowerman CI, et al. Farmer's lung: clinical, pathologic, and immunologic study of twenty-four patients. *Am J Med.* 1964;37:392.

Gudmundsson G, Hunninghake GW. Interferon-gamma is necessary for the expression of hypersensitivity pneumonitis. *J Clin Invest.* 1997;99:2386.

Jacobs RL, Andrews CP, Coalson JJ. Hypersensitivity pneumonitis: beyond classic occupational disease—changing concepts of diagnosis and management. *Ann Allergy Asthma Immunol.* 2005;95:115.

Kim HJ, Kim HY, Kim BK, et al. Engagement of glucocorticoid-induced TNF receptor costimulates NKT cell activation in vitro and in vivo. *J Immunol.* 2006;176(6):3507.

Pardo A, Barrios RM, Gaxiola M, et al. Increase of lung neutrophils in hypersensitivity pneumonitis is associated with lung fibrosis. *Am J Respir Crit Care Med.* 2000;161:1698.

Patel AM, Ryu JH, Reed CE. Hypersensitivity pneumonitis: current concepts and future questions. *J Allergy Clin Immunol.* 2002;108(5):661.

Reyes CN, Wenzel FJ, Lawton BR, et al. The pulmonary pathology of farmer's lung disease. *Chest.* 1982;81:142.

Schaaf BM, Seitzer U, Pravica V, et al. Tumor necrosis factor-alpha-308 promoter gene polymorphism and increased tumor necrosis factor serum bioactivity in farmer's lung patients. *Am J Respir Crit Care Med.* 2001;163:379.

Selman M, Pardo A, Barrera L, et al. Gene expression profiles distinguish idiopathic pulmonary fibrosis from hypersensitivity pneumonitis. *Am J Respir Crit Care Med.* 2006;173(2):188.

Tong Z, Chen B, Dai H, et al. Extrinsic allergic alveolitis: inhibitory effects of pentoxifylline on cytokine production by alveolar macrophages. *Ann Allergy Asthma Immunol.* 2004;92(2):234.

Travis WD, Colby TV, Koss MN, et al. *Diffuse Parenchymal Lung Diseases. Non-Neoplastic Diseases of the Lower Respiratory Tract.* Washington, DC: American Registry of Pathology and Armed Forces Institute of Pathology; 2001:115.

Vourlekis JS, Schwarz MI, Cherniak RM, et al. The effect of pulmonary fibrosis on survival in patients with hypersensitivity pneumonitis. *Am J Med.* 2004;116(10):662.

Allergic Bronchopulmonary Aspergillosis

21

Satoshi Yoshida, MD, PhD, FACP, FCCP, FAAAAI, FACAAI

Allergic bronchopulmonary aspergillosis (ABPA) is a hypersensitivity response to Aspergillus antigens in the lung, which is an uncommon but serious respiratory condition characterized by chronic airway inflammation and airway damage resulting from persistent colonization by and sensitization to the fungus *Aspergillus fumigatus*. The first cases of ABPA in the United States were identified more than 30 years ago, whereas the initial literature report in the United Kingdom was in 1952. The prevalence of ABPA is as high as 1% to 2% of patients with persistent asthma if screening is carried out, although even higher rates have been reported. Especially in corticosteroid-dependent asthma patients, it has been reported that ABPA might be complicated as high as 7% to 14%. In cystic fibrosis, the prevalence of ABPA ranges from 2% to 15%. ABPA is sometimes recognized in patients with allergic fungal sinusitis, although such an association is unusual. ABPA has been identified in patients with hyperimmunoglobulin E (IgE) syndrome and chronic granulomatous disease, which might create management dilemmas because of concerns about administration of prednisone. In patients with asthma, ABPA is sometimes diagnosed in the absence of the typical proximal bronchiectasis; in such cases, it is designated ABPA-seropositive. ABPA is often suspected (1) because of an episode of "pulmonary eosinophilia" or tenacious mucus plugging, (2) when a chest roentgenogram and an unexpected infiltrate is obtained, or (3) after skin testing and serologic testing.

PATHOGENESIS

Discussions on pathogenesis are available in greater detail in several additional references. After inhalation of spores of *A. fumigatus,* there is saprophytic growth in the hyphal form. It remains unclear what survival factors there might be in *A. fumigatus* or what abnormalities there might be in bronchial mucus that permit its growth in contrast to the clearing seen in all other patients with asthma who do not develop ABPA. The array of antibody production, cytokine generation, cellular proliferation (*A. fumigatus* can function as a growth factor for eosinophils in vitro), and effector molecules creates an intense immunologically mediated set of reactions. Many issues remain unclear, including how on histologic examination of patients with ABPA there can be, either individually or in combination, eosinophilic pneumonia, bronchocentric granulomatosis, granulomatous bronchiolitis, exudative bronchiolitis, *A. fumigatus* hyphae in microabscesses, lipid pneumonia, lymphocytic or desquamative interstitial pneumonia, pulmonary vasculitis, and bronchiolitis obliterans.

DIAGNOSIS

Classic criteria for the diagnosis of ABPA has been published by Rosenberg and colleagues in 1977, as mentioned in Table 21–1. Japanese allergist-immunologist or pulmonologists still usually use this criteria for the diagnosis of ABPA. Such cases have other features as well, including chest roentgenographic infiltrates, peripheral blood eosinophilia in the absence of oral corticosteroids, precipitating antibodies to *A. fumigatus,* and production of mucus plugs containing *A. fumigatus.* In such cases, the allergist-immunologist or pulmonologist should have little difficulty with the diagnosis. Failure of the chest roentgenographic or chest computed tomography (CT) infiltrates to clear over a 2-month period of prednisone therapy suggests noncompliance, another ABPA exacerbation, or possibly other diagnoses, such as cystic fibrosis. Proposed criteria for the diagnosis of ABPA in patients with cystic fibrosis are presented in Table 21–2, which is based on the work of a Consensus Conference of the Cystic Fibrosis Foundation. Of note, the prevalence of ABPA is higher

Table 21–1. Criteria for the diagnosis of allergic bronchopulmonary aspergillosis.

Primary
Episodic bronchial obstruction (asthma)
Peripheral blood eosinophilia
Immediate skin reactivity to *Aspergillus* antigen
Precipitate skin reactivity to *Aspergillus* antigen
Elevated serum immunoglobulin E concentrations
History of pulmonary infiltrates (transient or fixed)
Central bronchiectasis

Secondary
A. fumigatus in sputum (by microscopic examination)
History of expectoration of brown plugs or flecks
Arthus reactivity (late skin reactivity) to *Aspergillus* antigens

Table 21–3. Criteria for the diagnosis of allergic bronchopulmonary aspergillosis in patients with asthma.

Criteria for allergic bronchopulmonary aspergillosis (ABPA)-Central Bronchiectasis/Minimal Essential Criteria
1. Asthma/Yes
2. Central bronchiectasis (inner two-thirds of chest computed tomography field)/Yes
3. Immediate cutaneous reactivity to *Aspergillus* species or *Aspergillus fumigatus*/Yes
4. Total serum IgE concentration >417 kU/L (1000 (g/mL)/Yes
5. Elevated serum IgE: *A. fumigatus* and or IgG-*A. fumigatus*/Yes
6. Chest roentgenographic infiltrates/No
7. Serum precipitating antibodies to *A. fumigatus*/No

Criteria for the Diagnosis of ABPA-seropositive
1. Asthma/Yes
2. Immediate cutaneous reactivity to *Aspergillus* species or *A. fumigatus*/Yes
3. Total serum IgE concentration >417 kU/L (1000 µg/mL)/Yes
4. Elevated serum IgE-*A. fumigatus* and or IgG-*A. fumigatus*/Yes
5. Chest roentgenographic infiltrates/No

in patients with cystic fibrosis than in patients with persistent asthma. Table 21–3 presents another criteria proposed for the diagnosis of ABPA in patients with asthma. Some patients who seem to have had no history of asthma or cystic fibrosis and then present with chest roentgenographic infiltrates and lobar collapse are found to have ABPA. Some patients with ABPA have

Table 21–2. Criteria for the diagnosis of allergic bronchopulmonary aspergillosis in patients with cystic fibrosis.

Classic Case Criteria
• Clinical deterioration (increased cough, wheezing, exercise intolerance, increased sputum, decrease in pulmonary function)
• Immediate cutaneous reactivity to *Aspergillus* or presence of serum IgE-*Aspergillus fumigatus* Total serum IgE concentration >1000 kU/L
• Precipitating antibodies to *Aspergillus fumigatus* or serum IgG-*A. fumigatus*
• Abnormal chest roentgenogram (infiltrates, mucus plugging, or a change from earlier films)

Suggestions for Screening on Annual Phlebotomy for allergic bronchopulmonary aspergillosis (ABPA)
• Maintain clinical suspicion for ABPA.
• Annual total serum IgE determination: If it is >500 kU/L, test for immediate cutaneous reactivity to *Aspergillus* or by an in vitro test for serum IgE-*A. fumigatus*.
• If the total serum IgE is <500 kU/L, repeat if clinical suspicion is high.

From the ABPA Consensus Conference of the Cystic Fibrosis Foundation. Bethesda, Maryland; June 2001.

had histories of intermittent mild asthma (exercise-induced bronchospasm) before their ABPA was diagnosed. Conversely, the asthma might have been persistent, moderate, or severe (corticosteroid dependent).

STAGING

The five stages proposed by Patterson et al remain useful. These stages are not phases of a disease, and in each case the physician should attempt to determine the stage that is present. Table 21–4 lists the stages. Most patients who have classic findings and current chest roentgenographic or CT infiltrates are in stage III (recurrent exacerbation). Other patients with current infiltrates are in stage IV (corticosteroid-dependent asthma) or possibly stage I (acute) for first-time recognized infiltrates. High doses of inhaled corticosteroids have not prevented the emergence of infiltrates. Similarly, despite its widespread administration, the antifungal agent itraconazole has not prevented new infiltrates consistently. Patients who are in stage I or stage III with acute infiltrates should respond to prednisone administration, with clearing of the chest roentgenographic or CT infiltrates over 1 to 2 months, and they should become less symptomatic (reduced dyspnea and cough and improved spirometry results). Total serum IgE, if obtained serially, will decline

Table 21–4. Stages of allergic bronchopulmonary aspergillosis.

	Stage Description	Radiographic infiltrates	Total serum IgE
I	Acute	Lobes or middle lobe	Sharply elevated
II	Remission	No infiltrate and patient off prednisone for >6 mo	Elevated or normal
III	Exacerbation	Upper lobes or middle lobe	Sharply elevated
IV	Corticosteroid-dependent asthma	Often without infiltrates, but intermittent infiltrates might occur	Elevated or normal
V	Endstage	Fibrotic, bullous, or cavitary lesions	Might be normal

by at least 35% over 6 weeks. One should not attempt to administer prednisone indefinitely in an attempt to reduce the total serum IgE concentration into the normal range. Unless the patient enters stage II (remission) or stage V (endstage), it is doubtful that the total serum IgE concentration will return to normal ranges. Conversely, knowing the ranges of total serum IgE when there are no chest roentgenographic infiltrates will establish a baseline from which increases of 100% or greater can alert one to an exacerbation. Patients with fibrocavitary ABPA (stage V) can have extensive bronchiectasis resembling endstage cystic fibrosis. Infiltrates can be from *Pseudomonas aeruginosa* or *Staphylococcus aureus* pneumonias or from rare species that have colonized the bronchi. Response to prednisone is limited, and additional modalities, such as bronchial hygiene, coughing- or sputum-assist devices, inhaled RNAase, and antipseudomonal antibiotic coverage might be required. An earlier diagnosis of ABPA will result in fewer stage V patients. Noncompliant patients who refuse to take prednisone for infiltrates might develop a greater number of bronchiectatic areas that can eventually lead to stage V ABPA with a poor prognosis. Similarly, delays in diagnosis of ABPA are known to have resulted in patients presenting in stage V.

RADIOLOGY

CT scan with thin (1- to 2-mm) (HRCT; high-resolution CT scan) rather than conventional (10-mm) sections are extremely valuable in the diagnosis of ABPA. Proximal (central) bronchiectasis is defined as being present when there are bronchi that are dilated in comparison with the caliber of an adjacent bronchial artery in the inner two thirds of the lung CT field. Bronchiectasis is described as cylindrical when the bronchus does not taper and is 1.5 to more than 3 times the caliber of diameter of an adjacent artery. Bronchiectasis can also be varicoid or cystic. Ring shadows on chest roentgenograms are 1 to 2 cm in diameter; they represent dilated bronchi seen in an en face orientation. When the same dilated bronchus is visualized in a tangential (coronal) plane, it is called a parallel-line shadow. These findings are consistent with bronchiectasis. Some of the other findings include mucus plugs or mucoid impactions, bronchial wall thickening as occurs in asthma, atelectasis, lobar or whole lung collapse, pulmonary fibrosis, and cavities with or without air-fluid levels. Patients with ABPA can have cylindrical, varicose, and cystic bronchiectasis that involves multiple bronchi. When patients with asthma were examined, bronchial wall thickening was noted, and as many as 29% of patients had localized areas of cylindrical bronchiectasis. Typically, just one or two lobes are affected in patients with asthma.

LABORATORY FINDINGS

Laboratory assays depend on a number of factors; one of the most important is the source material used for sensitization of the solid phases. Antibody assays (and skin test results) are falsely negative when poorly reactive extracts are used. Furthermore, some laboratories do not use a specific positive control serum for each assay when panels are performed. In this scenario, it is possible that the positive control serum in an assay for IgE of *A. fumigatus* is a ragweed-positive serum. This positive serum might or might not have detectable IgE of *A. fumigatus* antibodies. Thus interpretation of a negative result in such an assay could be misleading, inasmuch as the assay could be insensitive and the technician unaware of this fact. Advances in the characterization and molecular detection of *A. fumigatus* allergens has led to the hope that certain reactive recombinant allergens might serve as superior source material. Depending on the conditions under which these fungi are grown, the reactivity might or might not be acceptable for precise use in laboratory assays. It is hoped that in the near future a sensitive and specific test will be developed that will involve the use of selected recombinant allergens and be available for widespread application. Sputum cultures might reveal *A. fumigatus* when plugs are expectorated. The patient often will stop producing plugs after the initial 2-month course of prednisone administration. CT examinations of the lung will show clearing of mucus plugs as well. Other patients expectorate plugs despite continued prednisone administration, and it is not always apparent that itraconazole has helped eliminate the plugs. Conversely, although demonstration of *A. fumigatus* is not required for the diagnosis of ABPA, some microbiology technicians do not report out *A. fumigatus* because they do not think the ordering physician is interested in a fungus that is so frequently recovered in the microbiology laboratory. However, generally speaking in patients with bronchiectasis, the isolation of mucoid strains of *Pseudomonas* suggests the diagnosis of cystic fibrosis, isolation of *A. fumigatus* suggests ABPA, and isolation of *Mycobacterium avium* complex suggests chronic infection with that organism, but isolating these organisms is not specific for these disorders.

TREATMENT

Table 21–5 presents the current recommended approach. Because the disease is a manifestation of a hypersensitivity reaction rather than an infection, treatment is aimed at immune modulation. The administration of oral prednisone to patients with ABPA is associated with the improvement of asthma and the presence of pulmonary infiltrates and eosinophilia, with reduction in serum levels of IgE, and probably reduced progression of bronchiectasis. The optimal dose is unknown, but 0.5 mg/kg/day is recommended, followed by a gradual taper and adjustment based on the patient's condition. The long-term use of corticosteroids is often necessary, but carries risk, including the development of invasive *Aspergillus* infection. Therefore, the antifungal agent itraconazole was tested in patients with ABPA as an adjunctive, steroid-sparing agent in two randomized placebo-controlled studies. The dose was 200 mg daily for another 16 weeks. Both studies spanned 16 weeks of treatment and showed reduced levels of markers of systemic immune activation (serum IgE level and eosinophil count). The study by Wark et al also showed reduced levels of markers of airway inflammation in induced sputum. Neither study showed significant changes in lung function, although Wark and colleagues showed that subjects receiving itraconazole experienced fewer exacerbations of disease requiring increased doses of corticosteroids. Therefore, although itraconazole appears to be promising as adjunctive treatment for patients with ABPA, long-term trials are needed to assess the clinical efficacy and safety in patients in different disease severity strata. There have been no randomized controlled trials to evaluate the use of antifungal therapies in patients with ABPA complicating cystic fibrosis. Optional effective antifungal agent for ABPA might be fluconazole, according

Table 21–5. Suggestions for initial treatment of allergic bronchopulmonary aspergillosis.

1. For new allergic bronchopulmonary aspergillosis (ABPA) infiltrates, administer prednisone 0.5 mg/kg/d for 1 to 2 wks, then on alternate days for 6 to 8 wks. Then attempt to discontinue prednisone by tapering by 5 to 10 mg every 2 wks.
2. Repeat the total serum IgE concentration in 6 to 8 wks, then every 8 wks for 1 yr to determine the range of IgE concentrations. Increases of more than 100% over baseline can signify a silent ABPA exacerbation.
3. Repeat the chest roentgenogram or CT of the lung after 4 to 8 wks to demonstrate that infiltrates have cleared.
4. Consider environmental sources of fungi (e.g., moldy basements, leaking roofs, water damage in walls) and recommend remediation.
5. Monitor pulmonary function tests.
6. If the patient cannot be tapered off prednisone despite optimal antiasthma treatment and avoidance measures, then he or she has evolved into stage IV (corticosteroid-dependent asthma). Try to manage with alternate-day prednisone as opposed to daily prednisone.
7. New ABPA infiltrates may be identified by:
   a. Cough, wheeze, or dyspnea with sputum production
   b. Unexplained declines in expiratory flow rates
   c. Sharp (more than 100%) increases in total serum IgE concentration
   d. Absent symptoms but new infiltrates on chest roentgenograms or chest CT examinations.
8. Diagnose and manage concomitant conditions such as allergic rhinitis, sinusitis, and gastroesophageal reflux disease.

to our clinical experiences. In addition, the American College of Chest Physicians proposed a new guideline for the treatment of the patients with chronic cough due to bronchiectasis including ABPA.

With early diagnosis and treatment, ABPA can enter a remission stage, a recurrent exacerbation stage, or perhaps a corticosteroid-dependent asthma stage. Patients who have endstage fibrocavitary lung disease often present in that stage without having been identified and treated previously. The other modalities for management of asthma should be instituted, and patients should be encouraged not to be overly pessimistic. The goal is to avoid progressive loss of lung function and maintain good respiratory status, which is achievable for many patients.

EVIDENCE-BASED MEDICINE

Diagnosis

For patients with suspected or proven asthma or cystic fibrosis who have pulmonary infiltrates and peripheral blood eosinophilia, allergen skin testing and in vitro tests, when correlated with history and other findings, can establish the diagnosis of ABPA.

Greenberger PA. Allergic bronchopulmonary aspergillosis. *J Allergy Clin Immunol.* 2002;110:685. Evidence grade: IV

Management

The optimal dose of corticosteroids is unknown, but 0.5 mg/kg/day is recommended, followed by a gradual taper and adjustment based on the patient's condition. The long-term use of corticosteroids is often necessary, but carries risk, including the development of invasive *Aspergillus* infection. Sixteen weeks of treatment with 200 mg of itraconazole daily showed reduced levels of markers of systemic immune activation (serum IgE level and eosinophil count). The study by Wark et al also showed reduced levels of markers of airway inflammation in induced sputum.

Wark P, Hensley M, Saltos N. Anti-inflammatory effect of itraconazole in stable allergic bronchopulmonary aspergillosis: a randomized controlled trial. *J Allergy Clin Immunol.* 2003;111:952. Evidence grade: Ib

BIBILIOGRAPHY

Greenberger PA, Patterson R. Allergic bronchopulmonary aspergillosis and the evaluation of the patient with asthma. *J Allergy Clin Immunol.* 1988;81:646.

Hinson KFW, Moon AJ, Plummer NS. Bronchopulmonary aspergillosis: a review and report of eight new cases. *Thorax.* 1952;7:317.

Lee TM, Greenberger PA, Patterson R, et al. Stage V (fibrotic) allergic bronchopulmonary aspergillosis: a review of 17 cases followed from diagnosis. *Arch Intern Med.* 1987;147:319.

Neeld DA, Goodman LR, Gurney JW. Computerized tomography in the evaluation of allergic bronchopulmonary aspergillosis. *Am Rev Respir Dis.* 1990;142:1200.

Patterson R, Greenberger PA, Lee TM. Prolonged evaluation of patients with corticosteroid-dependent asthma stage of allergic bronchopulmonary aspergillosis. *J Allergy Clin Immunol.* 1987;80:663.

Patterson R, Greenberger PA, Radin RC. Allergic bronchopulmonary aspergillosis: staging as an aid to management. *Ann Intern Med.* 1982;96:286.

Paul AG Allergic bronchopulmonary aspergillosis. *J Allergy Clin Immunol.* 2002;110:685.

Proceedings of the Cystic Fibrosis Foundation ABPA Consensus Conference; June 12–13, 2001; Bethesda, Md.

Ricketti AJ, Greenberger PA, Patterson R. Serum IgE as an important aid in management of allergic bronchopulmonary aspergillosis. *J Allergy Clin Immunol.* 1984;74:68.

Rosen MJ. Chronic cough due to bronchiectasis: ACCP evidence-based clinical practice guidelines. *Chest.* 2006;129(1 suppl):122S.

Rosenberg M, Patterson R, Mintzer R, et al. Clinical and immunologic criteria for the diagnosis of allergic bronchopulmonary aspergillosis. *Ann Intern Med.* 1977;86(4):405.

Stevens, D, Lee, J, Schwartz. A randomised trial of itraconazole in allergic bronchopulmonary aspergillosis. *N Engl J Med.* 2000;342,756.

Ward S, Heyneman L, Lee MJ, et al. Accuracy of CT in the diagnosis of allergic bronchopulmonary aspergillosis in asthmatic patients. *AJR Am J Roentgenol.* 1999;173:937.

Wark P, Hensley M, Saltos, N. Anti-inflammatory effect of itraconazole in stable allergic bronchopulmonary aspergillosis: a randomized controlled trial. *J Allergy Clin Immunol.* 2003;111:952.

Serum Sickness and Immune Complex Disease

22

Michael R. Nelson, MD, PhD

DISCOVERY

A patterned delayed reaction following heterologous hyperimmune serum treatments for diphtheria was observed and characterized by Clemens von Pirquet and Bella Schick in 1905. Patients experienced a progressive reaction consisting of lymphadenopathy, neutropenia, urticaria, and fever with an onset approximately 8 to 10 days following the injection of serum derived from horses hyperimmunized with diphtheria. They also recognized that the reaction occurred much earlier on repeated exposure. Using classic periodic serum sampling, they astutely described the appearance of new host antibodies and coincident decreases in horse serum components. This was followed by the appearance of a "toxic physiologic product" that represented a declaration just short of their suspicion of antigen-antibody complex formation and tissue deposition. Further characterization of heterologous serum reactions in humans and later in animal models have confirmed these initial observations that remain unchallenged today.

DEFINITION

Serum sickness today is regarded as a clinical syndrome resulting from immune complex formation and tissue deposition that activate an inflammatory cascade causing end-organ damage in affected tissues. Many triggers of serum sickness have been identified since the original description involving diphtheria antisera, but the final common pathway is immune complex mediated inflammation. Some authors have made the distinction between serum sickness and serum sickness–like reactions. Classic serum sickness results in the development of combined rash, fever, arthralgias, lymphadenopathy, edema, neuritis, and nephritis associated with administration of heterologous immune sera. Whereas some clinicians regard the appearance of this syndrome following nonimmunoglobulin medications as serum sickness, other refer to such delayed adverse events as "serum sickness–like reactions" caused by hapten or hapten-protein conjugates. Moreover, some clinicians use the term to refer to the delayed appearance of the less than full spectrum of organ system involvement associated with classic serum sickness. Regardless, the time course and likely involvement of immune complexes are central to the appearance of clinical disease.

EPIDEMIOLOGY

Serum sickness is a frequent occurrence following heterologous serum administration. In fact, antithymocyte and antilymphocyte globulin administration have become the modern-day human models of serum sickness given the high frequency and reproducibility of immune complex formation and development of serum sickness. In perhaps the most comprehensive description, Bielory et al in 1988 prospectively described the clinical progression of serum sickness in 30 of 35 (87%) bone marrow transplant patients receiving antithymocyte globulin for immunosuppression. Similarly, Tichelli and colleagues in Switzerland reported a 63% incidence (27 of 43) of patients treated with antilymphocyte globulin for severe aplastic anemia.

Heterologous serum is also used for the treatment of snake envenomation, and the postadministration course is frequently complicated by serum sickness. Tokish and colleagues reported a 1% readmission rate for serum sickness following therapy with snake antivenin, and LoVecchio et al describe a 61% (60 of 99) incidence of serum sickness in patients receiving Centruroides antivenom. Admittedly "liberal criteria" in the latter study and varying reporting bias in retrospective reviews highlight the difficulty of comparing serum sickness incidence data between studies of snake antivenins or any therapeutic antigen.

Humanized monoclonal antibodies that resemble "self" to the host immune system are significantly less prone than heterologous sera antibodies to evoke a serum sickness reaction. For example, Colombel and colleagues at the Mayo Clinic reported 14 of 500 patients (2.4%) with Crohn's disease receiving infliximab monoclonal therapy developed serum sickness–like reactions. Likewise, a 2.5% incidence of serum sickness–like reactions was observed in 971 sepsis patients infused with tumor necrosis factor (TNF-α) monoclonal antibody in a double-blind randomized controlled trial.

In general, the incidence of serum sickness following administration of antibiotics and other small molecular medications is much lower than antibody-based therapies. Heckbert et al reviewed the occurrence of serum sickness in their pediatric population receiving antibiotics in a large Massachusetts health care system. Twelve cases of serum sickness were identified in 11,523 child-years and in more than 24,962 prescribed antibiotic courses. Cefaclor is the most common antibiotic cause of serum sickness, with a reported rate of 1.8/100,000 compared to less than 1 in 10 million for cephalexin and amoxicillin in one study.

PATHOPHYSIOLOGY

Immune Complexes

The hallmark of human serum sickness is the in vivo development of immune complexes and tissue deposition following antigen exposure. The interaction of single antigen and single antibody molecules is technically an immunologic complex. However, the term *immune complex* refers to larger lattices of multiple antigen-specific antibodies, antigen molecules, and, in many instances, complement system components. This differentiation is highlighted by the realization that univalent and hapten antigens combine with a single antibody molecule but are unable to crosslink antibodies and unable to create classic immune complex lattices. In vivo immune complex formation occurs both intravascularly and directly in tissues.

The process of immune complex formation thus depends on many factors. One example is the concentration of antigen and antibody. Although antigen can and does bind to antibody combining sites with the appropriate specificity at any concentration, immune complexes rarely form under conditions of significant antigen or antibody excess. Rather, immune complexes are optimally formed within the so-called zone of equivalence where the concentrations of each are more closely matched (Fig. 22–1). Animal models and in vitro experiments have further revealed that slight antigen excess favors the formation of the large immune complexes. Clinically, the large complexes are more easily cleared within the reticuloendothelial system (especially hepatic) than smaller complexes formed at slight antibody excess. However, these smaller complexes tend to

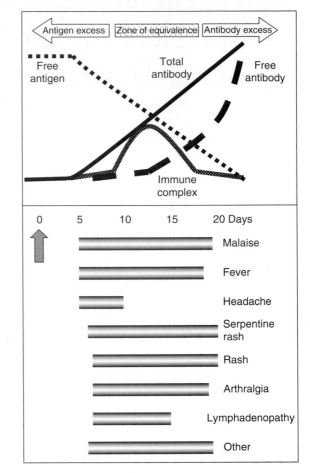

Figure 22–1. Schematic of serum sickness immune complex and symptom development. The top half of the figure depicts the induction of antigen-specific antibody production and immune complexes following an antigen stimulus on day 0 (arrow). The bottom half displays when typical symptoms appear in the context of immune system changes shown in the upper half. This estimation is based on Bielory's description of antithymocyte globulin induced serum sickness cohort. Other symptoms included blurred vision, arthritis, dyspnea, wheezing, hoarseness, and gastrointestinal complaints.

persist in vivo for longer periods and theoretically pose a higher risk for tissue deposition and end-organ damage. Another factor that affects immune complex formation is related to the nature of the antigen. The valency or number of epitopes on each antibody molecule is an important factor in immune complex genesis. Antigens with a limited number of epitopes are less likely to crosslink antibodies and thus may have a narrower zone of equivalence where immune complexes are formed. Alternatively, an example of antibody characteristics affecting immune complex formation is the affinity of the antibody for the antigen that may impact on the rate and/or size of immune complex formation.

End-Organ Damage Mediated by Immune Complexes

The formation of immune complexes alone is of little clinical significance whether in circulation or in host tissues. One reason for this is the existence of very effective clearance mechanisms led by the reticuloendothelial system. Following tissue deposition or formation, it is not until effector mechanisms of the humoral immune system are activated that end-organ damage occurs. This includes activation of the complement cascade and resultant inflammation from complement components serving as chemokines (C3a) and anaphylatoxins (mainly C3a and C5a). Perivascular cellular infiltration (neutrophils, lymphocytes, histiocytes) and local tissue changes in the form of cytotoxicity, fibrosis, and edema contribute to the development of tissue damage and end-organ effects of immune complex disease. The entire process from antigen or allergen presentation to immune complex formation and deposition followed by an inflammatory response defines the well-described Gell and Coombs type III hypersensitivity response, of which serum sickness is the prime example.

HUMAN DISEASE

Triggers

A multitude of agents are associated with the development of serum sickness. Table 22–1 reviews some of the more commonly described triggers. The vast majority represent therapeutic agents. Heterologous immune sera and antibiotics are the most common causative agents. Cefaclor likely represents the most commonly reported single antibiotic cause of serum sickness–like reactions.

Included in the list of therapeutic causes of serum sickness is the modern-day equivalent of von Pirquet and Schick's horse serum, antithymocyte (ATG) and antilymphocyte globulin (ALG). These heterologous serum immune globulins are derived from human lymphocyte inoculated horses (ATG) or rabbits (ALG) and administered as an immune suppressant for recipients of transplants and the treatment of aplastic anemia. This foreign antibody–enriched serum serves as a strong stimulator of the human host immune response on treatment. Human IgG or IgM recognizing horse or rabbit immunoglobulin molecules develops on exposure and results in the formation of immune complexes composed of the newly formed human immunoglobulin with the immunoglobulin components of infused ATG or ALG serving as the "antigen." In contrast to antibiotics

Table 22–1. Agents with reported serum sickness or serum sickness-like reactions.

Serum Sickness	Serum Sickness-Like Reactions
Allopurinol	Amoxicillin/clavulanate
Antithymocyte globulin	Ampicillin/sulbactam
Antivenins	Cefditoren
Bupropion	Ceftibuten
Carbamazepine	Cephalothin
Cefaclor	Ciprofloxacin
Cefoperazone	Demeclocycline
Cefoxitin	Doxycycline
Cefprozil	Lansoprazole/amoxicillin/clarithromycin
Ceftriaxone	Minocycline
Cephapirin	Penicillin G
Clopidogrel	Phenylbutazone
Diphtheria immune globulin	Infliximab
Fluoxetine ± olanzapine	Itraconazole
Insect stings and immunotherapy	Tetracycline
Levothyroxine	
Levofloxacin	
6-Mercaptopurine	
Nafcillin	
Phenytoin	
Pneumococcal vaccine	
Procarbazine	
Rituximab	
Streptokinase	
Sulfamethoxazole/trimethoprim	
Tetanus immune globulin	

and most oral medications that are comparatively rare causes of serum sickness, ATG and ALG frequently and reproducibly cause disease in humans. Other examples of heterologous serum products causing serum sickness are the group of anti–snake venom antidotes. Even hyperimmune globulin obtained from human donors used for treatment and prophylaxis of tetanus and diphtheria rarely causes serum sickness in recipients.

Whereas heterologous immune serum remains a common cause, the risk associated with newer antibody-based therapies is unknown. It stands to reason that the newer humanized monoclonal antibodies would be less likely to evoke an immune response and consequently be less prone to result in immune complex formation and serum sickness. For the most part, this appears to be the case. However, serum sickness is reported in association with a variety of recently introduced monoclonal therapies. For example, infliximab therapy for rheumatoid arthritis and Crohn's disease was complicated by serum sickness in 14 of 500 consecutively treated patients in one series at the Mayo Clinic.

An unusual cause of serum sickness–like reactions is multiple stings from winged stinging insects of the order Hymenoptera. In addition to natural stings, venom immunotherapy has also caused a serum sickness reaction in at least one patient. In both scenarios, delayed reactions result from the new generation of venom-specific IgG that complexes with venom proteins. The fact that this occurs during immunotherapy is intriguing given that patients by definition have preexisting antigen-specific IgE. It has been reported that IgE-containing immune complexes are not routinely formed. Such complexes would not activate complement and thus would be less likely to evoke the clinical features of overt serum sickness. It was not until the start of venom immunotherapy that antibody production shifted from IgE to IgG and resulted in the delayed onset of classic symptoms in the few reported affected patients. Rush immunotherapy giving multiple escalating doses over a shorter period of time may further increase the risk for this type of rare reaction.

In summary, a wide variety of so-called antigens can evoke immune complex formation and serum sickness. Most are therapeutic agents with classic examples of cefaclor, antithymocyte globulin, and other heterologous sera. Fortunately, serum sickness is a rare complication of administration of other implicated agents.

Symptoms and Signs

The clinical manifestations of serum sickness result from the tissue deposition of immune complexes formed initially in the intravascular or tissue extravascular fluid phase. The exact constellation of signs and symptoms varies from patient to patient and depends on many factors such as those just reviewed briefly in the pathophysiology description. There are thus distinct antigen, antibody, and immune complex characteristics that combine to determine when immune complexes form, where they are deposited, and which aspects of the host immune inflammatory response are activated (especially the complement system). Most of the data on symptom development have been acquired from animal models and observation of patients treated with heterologous serum. The most cited report is Bielory's prospective evaluation of serum sickness manifestations in 30 of 35 patients treated with ATG. Even within these "model" serum sickness subjects, there is wide variability in symptom expression that is more pronounced on comparing reactions induced by other triggers such as antibiotics.

Early signs and symptoms of serum sickness are usually related to the early systemic inflammatory response and can develop as early as the fifth day following antigen exposure. Most patients experience some form of malaise often coupled with fatigue. Many develop overt fever, including 100% of ATG-related serum sickness patients within 5 to 7 days in one study. The fever may also be accompanied by chills or rigors. Headache is also recognized as an early symptom.

Cutaneous eruptions are also frequently seen in serum sickness patients (93% in ATG-related serum sickness). The most common skin manifestation is a disseminated morbilliform rash that begins in the lower torso, axillary and inguinal regions. This is followed by gradual involvement of the back, abdomen, and chest. Polymorphous eruptions, flushing, edema, and palmar erythema have also been noted. Lesional skin biopsies reveal a small vessel lymphocytic and histiocytic perivascular infiltrate and only variable presence of immunoglobulin, immune complexes, and complement deposits. Perhaps the most characteristic rash and clinical sign of serum sickness is a serpiginous eruption at the interface of palmar and dorsal skin of the hand, as well as plantar and dorsal skin of the feet. More common in heterologous serum than drug reactions, this rash usually precedes the disseminated morbilliform eruptions. Progressive small vessel vasculitis can contribute to the conversion of an initially thin erythematous scalloped line into a hemorrhagic and purpuric one that can last for up to 2 weeks. Lesional skin histology often reveals a leukocytoclastic vasculitis involving venules and capillaries.

Urticarial eruptions can also be seen as a cutaneous finding in serum sickness. When present, urticaria is most often accompanied by the morbilliform rash, but it is rarely the sole delayed rash manifested by patients with serum sickness. Of note, the appearance of urticaria within the first 4 days following antigen exposure does not represent a risk factor for the development of serum sickness as observed in ATG-treated patients. Early urticarial reactions are more likely the result of immune mechanisms, such as type I IgE-mediated hypersensitivity.

Rheumatologic symptoms develop in a majority of affected patients ranging from arthralgias to myalgias and generalized bone pain. Arthralgias are most common, occurring in 20 of 20 evaluated ATG patients, with objective inflammatory arthritis occurring in 9 of these in one study. The knees, ankles, shoulders, wrists, lower thoracic and cervical spine, and temporomandibular joints are the most commonly affected anatomic sites. Delayed onset myalgias of the shoulder and thighs are also recognized as symptoms of serum sickness.

Less common manifestations include symptoms resulting from gastrointestinal, renal, lymphatic, and ocular organ systems involvement. Lymphadenopathy has been classically associated with serum sickness since Von Pirquet and Schick's original description. However, it is not seen in all affected patients. Enlarged lymph nodes when present are usually tender and have a distribution that is not necessarily related to the route of antigen exposure. Diffuse proliferative, membranous, necrotic glomerulonephritis and tubulointerstitial nephritis resulting from immune complex deposition have also been observed in severe cases of serum sickness. Relatedly, prospectively obtained serial laboratory studies also support asymptomatic renal involvement in a significant number of affected patients. Gastrointestinal complaints in the form of bloating, cramping, nausea, vomiting, and rarely diarrhea have also been observed in 67% of ATG-related serum sickness. Heme positive stools were noted in 2 of 30. Other signs and symptoms associated with serum sickness include blurred vision, ocular hemorrhage, and dyspnea.

DIAGNOSIS

The diagnosis of serum sickness and serum sickness–like reactions is largely a clinical one. Although supportive evidence can be obtained from laboratory studies such as the measurement of immune complexes, these results must be put in the context of the appropriately timed appearance of clinical signs and symptoms and cannot make the diagnosis alone. There are no well-accepted criteria for serum sickness diagnosis, making comparisons of cohorts from different studies difficult. Likewise, there has been no consensus on defining minimum specific signs, symptoms, or laboratory abnormalities that can be found in all patients.

Clinical

A diagnosis of serum sickness is suspected when typical clinical signs and symptoms develop approximately 5 to 7 days after a causative antigen presentation or sooner if a repeat administration. Although involvement of every described organ system is not required, the appearance of manifestations from multiple organ systems makes the diagnosis more likely. It is not surprising that there can be a delay in diagnosis during the acute evaluation of patients presenting with nonspecific symptoms who were exposed to less recognized or never before implicated causes of serum sickness. Patients and clinicians alike tend to focus on the acute clinical presentation that resembles a flulike illness or acute new-onset rheumatologic disorder, emphasizing the need to inquire about exposures the preceding week.

Laboratory

The hallmark of laboratory-based evaluation of serum sickness is the identification of circulating immune complexes. Table 22–2 presents an overview of assays designed to detect immune complexes in test sera. Some assays rely on physicochemical properties (size, density, temperature dependence, etc.) of precipitation that differ from monomeric antibody or antibody/antigen complexes. Other assays take advantage of the biochemical properties of immune complexes such as adherent complement proteins and conserved Fc portions of IgG and IgM molecules. The prototypic example of this assay type is the Raji cell assay. It utilizes a B cell Burkitt lymphoma cell line with surface receptors for components of typical circulating immune complexes, including IgG, C3, C3b, C3d, and C1q. After the addition of test sera, the complement and conserved antibody Fc portion sequences of immune complexes are recognized by the Raji cell surface receptors and detected after washing by the subsequent addition of labeled antihuman immunoglobulin conjugates. Raji cell complement receptors are believed to play a larger role than the Fc receptors. Another long-standing assay involves the use of a 750 kDa bovine or human protein that serves as a receptor for iC3b-containing immune complexes. In recognition of the difficulty working with cell lines and tissue-derived products, recent commercial assays use more readily available monoclonal or polyclonal antibodies directed against complement components (C1q, C3d, and C3dg) in enzyme-linked immunoabsorbent assay (ELISA) or radioimmunoassay-based test protocols. Some investigators consider those assays that focus on detection of immune complexes with incorporated complement components to be superior in the detection of physiologically relevant complexes. The rationale for this supposition is that activation of the complement system is required to produce the adherent split products.

All commercially available immune complex assays do so with generally good sensitivity and varying specificity. However, none of these detect specific immune complexes with a predefined antigen or antigen-specific antibody. Interfering monomeric IgG or IgM and aggregates of immunoglobulins in the absence of antigen contribute to lack of specificity for many assays and

Table 22–2. Immune complex detection.

Method	Assay	Basis	Interference
Direct physicochemical	Polyethylene precipitation	Exclusion of high molecular weight complexes from fluid phase	Monomeric IgG
	Sucrose density precipitation	Exclusion of high molecular weight complexes from fluid phase	Monomeric IgG, RF
	Cryoglobulin	Temperature (4°C) dependent precipitation (reversible)	Ig aggregates (without antigen)
Direct biochemical	C1q binding	ELISA based IC capture: C1q coated solid phase or labeled C1q precipitation	
	C3d binding	ELISA-based IC capture by C3d coated solid phase	
	Raji	B lymphoblastic Burkitt lymphoma cell with CR2 recognizing C3bi attached to many ICs	
	Conglutinin	Bovine 750kDa bovine/cattle protein that binds C3bi attached to many ICs	
	Antiglobulin	Monoclonal RF detection of polymeric Ig aggregates	
Indirect (Complement)	C3	IC activation of classical complement pathway	Acute-phase reactants, alternative pathway activation, inflammation, infection, vasculitis, sample handling, genetic deficiency
	C4	Same	Same
	CH50	Same	Same

IC, immune complex; Ig, immunoglobulin; RF, rheumatoid factor.

possibly falsely elevated results. It is also well recognized that no single immune complex assay should be relied on to detect all types of immune complexes. Given that each antigen-antibody reaction forms immune complexes of differing physicochemical and biochemical properties, the use of multiple assays of differing methodology will increase the yield of testing for immune complexes, a recommendation previously suggested by the World Health Organization.

Other laboratory abnormalities reflect organ-specific damage or signs of systemic inflammation. Periodic urinalysis during the course of serum sickness reveals reversible proteinuria followed by hematuria and hemoglobinuria in those patients with renal involvement. The urine sediment is rarely active, and some patients experience a decrement in renal function. Elevated hepatic transaminase levels have also been noted in acute serum sickness. Nonspecific markers of systemic inflammation are also abnormal, including C3, C4, CH50, erythrocyte sedimentation rate, and C-reactive protein.

Differential Diagnosis

The differential diagnosis is broad in light of the nonspecific constitutional symptoms and signs contributing to the diagnosis of serum sickness. Occurrences of bacterial and viral infections, vasculitis, connective tissue diseases, lymphoproliferative disorders, and paraneoplastic syndromes should also be considered. This is especially the case when no well-defined trigger heralded the onset of a patient's clinical presentation. Specific disorders with very similar presentations include systemic lupus erythematosus, juvenile rheumatoid arthritis, Henoch-Schönlein purpura, mononucleosis, adult Still's disease, Kawasaki disease, rheumatic fever, and shunt nephritis. The nonspecific systemic symptom development often observed in these disorders and formation of immune complexes in many of them should prompt clinicians to consider them in patients with relevant risk factors such as age and family history. It can also be hypothesized that subclinical systemic inflammatory disorders may be "unmasked" by the immune activation associated with immune complex activity.

NATURAL HISTORY

Figure 22–1 depicts the typical course of serum sickness. Approximately 6 to 7 days following antigen exposure, antigen-specific IgM and/or IgG antibody is first detectable. As the concentration of antibody rises, the zone of equivalence is reached and immune complexes begin to form. These events correspond with the onset of early symptoms of serum sickness, including malaise, fever, headache, and serpiginous erythema on days 6 to 8. As immune complex formation and tissue deposition proceeds, additional aspects of the clinical syndrome appear, namely arthralgias, morbilliform rash, lymphadenopathy, and other signs and symptoms. Laboratory abnormalities are also most commonly identified during the second week following antigen exposure. During the third and fourth weeks, antigen-specific antibody continues to rise creating an antibody excess state that is less favorable for immune complex formation. An activated reticuloendothelial clearance system, antibody excess, and host regulators of immune response all combine to downregulate the acute inflammation and promote the resolution of clinical symptoms. The addition of antiinflammatory therapy (i.e., corticosteroids) and removal of antigen accelerates clinical resolution. For the most part, organ involvement is reversible. However, prolonged untreated end-organ involvement such as glomerulonephritis could conceivably result in irreversible damage and ultimately impact on organ function. Figure 22–2 demonstrates immunofluorescent staining and electron microscopy of advanced glomerulonephritis due to immune complex mediated disease.

The course of serum sickness, however, is variable and depends on several factors related to antigen exposure and host factors. For example, the chronicity of antigen exposure can drastically affect the duration of symptoms and clinical findings. Continuous exposure from daily administered medications or agents with an extended half-life can result in protracted clinical disease when left untreated. An example of host factors affecting the course of serum sickness is underlying complement deficiencies. Deficiencies of complement components participating in the classical pathway may predispose patients to the early and more frequent development of immune complex mediated disease and thus the end-organ effects of serum sickness. This predisposition is attributed to impaired host ability to clear immune complexes from the circulation.

Patients experiencing anaphylaxis to a given antigen are at slightly increased risk of anaphylactic immediate-type reactions with future exposure. Aside from likely sensitization and IgE induction during the initial exposure, it is unknown why serum sickness patients are more likely to experience anaphylaxis than other asymptomatic sensitized individuals. One can hypothesize that the inflammatory milieu of serum sickness favors a Th2 response favoring IgE production and immunologic memory.

MANAGEMENT

The management of patients with serum sickness revolves around early detection, early removal of the precipitating antigen when possible, and early use of antiinflammatory medications when severe. Supportive therapy directed at treatment of organ-specific manifestations is also warranted.

Monitoring

Considerations in the management of patients suspected to have serum sickness include periodic physical exams and serial evaluation of urinalysis and renal function, as well as hepatic enzymes and function. Measurement of complement activation and/or C-reactive protein (or erythrocyte sedimentation rate) may also assist in following resolution of inflammatory processes or response to treatment. The serial measurement of immune complexes during the course of disease is of academic interest, particularly for less well-described triggers. However, once the presence of immune complexes is demonstrated in a patient suspected of having serum sickness, serial measurement is generally not indicated because the results rarely affect clinical decision making. For those patients with edema and/or renal involvement, monitoring fluid intake and output is also recommended.

Therapeutic Options

The acute management is directed toward trigger removal and selective use of antiinflammatory agents to limit the inflammatory effects on organ systems. Mild serum sickness can often be managed with antigen removal and supportive therapy only. The mainstay of antiinflammatory therapy for more pronounced serum sickness is systemic corticosteroids. Although no recommended dosing regimens are well established, 0.5 to 1 mg/kg for adults and 1 to 2 mg/kg for children have been used as reasonable starting doses. Nonsteroidal antiinflammatory agents and aspirin have also been used but mainly for supportive therapy of specific symptoms. Additional supportive therapy includes antihistamines for pruritic cutaneous eruptions and bronchodilators for dyspnea and wheezing.

If the trigger is a recently initiated medication, immediate discontinuation is recommended to remove the antigen, depleting the source for ongoing immune complex formation. Antigen removal is more difficult following single antigen administrations such as ATG and hyperimmune globulin. Antigens of this type (antibodies) can persist for weeks, although the half-life is likely

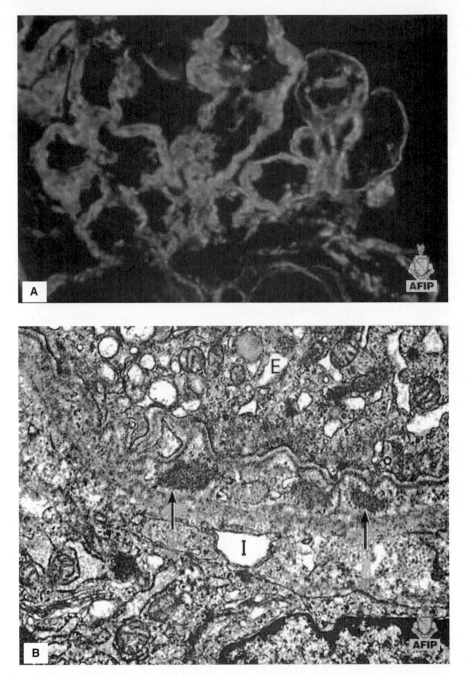

Figure 22–2. Kidney tubular basement membrane immune complex deposits. **A:** Immunofluorescence of predominantly peripheral capillary wall deposits of IgG-containing immune complexes. **B:** This patient had infectious endocarditis. Electron microscopy demonstrating immune complex deposits (arrows) in the kidney precipitated by amoxicillin treatment of infectious endocarditis. I, interstitium; E, tubular epithelial cell. (Reproduced, with permission, from *Atlas of Nontumor Pathology-Nonneoplastic Kidney Disease;* 21.2.3 Immune Complex Injury; Fig. 21–55; 1N04 Image no. 1047 and 10.2 Primary MPGN (Types 1, 2, and 3); Fig. 10–17; 1N04 Image no. 417.)

somewhat shorter than host immunoglobulin due to enhanced clearance of formed immune complexes. There have also been several reports of patients successfully managed with plasma exchange for progressive serum sickness uncontrolled by systemic corticosteroids.

PREVENTION

There are very few risk factors that can be identified for the primary prevention of serum sickness. However, ATG and ALG cause hypersensitivity reactions at such high frequency that package inserts include recommendations for preadministration skin testing for immediate-type hypersensitivity and consideration of prophylactic corticosteroids to mitigate immune complex mediated hypersensitivity reactions. Avoidance of known triggers of serum sickness for a given patients is also recommended. If repeat administration of a known trigger is necessary due to the absence of suitable alternatives and the benefits of readministration outweigh the risk, pretreatment with corticosteroids, nonsteroidal agents, and/or antihistamines can be considered. For example, 40 mg per day of prednisolone has been recommended for 2 days prior to and during 5 to 7 days after each infusion of infliximab in patients with previous delayed reactions.

Desensitization protocols used for type I IgE–mediated disease are not uniformly effective in preventing the occurrence of serum sickness. However, there may be a role in desensitizing patients to certain antigens to prevent the occurrence of anaphylactic reactions. For example, patients with serum sickness resulting from bee stings or immunotherapy benefit from cautious initiation (or resumption) of immunotherapy.

FUTURE DIRECTIONS AND EVIDENCE-BASED MEDICINE

There are several challenges facing clinicians in the identification and management of serum sickness as an adverse reaction to both new and old therapeutics. One major challenge is the development of consensus diagnostic criteria that will promote the standardized evaluation of diagnostic and therapeutic interventions.

Increased understanding of serum sickness pathogenesis will undoubtedly progress as animal models continue to provide details of the associated inflammatory process. For example, Alexander and colleagues, using a complement factor H knockout mouse model of chronic serum sickness glomerulonephritis, have recently uncovered a role for factor H in the regulation of immune complex and C3 deposition in kidney glomeruli. This and similar type findings may lead to the identification of new therapeutic targets of treatment and/or prevention.

There is also a need to identify improved diagnostic tests for serum sickness. Immune complex assays of increased sensitivity and new ones using more specific and early markers of disease will assist clinicians to confirm the diagnosis and perhaps reliably guide treatment. Further refinement of purified monoclonal/polyclonal antibody based assays will yield single or combinations of assays capable of detecting the full spectrum of immune complexes with high specificity. Given the increased recognition of the role lymphocytes and other cells play in the inflammatory cascade of serum sickness, study of newly introduced flow cytometry based assays of drug hypersensitivity in the context of serum sickness will also likely be explored.

Another area of interest is the identification of risk factors for serum sickness development. Currently, past association of certain medications with serum sickness complications is the only risk factor clinicians have to rely on. Only recently have studies begun to identify host factors that may predispose patients. As discussed earlier, certain complement deficiencies in animal models also favor the development of serum sickness following antigen exposure. It is also likely that there are other genetic polymorphisms associated with antigen immune system recognition, activation, and clearance or associated with medication pharmacokinetics or pharmacodynamics. Taking advantage of the knowledge of identified genotypes may permit the application of pharmacogenetics to minimize the risk of prescribed medications. The ability to predict which medications are at higher risk in which subsets of patients is of increasing importance in light of the introduction of record numbers of new medications to the market, including the burgeoning class of monoclonal antibody therapies. Infliximab, rituximab, and omalizumab are but a few examples of immunomodulating agents with postmarketing recognition of serum sickness and serum sickness–like reaction adverse events.

Novel approaches to drug design may also minimize the risk of serum sickness. Optimizing the "humanization" process of heterologous-based monoclonal antibody therapy has also contributed to lowering the risks of therapy. Cha et al described in 2002 a novel approach to designing a diphtheria antidote. The use of truncated recombinant heparin-binding epidermal growth factor–like growth precursor serves as a potent diphtheria toxin inhibitor in vitro and is a poor immunogen. Mutation of growth factor sequences is predicted to lessen the risk for potential mitogenic effects. This concept, however, presents new risks for other non–immune complex related adverse effects such as malignancy.

CONCLUSION

Serum sickness is a clinical syndrome characterized by the delayed presentation of systemic signs and symptoms following antigen exposure. Coincident with the development of antigen specific antibody and immune complexes, malaise, fever, arthralgias, rash, and lymphadenopathy typically begin to appear 5 to 7 days after the insult. However, there is wide variability in the expression of each associated clinical finding. The clinical syndrome is a manifestation of a type III hypersensitivity response involving immune complex formation and tissue deposition, activation of the complement system, and additional inflammatory pathways. Triggers are most often medications but can include such stimuli as insect stings. Rates of serum sickness adverse events for individual therapeutics vary widely and are especially high for heterologous serum derived products. The management of affected patients centers on early recognition, removal of the stimulus, and the addition of antiinflammatory medications, usually corticosteroids. The prognosis is generally favorable with full recovery without long-term sequelae in most patients. Future research designed to improved drug design, diagnostic tools, and risk assessment will lead to less morbidity from this condition.

BIBLIOGRAPHY

Abraham E, Wunderink R, Silverman H, et al. Efficacy and safety of monoclonal antibody to human tumor necrosis factor alpha in patients with sepsis syndrome. A randomized, controlled, double-blind, multicenter clinical trial. TNF-alpha MAb Sepsis Study Group. *JAMA* 1995;273(12):934.

Alexander JJ, Pickering MC, Haas M, et al. Complement factor h limits immune complex deposition and prevents inflammation and scarring in glomeruli of mice with chronic serum sickness. *J Am Soc Nephrol* 2005;16(1):52.

Bach S, Bircher AJ. Drug hypersensitivity reactions: from clinical manifestations to an allergologic diagnosis. *Allerg Immunol* 2005;37(6):213–8.

Benatuil L, Parra G, Rincon J, Quiroz Y, Rodriguez-Iturbe B. Expression of adhesion molecules in chronic serum sickness in rats. *Clin Immunol* 1999;90(2):196–202.

Berger W, Gupta N, McAlary M, Fowler-Taylor A. Evaluation of long-term safety of the anti-IgE antibody, omalizumab, in children with allergic asthma. *Ann Allergy Asthma Immunol* 2003;91(2):182–8.

Bielory L, Gascon P, Lawley TJ. Human serum sickness: a prospective analysis of 35 patients treated with equine anti-thymocyte globulin for bone marrow failure. *Medicine* 1988;67(1):40.

Cefaclor-associated serum sickness-like reaction. *CMAJ* 1996; 155(7):913.

Cha JH, Brooke JS, Chang MY, et al. T-cell reactions to drugs in distinct clinical manifestations of drug allergy. *J Invest Allergol Clin Immunol* 2001;11(4):275.

Cha JH, Brooke JS, Chang MY, et al. Receptor-based antidote for diphtheria. *Infect Immunol* 2002;70(5):2344.

Christiaans MH, van Hooff JP. Plasmapheresis and RATG-induced serum sickness. *Transplantation* 2006;81(2):296.

Clark BM, Kotti GH, Shah AD, Conger NG. Severe serum sickness reaction to oral and intramuscular penicillin. *Pharmacotherapy* 2006;26(5):705–8.

Colombel JF, Loftus EV Jr, Tremaine WJ, et al. The safety profile of infliximab in patients with Crohn's disease: the Mayo clinic experience in 500 patients. *Gastroenterology* 2004;126(1):19.

Cuzic S, Scukanec-Spoljar M, Bosnic D, Kuzmanic D, Sentic M. Immunohistochemical analysis of human serum sickness glomerulonephritis. *Croat Med J* 2001;42(6):618–23.

Dart RC, Seifert SA, Boyer LV, Clark RF, Hall E, McKinney P, McNally J, Kitchens CS, Curry SC, Bogdan GM, Ward SB, Porter RS. A randomized multicenter trial of crotalinae polyvalent immune Fab (ovine) antivenom for the treatment for crotaline snakebite in the United States. *Arch Intern Med* 2001;10;161(16):2030–6.

Dart RC, McNally J. Efficacy, safety, and use of snake antivenoms in the United States. *Ann Emerg Med* 2001;37(2):181–8.

Eichenfield AH. Minocycline and autoimmunity. *Curr Opin Pediatr* 1999;11:447.

Frank MM, Hester CG. Immune complexes and allergic disease. In: Adkinson NF, Yuninger JW, Busse WW, et al., eds. *Allergy: Principles and Practice.* 6th ed. St. Louis, Mo: Mosby; 2003:1006.

Gaig P, Garcia-Ortega P, Enrique E, Benet A, Bartolome B, Palacios R. Serum sickness-like syndrome due to mosquito bite. *J Investig Allergol Clin Immunol* 1999;9(3):190–2.

Heckbert SR, Stryker WS, Coltin KL, et al. Serum sickness in children after antibiotic exposure: estimates of occurrence and morbidity in a health maintenance organization population. *Am J Epidemiol* 1990;132(2):336.

IUIS/WHO Working Group. Laboratory investigations in clinical immunology: methods, pitfalls, and clinical indications. A second IUIS/WHO report. *Clin Immunol Immunopathol* 1988;49:478.

Jung LK. Serum sickness. *eMedicine* online publication, November 22, 2002. Available at: http://www.emedicine.com/PED/ topic2082. htm. Accessed September 6, 2006.

Knowles S, Shapiro L, Shear NH. Serious dermatologic reactions in children. *Curr Opin Pediatr* 1997;9(4):388.

Lambert PH, Dixon FJ, Zubler RH, et al. A WHO collaborative study for the evaluation of eighteen methods for detecting immune complexes in serum. *J Clin Lab Immunol* 1978;1:1.

Lundquist AL, Chari RS, Wood JH, Miller GG, Schaefer HM, Raiford DS, Wright KJ, Gorden DL. Serum sickness following rabbit antithymocyte-globulin induction in a liver transplant recipient: case report and literature review. *Liver Transpl* 2007;13(5):647–50.

Lock RJ, Unsworth DJ. Measurement of immune complexes is not useful in routine clinical practice. *Ann Clin Biochem* 2000;37:253.

LoVecchio F, Klemens J, Roundy EB, et al. The safety profile of infliximab in patients with Crohn's disease: the Mayo clinic experience in 500 patients. *Gastroenterology.* 2004;126(1):19.

LoVecchio F, Klemens J, Roundy EB, et al. Serum sickness following administration of Antivenin (Crotalidae) Polyvalent in 181 cases of presumed rattlesnake envenomation. *Wilderness Environ Med* 2003;14(4):220.

Mannick M. Serum sickness and pathophysiology of immune complexes. In: Rich RR, Fleisher TA, Shearer WT, et al., eds. *Clinical Immunology: Principles and Practice.* St. Louis, Mo: Mosby; 1996:1062.

Neukomm CB, Yawalkar N, Helbling A, et al. Immunohistochemical analysis of human serum sickness glomerulonephritis. *Croat Med J.* 2001;42(6):618.

Nangaku M, Couser WG. Mechanisms of immune-deposit formation and the mediation of immune renal injury. *Clin Exp Nephrol* 2005;9(3):183–91.

Platt R, Dreis MW, Kennedy DL. Serum sickness-like reactions to amoxicillin, cefaclor, cephalexin, and trimethoprim-sulfamethoxazole. *J Infect Dis* 1988;158(2):474.

Proctor L, Renzulli B, Warren S, Brecher ME. Transfusion Medicine Illustrated. Monoclonal antibody-stimulated serum sickness. *Transfusion* 2004;44(7):955.

Reisman RE, Livingston A. Late-onset allergic reactions, including serum sickness, after insect stings. *J Allergy Clin Immunol* 1989;84(3):331.

Roujeau JC, Stern RS. Severe adverse cutaneous reactions to drugs. *N Engl J Med* 1994;331(19):1272.

Schutgens RE. Rituximab-induced serum sickness. *Br J Haematol* 2006;135(2):147. Epub 2006 Jul 26.

Sexton DJ, Spelman D. Current best practices and guidelines. Assessment and management of complications in infective endocarditis. *Cardiol Clin* 2003;21(2):273–82.

Silverstein AM. Clemens Freiherr von Pirquet: explaining immune complex disease in 1906. *Nat Immunol* 2000;1(6):453.

Tanriover B, Chuang P, Fishbach B, et al. Polyclonal antibody-induced serum sickness in renal transplant recipients: treatment with therapeutic plasma exchange. *Transplantation* 2005;80(2):279–81.

Tatum AJ, Ditto AM, Patterson R. Severe serum sickness-like reaction to oral penicillin drugs: three case reports. *Ann Allergy Asthma Immunol* 2001;86(3):330–4.

Todd DJ, Helfgott SM. Serum sickness following treatment with rituximab. *J Rheumatol* 2007;34(2):430–3.

Waxman FJ, Hebert LA, Cornacoff JB, et al. Complement depletion accelerates the clearance of immune complexes from the circulation of primates. *J Clin Invest* 1984;74(4):1329.

Yancey KB, Lawley TJ: Circulating immune complexes and serum sickness. In: Rich RR, Fleisher TA, Shearer WT, et al., eds. *Clinical Immunology: Principles and Practice.* 2nd ed. New York: Mosby; 2001:59.1.

Yerushalmi J, Zvulunov A, Halevy S. Serum sickness-like reactions. *Cutis* 2002;69(5):395–7.

Complement Systems and Allergy Diseases

23

Marianne Frieri, MD, PhD

THE COMPLEMENT SYSTEM

Pathways and Physiologic Activities

The complement system consists of more than 30 plasma and cell membrane proteins both first discovered (C_1 to C_9) activated by antigen-antibody complexes, alternative pathway components (properdin, factor B and D), inhibitors (C_1, Factor 1, etc.), activated by microbial cell walls, and regulatory proteins (C_4 binding, Factor H, S protein) (Table 23–1).

Complement is part of the innate immune system and an important effector mechanism of humoral immunity. Tables 23–2A and 23–2B list the main physiologic activities, which illustrate host defense against infection, bridging innate and adaptive immunity. Removal of immune complexes and inflammatory products is performed by C1q and covalently bound fragments of C_3 and C_4. Initiators of activation pathways for the classical pathway include apoptotic cells, viruses, gram-negative bacteria, and C-reactive protein in addition to immune complexes (Table 23–3). Figure 23–1 illustrates the early steps of complement activation and classical pathways. The mannose-binding lectin or collectin, homologous to C_1q, is initiated by organisms with terminal mannose groups, and decreased levels have been noted in children with recurrent infections. The late steps of complement activation and the membrane attack complex (MAC) are shown in Figure 23–2.

BIOLOGIC PROPERTIES OF COMPLEMENT FRAGMENTS RELATED TO ALLERGIC DISEASES

Complement cascade activation leads to generation of biologically active fragments (Table 23–1). The products of C_3 and C_5 are small polypeptide anaphylatoxins that possess a variety of biologic properties. C_3a, C_4a, and C_5a release inflammatory mediators from mast cells, induce smooth muscle contraction, promote vascular permeability, and induce adhesion molecules on endothelial cells (Table 23–4). C_3a can also lead to mucus secretion by goblet cells, and C_3a and C_3a desArg can modulate synthesis of tumor necrosis factor alpha (TNF-α) and interleukin 1 beta (IL-1β) by mononuclear cells functioning to focus the production of proinflammatory cytokines. Such cytokines contribute to the pathophysiology of asthmatic inflammation. Therefore, anaphylatoxic peptides can trigger a variety of responses that contribute to allergic and inflammatory reactions. Elevated C_3a plasma levels have also been reported in patients with severe asthma, and levels of C_3a are increased by enzymatic activity of allergens generated when human serum is incubated with house dust and rye grass allergens. Anaphylaxis is an immediate systemic reaction due to rapid IgE-mediated release of potent mediators from tissue mast cells and peripheral blood basophils. Anaphylactoid reactions are immediate systemic reactions that mimic anaphylaxis but are not caused by IgE-mediated immune responses. Mast cell and basophil mediators may play a role in anaphylaxis and anaphylactoid reactions through tryptase, which may activate complement by cleavage of C3 (Table 23–1).

C_5a also plays an important role in recruiting phagocytic cells to sites of immune complex deposition in the lung, leading to enhanced oxidative and lipoxygenase activity with leukotriene B_4 (LTβ4) production. LTβ4, as well as other leukotriene mediators, are known to play important roles in asthma allergic rhinitis and cystic fibrosis. The presence of C_3a and C_5a in the lung can also induce respiratory distress through contraction of smooth muscle walls in bronchioles and pulmonary arteries. Animal studies have demonstrated the expression of C_3aR and C_5aR by cells in the lung, suggesting a role for these receptors during lung inflammation both in sepsis and asthma.

Table 23–1. Proteins of the human complement (C) system.

Component	Molecular Weight (=kd)	Normal (pg/mL)	Acute Phase[†] (% Increase)	Chromosomal Location
		Serum Levels		
Classical Pathway[*]				
C1q	460	70	13%	1p34–36.3
C1r	83	34		12p13
C1s	83	31	47%	12p13
C4	200	600	34%	6p21.3
C2	102	23		6p21.3
Alternative Pathway				
Factor D	25	2		19
Factor B	93	93	65%	6p21.1–21.3
Lectin Pathway				
MBL	288–576	2	Up to 1000%	10q11.2–21.0
MASP-1	97	6		3q27–28
MASP-2	80			1p36.23–36.31
MASP-3	105			3q27–28
Map 19	19			1p36.23–36.31
L-ficolin/P35	630	13.7		9
H-ficolin/Hakata antigen	630	15		
C3 and Terminal Components				
C3	185	1200	30%	19p 13.2–13.3
C5	190	75	55%	9q33
C6	128	45		5p 12–14
C7	120	55		5p 12–14
C8	163	68		1p32; 9q34.3
C9	79	60	49%	5p13
Control Proteins in Serum				
C1 inhibitor	105	150	21%	11q11–13.1
C4-binding protein	550	225		1q3.2
Factor H	150	550		1q3.2
Factor I	88	35		4q25
Properdin	223	5	–14%	Xp11.23–11.30
S protein	75	340		17q11
Clusterin	80	340		8p21
Anaphyloxin Inactivator	290	35		8p22–23, 10
		Ligands		
Membrane Receptor and Control Proteins				
DAF	70	C4b2a		1q3.2
MCFP	60	C3b		1q3.2
CD59	20	C8, C9		11p13–14
CR1	250	C3b, C4b		1q3.2
CR2	145	C3dg, C3d, EBV		1q3.2
CR3	250	iC3b, LPS, β-glucans		16p11–13.1, 21q22.3
CR4	245	iC3b, LPS		16p 11.2, 21q22.3
C3aR	100	C3a, C4a		12p13
C5aR	50	C5a		19q 13.3–13.4

[*]C-reactive protein (CRP; not shown) leads to classic pathway activation analogous to lectin pathway activation by MBL and ficolins.
[†]Acute-phase levels are estimates based on data.
DAF, decay-accelerating factor; EBV, Epstein-Barr virus; LPS, lipopolysaccharides; MASP, MBL-associated serine protease; MBL, mannan-binding lectin; MCP, membrane cofactor protein.
Data chiefly from Morley BJ, Walport MJ, eds. *The Complements Facts Book.* San Diego: Academic Press; 2000. Winkelstein, et al: Middleton's Allergy: Principles & Practice, 6ed., 2003. With permission from Elsevier.

Table 23–2A. Three physiologic activities of the complement system.

Activity	Complement Protein
Host Defense	
Opsonization	Covalently bound C_3; C_4
Chemotaxis and leukocyte activation	Anaphylatoxins (C5a, C3a; C4a); receptors on leukocytes
Lysis of bacteria and cells	Membrane attack complex (C5b–C9)

Modified from Walport MJ. *N Engl J Med.* 2001;344:1058.

CELLULAR RECEPTORS AND REGULATORS

Receptors for complement components are expressed on many cells. Important functions as listed in Table 23–5. Table 23–6 lists various inhibitors and regulators of complement activation and actions. C_5a also acts as potent chemoattractant for LFA integrins (CD11a/CD18) to enhance leukocyte movement into tissues at the site of infection. There are four cell membrane receptors for bound C_3, or CR1, CR2, Cr3, and Cr4, that are within two gene families (Table 23–5). CR1 or CD35 is found on mononuclear cells, neutrophils, mast cells, basophils, eosinophils, B and T lymphocytes and kidney podocytes. It functions in phagocytosis and clearance of immune complexes. CR2 or CD35 expressed on B cells and follicular dendritic cells, in addition to immature epithelial cells, is utilized by Epstein-Barr viruses (EBV) as a cellular receptor to promote cell entry.

CLINICAL ASSOCIATIONS

Tables 23–7 A to D are related to consequences of activation, the clinical effects of hereditary complement deficiencies related to infection, glomerulonephritis,

Table 23–2B. Interface of innate and adaptive immunity.

Augmentation of antibody responses	C3b; C4b bound to immune complexes; antigen receptor (AG); C3rc on B cells; antigen presenting cell (APC)
Enhancement of immunologic memory	C3b and C4b bound to immune complexes and to AG; C3rc on follicular dendritic cells

Modified from Walport MJ. *N Engl J Med.* 2001;344:1058.

Table 23–3. Activation pathways.

Pathway	Initiators
Classical	Immune complexes and apoptotic cells Several viruses and gram-negative bacteria C-reactive protein bound to ligand
Mannose-binding lectin	Microbes with terminal mannose groups
Alternative	Many bacteria, fungi, viruses, tumor cells

Modified from Walport MJ. *N Engl J Med.* 2001;344:1058.

angioedema, hemolysis, and systemic lupus erythematous (SLE). SLE can be associated with allergic diseases such as urticaria and can masquerade as atopy.

Complement deficiency can lead to increased susceptibility to pyogenic infections such as *Haemophilus influenzae* and *Streptococcus pneumoniae,* abnormality or function of the mannose-binding lectin, defective regulation of C_3 associated with membranoproliferative glomerulonephritis, or compromise of the lytic activity increasing neisserial infections (Table 23–7B). C_{3b} and iC_{3b}, which are covalently bound cleavage fragments of C_3, are the most significant opsonins for bacterial host defense. Mannose-binding lectin, as previously mentioned, is low in recurrent infections but also involved in tissue inflammation and necrosis. The mechanisms of entry used by various organisms involving complement are illustrated in Table 23–8. EBV uses glycoprotein 350/20, measles and picornaviruses employs hemagglutinin and capsid, and M tuberculosis uses C3 fragments.

A recent review has summarized the clinical manifestations and pathophysiology of congenital and acquired complement deficiency diseases and laboratory evaluation. Hereditary angioedema (HAE), an autosomal dominant disease, is a deficiency of the C_1 inhibitor with loss of regulation and failure to activate kallikrein. This disorder can lead to severe illness when it involves the intestinal submucosa or obstruction of the upper airway, leading to death by suffocation. Symptoms usually begin in adolescence, and edema of the gastrointestinal tract results in severe colicky abdominal pain, nausea, and vomiting. Urticaria is not part of the syndrome, and swelling can be triggered by trauma or psychological stress with increased frequency with angiotensin inhibitors. Over 100 mutations in the C_1-Inh gene have been described. Type 1 HAE is due to a mutation that prevents the transcription of the abnormal allele, whereas type 2 variant is due to a point mutation in the gene

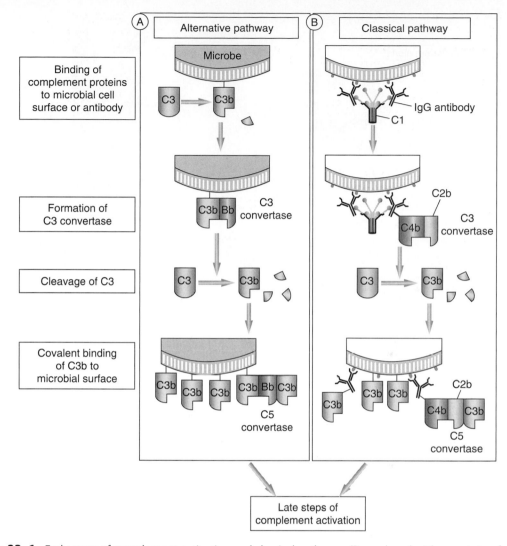

Figure 23–1. Early steps of complement activation and classical pathways. (Reproduced, with permission, from Elsevier 2005. Abbas, Lichtman. Cellular and Molecular Immunology. 5th ed.) [www.studentconsult.com.]

abolishing its activity as a serine protease inhibitor. Patients with the type 2 variant have normal or elevated antigenic levels but synthesize a dysfunctional protein with reduced or absent C_1-INH function.

A third type in women has clinical findings but normal C_1-INH levels and function. Acquired angioedema in older patients with lymphoproliferative or monoclonal gammopathies has consumption of C_1q. Laboratory features of HAE are decreased C_1-INH and C_2 and C4 levels. Treatment with infusion of C_1 inhibitor can be lifesaving for HAE.

Patients with complement deficiencies are also associated with various rheumatic diseases, such as SLE, anaphylactoid purpura, dermatomyositis, and vasculitis. Paroxysmal nocturnal hemoglobinuria is a rare disease characterized by intravascular hemolysis, hemoglobinuria, and venous thrombosis due to absence of decay accelerating factor (CD55) and inhibitor of the MAC (CD59).

Hemolytic uremic syndrome is due to factor H and I deficiency. Total deficiency of C_3 and Factor H mutations is associated with membranoproliferative glomerulonephritis. These patients have a complement-consuming

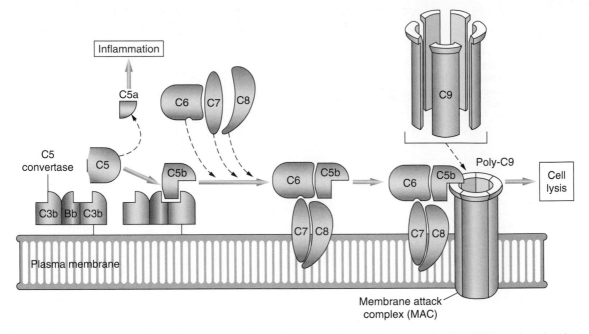

Figure 23–2. Late steps of complement activation and the membrane attack complex (MAC). (Reproduced, with permission, from Elsevier 2005. Abbas, Lichtman. *Cellular and Molecular Immunology.* 5th ed.) [www.studentconsult.com.]

antibody called nephritic factor also found in partial lipodystrophy.

Apoptosis has been linked with autoimmune diseases associated with complement deficiencies. C_1q can bind to cells undergoing apoptosis with facilitation of elimination. Clearance of apoptotic cells have occurred through reactivity with collectin receptors or phagocytic cells that interact with C_1q and mannose-binding lectin.

IMMUNOMODULATION OF AUTOIMMUNITY WITH INTRAVENOUS IMMUNE GLOBULIN AND MECHANISMS OF IMMUNOMODULATION

The mode of action of immune globulin involves modulation of the expression and function of Fc receptors with complement activation and the cytokine network. The

Table 23–4. Biological properties of complement.

Fragment	Cell Target	Function
C4a	Smooth muscle; endothelium	Contraction; increased vasopermeability
C5a	Skin mast cells, basophils, neutrophils, endothelium	Induce release of mediators, chemotaxis, increased vasopermeability
C3a	Smooth muscle; endothelium; mast cells	Induce release of mediators, chemotaxis, induce adhesion molecules, increased vasopermeability
C3b	Cells, bacteria	Opsonization
C3d	CR2 + B cells	B-cell activation

Basic immunology. In: *Medical Knowledge Self Assessment Program.* 3rd ed. Milwaukee, Wis: American Academy of Allergy Asthma and Immunology; 2003:1.

Table 23–5. Complement receptors.

Receptor	Ligands	Cell Distribution	Function
CR1, CD35	C3b, C4b, iC3b	Wide variety of cells	Phagocytosis Clearance of immune complexes
CR2, CD21	C3d/C3dg, iC3b	B cells, follicular dendritic cells	Coreceptor B-cell activation, Epstein-Barr virus receptor
CR3, CD11b/CD18	iC3b, ICAM-1	Monocytes, macrophages, neutrophils, NK cells (NK)	Phagocytosis Adherence
CR4, CD11c/CD18	iC3b	Monocytes, macrophages, neutrophils, NK	Phagocytosis Adherence
C5a receptor	C5a	Endothelial cells, mast cells; phagocytes	Binds C5a
C3a receptor	C3a	Endothelial cells, mast cells, phagocytes	Binds C3a

Basic immunology. In: *Medical Knowledge Self Assessment Program.* 3rd ed. Milwaukee, Wis: American Academy of Allergy Asthma and Immunology; 2003:1.

immunoregulatory effects of immune globulin that involve complement include blockade of Fc receptors on macrophages and other cells' inhibition of the Fcγ receptor IIB. The effect on inflammation includes decrease of complement-mediated damage and immune complex–mediated inflammation, induction of antiinflammatory cytokines, inhibition of endothelial cell activation, neutralization of bacterial toxins, and reduction in requirements of corticosteroids. Table 23–9 illustrates the effects on B cells and antibody production, T cells, and cell growth.

Immunomodulatory mechanisms and agents for the treatment of autoimmune diseases include antigen-specific tolerance using intravenous or mucosal antigen application, altered peptides, or vaccines. In addition to immunoglobulin treatment, immunomodulation may also involve a change in the cytokine balance; administration of agents that suppress regulatory cytokines, such as IL-10 and TGF-β that can occur in allergen immunotherapy; administration of agents that antagonize TNF-α; or stem cell transplantation.

Table 23–6. Inhibitors and regulators of complement activation.

Protein	Complement Targets	Action
C1 INH	C1r, C1s	Serine protease inhibitor, dissociates from C1r and C1s
Factor I	C4b, C3b	Cleaves C3b and C4b with Factor H
Factor H	C3b	Cofactor with Factor I in cleaving C3b; displaces Bb
C4 binding	C4b	Displaces C2 from C4b
Membrane cofactor protein (MCP, CD46)	C3b, C4b	Cofactor with Factor I mediated cleavage of C3b and C4b
CD59	C7, C8	Blocks C9 binding and prevents MAC formation
Decay-accelerating factor (DAF)	C4b2b, C3bBb	Dissociates C3 convertase

Basic immunology. In: *Medical Knowledge Self Assessment Program.* 3rd ed. Milwaukee, Wis: American Academy of Allergy Asthma and Immunology; 2003:1.

Table 23–7A. Clinical effects of hereditary complement deficiencies.

Complementary Deficiency	Consequence of Complement Activation
C3	Loss of opsonin and failure to activate membrane-attack-complex pathway
C3, properdin, membrane-attack-complex proteins	Failure to develop the membrane attack complex

Modified from Walport MJ. *N Engl J Med.* 2001;344:1058.

Table 23–7C. Clinical effects of hereditary complement deficiencies.

Complementary Deficiency	Consequence of Complement Activation
C1 inhibitor	Loss of regulation of C1 and activation of kallikrein
CD59	Failure to prevent membrane-attack complexes on autologous cells
C1q, C1r, C1s, C4, C2	Failure to activate the classical pathway
Factor H and Factor I	Failure to regulate activation of C3; severe secondary C3 deficiency

Modified from Walport MJ. *N Engl J Med.* 2001;344:1058.

Various autoimmune and inflammatory diseases benefiting from immune globulin are shown in Table 23–10. The immunomodulatory effects of immune globulin on B and T cells are illustrated in Figure 23–3.

AUTOIMMUNE URTICARIA

Patients with SLE also can present with chronic urticaria. A subpopulation of patients with chronic urticaria also possess IgG antibody directed to the α-subunit of high affinity type 1 IgE receptor. IgG can activate basophils, which depends on or is augmented by complement. SLE, a prototype of immune complex disease, and other autoimmune diseases are caused by a breakdown of tolerance and other factors. Factors that influence the pathogenesis of T cell–mediated autoimmune diseases are due to genetic susceptibility, activation of autoreactive T cells, or infiltration of target organs by T cells and damage to target organs by T-cell effector molecules or other cell populations. Breakdown to tolerance can occur in SLE, autoimmune diabetes, and multiple sclerosis.

COMPLEMENT THERAPEUTICS IN CLINICAL PRACTICE

Treatment of patients with congenital complement deficiencies focuses on the underlying problems of infection and autoimmunity. Recombinant complement components for a completely deficient patient are possible, and blood transfusion to replace missing components has been tried with some success in two SLE patients with C2 deficiency and several patients with Factor H deficiency. Renal transplantation might be a viable therapy specifically for atypical hemolytic uremic syndrome (HUS) patients with an MCP mutation.

Table 23–7B. Clinical effects of hereditary complement deficiencies.

Complementary Deficiency	Clinical Association
C3	Pyrogenic bacterial infections; could have a distinctive rash Membranoproliferative glomerulonephritis
C3, properdin membrane-attack-complex proteins	Neisserial infection

Table 23–7D. Clinical effects of hereditary complement deficiencies.

Complementary Deficiency	Clinical Association
C1 inhibitor	Angioedema
CD59	Hemolysis, thrombosis
C1q, C1r; C1s, C4, C2	Systemic lupus erythematosus
Factor H and Factor I	Hemolytic-uremic syndrome
	Membranoproliferative glomerulonephritis

Modified from Walport MJ. *N Engl J Med.* 2001;344:1058.

Table 23–8. Proteins of the complement system and entry into human cells.

Microorganism	Mechanism of Entry into Host Cell
Epstein-Barr virus	Glycoprotein 350/220
Measles	Hemagglutinin
Picornaviruses	Capsid
Mycobacterium tuberculosis	C3 fragments

Modified from Walport MJ. *N Engl J Med.* 2001;344:1058.

The success of animal studies led to clinical trials, with sCR1 being used for treatment of acute respiratory distress syndrome, myocardial infarction, lung transplantation, and post–cardiopulmonary bypass syndrome, and anti-C5 mAb in multicentered trials being used for myocardial infarction, post–cardiopulmonary bypass syndrome, rheumatoid arthritis, membranous nephropathy, and lupus nephritis.

The complement system as part of innate immunity provides an important effector system for host defense, clearance of immune complexes, and regulation or acquired immune reactions. The future of complement therapy may include targeted gene therapy or replacement with recombinant proteins for patients with complement deficiencies.

Table 23–9. Immunoregulatory effects of immune globulin.

B cells and production of antibodies
Control of bone marrow B-cell lines
Negative signaling via Fc-γ receptors
Selective downregulation and upregulation of
   antibody production
Neutralization by anti-idiotypes of circulating
   autoantibodies

T cells
Regulation of CD4-T-cell cytokine production
Neutralization of T-cell superantigens

Cells proliferation
Lymphocyte proliferation inhibition
Control of cell death

Modified from Kazatchkine MD, Kaven SV. Immunomodulation of autoimmune and inflammatory diseases with intravenous immune globulin. *N Engl J Med.* 2001;345(10):747.

Table 23–10. Autoimmune and inflammatory diseases benefiting from immune globulin.

Idiopathic thrombocytopenic purpura
Guillain-Barré syndrome
Chronic demyelinating polyradiculoneuropathy
Myasthenia gravis
Multifocal motor neuropathy
Corticosteroid-resistant dermatomyositis
Kawasaki disease
Prevention of graft-versus-host disease
Antineutrophil cytoplasmic vasculitis
Autoimmune uveitis
Multiple sclerosis

Modified from Kazatchkine MD, Kaven SV. Immunomodulation of autoimmune and inflammatory diseases with intravenous immune globulin. *N Engl J Med.* 2001;345(10):747.

Therapeutic complement inhibitor approaches have been considered for treatment of bulbous pemphigus, rejection of transplanted tissues, Alzheimer's disease because plaques contain high levels of classical and alternative pathway components as well as MAC components, immune-based fetal loss, HIV, and a great many other serious medical conditions. Other disorders that interface importantly with the complement system, in addition to SLE, include rheumatoid arthritis and related arthritides, including cryoglobulinemia.

Complement also can be an important factor in tissue necrosis after ischemia. In addition, myocardial infarction and stroke are associated with complement activation in the area of tissue infarction. Complement participates in internal homeostasis by removing damaged, neoplastic, or infected cells. Thus complement science is no longer thought to be just protein pathways involved in esoteric diseases but can be related to both autoimmune and cerebrovascular and myocardial disease.

EVIDENCE-BASED MEDICINE

According to Sackett (*BMJ.* 1996:312:71), "evidence based medicine is conscientious, explicit and judicious use of current best evidence in making decisions about care of individual patients. The practice of evidence based medicine means integrity, individual clinical experience with the best available clinical evidence from systematic research." This chapter has provided several references from the literature in terms of review articles and sections from textbooks that critically explain mechanisms and can also be applied to patient care, intervention, and outcome.

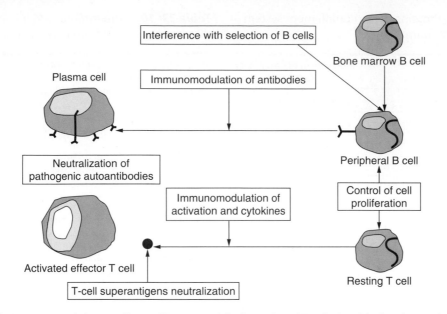

Figure 23–3. Immunomodulatory effects of immune globulin on B and T cells. (Modified and reproduced, with permission, from Kazatchkine MD, Frieri M., *Allergy and Asthma Proc.* 2002;23:319.

BIBLIOGRAPHY

Winkelstein J, Gewurz AT, Lint TF, et al. The complement system. In: Adkinson NE, Yunginger JW, Busse WW, eds. *Middleton's Allergy Principles and Practice.* 6th ed. Philadelphia: Mosby; 2003:66.

Walport MJ. Complement, first and second of two parts. *N Engl J Med.* 2001;344:1058.

Frieri M. Complement mediated diseases. *Allergy Asthma Proc.* 2002;23:319.

Frieri M. Basic immunology. In: *Medical Knowledge Self Assessment Program.* 3rd ed. Milwaukee, Wis: American Academy of Allergy Asthma and Immunology; 2003:1.

Frieri M. Asthma concepts in the new millennium-update in asthma pathophysiology. *Allergy Asthma Proc.* 2005;26:83.

Lieberman P. Anaphylaxis and anaphylactoid reactions. In: Adkinson NE, Yunginger JW, Busse WW, eds. *Middleton's Allergy Principles and Practice.* Vol 2. 6th ed. Philadelphia: Mosby; 2003:1497.

Petersen SV, Thiel S, Jensenius JC. The mannose-binding lectin pathway of complement activation: biology and disease association. *Med Immunol.* 2001;38:133.

Frieri M. Identification of masqueraders of autoimmune disease in the office. *Allergy Asthma Proc.* 2003;24(6):421.

Kaplan J, Anand P, Frieri M. Rash, drug hypersensitivity and autoimmunity in a 20 year old. *Ann Allergy Asthma Immunol.* 2005;95:111.

Wen L, Atkinson JP, Giclas PC. Clinical and laboratory evaluation of complement deficiency. *J Allergy Clin Immunol.* 2004;113:585.

Shum J, Frieri M. Evolution, apoptosis and autoimmune diseases. *Pediatr Allergy Asthma Immunol.* 1997;11:9.

Mansur A, Frieri M. Behcet's disease vs. Behcet's syndrome with some criteria of systemic lupus erythematosus. *Pediatr Allergy Asthma Immunol.* 1998;12:53.

Takabayashi T, Vannier E, Clark BD, et al. A new biologic role for C3a and C3a desArg: regulation of TNF-α and IL-1 beta synthesis. *J Immunol.* 1966;156:3455.

Kikuchi Y, Kaplan AP. Mechanisms of autoimmune activating basophils in chronic urticaria. *J Allergy Clin Immunol.* 2001;107:1056.

Kannradt T, Mitchison NA. Tolerance and autoimmunity. *N Engl J Med.* 2001;344:655.

Chaplin H. Review; The burgeoning history of the complement system 1888–2005. *Immunohematology.* 2005;21:85.

Food Allergy

Oscar L. Frick, MD, PhD

Peanut, tree nut, and shellfish allergies cause life-threatening anaphylaxis and thus present a significant public health problem. Foods can cause a spectrum of symptoms affecting several organ systems by both immunologic and nonimmunologic mechanisms. Such adverse reactions to foods may be toxic inherent in the food itself, like tyramine in aged cheeses and chocolate or caffeine in coffee, or toxic contaminants, such as histamine in scombroid fish or bacteria—*Salmonella, Shigella,* or *Campylobacter*—that cause food poisoning. Host factors such as lactase deficiency or idiosyncratic reactions are nonimmunologic.

Immunologic mechanisms are atopy, which is IgE antibody-mediated, causing urticaria and anaphylaxis, and they are the most common. Mixed IgE antibody and cellular immune mechanisms occur in atopic dermatitis and eosinophilic gastroenteropathies. IgA antibodies are involved in celiac disease. Cellular immunity is involved in inflammatory bowel diseases: regional enteritis (Crohn disease) and ulcerative colitis.

About 8% of infants and young children with immature gastrointestinal tracts are prone to develop food allergies, whereas in older children and adults, the incidence is about 2%.

Peanut allergy has tripled in the past two decades. Many people think they have a food allergy, although it cannot be substantiated by tests or diets.

MUCOSAL IMMUNITY AND TOLERANCE

Ingested foods are processed all along the gastrointestinal tract beginning with salivary ptyalin converting starch to maltose, by stomach acid and pepsin, and by intestinal trypsin and amylase and bile. Proteins are broken down to proteoses and amino acids for absorption and building host's tissues. Carbohydrates are broken down to sugars and fats to body lipids.

The gut-associated lymphoid tissue (GALT) is the mucosal immune system, consisting of M cells in Peyer patches that "sip" antigens and transfer them to macrophages in lamina propria, which then present antigens to T and B lymphocytes. Oral tolerance is effected by this mucosal immune system, which is able to distinguish pathogenic bacteria and viruses from the huge mass of commensal bacteria needed for digestion. Secretory IgA antibodies form a protective barrier that clumps incompletely digested proteins and harmful bacteria to be swept out in the stool. Mild anaphylaxis might have a physiologic function in increasing peristalsis to aid in removal of noxious materials from the gut.

Oral tolerance may be achieved by T-cell anergy in which intraepithelial cells (IELs) act as inefficient antigen-presenting cells (APCs) that present antigenic peptides to T cells as the first signal but lack the costimulatory second signals(CD-28 and ICAM-1) to effect an active immune response. Consequently, these partially activated T-cells become anergic or tolerant. Furthermore, there may be stimulation of T-regulatory cells secreting immunosuppressive cytokines, IL-10 and tumor necrosis factor beta (TNF-β).

Pathogenesis

The intestinal mucosa of infants and young children is immature and "leaky" to incompletely digested proteins, especially to the large volumes of milk (1 L/day in a 7-kg infant equals 10 L/day in a 70-kg adult). The secretory IgA antibody barrier develops slowly over months in infants. Food antigens cross the leaky gut to IgE-coated mast cells that release histamine, which separates the intraepithelial cells to enhance the gut permeability and presentation to IgE-forming B cells. As the intestinal barrier function matures, food allergens decrease, and many children "outgrow" their milk, egg and wheat allergies.

ALLERGENS

The most common food allergens are cow's milk, egg, wheat, soy, peanuts (in children) and tree nuts, fish, shellfish, and sesame seeds in adults. Specific allergenic epitopes in foods expressed as recombinant proteins

Table 24–1. Classical (class 1) food allergens.

Peanut	Ara h1, Ara h2, Ara h3	
Cow's milk	Caseins a, b, k	Bos d8
	β-Lactoglobulin	Bos d5
	α-Lactalbumin	Bos d4
	Bovine serum albumin	Bos d6
Egg	Ovomucoid	Gal d1
	Ovalbumin	Gal d2
Shrimp	Tropomyosin	Pen a1
Codfish	Parvalbumin	Gad c1
Lipid transfer proteins		
	Apple	Mal d1, Mal d4
	Peach	Pru p1, Pru p2, Pru p3
	Hazelnut	Cor a1, Cor a2

have been identified (Table 24–1). These are usually glycoproteins of mol wt 10 to 70 Kd that are heat and acid stable and protease resistant, enabling them to bypass denaturation by cooking and by gastric and upper intestinal digestion.

Cross-Reacting Food Allergens

In food plant and some animal families, there may be considerable cross-reactivity among allergens (Fig. 24–1). Patients should be made aware of these cross-reactions.

There is considerable public health concern about the potential allergenicity of genetically modified organism (GMO) foods. New GMO foods must be evaluated for these physical properties as well as comparison to 6 to 8 amino acids sequences of known food allergen recombinant epitopes. The original example was transgenically inserting methionine into methionine-poor soybeans from the methionine-rich S2-protein of Brazil nuts. Such transgenic soybeans bound IgE antibodies from Brazil nut–allergic patients, which precluded further development of such transgenic soybeans for animal feeds (or human consumption). This alerted public health authorities about the potential allergenicity in GMO foods.

CLINICAL MANIFESTATIONS

Anaphylaxis is the most serious food allergy because it can be life threatening. It causes about 300 deaths annually in the United States with foods implicated in about 40% of cases. Food allergens like peanut, tree nuts, and shrimp combine rapidly (within seconds) with IgE antibodies on ubiquitous vascular and tissue mast cells and circulating basophils to release massive amounts of histamine, PAF (platelet-activating factor), and leukotrienes.

Vascular endothelial cells are separated, allowing massive leakage of plasma into tissues that results in edema and circulatory collapse or shock. Smooth muscle cells become spastic, leading to bronchospasm, intestinal motility (diarrhea), and urination. Laryngeal edema closes the airway leading to anoxia, asphyxia, and death.

Exercise-induced anaphylaxis occurs if a person sensitized to a particular food allergen, like celery, exercises within 2 hours after ingesting that food.

Skin

Urticaria and *angioedema* commonly start in the face, eyelids, and lips and progress over the body and limbs. This is pruritic from histamine release and sometimes burning and painful from bradykinin formation. IgE antibodies and sometimes complement C4a and C2a anaphylatoxins contribute to symptoms. Handling or skin contact with food allergens may cause contact urticaria.

ATOPIC DERMATITIS

A chronic pruritic rash on face, limbs, and body usually begins in infancy and early childhood. This often clears by school age, although rashes may persist into adulthood. Due to the intense itching, the skin is damaged from scratching and secondarily infected with *Staphylococci*. Older lesions become lichenified, and discoloration may last for years.

Foods, especially egg and cow's milk, are common causes, as are other foods in about 40% of cases, with dust mites and animal danders causing another major portion of cases. IgE antibodies cause an immediate reddening and itching, which initiates a chronic inflammation with cellular infiltration with eosinophiles and T cells. Initially, these TH-2 cells elicit IL-4, IL-5, and IL-13 cytokines, but as chronicity occurs, TH-1 cell cytokines, IL-2, and IFN-γ perpetuate the inflammation.

Gastrointestinal Tract

Oral allergy syndrome (OAS) commonly from fruits or vegetables causes buccal, mucosal, and tongue itching and swelling but rarely proceeds further. This is due mostly to fruit and vegetable epitopes that cross-react with pollen allergens, like birch pollen Betv1, in birch pollen hayfever patients.

Vomiting, nausea, abdominal pain, and diarrhea are common symptoms of food allergy. Sometimes emesis is explosive. Infantile "colic" may be the first sign of an allergic child commonly due to cow's milk or a food in the nursing mother's diet. This may occur in 25% of colicky infants.

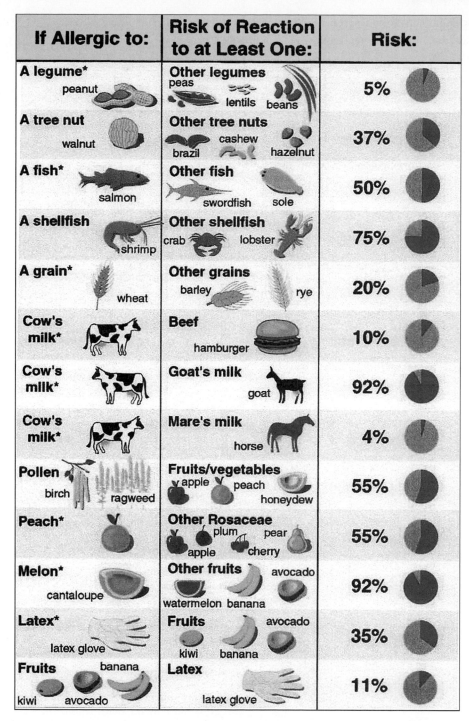

If Allergic to:	Risk of Reaction to at Least One:	Risk:
A legume* peanut	Other legumes peas lentils beans	5%
A tree nut walnut	Other tree nuts cashew brazil hazelnut	37%
A fish* salmon	Other fish swordfish sole	50%
A shellfish shrimp	Other shellfish crab lobster	75%
A grain* wheat	Other grains barley rye	20%
Cow's milk*	Beef hamburger	10%
Cow's milk*	Goat's milk goat	92%
Cow's milk*	Mare's milk horse	4%
Pollen birch ragweed	Fruits/vegetables apple peach honeydew	55%
Peach*	Other Rosaceae plum pear apple cherry	55%
Melon* cantaloupe	Other fruits avocado watermelon banana	92%
Latex* latex glove	Fruits avocado kiwi banana	35%
Fruits banana kiwi avocado	Latex latex glove	11%

Figure 24–1. Approximate rate of clinical reactivity to at least one other related food. The probability of reacting to related foods varieties, depending on numerous factors. Data derived from studies with double-blind placebo-controlled food challenges. (Reproduced, with permission, from Sicherer SH. Clinical implication of cross-reactive food allergens. J Allergy Clin Immunol. 2001;108(6):881.)

Eosinophilic Esophagitis and Gastroenteritis

Infiltration of the mucosa of the esophagus and of mucosa, muscle, and serosa of the gastrointestinal tract is being increasingly recognized. Diagnosis is made by endoscopy and biopsy. Eosinophils in more than 15/HPF constitutes gut eosinophilia. Peripheral blood may or may not express eosinophilia.

Symptoms in *esinophilia esophagitis* (EOE) resemble those of gastric reflux with nausea, vomiting, dysphagia, and epigastric pain (heartburn), especially in children. Most patients with EOE exhibit other signs of allergy—eczema, rhinitis, or asthma. A pH probe result is usually normal. A patient with gastroesophageal reflux and negative pH probe should have an endoscopy.

Food allergy, both IgE-mediated and cellular immunity, may be demonstrable by prick skin tests and atopy patch tests. Removal of positive foods may help in some cases; some may require an elemental diet for some weeks to quiet the inflammation. They usually respond to oral corticosteroids but relapse when withdrawn.

Patients with *eosinophilic gastroenteritis (EOG)* have vomiting, abdominal pain, and diarrhea. The serosal form may have eosinophilic ascites. They may respond to an elemental diet and corticosteroids.

Eosinophilic proctitis occurs in infants with flecks of blood in stool to bloody diarrhea. Implicated is cow's milk, soy, or a food in the mother's diet if nursing. Changing to protein hydrolysate alleviates the condition. Heiner syndrome in infants may also have melena and reflux with failure to thrive. Hemosiderosis in bronchial washings indicates regurgitation of milk into bronchi and lungs. Blood contains milk-precipitating IgG antibodies. With removal of cow's milk and substituting an elemental formula, the condition resolves in weeks.

Irritable Bowel Disease

Crohn disease and ulcerative colitis are beyond the scope of this chapter. But occasionally food hypersensitivity may be implicated.

Respiratory

Much less common symptoms from food allergy are rhinitis and asthma. Wheezing or cough from a food ingestion are rare, but increased sensitivity to inhaled methacholine after food challenge is a more subtle indication of food-induced bronchial inflammation.

Genitourinary

The bladder is another smooth muscle organ, so urinary urgency and enuresis have been attributed to food allergy. Anaphylaxis following coitus with a partner who had ingested walnuts or peanuts has been reported.

Central Nervous System

Headaches have been attributed to foods, but there are little published data. Most headaches may be due to chronic sinusitis secondary to allergic rhinitis. Tyramine in aged cheeses and chocolate may cause headaches, as may monosodium glutamate (MSG) in restaurant-served Asian foods.

DIAGNOSIS

Oral Food Challenges

The double-blind placebo-controlled food challenge (DBPCFC) is the gold standard in the diagnosis of food allergy. These are done in a controlled environment in a hospital or specialty clinic with emergency medications, equipment, and trained personnel at hand. Food in liquid or powdered form in a masking vehicle for blinding is given in a minute quantity and doubled every 15 to 30 minutes until allergic symptoms or signs occur. This indicates a positive reaction. If the maximum dose causes no symptoms, the test is negative.

Because this requires considerable staff and time, several alternative simpler procedures have been proposed. For example, if cow's milk allergy is suspected in an infant, cow's milk formula is mixed with placebo formula(1:2) to make it indistinguishable from placebo formula. At 30-minute intervals, 2, 10, 50, and 100 mL are given blindly. If no symptoms occur in the following 2 hours, then 60 mL per day for 4 days is given at home, watching for symptoms. If none occur, milk formula is resumed.

Prick Skin Tests

Prick skin tests are usually done in the initial workup with a screen testing with commercial extracts of the nine common foods—egg, cow's milk, wheat, peanut, tree nut, fish, seafood, and sesame seed—unless there is a history of anaphylaxis with one of these allergens, in which case an in vitro test is done. Various prick devices are available, but one should be standardized for use in a particular clinic. Positive reactions are a wheal larger than 3 mm, with wheal and erythema size recorded after 10 to 20 minutes. These are compared with the positive histamine control. A negative reaction is compared with a saline control. Certain food allergens are easily denatured. Therefore, pricking a fresh fruit or vegetable, then pricking the patient's skin (prick-to-prick method) yields more useful information. Intradermal skin tests with foods are contraindicated because of danger from anaphylaxis.

Positive prick tests give useful information about a food causing a current problem in about 40% of cases. So-called false-positive prick tests indicate sensitization, but clinically a problem may be past or may occur in the future. Properly done, negative skin prick tests are about 95% reliable that the food can be continued in the diet.

In Vitro Tests

In RAST (radioactive allergosorbent test) or ELISA (enzyme-linked sorbent allergen), food allergen is bound to a matrix that is bathed in the patient's serum. Food allergen-bound IgE antibodies are measured with a radioisotope-tagged or enzyme-tagged monoclonal anti-human IgE serum and developed with markers, such as alkaline phosphatase or horseradish peroxidase in ELISA. The CAP-RAST-FIEA (Pharmacia, Uppsala, Sweden) has been standardized so that above a given threshold the test correlated well with a DBPCFC (Table 24–2). If anaphylaxis is suspected, in vitro testing is mandatory. One may follow the course of a food allergy with subsequent in vitro tests at intervals to determine if the food sensitivity has decreased or disappeared and when it might be safe to cautiously reintroduce that food into the diet.

Basophil-Degranulation Tests

Several simplified versions of measurement of histamine release from sensitized basophils have been developed for clinical use.

Atopy Patch Tests

Dehydrated food is mixed one part with two parts petrolatum. This mixture (20 mg) is placed on a large (12-mm diameter) Finn chamber on Scanpor tape (Epitest, Tuusula, Finland) and applied to uninvolved skin of the back. Petrolatum in Finn chamber is a negative control. Occlusion time is 72 hours, and results are read 30 to 60 minutes after removal. The following scale is read: 1+ = redness and edema, 2+ = redness, edema, and a few papules, 3+ = redness, edema, and papules covering most of patch area, 4+ = papules spreading out side patch area or vesicles. This test may be useful in younger children with atopic dermatitis that has a cellular immune component.

Food Elimination Diets

Food elimination diets have been the major tool in diagnosis and management of food allergies for almost a century starting with the Rowe diets. Simpler elimination diets are available from the Food Allergy and Asthma Network (FAAN), www.foodallergy.org.

The suspect food in all its forms is removed from the diet completely for from 2 to 8 weeks to clear the food allergen from the patient's system. A simple symptoms scoring is recorded daily or at intervals. At the end of this period, the physician evaluates positive or negative improvement. Then a food challenge is done cautiously in a controlled setting with epinephrine at hand. The patient is given a minute quantity of the suspect food. If he had been eating the food daily he may have been partially desensitizing himself. During the elimination period, IgE antibodies may have built up, so that on reintroduction, anaphylaxis might occur. If the food is tolerated, next day larger increments of the food may be given at intervals to determine if symptoms recur. If not, the food can be continued in the diet. If positive, the food must be kept out of the diet for months or even years. Adequate nutrition must be maintained, especially

Table 24–2. Performance characteristics of 90% specificity diagnostic decision points generated in the retrospective study in diagnosing food allergy in 100 consecutive children and adolescents referred for evaluation of food hypersensitivity.

Allergen	Decision point (kU$_A$/L)	Sensitivity	Specificity	Efficiency	PPV	NPV
Egg	7	61	95	68	98	38
Milk	15	57	94	59	95	53
Peanut	14	57	100	84	100	36
Fish	3	63	91	87	56	93
Soybean	30	44	94	81	73	82
Wheat	26	61	92	84	74	87

NPV, negative predictive value; PPV, positive predictive value.
Sampson HA. Utility of food-specific IgE concentrations in predicting symptomatic food allergy. *J Allergy Clin Immunol.* 2001;107:891.

in growing children, where assistance of a dietitian may be helpful. Other methods include the following:

- **Radiography** with bowel contrast medium may detect ulcerations or irregularities in the bowel wall, especially in inflammatory bowel diseases.
- **Endoscopy and biopsy** of esophagus, stomach, intestine, and rectal mucosa for increased numbers of eosinophils and inflammation may be diagnostic in eosinophilic esophagogastroenteropathies.
- **Plasma histamine and/or tryptase** After a food challenge, plasma histamine and/or tryptase rise—histamine within minutes—but it is rapidly metabolized within an hour. Plasma tryptase elevation persists for many hours to days and may be useful in determining whether anaphylaxis caused an unexplained sudden death.

MANAGEMENT AND TREATMENT

Elimination Diet

Removing the offending food allergen is the treatment of choice and usually successful. If the food allergy is long-standing, there may be significant inflammatory damage to the gastrointestinal tract that may take months to heal.

Sometimes an elemental diet is necessary: The patient is given a protein hydrolysate (Nutramigen, Pregestimil, EleCare, Neocate, Alimentum, Vivonex) for 2 weeks to rest the gut. Then foods are gradually reintroduced one by one every 2 days, and the patient is observed for symptoms. In children, protein hydrolysate and a lamb and rice diet can be used as baseline and the diet gradually expanded.

The patient should be educated to recognize the first signs of anaphylaxis and to read food labels for high allergy-risk foods. Patient should have a written action plan for management of anaphylaxis for home, school, or work.

Pharmaceuticals

Self-injectable *epinephrine* (Epi-Pen; Dey Laboratories, Napa, CA) is mandatory in treating anaphylaxis. *Antihistamines* are the second line of drugs in the acute treatment of anaphylaxis. They are inefficient in managing food allergy symptoms, but hydroxyzine is helpful in alleviating the pruritus in atopic dermatitis and urticaria. *Antileukotrienes* have been reported to help occasionally but not consistently. *Cromolyn sodium* as a mast cell stabilizer has been helpful in individual cases but must be given in huge doses orally (100 to 200 mg) with each meal because only about 1% is absorbed.

New Experimental Approaches

Humanized anti-IgE antiserum: One study of TNX-109 showed increased tolerance permitting ingestion of

eight peanuts in peanut anaphylaxis patients. This is enough to lessen effects of an accidental ingestion of a peanut-containing product. Currently, another anti-IgE, omalizumab (Xolair; Genentech S, San Francisco, CA), is under investigation for effectiveness in peanut anaphylaxis.

Recombinant peptides as food allergen epitopes (e.g., peanut Ara h1, 2, or 3 coupled to a bacterial DNA CpG) are recognized by animal immune systems by initiating TH-1 and/or T reg suppression.

Heat-killed bacteria (*Listeria monocytogenes, Escherichia coli*) coupled to food allergens or epitopes have alleviated allergic reactions in murine and canine models.

Immunotherapy with conventional subcutaneous or sublingually administered cross-reacting pollen allergens has been successful in fruit-induced oral allergy syndrome in birch-sensitive patients. Immunotherapy with peas is being evaluated to minimize peanut allergy.

Chinese herbal mixture has been successful in patients with peanut allergy.

Hypoallergenic Foods

Different apple cultivars have either high or low Mal d1 content; this is the major apple allergen related to Bet v1. A hypoallergenic rice has been developed in Japan. A rice-based edible vaccine expressing multiple T-cell epitopes of cedar pollen has induced oral tolerance for inhibition of TH-2-induced cedar pollen allergy. This might be applied to food allergens.

EVIDENCE-BASED MEDICINE

From atopic and normal human cell cultures and animal models of food allergy, it is becoming clear that atopic dermatitis patients have deficiency in T-regulatory cells that suppress food-induced reactions and have increased apoptosis of TH-1 protective cells. Therapeutic approaches are tying to boost this suppressor T-regulatory cell capacity in atopic patients. The increase in allergies and anaphylaxis makes it imperative to educate the public and primary care physicians to properly treat, manage, and follow up anaphylaxis.

BIBLIOGRAPHY

Akdis M, Blaser K, Akdis CA. T regulatory cells in allergy: novel concepts in the pathogenesis, prevention and treatment of allergic diseases. *J Allergy Clin Immunol.* 2005;116:961.

Bock S, Lee W, Remigio I, et al. Studies of hypersensitivity reactions to foods in infants and children. *J Allergy Clin Immunol.* 1978;62:327

Bock SA, Sampson HA, Atkins FM, et al. Double-blind placebo-controlled food challenges (DBPCFC) as an office procedure: a manual. *J Allergy Clin Immunol.* 1988;82:986.

Frick OL, Teuber SS, Buchanan BB, et al. Allergen immunotherapy with heat-killed *Listeria monocytogenes* alleviates peanut and food-induced anaphylaxis in dogs. *Allergy.* 2005;60:243.

Frossard CP, Tropia L, Hauser C, et al. Lymphocytes in Peyer's patches regulate clinical tolerance in a murine model of food allergy. *J Allergy Clin Immunol.* 2003;113:958.

Grundy J, Matthews S, Bateman BJ, et al. Rising prevalence of allergy to peanut in children: data from two sequential studies. *J Allergy Clin Immunol.* 2002;110:784.

Li XM, Srivastava K, Grishin A, et al. Persistent protective effect of heat-killed *Escherichia coli* producing "engineered" recombinant peanut proteins in a murine model of peanut allergy. *J Allergy Clin Immunol.* 2003;112:159.

Mayer L. Mucosal immunity and gastrointestinal antigen processing. *J Pediatr Gastroenterol Nutr.* 2000;30:S4.

Nordlee JA, Taylor SL, Townsend JA, et al. Identification of a Brazil nut allergen in transgenic soybeans. *N Engl J Med.* 1996;334:688.

Rothenbart ME, Mishra A, Collins MH, et al. Pathogenesis and clinical features of eosinophilic esophagitis. *J Allergy Clin Immunol.* 2001;108:891.

Sampson HA. Utility of food-specific IgE concentrations in predicting symptomatic food allergy. *J Allergy Clin Immunol.* 2001;107:891.

Sampson HA. Adverse reactions to foods. In: Adkinson NF, Yunginger JW, Busse WM, et al., eds. *Middleton's Allergy, Principles and Practice.* 6th ed. Philadelphia: Mosby/Elsevier; 2003:1619.

Seidenari S, Guisti F, Bertoni L, et al. Combined skin prick and patch testing enhances identification of peanut-allergic patients with atopic dermatitis. *Allergy.* 2003;58:495.

Shreffler WG, Lencer DA, Bardina L, et al. IgE and IgG4 epitope mapping by microarray immunoassay reveals diversity of immune response to peanut allergen, Ara h 2. *J Allergy Clin Immunol.* 2005;116:893.

Sicherer SH. Clinical implications of cross-reactive food allergens. *J Allergy Clin Immunol.* 2001;108:881.

Simons FER. Anaphylaxis, killer allergy: Long-term management in the community. *J Allergy Clin Immunol.* 2006;117:367.

Insect Allergy

25

Donald F. German, MD, FAAAAI, FACAAI

Systemic reactions to insect stings have been known for millennia. The lore has it that the first recorded reaction to an insect sting was in ancient hieroglyphics; King Menes of Egypt apparently succumbed after a wasp sting in 2641 BC.

When stung, the majority of patients simply have an area of local pain and irritation lasting for a few hours; others may have persistent local swelling and discomfort that may last for days; and a few, like King Menes, have a systemic reaction. Studies demonstrate that sensitization is common after a sting. In the United States 30% of recently stung persons have transient evidence of IgE sensitivity to stinging insect venom, yet only 3.3% of adults have a history of a systemic reaction to a sting. It is estimated that there are at least 40 mortalities related to insect stings each year. Patients with previous systemic reactions are at increased risk of a similar reaction to a subsequent sting. Since the 1970s many advances have been made in knowledge of the natural history and treatment of insect sting reactions.

Stinging insects belong to the order Hymenoptera. Their sting deposits venom, which contains proteins and low molecular weight compounds. The venom causes much pain and provides the insect with a defense mechanism both for itself and its nest.

STINGING INSECTS, CLASSIFICATION, AND CHARACTERISTICS

Hymenoptera are classified into three main families: the *Apidae* (honeybees, bumblebees, and sweat bees), the *Vespidae* (comprised of two subfamilies, the Vespinae, which includes yellow jackets, yellow hornets, and white-faced hornets, and the Polistinae, which include the paper wasps), and the *Formicidae* (imported fire ants and harvester ants). All hymenoptera have an ovipositor, which is modified into a retractable stinger (Table 25–1).

The domesticated honeybee and the bumblebee are not aggressive and rarely sting unless they are markedly provoked. Their barbed stinger is attached to the venom sac, resulting in evisceration and death of the insect after stinging. The venom sac may contain approximately 50 μg of venom. Wild honeybees build their nests in the hollow of trees. Most honeybees are domesticated and are kept in boxed hives, which contain up to 2000 insects. Bumblebees are not aggressive. They build hives in the ground that contain 15 to 250 insects. When stimulated they are slow moving, giving time for the potential sting victim to escape. In attempts to improve honey production, the docile domesticated European honeybee was hybridized to the African honeybee. They escaped into the wilds of South America and migrated to Central America, Mexico, and now are found in Texas, Arizona, and Southern California. They are easily provoked and very aggressive. They have five times more guards at the hive entrance and will pursue an intruder 10 times farther (300 meters) than a European honeybee; pheromones are released at the time of the sting, which attracts other bees. The person may be subjected to multiple stings resulting in a toxic reaction, even death.

Members of the Vespinae subfamily (yellow jackets, yellow hornets, and white-faced hornets) are easily provoked and frequently sting. In much of the United States they cause most stings. They are capable of inflicting multiple stings because their stingers are without barbs. They are attracted to meat, fish, and sweets, and they often congregate in garbage and orchard areas and plague picnickers. The Polistinae subfamily includes wasps. Their nests, often found under eaves and windowsills of houses, contain 15 to 25 insects. They lack the aggressive tendencies of other vespids but will sting if provoked. They are an important cause of insect sting reactions in Gulf Coast states.

Formicidae include imported fire ants (IFAs), genus *Solenopsis,* and harvester ants, genus *Pogonomyrmex.* IFAs are the most important members of the family. They were inadvertently brought to the southeastern United States from South America but now have migrated throughout the southern United States. They live in the ground in nests that are slightly raised with

222

Table 25–1. Classification of stinging insects.

Class: Insecta
Order: Hymenoptera (ovipositor modified into
    a retractable stinger)
    Family: Apidae
        Genus: *Apis*
            Honeybee
        Genus: *Bombus*
            Bumblebee
    Family: Vespidae
        Genus: *Vespula*
            Yellow jacket
            Dolichovespula
            Yellow hornet
            White-faced (bald) hornet
            Vespa
            Hornet
    Family: Polistinae
        Genus: *Polistes*
            Paper wasp
    Family: Formicidae
        Genus: *Solinopsis*
            Imported fire ants
        Genus: *Pogonomyrmex*
            Harvester ants

a diameter of up to 2 feet containing thousands of insects. The ants bite, hang on with their jaws, and then rotate their bodies inflicting multiple painful stings with their well-developed posterior sting apparatus. The sting sites form a characteristic sterile pseudopustule 24 hours later, which may persist for a week. They are the most important cause of sting reactions along the Gulf Coast.

VENOMS

Honeybee venom is collected when the insect stings through a membrane beneath electrically charged plates at the hive entrance. Vespid venoms are obtained by collecting, then freezing an entire nest. The venom sack is extracted from each of the insects. The products ultimately are processed, standardized, and lyophilized. Formicidae venoms are not commercially available; hence a whole-body extract (WBE) is used both for testing and immunotherapy (Table 25–2).

The major allergens found in Apidae venom are phospholipase A2 (PLA2), which is the most common sensitizer, and hyaluronidase. Other important allergens include acid phosphatase, allergen C, and melittin, which are both unique to honeybee and make up almost half of the protein in the venom. Apidae venom is standardized on the basis of PLA2 content.

Important Vespidae allergens include hyaluronidase, which minimally cross-reacts with that of apids, phospholipase A1 (PLA1), which is the most common sensitizer but lacks identity with Apidae PLA2 and antigen 5, which is unique to vespids. Vespid allergens have varying degrees of intergenus identity ranging from 60% for phospholipases and antigen 5 to 80% for hyaluronidase. Vespid antigens are standardized on the basis of hyaluronidase content. Both apid and vespid venoms contain a number of nonallergenic toxic substances, some of which include kinins, vasoactive amines, chemotactic peptides, mast cell activators, and pheromones.

Formicidae venoms are not commercially available. Studies show that nonallergic alkaloids, which comprise almost all of the venom, are responsible for the characteristic pseudopustule formation that occurs 24 hours after a sting. The protein content of IFA (*Solinopsis invicta*) is less than 1%. Four important allergens have

Table 25–2. Important Hymenoptera venom allergen components.

Insect Genus	Allergen	Comments
Apis	Phospholipase A2	Does not cross-react with vespid phospholipase A1
	Hyaluronidase	
	Melittin	Unique to *Apis*; 40–50% of venom
	Acid phosphatase	
Vespula and Vespa	Phospholipase A1	Does not cross-react with *Apis* phospholipase A2
	Hyaluronidase	Very minimal sequence identity to *Apis* venom
	Acid phosphatase	
	Antigen 5	Unique to vespid venom, extensive sequence identity among species
Solinopsis	Sol i 1 phospholipase	
	Sol i 2	
	Sol i 3 Antigen 5 like protein	Has 50% sequence identity to vespid Antigen 5
	Sol i 4	

been identified: Sol i 1 (a vespid-like phospholipase), Sol i 2, Sol i 3 (which shares partial identity with vespid antigen 5), and Sol i 4. There is a high degree of radioallergosorbent (RAST) cross-reactivity among various fire ant species. IFA WBE contains significant quantities of relevant venom antigens. Harvester ants occasionally cause allergic reactions. Their venom contains lipase, a phospholipase, esterases, hyaluronidase, and a number of nonallergenic toxic substances.

INSECT STING REACTIONS, CLASSIFICATION

Stinging insect reactions are classified into normal, toxic, local, systemic, and unusual. The venoms are highly allergenic (Table 25–3).

Normal Reaction

Typically pain, erythema, and slight swelling may occur at the sting site. Pain is the predominant symptom. A small sterile pseudopustule occurring at the sting site 24 hours later characterizes an IFA sting.

Toxic Reaction

Toxic reactions occur as a result of multiple simultaneously occurring stings. The introduction of large quantities of potent venom proteins and nonprotein compounds may result in hypotension, shock, vascular collapse, and death. It is estimated that a 70-kg healthy person would have to sustain 1500 stings simultaneously to cause death.

Local Reactions

Local reactions are characterized by induration, erythema, and initially pain, often followed the next day by itching contiguous to the sting site. Usually these occur 12 to 24 hours after the sting, peaking within 48 hours, and persisting for 7 days or longer. They are associated with IgE sensitization. Local reactions often recur after a subsequent sting. Upto ten percent of patients exhibit a systemic reaction at the time of a future sting.

Systemic Reactions

The incidence of systemic reactions to winged hymenoptera in the United States is 3.3% in adults and 1% in children. In the southeastern United States, systemic reactions to IFA stings occur in 0.6% to 1%. In two thirds of patients, systemic reactions occur within 10 minutes after a sting.

Generally, the sooner the reaction occurs the more severe it is. Systemic reactions are mediated by IgE antibody and vary from localized urticaria to anaphylaxis and death. Cutaneous reactions as the only manifestation of a systemic reaction are seen in 15% of adults and 60% of children. Systemic reactions are relatively consistent from one sting episode to another. Honeybee reactions are more severe and longer lasting, but yellow jacket reactions are more common. Most anaphylactic deaths occur in adults. Fatal reactions are often caused by respiratory obstruction and circulatory collapse. Risk factors for a severe systemic reaction include older age, history of asthma, sensitization to honeybee, and mastocytosis.

Unusual Reactions

Serum sickness, which is associated with IgE sensitivity occurring 7 to 10 days after a sting, has been reported. Other reported unusual reactions include persistent cold urticaria, acute encephalopathy, Guillain-Barré syndrome, nephrotic syndrome, and acute renal failure.

NATURAL HISTORY OF SENSITIVITY

Sensitization to venom after a sting may occur at any age. In the United States, 1% of children and 3.3% of adults have a systemic reaction to an insect sting. Even

Table 25–3. Stinging insect reactions.

Normal	Transient pain and local erythema clearing within 24 h; fire ant sting causes painful sterile pseudopustule at 24 h
Local	Local swelling and itching contiguous with the sting site, peaking within 24–48 h and persisting for up to a week or longer

Systemic
  Cutaneous
  Moderate to severe
    generalized
	
	Urticaria as sole manifestation
	Immediate cardiovascular, respiratory, and or other organ
	    system involvement

Unusual	Serum sickness, Guillain-Barré syndrome, encephalopathy, nephrotic syndrome, acute renal failure, cold urticaria
Toxic	Direct toxic effect of venom from multiple simultaneously occurring stings

after an uneventful sting, more than 30% develop a positive venom skin test that is usually transient; venom skin tests return to negative in 30% after 2 to 3 years, and 50% after 5 years. In one study, 17% of adults who were sensitized but had no reaction after a sting had a systemic reaction up to 10 years later. Ten percent of persons with a history of a large local reaction have a systemic reaction 10 to 20 years later.

In untreated patients with a history of a mild to moderate systemic reaction, the risk of a subsequent reaction gradually declines from a high of 50% after a recent sting to 10% to 20% a decade later. Children with a cutaneous systemic reaction have a 10% chance of a systemic reaction for 1 to 9 years and a 5% chance 10 to 20 years after an initial reaction, but only a 1% to 2% chance of a more severe reaction. Little is known about the natural history of IFA sensitivity; however, none of a group of patients younger than 17 years who initially experienced a cutaneous systemic or large local reaction developed a more severe reaction to a subsequent sting.

DIAGNOSIS

History is important in determining the type and severity of the reaction. The presence and location of a nest at the site where the sting occurred, the time of year of the sting, and a stinger left at the sting site may help with identification, but this is often thwarted with error. Ideally, it would be helpful if the sting victim would bring in the offending insect. Testing is recommended for all individuals who have had a systemic reaction to an insect sting to determine the presence of venom-specific IgE. The exception is children younger than 17 years who have experienced only a cutaneous systemic reaction to a honeybee or vespid sting. Children who have had a cutaneous systemic reaction to an IFA or harvester ant and live in an area where these ants are endemic should be considered for testing and immunotherapy.

Extensive cross-reactivity exists among vespid venoms, particularly the yellow jacket, yellow hornet, and white-faced hornet so many investigators recommend testing with all venoms. Others recommend testing with the venom of the most likely stinging insect. To maximize the chance of a positive test, there should be an interval of 3 to 4 weeks from the time of the sting.

For flying hymenoptera, skin *prick* tests are first performed with specific venoms at a concentration of 0.1 to 1.0 µg/mL depending on the history of the severity of the reaction. If this is negative, *intradermal* tests are performed at an initial concentration of 0.001 µg/mL and then repeated at increasing 10-fold increments every 20 minutes until a venom concentration of 1.0 µg/mL or a positive reaction is reached. *Intradermal* testing with venom at concentrations greater than 1.0 µg/mL may cause nonspecific irritant reactions and are not diagnostic.

The sting of an IFA results in a sterile nonimmunologic pseudopustule secondary to alkaloids in the venom 24 hours later. The diagnosis and treatment of IFA sensitivity is compromised by the lack of a commercially available venom antigen or a standardized WBE. Antigen quality varies among manufacturers. Skin tests with WBE are used for diagnosis. A skin *prick* test is initially performed at a concentration of 1:1000 weight/volume (w/v). If negative, *intradermal* testing is performed beginning at a concentration of 1:1,000,000 w/v and increased at 10-fold increments until reaching a 1:1000 w/v level or there is a positive reaction.

For all hymenoptera, if there is a strong suggestion of a systemic reaction and the skin test is negative, an in vitro test (e.g., RAST) for venom-specific IgE should be performed. Skin testing is preferred and may be positive in 20% of patients who have a negative RAST, whereas a RAST is positive in 10% of skin test–negative patients. These tests supplement each other. If both the skin and the in vitro tests are negative and there is a strong suspicion of a systemic reaction, tests should be repeated after a 2- to 6-month interval.

TREATMENT OF INSECT STING REACTIONS

Normal reactions and local reactions are treated with cold compresses, oral antihistamines, and nonsteroidal antiinflammatory agents (NSAIDs). Large local reactions may require use of a short course of oral corticosteroids. Patients should be instructed regarding stinging insect avoidance. They should wear shoes and long pants when outdoors, especially in grass or brush areas. IFA-sensitive patients should wear socks. Dark-colored clothing and flowery prints attract stinging insects, whereas khaki color does not. Fragrances should be avoided. Foods, especially sweets, meats, seafood, and sweet drinks, attract vespids to garbage cans, fruit orchards, and outdoor eating areas. Patients who have had a systemic reaction should obtain a medical alert bracelet or necklace and should be considered for immunotherapy. Insect repellants are of no proven value.

Epinephrine should be available for self-administration for all who have had a systemic reaction to an insect sting, and rarely for some who have had large local reactions. It should be used for any systemic reaction more than urticaria. In some studies more than 20% of patients experiencing a systemic reaction require a second dose of epinephrine. Two products are available: the Epi-Pen, which can be prescribed as a dual pack, and the Twinject, which contains two separate doses of epinephrine for intramuscular administration. Both are available in a pediatric dose of 0.15 mL of 1:1000 aqueous epinephrine for patients less than 30 kg, and a standard dose of 0.3 mL for patients weighing more than 30 kg.

IMMUNOTHERAPY

Immunotherapy is indicated for all patients with a history of systemic reaction to an insect sting who have IgE sensitivity to venom antigens. It is not recommended for patients with a history of large local reactions where the risk of a subsequent systemic reaction is no more than 10%; it is not effective in reducing the incidence of large local reactions. It is generally not indicated for children 16 years and younger who have only a cutaneous systemic reaction to the sting of a flying hymenoptera. It should be administered under the direction of a knowledgeable physician at a medical entity where appropriate personnel and equipment are available to treat anaphylaxis. Informed consent should be obtained and documented.

An exception is the use of IFA WBE immunotherapy. Moffitt et al, in a survey of allergists living in IFA endemic areas, reported that 29% would consider immunotherapy for children younger than 17 years and 79% for adults if they have had only a cutaneous systemic reaction to an IFA sting and live in an endemic area (Table 25–4).

The classic study by Hunt, Valentine, and Sobotka and subsequent studies by others demonstrate that venom immunotherapy reduces the rate of systemic reaction to 5% or less. Venom immunotherapy for children is particularly beneficial. Children with a history of a moderate to severe systemic reaction who received a mean of 3.5 years of venom immunotherapy had a 5% incidence of a systemic reaction during a mean follow-up period of 18 years, compared to 32% for a similar group who did not receive immunotherapy. According to Riesman, patients who experience a serum sickness reaction to an insect sting may be candidates for immunotherapy.

The choice of venom depends on a number of factors including the test reaction to specific insects; there is often much cross-reactivity among the vespids. Identification of the insect is often helpful but is often flawed. Some allergists treat only with specific venoms if the insect can be identified. Others recommend treatment with all venoms to which the patient demonstrates sensitivity. Generally, venom immunotherapy is administered at weekly intervals beginning with a dose of 0.05 to 0.1 μg and ultimately achieving a dose of 100 μg for each venom used. Reisman advocates a maintenance dose of 50 μg, which is equivalent to the amount found in a venom sac; however, in one study patients receiving a 50-μg dose had only 79% protection from a systemic reaction. For multiple vespid sensitivity, a mixed vespid venom (a mixture of yellow hornet, white-faced hornet, and yellow jacket venom, which contains 100 μg of each, or a total of 300 μg) is available. The target dose is reached in 16 to 18 weeks. Modified "rush" regimens have been successfully employed, enabling patients to achieve the target dose in days to 4 to 6 weeks with no significant difference in morbidity from the conventional regimen. Once the target dose has been reached, the interval may gradually be increased to every 4 weeks for the first year, 6 weeks in the second and third year, and 6 to 8 weeks thereafter. In the small minority of patients who still have systemic stinging insect reactions at a 100-μg dose of venom, the dose of venom needs to be increased by 50% to 100% (Table 25–5).

Uncontrolled studies have demonstrated the effectiveness of immunotherapy with IFA WBE. Freeman reported that only 1 of 47 patients receiving IFA WBE immunotherapy experienced a systemic reaction, whereas all 6 not receiving immunotherapy had a systemic reaction with a subsequent sting. Investigators

Table 25–4. Indications for Hymenoptera venom immunotherapy.

Sting Reaction	Skin Test or RAST for Venom	Immunotherapy Indicated
Local	Positive or negative	No
Systemic (cutaneous only) Child <17 y	Positive or negative	No
Systemic (cutaneous only) Patient >16 y	Positive	Yes (United States) No (Europe)
Systemic (moderate to severe, other than just cutaneous)	Positive	Yes
Unusual immunologic	Positive	Uncertain*
Toxic	Positive or negative	Not indicated

*Reisman recommends immunotherapy for serum sickness reaction.
RAST, radioallergosorbent test.

Table 25–5. Weekly dosage schedule for single Hymenoptera venom immunotherapy.

Dose	1 µg/mL	Dose	10 µg/mL	Dose	100 µg/mL
1	0.05 mL	5	0.05 mL	9	0.05 mL
2	0.10 mL	6	0.10 mL	10	0.10 mL
3	0.20 mL	7	0.20 mL	11	0.20 mL
4	0.40 mL	8	0.40 mL	12	0.40 mL
				13	0.60 mL
				14	0.80 mL
				15	1.00 mL

Mixed vespid contains three times the venom protein per mL shown here.
Adapted from insect venom package insert.

recommend beginning with a concentration of 1:100,000 w/v of WBE and increasing weekly to a maximum tolerated level varying from 0.5 mL of 1:100 w/v to 0.5 mL of 1:10 w/v WBE; the interval then is gradually increased to every 4 to 6 weeks. Unblinded retrospective studies suggest it is effective.

Reactions to Immunotherapy

Reactions to immunotherapy vary from local to systemic. Systemic reactions occur in approximately 10% of patients. Risk factors include female sex, history of atopy, mastocytosis, and honeybee venom immunotherapy. Concomitant β-blocker therapy, and possibly ACE inhibitor therapy, are associated with increased risk; when possible, alternative medications should be prescribed.

Systemic reactions require a temporary reduction in dose. Depending on the degree, local reactions may be managed by decreasing the dose or the interval between injections, premedicating with antihistamines, or all these. Splitting the dose between two injection sites is helpful, especially when using mixed venom antigens. Venom immunotherapy is safe in pregnancy; however if pregnancy occurs, the dose should be maintained and initiation of immunotherapy should be deferred. Regular review of interval history, medications, antigen dosing, and insect sting reactions while on treatment helps identify potential problems.

Duration of Immunotherapy

The duration of immunotherapy is controversial. The package insert for stinging insect venoms immunotherapy recommends that it be continued indefinitely. But guidelines for discontinuing immunotherapy continue to evolve. It has been suggested that immunotherapy may be discontinued when skin and in vitro tests revert to negative; however, this only occurs in 25% of patients after 5 years of treatment. The 2004 Practice Parameter Update of the AAAAI and the ACAAI recommends continuation for 3 to 5 years for patients with a mild to moderate systemic reaction. In a 5- to 10-year follow-up study, 16.7% of patients who discontinued immunotherapy after 5 or more years sustained a mild to moderate systemic reaction to a subsequent sting. The risk is greater in those who have had a systemic reaction to immunotherapy, continue to have a positive skin test, and are sensitive to honeybee venom. Patients who have had a history of a severe anaphylactic episode should receive immunotherapy indefinitely or until there is no evidence of skin or IgE in vitro test reactivity.

In contrast with other stinging insects, there are no data concerning the duration of IFA WBE immunotherapy. Thirty-six percent of allergists discontinue therapy after 4 to 5 years, and 45% after a negative test.

BITING INSECT HYPERSENSITIVITY

Biting insects use their developmentally unique needle-like proboscis to obtain a blood meal. This is inserted directly into a dermal capillary or a pool of extravasated blood. At the same time they inject saliva, which contains both proteins and low molecular weight compounds. The secretions have anticoagulant, vasodilatory, and, in some cases, anesthetic activity. Often the victim is totally unaware of the bite. The bites of many insects result in a reaction varying from a small papule to an area of marked swelling and even necrosis. Many of these reactions have yet to be shown to have an immunologic origin; others, in particular flea and mosquito bite reactions, have been well studied and have an immunologic origin; their oral secretions are responsible for sensitization and allergic reactions. Although rare, there are credible reports of anaphylactic reactions, most commonly to the bite of the kissing bug (*Triatoma* sp.), but also rarely to the mosquito, blackfly, deerfly, and horsefly. Anaphylaxis due to the bite of a tick (an arachnid) has been reported.

Insect Bite Reactions

Reactions to insect bites vary greatly. Five stages of bite reactivity have been demonstrated. Stage I is the stage of induction in which there is no observable reaction. Stage II is the stage of delayed reactivity in which an erythematous papule develops at 18 to 24 hours. Stage III is the stage of immediate followed by delayed reactivity. Stage IV is the stage of immediate reactivity. Stage V is the stage of nonreactivity (Table 25–6).

In a study by Feingold et al, guinea pigs, subjected to cat fleabites for 5 consecutive days and then twice weekly for 14 weeks, initially demonstrated no reaction. On day 6 they developed an erythematous papule at 18 to 24 hours after the bite. On day 9, they developed an immediate reaction 20 to 60 minutes after a bite that cleared in 4 hours, followed by a delayed reaction at 18 to 24 hours; this immediate and delayed sequence persisted for the next 7 weeks. At 9 weeks only the immediate reaction was evident. At 13 weeks the bite sites became completely nonreactive. For the next 5 months the animals were challenged every few weeks and exhibited no reaction. Peng and Simmons reported similar sequence in a human subject and a rabbit subjected to multiple mosquito bites every 2 weeks over a period of 49 weeks; in the human subject there was a loss of skin reactivity at 26 weeks, which persisted until the end of the study at 49 weeks. This loss of reactivity is observed in longtime residents living in areas of heavy endemic flea or mosquito bite exposure and possibly accounts for those patients who say they are "never bitten."

Thus the response to the bite depends on the victim's state of reactivity. In rare cases a systemic reaction may occur. Papular urticaria, which may persist for weeks, is seen most commonly with fleabites; it is hypothesized that it is the result of antibody reacting with residual antigen at bite sites in a previously unsensitized person. Simons and Peng have described "skeeter syndrome," characterized by large local reactions involving an entire body part developing within hours after a mosquito bite. Bite victims who have immune aberrations such as Epstein-Barr virus, hematologic malignancies, and AIDS are at increased risk for mosquito bite reactions. There are no reports of retroviral transmission by biting insects.

Antigens

The antigens involved in the immune response generally are proteins found in the saliva. Up to 74 protein antigens have been identified in a study of various mosquito species; some are shared, and others are species specific. Because of difficulties obtaining pure salivary antigens, cloned recombinant antigens have been developed, in particular for the *Aedes aegypti* mosquito; at least three (rAed a 1, rAed a 2, rAed a 3) possess immune activity in humans. The dominant salivary antigen for the cat flea is a hapten with a MW of 500 d, which binds with a carrier protein possibly found in collagen to form an immunogen; salivary protein antigens have also been isolated but apparently do not play a part in the human fleabite response.

Immune Response to Insect Bites

Studies of immunologic changes seen with mosquito bites demonstrate increases in antigen-specific IgG and IgE levels that mirror the development of the delayed and immediate reaction. There is no demonstrable antibody activity in stage I, and almost total loss of specific IgE in the stage V nonreactive state. Histopathology studies of

Table 25–6. Sequence of guinea pig allergic response to repetitive cat fleabites.

Stage	Type of Response	Time of Onset
I	Induction	No reaction
II	Delayed reaction	Reaction at 18–24 h
III	Immediate followed by delayed reaction	Immediate followed by delayed reaction
IV	Immediate reaction	Immediate reaction
V	No reaction	No reaction

Adapted from Feingold B, Benjamin E, Michaela D. The allergic response to insect bites. *Annu Rev Entomol.* 1968;13:137.

the various stages of mosquito and flea bite reactions determined by biopsies at 20 minutes and 24 hours revealed the following: stage I, no observable microscopic changes in either biopsy; stage II, no change at 20 minutes but an intense mononuclear and lymphocytic infiltration of the dermis and epidermis at 24 hours; stage III, at 20 minutes edema and neutrophilic and massive eosinophils infiltration followed at 24 hours by the typical mononuclear infiltrate of the delayed reaction; stage IV, at 20 minutes edema and neutrophilic and massive eosinophilic infiltration, and at 24 hours only a minimal mononuclear infiltrate; stage V, biopsies at 20 minutes and 24 hours revealed a negligible cellular response.

Diagnosis

The clinical diagnosis of insect bite reactions depends on many factors. Knowledge of the type of biting insects found in a given locale and at a given time is helpful. For example, mosquitoes are common in temperate climes during warmer months; in tropical climes they are found year round; exposure is worse at dawn and dusk, but there are exceptions. Black flies, found in Canada and the northern United States, and horseflies, common throughout much of the United States, inflict painful bites. Mosquitoes, black flies, and stable flies bite exposed areas. *Triatoma* (kissing bugs), found in Texas, the Southwest, and California, bite at night. There are reports of anaphylaxis and even death as the result of *Triatoma* bites; this could be the result of unique characteristics of the antigens in the saliva, possibly the greater volume of antigen administered at the time of the bite, the frequency of the bites leading to a higher titer of specific IgE, and/or to unique characteristics of the individual. Fleabites occur often in clusters under clothing, particularly where it constricts, such as a waistband or the top of stockings; flea exposure is greatest in the late spring and during the summer but may be year round, especially if there are pets in the environment.

In a few cases, salivary antigens have been identified. But because of the difficulties collecting salivary antigens, the small amount of antigen available, and the lack of a commercial supply, there is no practical way to test with purified antigens; hence WBE has been used both for testing and treatment. The available WBE antigens have limited in vitro and in vivo test reliability.

Treatment

The ideal treatment is bite avoidance. In the case of mosquitoes and other flying insects, screening and netting are helpful. Elimination of standing water in the area of the home is important. Wetlands pose a special hazard. Bite-sensitive individuals should wear clothing with long sleeves and pants, and socks when outdoors at times when the insects are present. For special outdoor situations, permethrin-impregnated clothing is available. Insect repellants containing 20% DEET (N,N-diethyl-meta-toluamide) are effective. Caution must be taken when DEET is used for young children; it is neurotoxic and has caused convulsions when applied in high concentrations on large surfaces. There are no known effective oral insect repellants. Appropriate use of insect sprays and so-called bug bombs is often effective in controlling fleas and *Triatoma*; the use of bug bombs 14 days apart will destroy not only the adults but also the ova and pupae. Use of flea collars or topical insect repellants for pets is effective. For local bite reactions, cool compresses, topically applied menthol-containing products, and corticosteroids, sedating antihistamines, and possibly NSAIDs may be helpful. Persons with a history of a systemic reaction to a bite should carry an emergency epinephrine kit. Reports of success of WBE immunotherapy to treat patients with a history of a systemic reaction to a biting insect are anecdotal and uncontrolled. In a small uncontrolled study, immunotherapy with *Triatoma* salivary gland extract has been effective in treating anaphylaxis. Anecdotal reports of the value of mosquito WBE immunotherapy have been inconsistent. Uncontrolled studies to treat dogs sensitive to cat fleabites with purified salivary antigens is have been shown to be effective. In some cases the favorable results that have been reported may be a manifestation in the natural course of insect bite sensitivity rather than the effect of immunotherapy.

THE FUTURE

An important goal for the future is the development of relevant recombinant insect venom and salivary antigens. This has the potential of opening new vistas, particularly for diagnosis and treatment of insect hypersensitivity reactions. A major drawback will be cost.

EVIDENCE-BASED MEDICINE

Golden B, Kagey-Sobotka A, Norman P, et al. Outcomes of allergy to insect stings in children, with and without venom immunotherapy. *N Engl J Med.* 2004;351:668.

This article demonstrates the effectiveness of immunotherapy for stinging insects in children. The study conducted by telephone and mail reports the results of a mean 18-year follow-up of a group of patients who at time zero suffered a systemic reaction to an insect sting and who were later stung. Systemic reactions occurred in 19 of 111 (17%) who did not receive immunotherapy and 2 of 64 (3%) who received a mean of 3.5 years of immunotherapy.

Golden D, Kagey-Sobotka A, Lichtenstein L. Survey of patients after discontinuing immunotherapy. *J Allergy Asthma Immunol.* 2000;105:385.

This is a report of a 5- to 10-year follow-up of 74 patients who had discontinued stinging insect immunotherapy after at least 5 years of treatment. Up to 16.7% suffered a subsequent systemic reaction. The reactions were similar in severity and type as the original reaction. In some cases patients lost evidence of venom skin test reactivity.

Peng Z, Simons FE. A prospective study of naturally acquired sensitization and subsequent desensitization to mosquito bites and concurrent antibody responses. *J Allergy Clin Immunol*. 1998;101:284.

This is the first prospective study in a human subject of the immunologic sequence to repeated mosquito bites ultimately resulting in acquired desensitization.

BIBLIOGRAPHY

Engler R. Mosquito bite pathogenesis in necrotic skin reactors. *Curr Opin Allergy Clin Immunol*. 2001;1:349.

Feingold B, Benjamini E, Michaeli D. The allergic response to insect bites. *Annu Rev Entomol*. 1968;13:137.

Freeman T. Hymenoptera hypersensitivity in an imported fire ant endemic area. *Ann Allergy Asthma Immunol*. 1997;78:369.

Freeman T. Hypersensitivity to hymenoptera stings. *N Engl J Med*. 2004;351:1978

Golden D, Kagey-Sobotka A, Lichtenstein L. Survey of patients after discontinuing immunotherapy. *J Allergy Asthma Immunol*. 2000;105:385.

Golden B, Kagey-Sobotka A, Norman P, et al. Outcomes of allergy to insect stings in children, with and without venom immunotherapy. *N Engl J Med*. 2004;351:668.

Golden B. Insect sting allergy and venom immunotherapy: a model and a mystery. *J Allergy Clin Immunol*. 2005;115:439.

Hunt K, Valentine M, Sobotka A. A controlled trial of immunotherapy in insect hypersensitivity. *N Engl J Med*. 1978;299:156.

Levine MI, Lockey RF, eds. *American Academy of Immunology Monograph on Insect Allergy*. 4th ed. Pittsburgh: David Lambert Associates; 2003.

McCormack D, Salata K, Hershey J, et al. Mosquito bite anaphylaxis: immunotherapy with whole body extracts. *Ann Allergy Asthma Immunol*. 1995;74:39.

Moffitt J, Barker J, Stafford C. Management of imported fire ant allergy: Results of a survey. *Ann Allergy Asthma Immunol*. 1997;79:125.

Moffitt J, Venarske D, Goddard J, et al. Allergic reactions to triatoma bites. *Ann Allergy Asthma Immunol*. 2003;91:122.

Moffitt J, Golden D, Reisman R, et al. Stinging insect hypersensitivity: a practice parameter update. *J Allergy Clin Immunol*. 2004;114:869.

Nguyen S, Napoli D. Natural history of large local and generalized reactions to imported fire ant stings in children. *Ann Allergy Asthma Immunol*. 2005;94:387.

Peng Z, Simons FE. A prospective study of naturally acquired sensitization and subsequent desensitization to mosquito bites and concurrent antibody responses. *J Allergy Clin Immunol*. 1998;101:284.

Reisman R. Insect stings. *N Engl J Med*. 1994;331:523.

Latex Allergy

Donald F. German, MD, FAAAAI, FACAAI

Latex allergy is a disorder associated with the presence of allergy symptoms and signs, varying from dermatitis to anaphylaxis on exposure to natural rubber latex, and the demonstration of IgE sensitivity to this substance.

HISTORY

Latex sensitivity was first reported in 1927 in Germany, but it was not until 1979 that the first skin test proven report of an allergic reaction, contact urticaria, to a natural rubber product was published in the English literature. Anaphylaxis was first reported in 1984 in two nurses who underwent surgical procedures; both had a positive skin test and radioallergosorbent test (RAST) to latex. In 1989 reports appeared of latex-induced anaphylaxis in children with spina bifida who had multiple surgeries.

In 1991 there was a report of six anaphylactic reactions including one fatality due to the latex balloons of barium enema catheters. In that same year because of these and other reports of allergic reactions in medical care settings, the Food and Drug Administration (FDA) issued a warning concerning the risks of latex allergy.

EPIDEMIOLOGY

It is important to distinguish between the prevalence of IgE *sensitization* and the prevalence of type I (IgE)-mediated *allergic reactions* to latex antigens. There are reports of both in the general population and in occupational settings, especially health care workers. The prevalence of latex sensitization by skin testing in adults is approximately 1%. Turjanmaa (1997) was the first to report the prevalence of latex sensitivity in hospital personnel, noting a higher prevalence (6.2%) in subjects regularly exposed to latex gloves. Sussman (1998) reported that 12.1% of 1351 health care workers exhibited sensitivity. In addition to health care workers, persons who are employed in the rubber industry, housekeepers, and hairdressers are at higher risk. The presence of atopy is a major risk factor for sensitization. Latex sensitization increases in relation to the frequency

and duration of exposure to latex. Multiple surgeries increase the risk of sensitization. Up to 64% of patients who have had multiple procedures because of spina bifida or congenital urogenital abnormalities are sensitized to latex, and many of these have experienced severe, even life-threatening reactions. A group of dental hygiene students followed during their 3 years of training had, a cumulative incidence rate of sensitization of 6.4%; rhinoconjunctivitis, 1.8%; and asthma, 4.5%. Many reasons have been offered as a cause for the increase in latex sensitivity; however, there is probably no one factor (Table 26–1).

There are a paucity of studies of the prevalence of IgE proven allergy to natural rubber latex. The prevalence of subject-reported upper respiratory allergy symptoms was 7.8% in a pooled population of 3567 health care workers and 1.4% for asthma in this same group. In a questionnaire survey, the annual incidence rate for contact urticaria was estimated to be 1.9 per 10,000 health care workers. The prevalence of anaphylaxis during surgical procedures varies from 1 in 5000 to 1 in 10,000. In the past decade with the recognition of latex allergy and efforts made to reduce exposure to latex allergens, there has been a reduction in the incidence of latex sensitization and allergy in health care workers in developed countries.

NATURAL RUBBER LATEX PRODUCTS, PRODUCTION, AND ALLERGENS

Natural rubber latex is harvested by tapping the Hevea brasiliensis tree. Milky latex, which defends against pathogens and insects and promotes wound healing, flows from the site. Initially, the fluid is treated with ammonia to prevent coagulation. It is then centrifuged isolating the rubber phase at the top. The majority of the latex is coagulated, washed, and sulfur heat vulcanized at high temperature. The resultant "*dry* product" is formed into rubber crumbs or sheets. These products have very low levels of latex antigen. The remaining latex liquid is compounded with various low molecular weight

Table 26–1. Reasons for increased sensitivity to latex allergens.

1. Institution of universal precautions.
2. Change from offshore production of latex gloves to production at country of origin of latex collection, resulting in less time for degradation of native latex proteins by ammonia anticoagulant.
3. Increased latex protein contamination of the cornstarch slurry.
4. Increased use of latex gloves when there is no indication.
5. Increased tapping of rubber to increase latex production may lead to increased generation of antigenic proteins.

accelerators, preservatives, and antioxidants (thiurams, carbamates, benzothiazoles, thioureas) (Table 26–2). Porcelain molds of the product to be produced (e.g., gloves, condoms, and balloons) are coated with a cornstarch-coagulant mix and then dipped into the compounded latex liquid. The latex-coated molds are removed from the latex compound, oven heated to complete formation of the *"dipped"* product, washed several times to leach out soluble latex proteins, and then sulfur heat vulcanized. Gloves are then dipped into a cornstarch slurry. The powdered gloves are stripped from the molds. Omitting the cornstarch application and using a chlorination wash produces powder-free gloves, which have a much lower quantity of water-soluble latex proteins.

Raw natural rubber latex contains 1% to 2% protein. More than 50 latex peptides have been described that induce IgE sensitization. Each varies in stability, bioavailability, and antigenicity. The International Allergen Nomenclature Committee has designated 13 of the proteins as major and minor allergens. Some are more likely to induce sensitization in specific groups of patients. Spina bifida patients are likely to be sensitized to Hev b 1 (rubber elongation factor), Hev b 3, Hev b 5, Hev b 6, and Hev b 13; health care workers are more likely to be sensitized to Hev b 2, Hev b 5, Hev b 6, and Hev b 13 (Table 26–3). Significant cross exists between latex allergens and several fruits, most commonly chestnut, avocado, potato, tomato, kiwi, banana, and tropical

Table 26–2. Classes of additives used in the fabrication of "dipped" rubber latex products.

Benzothiazoles
Carbamates
Thiazoles
Thiurams

fruits (e.g., papaya, pineapple, mango, passion fruit, jack fruit, and star fruit) resulting in the latex/food allergy syndrome (Table 26–4).

PATHOGENESIS

Sensitization depends on the characteristics of the subject, the state of the integument, the quality of the antigen, and the degree, route, and duration of exposure. Atopy is an important risk factor. Latex allergens adsorbed onto cornstarch particles on dipped rubber products are the most common source of exposure. Repeated exposure facilitates sensitization. To induce sufficient IgE sensitization, amounts of latex allergens must come in contact with the immune system. The most important sites of exposure are through the skin and respiratory tract and, to a lesser degree, the eyes and the gastrointestinal and genitourinary tracts.

Persons employed in certain occupations or those with a history of repeated surgeries are especially vulnerable. Health care personnel, particularly those working in surgical areas, are at increased risk for sensitization. The estimated threshold level of aerosolized latex antigen necessary for inhalant sensitization is 0.6 ng/m^3. This is at least 100-fold less than levels found in operating suites where powdered latex gloves are used. In past years many latex gloves contained very high levels of latex allergens. The latex content of gloves has been drastically reduced in recent years. In the early 1990s, the soluble latex antigen content for many gloves was 100 to 1000 μg or even higher per square decimeter. The current recommendation for residual latex protein in gloves is 10 μg or less per square decimeter.

Once sensitized, the subject is at risk for latex allergy. Not all subjects who are exposed to latex develop sensitivity, and not all who are sensitized develop allergic symptoms. Atopy is a risk factor. The most common problem is an IgE-mediated allergic dermatitis. This must be distinguished from irritant dermatitis, and contact dermatitis due to the antioxidants, preservatives, and accelerators compounded in the formation of "dipped" products. Other manifestations of IgE allergy include local and systemic urticaria, rhinoconjunctivitis, bronchial asthma, and anaphylaxis.

DIAGNOSIS

The diagnosis of latex allergy depends on the presence of clinical findings confirmed by objective testing for latex sensitivity. A detailed history of the type of symptoms and clinical findings and their temporal relation to latex exposure is key. Some risk factors for potential sensitization include the presence of hand dermatitis, atopy, frequent surgeries, the presence of spina bifida, food allergy (in particular to kiwi, avocado, banana, potato, and chestnut) (Table 26–5), and occupational

Table 26–3. Important latex allergens.

| Allergen | M.W. kDa | Description | Importance as an Allergen | | Cross-Reactivity with Other Allergens |
			HCW	Spina Bifida	
Hev b1	14.6	Elongation factor	+++	++++	Papain
Hev b2	35.1	Gluconase	++++	++	Bell pepper
Hev b3	22.3		++	++++	
Hev b4	50–57		++	++	
Hev b5	16		++++	++++	Kiwi
Hev b6	4.7, 14	Prohevlin	++++	+++	Avocado, kiwi, banana
Hev b7	43–46	Patatin-like protein	++	++	Potato
Hev b8	14	Profilin	++	++	Banana, celery, bell pepper, pineapple, ragweed
Hev b9	46.9	Encolase	+/–	–	Tomato Alternaria Cladosporium
Hev b10	22.9		–	+/–	Aspergillus fumigatus
Hev b11	31.6,33	Chitinase	?	?	Avocado, banana, chestnut
Hev b12	9.3		?	?	Peach
Hev b13	42.9	esterase	++++	++++	

HCW, health care worker.

exposure (including those employed as rubber industry workers, cosmetologists, housekeepers, and health care workers, especially those assigned to surgical units). Local pruritus, dermatitis, or edema after a gynecologic or dental procedure or after blowing balloons suggest latex sensitization.

Confirmatory testing is necessary to establish the diagnosis. In the United States, skin testing is thwarted by the lack of an FDA-approved commercially available extract. Often an in vitro test for natural rubber latex specific IgE is performed. Three tests are currently available, CAP RAST, AlaSTAT, and HY-TEC; there is relatively close agreement among the tests, but the incidence of a false-negative result varies from 25% to 27%. High titers are very confirmatory of latex sensitivity. If in vitro tests are negative, many allergists perform percutaneous and intracutaneous testing using various dilutions of an antigen prepared by incubating pieces of powdered latex gloves in a diluent solution. If there is a strong suspicion of latex sensitivity and these tests are negative, a modified "glove-use"

Table 26–4. Common foods associated with food/latex allergy syndrome.

Avocado
Banana
Chestnut
Hazelnut
Potato
Tropical fruits: passion fruit, mango, papaya, pineapple, jack fruit, star fruit

Table 26–5. Risk factors for latex sensitization.

1. Occupation (health care workers, rubber industry workers, housekeepers
2. Repeated surgeries
3. Atopy
4. Hand dermatitis
5. Spina bifida
6. Food allergy (avocado, chestnut, banana, kiwi, potato, tropical fruits)

test described by Hamilton may be employed; a bifurcated needle is used to make three scratches through saline on the moistened hand; then a latex glove is placed on the hand for up to 30 minutes. The area over the scratch sites is rubbed repeatedly; finally, the patient is observed for any cutaneous or respiratory symptoms. For most practitioners these tests are compromised by not knowing the concentration of latex allergen in the glove; many newly manufactured gloves have very low levels of allergen. A work challenge monitoring the patient for symptoms and signs and following pulmonary function or peak flow has also been employed. Despite all this, there are still rare patients who have a convincing history and negative tests.

Patients who have dermatitis as the sole manifestation of latex glove use and yet have negative tests for natural rubber latex protein may have nonallergic irritant dermatitis, the most common reaction, or delayed allergic contact dermatitis. They may benefit from patch testing to the low molecular weight compounds used in the fabrication of dipped latex products. Thiurams and benzothiazoles are the most common reactants (Table 26–2).

MANAGEMENT

Avoidance of natural rubber latex exposure is the primary goal of treatment. Sensitive patients need to be instructed regarding potential sources of contact and avoidance. Their health care providers need to be informed of the sensitivity. When traveling to foreign countries, they should carry a supply of nonlatex sterile surgical gloves. If clinically sensitive the subject should avoid foods associated with the latex/food allergy syndrome. If there is no prior experience with these foods, the latex-sensitive patient should be warned of the potential of a reaction. Patients with a history of an anaphylactic reaction to latex or who have more than a cutaneous reaction to a cross-reacting food should carry epinephrine for emergency use.

Surgical and other health care procedures pose a special hazard for latex-sensitive patients. Latex allergy is the second most common cause of intraoperative anaphylaxis. Latex aeroallergen content in the operating room gradually increases during the workday; this depends on the number of powdered latex gloves used and the amount of activity. A so-called latex-safe environment should be provided for the sensitive patient undergoing surgery. The operating room should be wiped down, the patient should be scheduled for the first case of the day, powdered latex products should not be used, and latex products should not come in contact with the patient; when possible, products to be used parenterally should be drawn from unit dose vials and administered through nonlatex ports. The avoidance procedures should be carried through postoperative and hospital care. Both the patient and the hospital room should have latex precaution labels. Latex avoidance procedures should be instituted for all patients with spina bifida at birth. Protocols using antihistamines and glucocorticoids preoperatively have been proposed; they have not met with consistent success and are not recommended. In addition to the problem with dipped rubber products, there are rare reports of sensitivity to solutions drawn through "dry" latex ports used in multidose vials. The FDA now requires that all medical devices containing natural rubber latex or their packages be labeled.

Occupational latex allergy has been a recognized problem since the 1980s. The prevalence of occupational latex sensitivity is highest in health care workers, particularly in women. A number of studies have shown that the highest prevalence is in medical personnel working in areas where powdered latex gloves are used a lot. Not uncommonly, the initial presentation in health care workers occurs at the time of labor or surgery. The incidence of latex sensitivity in this group seems to be leveling off, probably because of a change in the quality and decreased frequency of exposure to powdered latex gloves. The amount of latex protein in powdered latex gloves has markedly decreased. When possible there has been a conversion to low-protein powder-free latex or nitrile gloves. Vinyl gloves should be used when barrier protection is not necessary. Latex-sensitive health care personnel must discontinue their use of latex gloves, and if necessary for barrier protection use nitrile gloves; they should be assigned to well-ventilated areas where other personnel are using powder-free latex gloves. By making these accommodations, these personnel can return to work successfully.

THE FUTURE

Manufactures continue to make improvements in reducing the concentration of latex allergens in natural rubber products. There has been and will continue to be a reduction in the use of rubber stoppers for multidose vials. The development of recombinant latex allergens has permitted more specific identification of the offending latex protein and has the potential of offering an avenue to immunotherapy. There are anecdotal reports of success using either subcutaneous or sublingual latex immunotherapy; however, controlled studies utilizing natural rubber latex or specific latex antigens need to be conducted. Although the prevalence of latex sensitivity is falling in developed countries, there is a risk of an increase in developing countries with their increased use of powdered latex gloves.

EVIDENCE-BASED MEDICINE

Noted here are two evidence-based references prospectively addressing latex sensitization and allergy, one in children undergoing surgery, and the other in a group of dental hygiene students.

Houribane J, Allard WJ, McEwan A, et al. Impact of repeated surgical procedures on the incidence and prevalence of latex allergy: a prospective study of 1263 children. *J Pediatr.* 2002;140:479.

The purpose of this study was to determine prospectively the prevalence of latex sensitivity and allergy in a group of 1263 children, mean age 6 years, who underwent their first surgery. RAST and skin testing for latex was performed before and after surgery. One hundred and fifty-six repeat surgeries were performed. Fifty patients developed latex sensitivity. Six developed latex allergy. Latex allergic and sensitive patients had more frequent subsequent surgeries, were older, had a higher rate of atopy, and a higher incidence of allergy to kiwi, banana, and peanut.

Archambault S, Malo J, Infante-Rivard C, et al. Incidence of sensitization, symptoms, and probable occupational rhinoconjunctivitis and asthma in apprentices starting exposure to latex. *J Allergy Clin Immunol.* 2001;107:921.

This is a prospective study of dental hygiene students from the start to the completion of their training 3 years later. One hundred and ten, mean age 21.4 years, had an initial evaluation and at least one follow-up visit. Each completed an initial questionnaire, had skin tests for aeroallergens and latex, and pulmonary function tests with methacholine challenge at time 0 and at 20 and 32 months. Initially none were latex sensitive. Seven (6.4%), all of whom were atopic, developed skin test reactivity to latex. Six (6.4%) of these developed cutaneous symptoms; 5 (4.5%) demonstrated increased responsiveness to methacholine; 2 (1.8%) developed symptoms of rhinoconjunctivitis on later exposure.

BIBLIOGRAPHY

Ahmed D, Sobczak S, Yunginger J. Occupational allergies caused by latex. *Immunol Allergy Clin North Am.* 2003;23:205.

Archambault S, Malo J, Infante-Rivard C, et al. Incidence of sensitization, symptoms, and probable occupational rhinoconjunctivitis and asthma in apprentices starting exposure to latex. *J Allergy Clin Immunol.* 2001;107:921.

Hamilton R, Adkinson N. Natural rubber skin testing reagents: safety and diagnostic accuracy of nonammoniated latex, ammoniated latex, and latex rubber glove extracts. *J Allergy Clin Immunol.* 1996;98:872.

Kujala V. A review of the current literature on epidemiology of immediate glove irritation and latex allergy. *Occup Med.* 1999;49:3.

Leynadier F, Herman D, Vervolet D, et al. specific immunotherapy with standardized latex extract versus placebo. *J Allergy Clin Immunol.* 2000;106:585.

Norman P, Fish J, Lowery A, et al., eds. Natural rubber latex sensitivity. *J Allergy Clin Immunol.* 2002;110(suppl 2):S1.

Poley G, Slater J. Latex allergy. *J Allergy Clin Immunol.* 2000; 105:1054.

Reines H, Seifert P. Patient safety: latex allergy. *Surg Clin North Am.* 2005;85:1329.

Saxon A, Ownby D, Huard T, et al. Prevalence of IgE to natural rubber AlaSTAT testing, *Ann Allergy Asthma, Immunol.* 2000;84:199.

Sussman G. Lessons learned from latex allergy. *Ann Allergy Asthma Immunol.* 2003;91:510.

Tilles S. Occupational latex allergy: controversies in diagnosis and prognosis. *Ann Allergy Asthma Immunol.* 1999;83:640.

Turjanmaa K, Alenius H, Reunala T, et al. Recent developments in latex allergy. *Curr Opin Allergy Clin Immunol.* 2006;2:407.

Wagner S, Breiteneder H. Hevea brasiliensis latex allergens: current panel and clinical relevance. *Int Arch Allergy Immunol.* 2006;136:90.

Yunginger J. Natural rubber latex. In: Adkinson NF, Yunginger J, Busse W, et al., eds. *Middleton's Allergy Principles and Practice.* 6th ed. Philadelphia: Mosby; 2003:1487.

Yeang H. Natural rubber latex allergens: new developments. *Curr Opin Allergy Clin Immunol.* 2004;4(2):99.

Zeiss C, Gormaa A, Murphy F, et al. Latex hypersensitivity in Department of Veterans Affairs health care workers: glove use, symptoms, and sensitization. *Ann Allergy Asthma Immunol.* 2003;91:539.

Drug Allergy

Schuman Tam, MD, FACP, FAAAAI

Adverse drug reaction is a noxious and unintended response to a drug. Adverse drug reactions are separated into two major types: type A, which is dose dependent and predictable, and type B, which is dose independent and unpredictable. The majority of adverse drug reactions are type A (e.g., bleeding secondary to warfarin). Type B reactions, which include hypersensitivity drug reaction, comprise about 10% of all adverse drug reactions. Drug allergy is considered a hypersensitivity reaction for which a definite immunologic mechanism, either IgE or T cell mediated, is demonstrated. An example is type I IgE-mediated allergic reaction to penicillin. True overall incidence of adverse drug reactions is unknown for the general population. Based on a meta-analysis of 39 prospective studies performed in the United States between 1966 and 1996, Lazarou et al estimated that the overall incidence of serious adverse drug reactions was 6.7% of hospitalized patients and of fatal adverse drug reactions was 0.32% of hospitalized patients. They estimated that in 1994, fatal adverse drug reaction ranked between the fourth and sixth leading cause of U.S. deaths. Based on the analysis of eight prospective studies, Lazarou estimated that type A adverse drug reaction comprised 76% of the cases, and type B reactions comprised 24% of the cases. In Singapore, a 2-year prospective study performed by Thong, using a network-based electronic notifications system for which each case was verified by a trained allergist, detected the incidence of drug allergy as about 4.2 per 1000.

CLASSIFICATION

Type A Drug Reaction

DESCRIPTION

The majority (85% to 90%) of adverse drug reactions are type A. It is dose dependent and predictable.

SUBTYPES AND EXAMPLES

Overdose: For example, hepatic failure secondary to high-dose acetaminophen.

Side effects: For example, bleeding or ecchymosis secondary to warfarin; nausea secondary to erythromycin.

Drug interactions: Concurrent usage of erythromycin and warfarin can increase the international normalized ratio (INR) and thus can increase the risk of bleeding.

Type B Drug Reaction

DESCRIPTION

The reactions are restricted to a small subset of the general population. They are dose independent and unpredictable.

SUBTYPES AND EXAMPLES

Intolerance: Psychological disturbance after being on steroids.

Idiosyncrasy (genetically determined drug reactions/ pharmacogenetics): Patients who are homozygous for the arginine 16 allele (about a sixth of the U.S. asthmatic population) of the β_2-adrenergic receptor may have declines in airflow and asthma control when they utilize β_2-agonists regularly.

Immunologic drug reaction (drug allergy): Discussed in detail later.

IMMUNOLOGIC DRUG REACTION (DRUG ALLERGY)

Immunologic Drug Reaction Based on Gell and Coombs Classification

TYPE I IgE-MEDIATED ANAPHYLACTIC REACTION

Mechanism: A complete antigen with multivalent epitopes, like an antibiotic, binds IgE antibodies on mast cells. If the antigen is small, it is called a hapten; it binds to an endogenous carrier protein to become a complete antigen with multiple epitopes. The binding pulls the IgE antibodies on the surface of mast cell together. The process leads to degranulation of mast cells. Degranulation of mast cells releases mediators, including histamine, that can cause the typical presentation of an allergic reaction.

Clinical manifestations: The mediators released from the mast cells can cause urticaria, angioedema, and/or anaphylaxis with bronchospasm and/or hypotension. They can occur early or late in a course of therapy and even can persist for weeks or months after drug withdrawal.

Types of complete allergens: Foreign macromolecules (e.g., insulin, and vaccines), and functionally multivalent chemicals (e.g., succinylcholine).

Types of incomplete antigens (haptens): The small antigens require binding to carrier protein before being able to elicit an immune response (e.g., penicillin, antithyroid drugs, and quinidine).

Metabolism to haptenic form: Some drugs, in their native forms, are unreactive with macromolecules. They must be converted into reactive intermediates during drug metabolism. The intermediates then can be haptenated to become complete antigens that are capable of inducing type I IgE-mediated allergic reactions (e.g., acetylation and oxidation of sulfonamides to form N4-sulfonamidoyl hapten).

TYPE II IgG/IgM ANTIBODY AND COMPLEMENT MEDIATED REACTION

Mechanism: Specific IgG or IgM antibody binds to a drug antigen located on cell membranes. In the presence of complement, the antibody-antigen complex is cleared by the monocyte-macrophage system and destroyed.

Clinical manifestation: Drug-induced hemolytic anemia and thrombocytopenia.

TYPE III IMMUNE COMPLEX REACTION

Mechanism: Soluble complexes of a drug or its metabolite in slight antigen excess bind with IgG or IgM antibodies. Immune complexes are deposited in blood vessel walls and cause injury by activating the complement cascade.

Clinical manifestations: Fever, urticaria (usually persists more than 1 day, and microscopically shows leukocytoclastic vasculitis), erythema multiforme, lymphadenopathy, and arthralgia. Symptoms typically appear 1 to 3 weeks after the last dose of an offending drug, although they can appear while the patient is taking the drug and subside when the drug is cleared from the body. The antigens can be any drug, including penicillin and cephalosporins.

TYPE IV DELAYED HYPERSENSITIVITY REACTION

Mechanism: The reaction is mediated by drug-specific T lymphocytes. It typically occurs 2 to 3 days after exposure.

Clinical manifestations: Contact dermatitis secondary to neomycin and topical antihistamine, and maculopapular eruption (morbilliform eruption) secondary to antibiotics.

PSEUDOALLERGIC DRUG REACTION

Mechanism: This drug reaction cannot be classified under the Gell and Coombs classification as outlined earlier but can manifest similarly to an immunologic drug reaction. This type of reaction is also called an anaphylactoid reaction.

Clinical manifestations: Similar to type I IgE-mediated allergic reaction as previously described, with urticaria, angioedema, bronchospasm, and/or cardiovascular collapse.

Important Examples—

1. *Radiocontrast media–induced anaphylactoid reaction:* Adverse reactions are attributable to contrast's hypertonicity, which augments basophil and mast cell histamine release. The release of histamine, upon binding to histamine receptors, can cause typical type I like reactions. Allergy to seafood's is not a risk factor for anaphylactoid reaction to radiocontrast media. Usage of newer nonionic contrast media, which are almost isotonic, can reduce but not eliminate this pseudoallergic reaction. Addition of steroid and antihistamine preoperatively can help decrease the risk of reaction further (see later). Risk factors include atopic background, underlying cardiovascular disease, and a previous history of radiocontrast reaction.

2. *Opiate-induced urticaria:* Narcotics such as morphine can induce direct mast cell degranulation without involving the IgE-antigen process. Manifestation includes pruritus, urticaria, and occasionally wheezing. Management includes usage of non-narcotic medications, premedication with antihistamine, and graded challenge.

3. *Vancomycin-induced red man syndrome*: The mechanism is nonspecific non–IgE-mediated histamine release. Patients present with diffuse erythema, pruritus, and/or hypotension. Management includes slowing the rate of vancomycin infusion to about 2 hours and preadministration with an H1 blocker.

4. *Colloid volume expanders*: Examples include dextran and human serum albumin. The mechanism is believed to be hyperosmolar-dependent histamine release. Manifestation is similar to reaction to radiocontrast media.

5. *Aspirin (ASA)/nonsteroidal antiinflammatory drug (NSAID)*:

1. ASA/NSAID-induced asthma/rhinitis.
   a. Mechanism: Blockage of cyclooxygenase enzyme leads to overproduction of leukotrienes. The presentation is like an allergic reaction, but no IgE antibody is involved.
   b. Clinical manifestation: asthma and rhinitis after taking ASA or NSAID. Patient reacting to one type of NSAID medication tends to react to other types of NSAID.

2. ASA/NSAID-induced urticaria and angioedema.
   a. Mechanism: Blockage of cyclooxygenase enzyme leads to overproduction of leukotrienes.
   b. Clinical manifestation: Patient has underlying idiopathic urticaria/angioedema that can be further aggravated by ASA/NSAID usage. Patient, who reacts to one type of NSAID medication, tends to react to other types of NSAIDs.

3. ASA/NSAID single drug—induced anaphylaxis.
   a. Classification: This is not a pseudoallergic reaction; it is a true IgE-mediated allergic reaction.
   b. Mechanism: IgE-mediated allergic reaction to a specific NSAID or ASA. The reaction is specific to the NSAID drug in question but cross reaction with other drugs in the NSAID is rare, unless the structure of the two NSAIDs are very similar.
   c. Clinical manifestation: The patients do not have underlying chronic idiopathic urticaria that predisposes patients to cross reactions with other NSAIDs. The history usually indicates that the patient has never had allergic reactions to other NSAIDs (not the one that causes the reaction). Therefore, this patient has a single drug reaction without cross reaction with other NSAIDs. This suggests the mechanism of the reaction is not by blocking the common cyclooxygenase pathway. The single drug reaction suggests specific IgE-mediated reaction to a specific NSAID. The classic allergic symptoms are urticaria, angioedema, wheezing, and hypotension.
   d. For organizational purposes, ASA/NSAID single drug—induced anaphylaxis is listed under pseudoallergic drug reaction. However, immunologically, this unique type of NSAID reaction, mediated by IgE, should be listed under type I IgE-mediated allergic reaction.

DIAGNOSIS OF DRUG REACTION/ALLERGY

Clinical Assessment

A detailed history is the most important tool in the diagnosis of drug reaction. Keep in mind the classification of the drug reaction as mentioned earlier and as summarized diagrammatically in Fig. 27–1. It is important to know the pharmacologic property of the drug in question to distinguish between type A and type B reactions. Next, it is helpful to know if the patient has taken the medication in the past. If he or she has taken the medication in the past and now has a reaction, the patient may have been sensitized to the drug previously, causing the current immunologic IgE-mediated allergic reaction. Next, it is important to know the clinical manifestation of the timing of the reaction. Does the patient have a typical IgE-mediated reaction, like urticaria, angioedema, hypotension, or bronchospasm? If you have a chance to examine the patient when he or she has the allergic reaction, it will be helpful. Sometimes, one has to rely on examination record from another physician who examined the patient at the time of the reaction. Immediate type I IgE-mediated allergic reactions occur within minutes to hours after the administration of the drug. Delayed type IV T–cell-mediated drug reactions occur days to weeks after the administration of the drug and may present with maculopapular, bullous, and pustular exanthem. It is important to know when a reaction occurs relative to the timing of the administration of the drug. One also has to consider other concurrent administered drugs and render a decision whether the reaction is caused by another drug. Therefore, temporal association between initiation of drug therapy and onset of allergic reaction is essential. It will also be important to know if the drug in question is the only drug available for the patient and if the patient requires using the medication without alternative. This will help a physician decide whether to proceed with desensitization. For example, a patient with type I diabetes mellitus has to take insulin for survival. In this situation, one has to continue using the medication by desensitization and/or premedication with antihistamine.

Diagnostic Investigation

SKIN TESTING

Not all drugs can be reliably skin tested. Frequently, the reaction to a drug can be secondary to the metabolite of the drug in question. In addition, false-positive and false-negative predictive values of skin testing of many drugs are not known. Therefore, a positive skin testing may be helpful with confirmation by history. A negative skin testing for a certain drug may be a false-negative finding. An exception to that is penicillin (PCN) skin

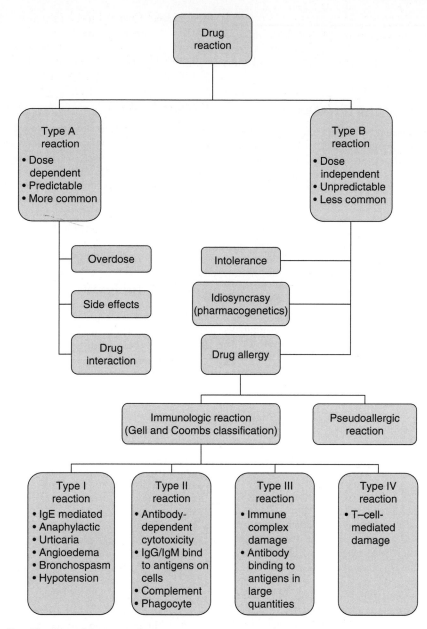

Figure 27–1. Classification of drug reactions.

testing using the major and minor determinants of PCN. Allergic reactions observed in retreatment of history positive, skin test negative patients have virtually all been mild and self-limited; no life-threatening false-negative reactions have been reported. The theoretic risk of a course of penicillin resensitizing the patient with a positive history but a negative skin test response is low and on the order of 3% or less. Thus once a patient with a positive history is shown to have a negative skin test response and tolerates a course of penicillin or a β-lactam drug, future administration of such agents would not require additional skin testing.

SERUM TRYPTASE

Tryptase is released by mast cells and an indication of mast cell degranulation like that seen in anaphylaxis. Measurement taken within 4 hours of the reaction is helpful to confirm mast cell degranulation or anaphylaxis.

COMPLEMENTS

CH50, C3, and C4 measurements are helpful to determine if the complement system is activated like what one would expect in type II and type III immunologic drug reactions.

Graded Drug Challenge (Test Dosing)

When skin testing is not available, one may have to perform graded drug challenge under physician observation in case of anaphylaxis. This will help determine if the patient can safely tolerate the medication in question when diagnostic testing to determine the possibility of true drug allergic reaction is not available, the history is not definite for drug allergy, and/or the patient has to continue the medication without alternatives. The principles of incremental test dosing are to administer sufficiently small doses that would not cause a serious reaction initially and increase by safe increments, usually by 10-fold, every 20 to 60 minutes over a few hours or a few days. The procedure is not a true desensitization because the dose is increased more rapidly compared to desensitization. The intent of graded drug challenge is to assure that the patient can tolerate a small dose without allergic reaction before administering a higher dose safely. Repeated drug administration is contraindicated after any life-threatening reaction that is not medicated by IgE mechanism (e.g., drug-induced hemolytic anemia, immune complex reaction, and Stevens-Johnson syndrome).

MANAGEMENT

General Considerations

Based on the algorithm shown diagrammatically in Figure 27–1, one should be able to derive the correct type or classification of a drug reaction. If the patient has a type A reaction because of an overdose, dosage adjustment is all that is necessary. If the reaction is secondary to drug interaction, dose adjustment of the drug in question or the interacting drug will be sufficient. If the patient has a type B reaction secondary to intolerance, an alternative drug should be administered if clinically indicated. If the drug is the only medication most appropriate for the patient, the medication can be given without a type I IgE-mediated allergic reaction (the reaction is intolerance and not an allergic reaction). However, the patient may need to be warned regarding the reaction, which is not life threatening. If the patient's reaction is a type B reaction secondary to drug allergy, one has to determine if the drug has to be given without alternative. If the reaction is a type I IgE-mediated allergic reaction, desensitization will be necessary so the essential drug, can be given to the patient. Type II, type III, and type IV reactions cannot be

desensitized. One has to be prepared to stop the medications if these reactions recur. If the patient has had Stevens-Johnson syndrome in the past, the responsible drug should not be readministered. Desensitization does not work for Stevens-Johnson syndrome.

Desensitization

A specific drug that a patient is allergic to via the type I reaction can be desensitized, provided the medication is the one the patient needs without alternative, because the procedure is dangerous. In other words, the benefit of administering the medication via desensitization is higher than the risk of complications associated with the desensitization. The best described desensitization is penicillin desensitization. The other drugs can be desensitized using the same principle. Table 27–1 shows an example of penicillin desensitization.

Special Considerations

INSULIN ALLERGY

Systemic reactions to insulin are IgE mediated and characterized by urticaria, angioedema, shortness of breath, wheezing, and hypotension. Patient can have a mild form of reaction with rash only. Treatment may include antihistamine for symptomatic relief until the reaction disappears. Systemic life-threatening allergic reactions may occur. In situations in which insulin is crucial to the patient's health, insulin should not be discontinued after a systemic reaction, if the last dose of insulin is given within 24 hours. Rather, the dose should be reduced to about a tenth of the dose that caused the systemic reaction. The dose should then be slowly increased by 2 U per injection until a therapeutic dose is achieved. After that, the patient should receive insulin as least daily, to keep him or her desensitized to the insulin. A lower dose may be given if the patient's blood glucose level is low.

If the patient who is allergic to insulin has not received insulin for more than 24 hours, one may have to put the patient through the insulin desensitization protocol. The physician should be prepared to treat anaphylaxis and hypoglycemia during the desensitization procedure. Rapid desensitization like PCN desensitization in the intensive care unit may be necessary if the patient requires insulin urgently. If requirement for insulin is not critical, one can desensitize the patient via a modified protocol over a 6-day period with three doses each day. A copy of the *Drug Allergy and Protocols for Management of Drug Allergies*, published by Grammer and Greenberger, is suggested.

MEASLES, MUMPS, RUBELLA VACCINE ALLERGY

Skin testing for the measles, mumps, rubella (MMR) vaccine is indicated for the patient who has had a prior

Table 27–1. PCN desensitization.

Requires the following penicillin concentrations: 100 U/mL (0.0625 mg/mL); 1000 U/mL (0.625 mg/mL); 10,000 unit/mL (6.25 mg/mL); 40,000 U/mL (25 mg/mL); 1,000,000 U/mL.
PCN:VK: 125 mg = 200,000 U
No more than double the previous dose each time every 15 minutes. Decrease dose by a third if allergic reaction and continue to increase the dose.
IV access and urgent medication available as indicated above. Double dose every 15 minutes IV. Increase dose in doses that are no more than double the previous dose at each administration. If a systemic reaction occurs, treat with epinephrine, 0.3 mg IM, of 1:1000. Then reduce the dose to a third the previous dose and slowly continue cautious increase in doses.

Time (min between doses)	Dose	Units/mg	Concentration (Units/mL)	Volume (mL)	Total Dose (U/mg)
0	1	50 U/0.03 mg (IV/PO)	100 U/mL (0.0625 mg/mL)	0.5	50 U/0.03 mg
15	2	100 U/0.06 mg (IV/PO)	100 U/mL (0.0625 mg/mL)	1	150 U/0.09 mg
30	3	200 U/0.13 mg (IV/PO)	100 U/mL (0.0625 mg/mL)	2	350 U/0.22 mg
45	4	400 U/0.25 mg (IV/PO)	100 U/mL (0.0625 mg/mL)	4	750 U/0.47 mg
60 (1 h)	5	800 U/0.5 mg (IV/PO)	100 U/mL (0.0625 mg/mL)	8	1,550 U/0.97 mg
75	6	1,600 U/1 mg (IV/PO)	1000 U/mL (0.625 mg/mL)	1.6	3,125 U/1.97 mg
90	7	3,200 U/2 mg (IV/PO)	1000 U/mL (0.625 mg/mL)	3.2	6,350 U/3.97 mg
105	8	6,400 U/4 mg (IV/PO)	1000 U/mL (0.625 mg/mL)	6.4	12,750 U/7.97 mg
120 (2 h)	9	12,800 U/8 mg (IV/PO)	1000 U/mL (0.625 mg/mL)	12.8	25,550 U/15.97 mg
135	10	25,000 U/15.6 mg (IV/PO)	10,000 U/mL (6.25 mg/mL)	2.5	50,550 U/31.57 mg
150	11	50,000 U/31.3 mg (IV/PO)	10,000 U/mL (6.25 mg/mL)	5	100,550 U/62.9 mg
165	12	100,000 U/62.5 mg (IV/PO)	10,000 U/mL (6.25 mg/mL)	10	200,550 U/125 mg
180 (3 h)	13	200,000 U/125 mg (IV/PO)	40,000 U/mL (25 mg/mL)	5	400,550 U/250 mg
195	14	400,000U/250 mg (IV/PO)	40,000 U/mL (25 mg/mL)	10	800,550 U/500 mg
210	15	800,000/500 mg (IV/PO)	40,000 U/mL (25 mg/mL)	20	1.6 MU/1000 mg
225	16	800,000 (IV)	40,000 U/mL	20	2.4 MU/
585	17	1,000,000 (IV)	40,000 U/mL	25	3.4 MU/

After dose 17, then q6h without dose interruption.
IV, intravenous; PO, by mouth.

reaction to MMR or who has had a prior reaction to gelatin, which is also a stabilizer present in MMR. The risk for serious allergic reaction to the MMR in egg-allergic patients is extremely low, and the vaccine may be administered to egg-allergic individuals.

INFLUENZA VACCINE ALLERGY

Skin testing for influenza vaccine is indicated for the patient who has had a prior reaction to influenza vaccine or who has had an allergic reaction to egg. If skin testing is positive for the influenza vaccine, influenza vaccine desensitization is indicated if the administration of flu vaccine is essential (Table 27–2). Administration of yellow fever vaccine is also contraindicated in patients with egg allergy.

TETANUS ALLERGY

If an immediate type I allergic reaction occurs after tetanus immunization, a subsequent tetanus booster can be administered pending skin testing results and possible desensitization. If the skin testing is negative, 0.1 mL intramuscularly (IM) can be given, then 0.4 mL IM

Table 27–2. Influenza vaccine skin testing and desensitization protocol and record.

Influenza Vaccine (INV)	Time Adm.	Injection Site	VS BP/P	Prick	ID	IM
Diluent control						Not applicable
Histamine					N/A	Not applicable
1:10 Dilution of INV					N/A	Not applicable
1:100 dilution of INV				N/A		Not applicable
0.50 mL 1:1 INV (**negative skin testing "prick & ID" to INV**)			BP: HR: PF:	N/A	N/A	Local Rx: Auscultation:
0.05 mL 1:100 INV (0 min) (Positive skin testing to INV)			BP: HR: PF:	N/A	N/A	Local Rx: Auscultation:
0.05 mL 1:10 INV (at 15 min) (Positive skin testing to INV)			BP: HR: PF:	N/A	N/A	Local Rx: Auscultation:
0.05 mL 1:1 INV (at 30 min) (Positive skin testing to INV)			BP: HR: PF:	N/A	N/A	Local Rx: Auscultation:
0.10 mL 1:1 INV (at 45 min) (Positive skin testing to INV)			BP: HR: PF:	N/A	N/A	Local Rx: Auscultation:
0.15 mL 1:1 INV (at 60 min) (Positive skin testing to INV)			BP: HR: PF:	N/A	N/A	Local Rx: Auscultation:
0.20 mL 1:1 INV (at 75 min) (Positive skin testing to INV)			BP: HR: PF:	N/A	N/A	Local Rx: Auscultation:

1. Amount of dilution is designated as 1:1 (undiluted), 1:10 (10-fold dilution), 1:100 (100-fold dilution) using saline.
2. Result is histamine equivalent prick.
3. Treat generalized reaction with epinephrine, antihistamine, and steroid.
4. If reaction limited to lung, use epinephrine and/or bronchodilator.
5. Observe all patients for 45 minutes after the last dose.
6. Abbreviations: INV=influenza vaccine; N/A=not applicable; Rx=reaction; BP=blood pressure; HR=heart rate; PF=peak flow measurement; VS=vital sign; prick=prick skin testing result; ID=intradermal skin testing result; IM=intramuscular injection; Time adm=time when skin testing or injection is performed.

From Murphy KR, Strunk RC. Safe administration of influenza vaccine in asthmatic children hypersensitive to egg proteins. *J Pediatr.* 1985;106(6):931.

30 minutes later if the patient tolerates the previous dose. If skin testing is positive, tetanus desensitization is indicated starting from 1:1000 diluted tetanus vaccine. The rate of immunization can be given at weekly or biweekly intervals. For each administration day, up to five doses can be given every 20 minutes (Table 27 3).

RADIOCONTRAST ANAPHYLACTOID REACTION

If radiocontrast administration is medically indicated without other alternatives, premedication is indicated in addition to the usage of a lower osmolality radiocontrast (Table 27–4).

Table 27–3. Tetanus desensitization protocol.

	1:1000 diluted dT	1:100 diluted dT	1:10 diluted dT	Undiluted dT
0 min	0.05 mL	0.05 mL	0.05 mL	0.05 mL
20 min	0.1 mL	0.1 mL	0.1 mL	0.1 mL
40 min	0.2 mL	0.2 mL	0.2 mL	0.15 mL
60 min	0.3 mL	0.3 mL	0.3 mL	0.2 mL
80 min	0.5 mL	0.5 mL	0.5 mL	

Note: May need to repeat the dose or to lower the dose if the patient has an allergic reaction.
dT, diphtheria-tetanus toxoid.

LOCAL ANESTHETIC REACTION

True type I IgE-medicated allergic reaction has not been documented. Nevertheless, skin testing and test dosing protocol are usually employed to ensure that the patient can tolerate the anesthetic (Table 27–5).

NSAID REACTION

If a patient has single drug—induced anaphylaxis as discussed earlier, he or she can tolerate another NSAID of a different structure. The first dose, however, should be given in a doctor's office, in case of anaphylaxis. If the reaction is a class effect, the patient may have to avoid all NSAIDs. If clinically indicated, ASA/NSAID desensitization can be performed by a specialist in the hospital.

MUSCLE RELAXANT REACTION

Muscle relaxant allergic reaction accounts for 60% to 70% of anaphylactic reactions during general anesthesia. Other causes to consider include latex, opioids, and antibiotics. A different muscle relaxant, especially one to which the patient has a negative skin test, should be used. It is preferable to use agents with lower histamine-releasing abilities, like atracurium and pancuronium. In any case, histamine release occurs commonly during anesthesia and surgery in response to various opiates, induction agents, and muscle relaxants. H1 and H2 antagonists given simultaneously decrease the effect of histamine release and the frequency and severity of these reactions. Premedicating patient with a steroid (prednisone, 50 mg PO [by mouth], 13 hours; prednisone, 50 mg PO, 7 hours; and hydrocortisone, 200 mg intravenously [IV] 1 hour prior to general anesthesia), an H1 receptor antagonist (diphenhydramine, 50 mg IV, 1 hour before general anesthesia), and an H2 receptor antagonist (Ranitidine, 50 mg IV, 1 hour before general anesthesia) is recommended. Decreasing the rate of muscle relaxant administration may avoid cardiovascular collapse.

EVIDENCE-BASED MEDICINE

Absence of Cross-Reactivity Between Sulfonamide Antibiotics and Sulfonamide Nonantibiotics

There is an association between sulfonamide antibiotics hypersensitivity and a subsequent allergic reaction after the receipt of sulfonamide nonantibiotics. However, this association appears to be due to a predisposition to allergic reactions rather than to a cross reactivity of sulfonamide-based drugs. In a retrospective study performed by Strom et al in the United Kingdom, of the 969 patients with prior allergic reaction to sulfonamide antibiotics, about 10% had an allergic reaction after subsequent usage (within 30 days) of a sulfonamide nonantibiotic. For those patients who had no allergic reaction to sulfonamide antibiotics, only 1.6% had an allergic reaction after receiving a sulfonamide nonantibiotic. However, the chance of a subsequent allergic reaction to penicillin was even greater among patients who had an allergic reaction to sulfonamide antibiotics (14%). The risk of

Table 27–4. Radiocontrast pretreatment.

	Steroid	Antihistamine	Contrast Agent
Nonemergent	Prednisone, 50 mg PO, 13 hours, 7 hours, and 1 hour before procedure	Diphenhydramine, 50 mg PO, 1 hour before procedure	Low osmolality
Emergent	Hydrocortisone, 200 mg IV, immediately and q4h until procedure completed	Diphenhydramine, 50 mg IV, 1 hour before procedure	Low osmolality

Table 27–5. Local anesthetic skin testing and test dosing protocol.

	Time Adm.	Site	VS BP//P	Prick Test Result	Subcutaneous Challenge Result
Diluent control					N/A
Histamine					N/A
LA (undiluted) 0 min					N/A
LA (0.1 ml of 1:100) at 15 min				N/A	
LA (0.1 ml of 1:10) at 30 min				N/A	
LA (0.1 ml of 1:1) at 45 min				N/A	
LA (1 ml of 1:1) at 60 min				N/A	
LA (2 ml of 1:1) at 75 min				N/A	

Local Anesthetic (LA) for Testing: 1% Lidocaine HCL injection, USP 10 mg/mL (preservative free).
LOT #:_____ EXP: _____

1. Local anesthetics used should be the same type to be used in the actual procedure.
2. Local anesthetics should have no epinephrine and no preservative.
3. Amount of dilution is designated as 1:1 (undiluted), 1:10 (10-fold dilution), 1:100 (100-fold dilution) using normal saline.
4. Prick test result: both the diameter in millimeter of the erythema and the diameter in millimeter of the wheal are recorded.
5. Subcutaneous challenge result: both the diameter in millimeter of the erythema and the diameter in millimeter of the wheal are recorded; systemic reaction, if occurs, will be recorded.
6. Abbreviations: Time adm.=time when skin testing or the subcutaneous injection is performed; Site=the site of injection or skin testing; VS=vital sign; BP=blood pressure; P=pulse or heart rate.

INTERPRETATION
1. This patient has received 3 mL of the respective local anesthetic ( ) with no reaction and is at no greater risk for a subsequent allergic reaction than the general population (for the same type of local anesthetic tested without epinephrine and preservative).
2. Others:

_____
Dr.

an allergic reaction after receipt of a sulfonamide nonantibiotic was lower among patients with a history of sulfonamide antibiotics hypersensitivity than among patients with a history of penicillin hypersensitivity (odd ration 0.6; 95% confidence interval, 0.5–0.8). Therefore, the association between hypersensitivity after the receipt of sulfonamide antibiotics and subsequent allergic reaction after the receipt of a sulfonamide nonantibiotic is due to a predisposition to allergic reactions in general rather than a cross reactivity with sulfonamide-based drugs. Although a history of allergy to sulfonamide antibiotics increases the risk of allergic reaction to sulfonamide nonantibiotics (such as furosemide, dapsone, glyburide, glipizide, etc.), the risk is not unique to sulfonamide antibiotics. Patients who are allergic to sulfonamide have an increased risk of allergic reaction to penicillin. Patients who have a history of allergic reaction to penicillin have a higher risk of having an allergic reaction to sulfonamide nonantibiotics

than among patients who have had a prior allergic reaction to sulfonamide antibiotics. The association, at least for sulfonamide antibiotics and sulfonamide nonantibiotics, may be a general disposition to allergic reactions among certain patients rather than a specific cross reactivity with drugs containing the sulfa moiety. Patients with a history of allergic reaction to drugs may be at an increased risk of allergic reaction to other drugs that are structurally distinct.

The Risk of a Course of Penicillin Resensitizing the Patient with a Positive History But Negative Skin Test Response Is Low

Prior to 2003, skin testing for penicillin was usually performed immediately before the administration of PCN to PCN-sensitive patients because PCN allergy was not believed to be a permanent condition. It was believed that a negative PCN skin testing would not guarantee that the patient would not have an allergy to the antibiotics a few weeks or a few months or a few years later, because of the possibility of resensitization. Published in the *Journal of Allergy and Clinical Immunology* in 2003, Macy et al reviewed medical records for penicillin use and associated adverse reaction in 568 penicillin skin test-negative individuals who had histories of penicillin reactions prior to PCN skin testing and who had received at least one course of oral penicillin after PCN skin testing. The mean length of follow-up was about 4 years. The mean penicillin exposure was about four courses. There were 71 (about 3%) reactions with 2236 total penicillin courses. There were no serious reactions. Repeated skin testing was done in 33 subjects who had PCN reactions after prior PCN skin testing; only 1 subject was positive on repeated penicillin skin testing. The authors conclude that penicillin use after negative penicillin skin testing done in advance of need is safe, and resensitization is rare. Thus, once a patient with a positive history is shown to have no allergy by skin testing using the major and minor determinants, future administration of PCN or β-lactam drugs would not require repeated skin testing.

RECENT ADVANCES

The Role of T Cells in Drug Reaction

T cells play a key role in the development of a type IV drug reaction. T cells are directly responsible for the tissue damage that results from T–cell-mediated cytotoxicity and release of proinflammatory cytokines. Both CD4 and CD8 T cells accumulate at the dermoepidermal junction and in the superficial dermis and express perforin and granzyme B. CD4 T cells isolated from the lesional skin kill with a perforin-dependent mechanism of autologous keratinocytes in the presence of the specific drug. In comparison, cellular infiltrate of bullous exanthem comprises a higher number of cytotoxic CD8 T cells, found in the dermis and in the epidermis in close contact with keratinocytes. CD8 T cells isolated from the skin of patients affected by toxic epidermal necrolysis developed after assumption of cotrimoxazole and carbamazepine were found to be highly cytotoxic for keratinocytes in the presence of the causative drugs. With recent researches, we may be closer to understanding the immunopathologic mechanism of a type IV allergic drug reaction.

Noncovalent Interactions of Drugs with Immune Receptors May Mediate Drug-Induced Hypersensitivity Reactions

In classic delayed-type hypersensitivity, an antigen-presenting cell has to take up the antigen and process it and subsequently present the peptide in the context of HLA (covalently linked to the HLA) and present it to the T cell via the T-cell receptor. In recent years, evidence has become stronger that not all drugs need to bind covalently to the MHC or HLA-peptide complex to trigger an immune response. Rather, some drugs may bind reversibly to the MHC or possibly to the T-cell receptor, eliciting immune reactions. The noncovalent drug presentation leads to the activation of drug-specific T cells. In some patients with hypersensitivity, such a response may occur within hours. Thus the reaction to the drug may not be the result of classic delayed-type hypersensitivity. This is called the p-i concept: pharmacologic interaction of drugs with immune receptors. This was first verified for sulfamethoxazole-specific T-cell clones and further confirmed for lidocaine, mepivacaine, celecoxib, carbamazepine, and, most recently, quinolone-reactive T cells. The type IV T–cell-mediated drug reactions appear more complex based on recent researches than how they were described in the past. An allergic drug reaction occurring within a few hours after drug administration may be T-cell mediated rather than IgE-mast cell mediated.

Diagnostic Testing for T-Cell-Mediated (Type IV) Drug Reaction

Drug-specific T cells, which are involved in the type IV drug reaction, may be detected by in vitro lymphocyte transformation and in vivo patch testing, which are used in Europe but not approved for use in the United States. Because a metabolite may be the one responsible for stimulating the T cells, the testing of the parent drug may have low negative and low positive predictive values. When studies are performed to validate the predictive values of the testing systems, they possibly will become useful to physicians in the future.

BIBLIOGRAPHY

Adkinson NF. Drug allergy. In: Adkinson NF, Yunginger JW, Busse WW, et al., eds. *Middleton's Allergy, Principles & Practice.* 6th ed. St. Louis, Mo: Mosby-Year Book; 2003:1679.

Thong B, Leong K-P, Tang, C-Y, et al. Drug allergy in general hospital: results of a novel prospective inpatient reporting system. *Ann Allergy Asthma Immunol.* 2003;90:342.

Gerber BO, Pichler J. Noncovalent interactions of drugs with immune receptors may mediate drug-induced hypersensitivity reactions [Article 19]. *The AAPS Journal* 2006;8(1):E160. Available at: http://www.aapsj.org.

Gomes ER, Demoly P. Epidemiology of hypersensitivity drug reactions. *Current Opin Allergy Clin Immunol.* 2005;5:309.

Grammer LC, Greenberger PA. *Drug Allergy and Protocols for Management of Drug Allergies.* 3rd ed. Providence, RI: OceanSide Publications; 2003.

Greenberger PA. Drug allergy. *J Allergy Clin Immunol.* 2006;117:S464.

Gruchalla RS, Pirmohamed M. Antibiotic allergy. *N Engl J Med.* 2006;354:601.

Israel E, Chinchilli VM, Ford JG, et al. Use of regularly scheduled albuterol treatment in asthma: genotype-stratified, randomised, placebo-controlled, cross-over trial. *Lancet.* 2004;364:1505.

Kelso JM. The gelatin story. *J Allergy Clin Immunol.* 1999;103:200.

Lazarou J, Pomeranz BH, Corey PN. Incidence of adverse drug reactions in hospitalized patients. *JAMA.* 1998;279:1200.

Macy E, Mangat R, Burchette M. Penicillin skin testing in advance of need: Multiyear follow-up in 568 test result-negative subjects exposed to oral penicillins. *J Allergy Clin Immunol.* 2003;111:1111.

Stevenson D. Classification of allergic and pseudoallergic reactions to drugs that inhibit cyclooxygenase enzymes. *Ann Allergy Asthma Immunol.* 2001;87:177.

Strom BL, Schinnar R, Apter AJ, et al. Absence of cross-reactivity between sulfonamide antibiotics and sulfonamide nonantibiotics. *N Engl J Med.* 2003;349:1628.

Cavani A, Pita OD. The role of T cells in drug reaction. *Curr Allergy Asthma Reports.* 2006;6:20.

Smoke, Pollution, and Allergies

Haig Tcheurekdjian, MD and Massoud Mahmoudi, DO, PhD

The development and exacerbation of allergic disease is a multifaceted process involving an interplay between genetic and environmental factors. Airborne pollutants are a nearly ubiquitous environmental hazard that have long been recognized as contributors to poor health outcomes in many disease processes. Recently, airborne pollutants have been implicated in the manifestations of allergic disease, especially those affecting the airways, such as asthma. The role of pollution in allergic disease is complex, and its effects vary based on a number of factors including the type of pollution and the attributes of the individual exposed to the pollution.

CHARACTERISTICS OF POLLUTANTS

Indoor Versus Outdoor Pollution

Pollution is generally categorized as being either indoor or outdoor pollution, although the two types overlap. Most people spend the majority of their time indoors whether they are at home, school, or work; therefore, exposure to indoor pollutants is a significant problem. Common sources of indoor air pollutants are tobacco smoke, appliances (e.g., gas stoves, fireplaces), and building and renovating materials such as paint. Fortunately, some of these sources are being diminished, such as through bans on indoor smoking. Nonetheless, the levels of many indoor pollutants may be up to two to five times higher than those found outdoors, and indoor levels can even reach a thousand times higher than outdoor levels immediately after certain activities such as paint stripping. Exposures to indoor pollutants may also be prolonged due to the more energy-efficient, airtight building designs being used today that do not allow air to circulate as efficiently between the indoor and outdoor environments. Although these building designs bring benefits such as a reduction in heating and cooling expenditures, they also do not allow pollutants generated indoors to escape to the outdoors.

Outdoor air pollution has been the subject of intense research because of its public health implications and the potential health benefits that can be achieved on a national scale if exposures to these pollutants are reduced. To this end, the U.S. Environmental Protection Agency (EPA) has set National Ambient Air Quality Standards (NAAQS) that identify and set the national standards for acceptable levels of major outdoor pollutants that are considered to be harmful to health. Four of the six pollutants identified in the NAAQS are known contributors to the exacerbation of asthma or allergic disease (Table 28–1). The NAAQS is currently under review by the EPA, and changes to these standards may soon be implemented.

Pollution is frequently a complex mixture of various pollutants; therefore, its effects are significantly more complex than those of a single pollutant listed by the NAAQS. For example, diesel exhaust contains numerous pollutants, including particulate matter, nitrogen dioxide, and carbon monoxide, that may act in concert to initiate or worsen disease.

Actions of Pollution

In general, pollution can interact with allergic disease in three ways: by contributing to the development of disease, by exacerbating established disease, or both (Figure 28–1). On one hand, a single pollutant may act alone in all of these processes, as seen with tobacco smoke that contributes to both the development of asthma in exposed children and the exacerbation of asthma in individuals who already have the disease. On the other hand, pollutants may act in concert to initiate and exacerbate disease. For example, a child may develop asthma secondary to exposure to tobacco smoke and then develop an asthma exacerbation on exposure to high levels of ozone.

The actions of pollutants are multiple. They can operate nonspecifically to worsen allergic disease, such as acting as simple irritants to worsen allergic rhinitis symptoms (see Chapter 6), or they can act more specifically by contributing to allergic inflammation through the promotion of T helper (Th) type 2 immune responses and the downregulation of Th1 responses (see Chapter 1), both of which can promote the expression of allergic disease.

Table 28–1. Outdoor pollutants identified by the National Ambient Air Quality Standards.

Known Contribution to Asthma or Allergic Disease	Major Sources
Nitrogen dioxide	Primary: fossil fuel use by automobiles Secondary: fossil fuel use by power plants, industrial plants, commercial plants.
Ozone	Precursors produced by fossil fuel use by automobiles and industrial emissions
Particulate matter	Primary: fossil fuel use by power plants and automobiles Secondary: construction sites, fires, unpaved roads
Sulfur oxides	Primary: fossil fuel use by power plants Secondary: petroleum refineries, cement manufacturing, metal-processing facilities, locomotives, large ships
No Known Contribution to Asthma or Allergic Disease	**Major Sources**
Carbon monoxide	Primary: fossil fuel use by automobiles Secondary: fossil fuel use by non–road vehicles (construction boats, etc), chemical processing
Lead	Primary: metal-processing plants Secondary: fossil fuel use by power plants, waste incinerators

CHARACTERISTICS OF INDIVIDUALS

The health effects of pollution are not only caused by the specific features of the pollutant but are also due to features of the exposed population. The age of the exposed individual is one of the most important factors contributing to the effect of pollutants. The time period beginning in fetal life and extending throughout childhood is a period of marked vulnerability as the respiratory tract and immune system are developing and maturing. Furthermore, children usually have higher exposures to

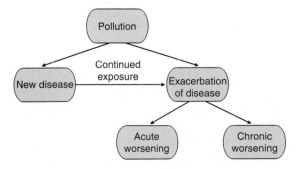

Figure 28–1. Effects of pollution on allergic disease.

outdoor pollutants because they spend a larger portion of their time outdoors compared to adults. Children also have a higher minute ventilation than adults, leading to increased exposure to inhaled pollutants.

Respiratory Tract Development

The respiratory tract is only partially developed at birth and undergoes rapid changes postnatally. Development of the paranasal sinuses has only begun at birth with the presence of rudimentary ethmoid sinuses and early pneumatization of the maxillary sinuses. Complete development and pneumatization of all the sinuses does not occur until adolescence. Likewise, the lungs undergo significant changes after birth. Although the lungs are functional at birth, they are structurally immature with only a fraction of the alveoli that will be present in adulthood. During the first 4 years of life, significant septation of the lung parenchyma occurs with the number of alveoli increasing by greater than 10-fold. Pulmonary development continues to progress throughout adolescence with complete development being attained only in early adulthood. Because of the immaturity of the respiratory tract in utero and during childhood, exposure to pollution during this time has the ability to alter normal pulmonary development, potentially leading to adverse consequences for an individual's entire life. These adverse effects are not theoretical but are well-described events discussed later in this chapter.

Immune System Development

Similar to the respiratory tract, the pediatric immune system is immature at birth and undergoes significant changes in the first few years of life. The healthy adult immune system maintains a fine balance between Th1 immune responses, which are important in cell-mediated immunity, and Th2 immune responses, which are important in humoral immunity and the development of allergic diseases. Compared to adults, infants naturally have a Th2 polarized immune system that later matures into an immune system that produces balanced Th1 and Th2 responses. Furthermore, atopic children maintain this Th2 polarization for a longer period of time compared to nonatopic children, indicating the central role of the Th phenotype in allergic disease. Because the immune system continues to mature throughout early childhood, this is a time period during which children may be at heightened risk for the inappropriate skewing of immune responses towards the allergic Th2 phenotype.

SPECIFIC POLLUTANTS

In the following sections, we review the evidence implicating the role of various pollutants in the development of allergic disease and asthma. Tobacco smoke and diesel exhaust, two pollutants with complex mixtures of various compounds, are discussed first, followed by the discussion of the four key pollutants affecting allergic disease identified in the NAAQS.

Tobacco Smoke

Exposure to tobacco smoke can occur through an active or passive process. Active exposure is through smoking a cigarette or other tobacco product. Passive exposure occurs by inhaling sidestream smoke (smoke released from the burning end of the cigarette) or inhaling smoke exhaled by the active smoker. This is referred to as secondhand smoke or environmental tobacco smoke (ETS).

ETS consists of a complex combination of hundreds of chemicals and pollutants. Exposure to ETS has been linked to numerous health problems affecting every age group from infancy through adulthood. These health problems include intrauterine growth retardation, sudden infant death syndrome, asthma, otitis media, pneumonia, chronic obstructive pulmonary disease, cardiovascular disease, and cancer. In regard to allergic disease, ETS both causes and exacerbates allergic diseases and asthma.

DISEASE DEVELOPMENT

Children born to mothers who smoked during their pregnancy have approximately twice the risk of developing asthma during the first year of life compared to children not exposed to tobacco smoke during pregnancy. The effect of intrauterine exposure to tobacco smoke on asthma appears to be dose dependent; the greater the number of cigarettes smoked by the pregnant mother, the greater the risk of the exposed child developing asthma. ETS exposure also increases both total and allergen-specific serum IgE levels, potentially contributing to the development of other allergic diseases. It is estimated that up to 26,000 cases of childhood asthma in the United States are secondary to exposure to ETS.

DISEASE EXACERBATION

Exposure to ETS is clearly linked to exacerbations of asthma. Various studies have demonstrated that children exposed to ETS have nearly twice the number of asthma exacerbations as those who have not been exposed. This amounts to approximately 1 million asthma exacerbations in children in the United States that are secondary to ETS exposure. Maternal smoking has been linked to a higher risk of asthma exacerbation compared to paternal smoking, and the effect on the number of exacerbations appears to be dose dependent (i.e., the more ETS exposure, the greater the number of asthma exacerbations). Asthma control in adults is also adversely affected by ETS. Adults with ETS exposure require greater amounts of asthma medications such as maintenance corticosteroids and bronchodilators, and they have lower measurements of lung function compared to unexposed adults.

ETS can also exacerbate allergic rhinitis and allergic conjunctivitis. ETS can act as an ocular irritant. In fact, ocular irritation is one of the most commonly reported effects of ETS by nonsmokers. The effects of ETS on the eye may be secondary to its ability to disrupt the thin protective film of tear on the cornea. This is supported by experiments that document instability of the tear film after exposure to ETS and an increase in blinking and lacrimation (tearing), both of which act to reestablish the protective film of tear on the cornea.

Rhinitis symptoms also develop in many individuals on exposure to ETS. ETS exposure can lead to the development of rhinorrhea and nasal congestion, and these symptoms coincide with objectively measured endpoints such as nasal airway resistance. Although these symptoms can occur in any individual on exposure to ETS, they tend to be found predominantly in atopic individuals.

Although different disorders of the respiratory tract have traditionally been thought of as isolated diseases, it is becoming increasingly evident that disease activity in one part of the respiratory tract can adversely affect other parts. In other words, the respiratory tract may be envisioned as a unified system instead of as a combination of different components (i.e., nose, sinuses, lungs, etc.). For example, an episode of acute sinusitis, a disorder of the upper respiratory tract, can contribute to the development of an asthma exacerbation, a disorder of the lower respiratory tract. This concept of a unified respiratory system also extends to the effects of ETS, in that the effects of ETS that do not immediately affect the lungs or nasal cavity may still lead to exacerbations of allergic rhinitis or asthma. For example, the incidence of otitis media, adenoid hypertrophy, tonsillitis, and bronchitis are higher in children exposed to ETS in the home compared to those that are not. Secondary to the effects of the unified respiratory system, these disorders may contribute to the exacerbations of allergic rhinitis and asthma.

Diesel Exhaust

The burning of fuel by motor vehicles is one of the largest sources of airborne pollutants, and diesel exhaust accounts for a large portion of this pollution. Diesel exhaust consists of diesel exhaust particles (DEPs) and gaseous combustion products. DEPs are carbon particles of 0.1 μm or less to which numerous chemicals produced in the combustion process or already present in the atmosphere can attach. Gaseous combustion products include nitrogen dioxide, carbon monoxide, and hydrocarbons that are precursors to ozone production.

Like ETS, diesel exhaust has been linked to numerous adverse health outcomes, including leukemia, lymphoma, lung cancer, and wheezing. In regard to allergic disease, diesel exhaust is associated with both the development and exacerbation of asthma, the promotion of sensitization to new allergens, and the enhancement of the allergic response to antigen.

DISEASE DEVELOPMENT

There are significant epidemiologic and clinical research data indicating that exposure to diesel exhaust leads to the development of allergic disease. Accurate measurement of diesel exhaust exposure is difficult; therefore, studies have used proximity to automobile traffic and similar measures as a proxy for the measurement of diesel exhaust exposure. Infants exposed to traffic-related pollutants have 2.5 times the prevalence of wheezing compared to a nonexposed population. Of note, it is the proximity to traffic and the type of traffic (stop-and-go bus and truck traffic) that are the most significant risk factors for the development of disease, not the volume of traffic. Likewise, older children with exposure to traffic-related pollution have a prevalence of asthma twice as high as that compared to an unexposed population. As with asthma, exposure to traffic-related pollution also leads to the development of allergic disease. There is a 2.5 times increased prevalence of allergic disease in children with high exposure to traffic-related pollutants compared to children with low exposure. Furthermore, increased rates of allergic sensitization are found in individuals exposed to higher amounts of traffic-related pollutants.

From a mechanistic standpoint, numerous studies have investigated the methods by which diesel exhaust induces the development of allergic disease. When atopic individuals are given an intranasal challenge of a new allergen plus DEPs, they produce IgE specific to the allergen and upregulate Th2 cytokine production. But atopic individuals challenged with new allergen alone do not produce allergen-specific IgE, and there is no change in Th2 cytokine production. It has also been demonstrated that challenging individuals with DEPs plus ragweed induces B lymphocytes producing ragweed-specific immunoglobulin to switch from the production of IgM to the production of IgE. This switch did not occur with the challenge was with ragweed alone. Therefore, diesel exhaust promotes the development of new allergic disease by inducing the immune system to produce Th2-polarized responses to new allergens and inducing the production of allergen-specific IgE.

DISEASE EXACERBATION

In addition to being associated with the development of disease, exposure to traffic-related pollution is also associated with exacerbations of asthma. The role of diesel exhaust in the exacerbation of asthma is described in detail in the sections later that discuss the individual pollutants that are products of combustion (i.e., particulate matter, nitrogen dioxide, ozone). In general, increased exposure to traffic-related pollution increases the risk of asthma exacerbations for both children and adults.

Multiple mechanisms by which diesel exhaust exacerbates allergic disease have been elucidated. In individuals sensitized to an allergen, challenge with that particular allergen plus DEPs leads to the augmented production of IgE and Th2 cytokines and downregulation of Th1 cytokines. This shift in immunoglobulin and cytokine production is a potent promoter of allergic inflammation. Furthermore, DEPs augment mast cell degranulation leading to the release of increased amounts of mast cell mediators. DEPs also alter the secretion pattern of various cytokines, leading to alterations of cellular infiltration of tissues, such as the respiratory epithelium. This may promote allergic inflammation, leading to disease exacerbation.

Nitrogen Dioxide

Nitrogen dioxide (NO_2) is a precursor to smog and ozone. It is both an important outdoor and indoor pollutant. Most NO_2 is produced by the burning of fossil fuels by automobiles, but other important outdoor sources include fossil fuel combustion by power plants and other industrial sources. Stoves that burn natural gas are a major indoor source of NO_2.

The results of studies evaluating the role of NO_2 in allergic disease have been conflicting, although a number of studies indicate it plays a role in the exacerbation of established disease. Indoor exposure from appliances using natural gas is associated with an increased incidence of coughing and wheezing, and outdoor exposure is linked to asthma exacerbations and diminished pulmonary development. NO_2 also augments the allergic response to allergen when subjects are pretreated with NO_2. In addition to these direct effects, NO_2 also reacts with sunlight and hydrocarbons in the atmosphere to produce ozone, another important pollutant.

Ozone

Ozone (O_3), which is naturally found in the upper parts of the atmosphere, has the beneficial effect of protecting the earth's surface from ultraviolet radiation produced by the sun. But O_3 is toxic when it is present near ground level. As described earlier, ground-level O_3 is produced primarily by the interaction of sunlight with by-products of fossil fuel combustion, namely NO_2 and hydrocarbons. O_3 is a well-studied pollutant and is associated with numerous adverse health outcomes, including both the development and exacerbation of asthma.

DISEASE DEVELOPMENT

A well-conducted study investigated the role of O_3 and other air pollutants on the incidence of asthma in children in Southern California. Over 3500 children without asthma were followed prospectively for up to 5 years to determine if O_3 exposure had an effect on the prevalence of asthma. The investigators discovered that children who spent a large amount of their time playing outdoor sports in areas with high O_3 levels had greater than three times the risk of developing asthma than children who did not play outdoor sports. Outdoor sports activity had no effect on the development of asthma in areas with low O_3 levels, indicating that increased exposure to O_3 was the cause of the increased risk of asthma.

DISEASE EXACERBATION

The exacerbation of asthma secondary to exposure to O_3 is well documented in numerous studies. Hospital admissions for respiratory symptoms and emergency department visits for asthma exacerbations increase during periods of elevated O_3 levels. The use of asthma medications also increases by nearly two times during periods of elevated O_3 levels compared to periods of time with low levels. An interesting event highlighting the effect of O_3 on asthma exacerbations in children occurred during the 1996 Summer Olympics in Atlanta, Georgia. During the Olympics, the city instituted citywide alternative traffic measures, including expanded public transportation services and closure of the downtown area to private automobiles in an effort to decrease traffic congestion. These efforts led to a 28% decrease in O_3 levels associated with a greater than 40% decrease in emergency department visits

and hospitalizations secondary to asthma exacerbations. This study not only highlights the adverse effects of high levels of O_3 but also demonstrates that reasonable changes in public policy can have a large positive impact on public health.

Of note, there may be up to a 2-day interval between O_3 exposure and an increase in asthma exacerbations, indicating that the effects of O_3 on the respiratory system are more complex than just an irritant or bronchoconstrictive effect. This has been borne out in a number of studies involving challenges with O_3. O_3 exposure does lead to a rapid decrease in pulmonary function, but it also leads to pulmonary neutrophilic inflammation lasting for up to 1 day after exposure. This mix of bronchoconstriction plus tissue inflammation describes mechanisms by which O_3 exposure can lead to both early and delayed respiratory symptoms.

Particulate Matter

Particulate matter (PM) consists of tiny, solid particles or liquid droplets suspended in the air which are thus respirable. PM is classified by the EPA as smaller than 0.1 μm, smaller than 2.5 μm, smaller than 10 μm, and smaller than 10 μm in diameter. PM larger than 10 μm in diameter is not of significant concern in older children and adults because it is filtered out by the upper respiratory tract during nasal breathing. These particles may pose a problem for younger children because they are frequent mouth breathers, and the particles can therefore deposit in the lower respiratory tract. PM smaller than 0.1 μm is found in relatively low levels in the environment because these particles tend to agglomerate quickly after production, yielding PM of larger sizes. However, PM smaller than 10 μm and smaller than 2.5 μm are considered significant pollutants because they are of a size that can easily penetrate the upper respiratory tract and deposit in the lungs, particularly PM smaller than 2.5 μm. Furthermore, PM smaller than 2.5 μm can remain airborne for many days, allowing it to be carried for many miles from its source of production.

PM is a major product of fossil fuel combustion. PM is not a homogeneous pollutant but rather a combination of numerous constituents including metal ions, hydrocarbons, sulfates, nitrates, crustal materials (i.e., soil and ash) and biologic contaminants. Furthermore, the composition of PM varies on a national scale due to its production from different sources in different locations. Because of this heterogeneous composition, it has not been possible to identify the specific components that lead to adverse health outcomes.

DISEASE DEVELOPMENT

There are limited data on the effects of PM on the development of allergic diseases and asthma. One study has shown that increasing exposure to PM smaller than 10 μm is associated with an increased risk of developing allergic rhinitis. Further investigation is required to elucidate further the role of PM in the development of allergic disease.

DISEASE EXACERBATION

Exposure to high levels of PM is associated with adverse outcomes in asthma. Elevated ambient PM levels are associated with an increased number of hospitalizations secondary to asthma exacerbations in studies conducted in a number of countries. Elevated PM levels also lead to worsening asthma control as evidenced by increased nighttime symptoms, increased variability in peak expiratory flow rates, and lower forced expiratory volumes in 1 second. These effects may be more prominent in more severe asthmatics, defined as those requiring inhaled corticosteroids. PM exposure also leads to an increased need for asthma medication use and to increased hospitalizations secondary to respiratory infections.

Sulfur Oxides

Sulfur dioxide (SO_2) is the primary sulfur oxide implicated in causing adverse outcomes in respiratory diseases. Although SO_2 is primarily produced by power plants powered by fossil fuels, it is also a by-product of numerous industrial processes; therefore, significant occupational exposures can occur in addition to environmental exposures.

DISEASE DEVELOPMENT

Occupational exposures to SO_2, such as in petroleum refineries, can lead to exposure to very high levels of the gas, which is associated with nearly six times the risk of being diagnosed with asthma as compared to a nonexposed population. Exposure to the much lower levels of SO_2 found in the atmosphere is also associated with allergic disease and asthma. In school-age children in France, a positive association was found between increasing levels of SO_2 exposure and the odds of being diagnosed with asthma or allergic rhinitis.

DISEASE EXACERBATION

Studies evaluating the effects of SO_2 on asthma exacerbations have yielded mixed results, but a number of studies showed an increased risk of asthma exacerbations with exposure to high levels of SO_2. Increased numbers of emergency department visits due to asthma exacerbations have also occurred during periods of time with elevated ambient SO_2 levels, but numerous studies have found no correlation. A well-conducted study of children from birth to 14 years of age showed that exposure to elevated SO_2 levels increases the rate of hospitalization for asthma exacerbations. Although there was an

increased risk of hospitalization on the day of exposure, this risk continued to increase until 3 days after exposure. As with O_3, this lag period until the onset of symptoms in certain individuals indicates that the effects of SO_2 on asthma exacerbations are complex and likely involves both bronchospastic and immunologic effects.

Much of the difficulty in finding associations between SO_2 exposure and asthma outcomes has been due to the difficulty in separating the effects of SO_2 from other pollutants. Furthermore, ambient SO_2 can lead to the formation of sulfuric acid aerosols, which may themselves contribute to asthma exacerbations, leading, in turn, to difficulties in gauging the true effects of SO_2.

In studies where individuals are intentionally challenged with SO_2, exposure leads to bronchospasm and drops in measurements of pulmonary function. These findings are accompanied by symptoms of wheezing and dyspnea. Furthermore, exposure to other pollutants, such as O_3, can increase the severity of adverse effects that asthmatics experience on exposure to SO_2.

CONCLUSION

Indoor and outdoor pollutants can lead to both the development and exacerbation of allergic diseases and asthma. The effects of these pollutants can occur in utero or in early childhood, potentially leading to lifelong morbidity from allergic disease or asthma. Furthermore, these pollutants can lead to exacerbations of disease throughout an individual's life. Public policy changes to curb the adverse effects of airborne pollutants can lead to significant public health benefits by decreasing the morbidity associated with allergic and respiratory diseases.

EVIDENCE-BASED MEDICINE

The adverse effects of exposure to PM on respiratory and cardiovascular diseases was recently investigated by Dominici and associates. They evaluated the effect of PM smaller than 2.5 μm on the rate of hospital admissions secondary to respiratory and cardiovascular diseases. A strength of this study was the assessment of pollutant levels and associated morbidity from across the entire United States and not just a particular geographic area. The primary results of this study showed that exposure to increasing levels of PM leads to increasing rates of hospitalization for all cardiovascular and pulmonary outcomes measured (including respiratory infections and exacerbations of chronic obstructive pulmonary disease). Although allergic diseases were not specifically measured, the study's importance lies in the fact that it shows a robust association between PM exposure and adverse cardiopulmonary outcomes for the entire nation.

Gauderman and associates investigated the effects of air pollution on pulmonary development in children. The investigators followed nearly 2000 fourth-grade children over an 8-year period to determine whether exposure to air pollution in Southern California adversely affected pulmonary development. The investigators followed children until approximately 18 years of age, which is when pulmonary maturity is nearly complete in both males and females and after which further significant pulmonary development is unlikely. This study established that children exposed to higher levels of air pollutants (primarily NO_2, PM smaller than 2.5 μm, and acid vapors) were at a greater risk of poor pulmonary development compared to those exposed to low levels. In fact, there were five times as many children with abnormal pulmonary function living in areas with high levels of air pollution compared to children living in areas with low levels of air pollution. This study, therefore, provides strong evidence that exposure to air pollution in childhood can lead to poor pulmonary development that will likely persist throughout an individual's entire life.

Indoor air pollution is also a significant source of morbidity, and the effects of indoor NO_2 on asthma were evaluated by Phoa and associates. In this study, the effect of NO_2 exposure from unvented natural gas heaters on multiple asthma outcomes was assessed. The enrolled 1300 children, from 8 to 11 years of age, underwent medical interviews, prick skin testing to multiple allergens, and bronchoprovocation testing to assess airway hyperresponsiveness. The investigators found that children exposed to unvented natural gas heaters in the first year of life had 1.5 times the risk of having airway hyperresponsiveness and recent wheeze. They also reported having asthma twice as much as the unexposed children. Current exposure to unvented natural gas heaters had no effect on the asthma outcomes measured. This study is important because it demonstrates that early life exposure to NO_2-producing natural gas heaters can have pulmonary effects lasting for at least 11 years after exposure. This highlights the importance of exposures that occur early in life at a time when the respiratory tract and immune system are continuing to develop and mature.

BIBLIOGRAPHY

Dominici F, Peng RD, Bell ML, et al. Fine particulate air pollution and hospital admission for cardiovascular and respiratory diseases. *JAMA.* 2006;295:1127.

Eisner MD, Klein J, Hammond SK, et al. Directly measured second hand smoke exposure and asthma health outcomes. *Thorax.* 2005;60:814.

Friedman MS, Powell KE, Hutwagner L, et al. Impact of changes in transportation and commuting behaviors during the 1996 Summer Olympic Games in Atlanta on air quality and childhood asthma. *JAMA.* 2001;285:897.

Gauderman WJ, Avol E, Gilliland F, et al. The effect of air pollution on lung development from 10 to 18 years of age. *N Engl J Med.* 2004;351:1057.

Lewis TC, Robins TG, Dvonch JT, et al. Air pollution-associated changes in lung function among asthmatic children in Detroit. *Environ Health Perspect.* 2005;113:1068.

Lwebuga-Mukasa JS, Oyana T, Thenappan A, et al. Association between traffic volume and health care use for asthma among residents at a U.S.-Canadian border crossing point. *J Asthma.* 2004;41:289.

McConnell R, Berhane K, Gilliland F, et al. Asthma in exercising children exposed to ozone: a cohort study. *Lancet.* 2002;359:386.

Millstein J, Gilliland F, Berhane K, et al. Effects of ambient air pollutants on asthma medication use and wheezing among fourth-grade school children from 12 Southern California communities enrolled in The Children's Health Study. *Arch Environ Health.* 2004;59:505.

Miyake Y, Miyamoto S, Ohya Y. Association of active and passive smoking with allergic disorders in pregnant Japanese women: baseline data from the Osaka Maternal and Child Health Study. *Ann Allergy Asthma Immunol.* 2005;94:644.

Penard-Morand C, Charpin D, Raherison C, et al. Long-term exposure to background air pollution related to respiratory and allergic health in schoolchildren. *Clin Exp Allergy.* 2005;35:1279.

Phoa LL, Toelle BG, Ng K, et al. Effects of gas and other fume emitting heaters on the development of asthma during childhood. *Thorax.* 2004;59:741.

Ryan PH, LeMasters G, Biagini J, et al. Is it traffic type, volume, or distance? Wheezing in infants living near truck and bus traffic. *J Allergy Clin Immunol.* 2005;116:279.

Senechal S, de Nadai P, Ralainirina N, et al. Effect of diesel on chemokines and chemokine receptors involved in helper T cell type 1/type 2 recruitment in patients with asthma. *Am J Respir Crit Care Med.* 2003;168:215.

Sick Building Syndrome

Massoud Mahmoudi, DO, PhD

Exposure of building occupants to an unhealthy and hazardous environment may cause various symptoms collectively known as "sick building syndrome." Any chemical, gas, fumes, or smoke may potentially cause sickness or illness in occupants of such buildings, but the term *sick building syndrome* is usually used to refer to nonspecific symptoms resulting from exposure to molds or bacteria and their toxins or products. Many articles have associated the black mold *Stachybotrys chartarum*, also known as *Stachybotrys atra,* to this syndrome. However, the cause and effect has never been confirmed.

IS SICK BUILDING SYNDROME AN ALLERGIC CONDITION?

Although sick building syndrome is not an allergic condition, some of the symptoms mimic those of allergic rhinitis and allergic asthma. The affected individuals suffer from irritation and the effects of inhaled organisms or their toxic by-products. Individuals with preexisting allergic rhinitis or asthma may experience exacerbation of their symptoms; those without such conditions remain at risk for developing indoor allergies.

ETIOLOGY OF SICK BUILDING SYNDROME

Although no single organism or substance has been identified as a cause of this syndrome, mold exposure and specifically *S. chartarum* are mentioned more than any other organisms in the literature. The toxicity of this mold is due to the production of potent and lethal toxins known as stachybotryotoxin. Other factors, such as poor building ventilation, polluted indoor air with chemicals such as detergents, pesticides, or others may also contribute to these nonspecific health problems.

STACHYBOTRYS CHARTARUM AND HUMAN DISEASES

In 1931 a disease of unknown etiology caused mortality of the horse population in several villages in Ukraine. The etiology of this disease remained unknown until 1938 when investigators associated the disease with *S. chartarum*. It turned out that the straws fed to animals were contaminated with *Stachybotrys* toxin.

In the 1990s, the Center for Disease Control and Prevention (CDC) published a series of reports on "infant pulmonary hemorrhage/hemosiderosis" occurring in different regions of the United States; the reports noted that the affected individuals were living in unhealthy moldy environments. However, the link between *S. chartarum* and the infant pulmonary hemorrhage was never established.

WHERE ARE THE MOLDS FOUND?

Molds typically live in outdoor environments. They generally get indoors through open doors or windows. They can also attach themselves to hair, clothing, or pets and find their way indoors. When they get indoors, they settle on wet and damp surfaces. They need a humid environment and a constant source of moisture such as water leakage from a pipe or roof to grow. *S. chartarum*, specifically, uses materials that are rich in cellulose and low in nitrogen content as a nutrient source. Therefore, any object with such nutrients is subjected to mold contamination. Some examples of household materials of this category include insulation and paper products such as wallpapers. Any damp area of the house with enough moisture can support the growth of the molds. Places such as basements and bathrooms are particularly the target of such growth.

IDENTIFICATION OF MOLDS IN THE BUILDING

Damp and water-damaged buildings should be inspected for the presence of mold and bacteria. Occupational health inspectors need to visit the site and inspect the entire building. The following areas need specific attention:

1. Water-damaged areas: These are places where water leakage from a damaged pipe has caused destruction

of wood, wall, or the flooring. Several areas such as bathrooms, areas under sinks, wallpapers, and flooring covers should be inspected. Areas under the carpet, linoleum, or hardwood may all be potential areas of mold growth.

2. Humidity: Areas with higher humidity such as basements need to be inspected for visible mold growth.

3. Heating ventilation air-conditioning (HVAC) systems: This system may also be a potential source of mold contamination. Therefore these units/parts need to be inspected.

Inspectors take samples of obvious mold growth and other suspicious areas such as furniture or walls in the absence of visible molds. Then they grow the sample in the appropriate culture medium in the laboratory. After growth, the colonies are subjected to staining and microscopic evaluation. Identification is based on morphologic characteristics of the grown mold.

Serologic methods, such as the use of serum immunoglobulin E (IgE) and serum immunoglobulin G (IgG), against molds such as *S. chartarum* and their antigenic components are also reported. Use of monoclonal antibody has had some success for the identification of molds, but cross-reactivity among fungi make species-specific identification a challenge.

Other methods of mold identification, such as polymerase chain reaction (PCR), have also been used. A recent study introduced a multiplex polymerase chain reaction that has the capability of identifying *S. chartarum*, *Aspergillus versicolor*, *Penicillium purpurogenum*, and *Cladosporium* species within an 8-hour period.

Identification of fungi helps assess causal effect and their relationship with sick building syndrome, developed in water-damaged building. Table 29–1 summarizes the recommended areas of sampling for mold and bacteria and other organisms in water-damaged buildings.

SYMPTOMS

The reported symptoms of sick building syndrome are nonspecific and may affect one or more of the following: head, eyes, nose, sinuses, throat, chest, gastrointestinal system, skin, cognition, and senses. Table 29–2 lists examples of reported symptoms.

CHARACTERISTICS OF A HEALTHY BUILDING ENVIRONMENT

A healthy building is an environment free of physical, biological, and psychosocial stressors. Such a building environment has the following characteristics (Table 29–3):

1. Free of environmental contaminants such as bacteria, fungi, and their by-products.

2. Free of pollutants such as smokes, fumes, gas, and chemical vapors.

Table 29–1. Recommended areas of sampling for mold and other organisms in a water-damaged building.

Sampling Location	Examples
Obvious mold growth	Walls, wallpapers, flooring, and bathtubs.
Water-damaged area	These are water-damaged areas and may or may not have visible mold growth.
Areas of high humidity	Bathrooms, basements, crawl spaces.
Heating ventilation air-conditioning system (HVAC)	Each unit or part of HVAC system with or without visible mold growth.
Any reported area of the building by affected individuals	Furniture, desk or tables, countertops, and various parts of the building with or without obvious mold growth.

3. Free of infestations such as cockroaches, ants, rats, and others.

4. Free of pets: Too many pets can cause health hazards such as exacerbation of allergy and asthma symptoms.

5. Good ventilation: Poor ventilation may trigger asthma symptoms.

Table 29–2. Examples of reported symptoms in sick building syndrome.

Head	Headaches, dizziness
Eyes	Irritation, pruritus, watery
Nose	Congestion, blockage
Sinuses	Congestion
Throat	Irritation
Skin	Dry, pruritus
Respiratory	Cough, shortness of breath, wheezing
Gastrointestinal	Nausea, vomiting, diarrhea, constipation
Senses	Sensitivity to odor
Constitutional	Fatigue
Cognition	Difficulty concentrating

Table 29–3. Characteristics of a healthy building.

Parameter	Examples	Comment
Contaminants	Bacteria, fungi or their by-products, animal dander or pollens	The building should be free of such contaminants. The fungi, animal dander or pollens can cause or exacerbate allergic rhinitis and asthma; bacterial or fungal toxins may cause nonspecific symptoms.
Pollutants	Smoke, fumes, gas vapors	Such pollutants can trigger asthma or cause irritation of the upper respiratory tract.
Infestation	Cockroaches, rats, and others	Such infestations not only trigger or exacerbate allergic rhinitis or asthma, but they also may cause irritation of the respiratory system.
Pets	Cats, dogs, rabbits, and others	These are triggers of allergic diseases such as allergic rhinitis and asthma.
Ventilation	Heating ventilation air-conditioning system (HVAC)	The HVAC system should be free of contaminants.
Light	Different light sources used in the building	Too bright or too dark areas may cause physical stress.
Humidity	Damp areas in basements, bathrooms, etc.	Keeping humidity below 55% helps control dust mites, fungi, and cockroaches.
Temperature	Too high or too low temperature	Too high or too low temperature can cause discomfort for building occupants.
Work stress	Job demand, workload, job performance	Work stress can affect well-being of the office worker.

6. Good lights throughout the building.

7. High or low humidity: Humidity below 55% is recommended for people with dust mite or mold allergy.

8. Suitable temperature: High or low temperatures can affect the building occupants and may cause health problems in addition to work performance.

9. Stress-free work environment: Work stress can affect the health of building occupants.

HOW TO PREVENT SICK BUILDING SYNDROME

The following strategies are suggested:

1. Avoidance: The best strategy is to avoid living in an unhealthy environment; to do that, one should inspect the residence before moving in. This is also true for the office building and any work environment.

2. Plumbing inspection: This is perhaps the most important part of building inspection. Residents should look for water-damaged areas and then look for the possible sources. Damaged pipes need to be fixed or replaced. After fix and repairing the source, the damaged areas, such as carpets, wallpaper, ceilings, floors, and others, should also be replaced.

3. Controlling humidity: Humidity should be kept below 55%, which can be achieved by using a dehumidifier. In addition to molds, such low humidity can also control dust mites and cockroach populations.

4. HVAC system: This system can get contaminated with molds/bacteria and their toxins. Circulating air from this system can distribute such contaminants to other sites of the building. The contaminated parts of HVAC system should be identified and replaced. If any of the units are damaged beyond repair, the entire unit should be replaced.

5. Washing, disinfecting, and maintaining a healthy environment: This not only helps remove the organisms but also helps maintain a healthy environment.

6. Preventing entrance of outdoor molds: To prevent entrance of outdoor molds to the indoor environment, windows and doors should be kept closed.

MANAGEMENT OF SICK BUILDING SYNDROME

The best solution for the affected individuals is moving to a new environment, that is, a new or different building. Those who live in apartment complexes should move to a different unit, ideally to a different building complex because other units of the same building may also have mold contamination. Individuals who suffer from sick building syndrome usually do better after moving to a healthy environment. If the symptoms persist in the new environment, other causes should be considered and investigated.

EVIDENCE-BASED MEDICINE

We have considered sick building syndrome as a biologic phenomenon. However, it is important to consider other factors contributing to the existence of such nonspecific symptoms. A series of recent publications have reviewed other parameters that may play roles in development of sick building syndrome; they include physical factors, such as light, temperature, and humidity of the buildings, and psychosocial factors, such as work stress affecting the occupants.

In a cross-sectional study, Marmote et al reviewed self-reported questionnaire from 4052 participants, 42 to 62 years of age, who were office occupants of 44 buildings in London. The obtained data were used to investigate the relationship of sick building syndrome with the physical and psychosocial work environment. The authors noted that the psychosocial work environment had more effect on the symptoms than the physical environment of the work area and the office buildings.

When managing the affected individuals, obtaining information such as past history of allergic diseases, family history of atopy, detailed history of the working environment including physical, such as light, temperature, ventilation; biological, such as fungal or bacterial contamination; and psychosocial factors, such as work-related stress, are crucial for better identification, diagnosis, and management.

BIBLIOGRAPHY

Dean TR, Roop B, Betancourt D, et al. A simple multiplex polymerase chain reaction assay for the identification of four environmentally relevant fungal contaminants. *J Microbiol Methods.* 2005;61:9.

Hardin BD, Kelman BJ, Saxon A. American College of Occupational and Environmental Medicine (ACOEM) evidence-based statement. Adverse human health effects associated with molds in indoor environment. *J Occup Environ Med.* 2003; 45:470.

Mahmoudi M., Gershwin E. Sick building syndrome. III. *Stachybotrys chartarum. J Asthma.* 2000;37(2):191.

Marmot AF, Eley J, Stafford M, et al. Building health: an epidemiological study of "sick building syndrome" in the Whitehall II study. *Occup Environ Med.* 2006;63:283.

Schmechel D, Simpsom JP, Beezhold D, et al. The development of species-specific immunodiagnostics for *Stachybotrys chartarum*: the role of cross-reactivity. *J Immunol Methods.* 2006; 309:150.

Allergy in the Elderly

Marianne Frieri, MD, PhD

CHRONIC RHINITIS AND SINUSITIS

Inflammatory and noninflammatory nonallergic rhinitis is more prevalent in the fifth decade and later in life. The elderly frequently have atrophic and medication-related rhinitis. Adults comprise the largest group with seasonal or perennial allergic rhinitis or both. In a survey by allergy immunology specialists of older adults, 6% are older than 70 years, and individuals in their 80s represent the fastest growing population in the United States.

There are many triggers for allergic rhinitis, but skin test reactivity decreases with age and symptoms tend to be milder. The elderly have variable nasal physiologic function and frequently have a dry nasal mucosa but complain of severe congestion, lack turbinate edema, and have negative skin tests. Structural changes can develop with aging due to atrophy of collagen and alterations in nasal cartilage. Other types of rhinitis in the elderly include idiopathic rhinitis and rhinitis due to granulomatous, collagen vascular diseases and neoplasia.

The elderly often consume multiple medications, especially for chronic cardiac and gastrointestinal disorders. Rhinitis due to medications is a condition for elderly patients on chronic β-blockers, diuretics, and antireflux therapy. Chronic nasal congestion can also lead to overuse of topical sympathomimetics, resulting in the development of rhinitis medicamentosa or, with oral α-adrenergic agonists, with hypertension or sleep disturbances.

Chronic sinusitis, an inflammatory process, also contributes to the cough common in elderly asthmatics and affects more than 30 million Americans. Chronic or persistent sinusitis can overlap with recurrent sinusitis and be associated with anatomic abnormalities, rhinitis, aspirin sensitivity, and nasal polyps that can occur in the elderly. Treatment consists of hydration, nasal lavage, antibiotics, and topical corticosteroids.

ASTHMA IN THE ELDERLY

The prevalence of asthma in older adults is approximately 5%, but the increased burden will increase. Evidence-based literature suggests asthma in older patients is often underdiagnosed and underrated, and older asthmatics have greater morbidity, mortality with a higher risk of hospitalization, and a lower quality of life. In addition, the elderly are more likely than younger patients to be poor perceivers of airway obstruction. Mishra reviewed asthma in the elderly and discussed the goals of treatment as maintaining desired level of activity, optimizing pulmonary function, controlling chronic symptoms, preventing and treating exacerbations, promoting prompt recognition, eliminating the need for emergency department or hospital visits, avoiding aggravating other medical conditions, and minimizing adverse effects from medications. A review chapter on asthma in the elderly by Barbee discussed a historical review of chronic obstructive pulmonary disease, which can overlap with asthma; the natural history of asthma in the elderly; changes in pulmonary function with age, which includes lowered forced expiratory volume in 1 second (FEV_1), FEV_1/FVC, diffusing capacity of lung for carbon monoxide (D_{LCO}), PO_2, muscle strength, and increased residual volume (RV). In addition, clinical characteristics, diagnosis, and comorbid disease, differential diagnosis, management, and education are discussed. There is a large overlap in the symptoms of chronic obstructive pulmonary disease (COPD) and asthma, but they have different risk factors and clinical course, and the differential diagnosis is an important step for successful management. Elderly patients with asthma may have airway remodeling and nonreversible disease associated with matrix changes reminiscent of COPD. The elderly woman with asthma and COPD needs special attention because it is more common in women. Coexisting diseases can occur with asthma, such as hypertension, coronary artery disease, diabetes, glaucoma, osteoporosis, and nicotine dependence, that can complicate the diagnosis. Advanced age is also a risk factor for asthma mortality.

OTHER ALLERGIC CONDITIONS

Acquired Angioedema, Anaphylaxis, Food and Drug Allergy

Chronic angioedema due to the acquired C1-INH deficiency can occur in the elderly, who can have adenocarcinoma of the colon or lymphoproliferative disease with antiidiotypic antibodies of monoclonal paraproteins. A depressed C1q complement component with a decreased C1 esterase inhibitor or CH50 in an older individual should raise a high suspicion for a lymphoproliferative disorder. Therapy with angiotensin-converting enzyme (ACE) inhibitors in the elderly can also lead to facial angioedema even after long-term therapy.

Anaphylaxis is an immediate systemic reaction due to rapid IgE-mediated release of potent mediators from tissue mast cells and peripheral blood basophils. Anaphylactoid reactions are immediate systemic reactions that mimic anaphylaxis but are not caused by IgE-mediated immune responses (Table 30–1). Cardiovascular abnormalities that can occur in the elderly also develop during anaphylaxis. Because the differential diagnosis could include myocardial infarction, it is important to note that arrhythmias and coronary artery vasospasm with ischemia can occur during exercise-induced anaphylactic events without the presence of intrinsic coronary artery obstruction. The capillary leak syndrome is a rare disorder usually associated with monoclonal gammopathy that can occur in the elderly. Table 30–2 lists the clinical findings associated with both anaphylaxis and anaphylactoid reactions. Systemic symptoms suggestive of anaphylaxis can occur with hypotension, angioedema, and gastrointestinal signs. Other disorders in the differential diagnosis of anaphylaxis include flushing disorders, which can occur with systemic mastocytosis; idiopathic anaphylaxis; or the carcinoid syndrome (Table 30–3). In older adults, systemic mastocytosis can result in leukemia, lymphoma, or carcinoma. Carcinoid-like symptoms can also be produced by oat cell carcinoma of the lung, medullary carcinoma, pancreatic tumors such as insulinoma, glucagonoma, vasoactive intestinal polypeptide-secreting tumors, and gastrinoma.

Table 30–1. Causes of anaphylaxis/anaphylactoid reactions.

Immunoglobulin E–mediated reactions
Foods
Antibiotics and other drugs
Foreign proteins (insulin, seminal proteins, latex, chymopapain)
Immunotherapy
Hymenoptera stings
Exercise plus food ingestion

Complement-mediated reactions
Blood; blood products

Nonimmunologic mast cell activators
Opiates (narcotics)
Radiocontrast media
Vancomycin (red man syndrome)
Dextran

Modulators of arachidonic acid metabolism
Nonsteroidal antiinflammatory agents
Tartrazine (possible)
Sulfiting agents
Idiopathic causes
Exercise
Catamenial anaphylaxis
Idiopathic recurrent anaphylaxis

From Kaliner MA. Anaphylaxis. In: Frieri M, Kettelhut B, eds. *Food Hypersensitivity and Adverse Reactions.* New York: Marcel Dekker; 1999:257, and Frieri M. Anaphylaxis. In: *Expert Guide to Critical Care.* Philadelphia: American College of Physicians. In press.

Table 30–2. Clinical findings in anaphylaxis and anaphylactoid reactions.

System	Signs	Symptoms
Cutaneous	Flushing, urticaria, angioedema	Flushing, pruritus
Cardiovascular	Tachycardia, hypotension, shock, syncope, arrhythmias	Faintness, palpitations, weakness
Gastrointestinal	Abdominal distension, vomiting, diarrhea	Bloating, nausea, cramps, pain
Respiratory	Rhinorrhea, laryngeal edema, wheezing, bronchorrhea, asphyxiation	Nasal congestion, shortness of breath, difficulty in breathing, choking, cough, hoarseness, lump in throat
Other	Diaphoresis, fecal or urinary incontinence	Feeling of impending doom, conjunctivitis, genital burning, metallic taste

From Kaliner MA. Anaphylaxis. In: Frieri M, Kettelhut B, eds. *Food Hypersensitivity and Adverse Reactions.* New York: Marcel Dekker; 1999:257.

Table 30–3. Differential diagnosis of anaphylaxis and anaphylactoid reactions.

Anaphylaxis
Immunoglobulin E mediated
Complement mediated
Nonimmunologic mast cell degranulation
Idiopathic
Exercise related
Sulfiting agents
Idiopathic causes
Nonsteroidal antiinflammatory drug reactions
Vasovagal collapse
Hereditary angioedema
Serum sickness
Systemic mastocytosis and urticaria pigmentosa
Pheochromocytoma
Carcinoid syndrome
Panic reactions
Münchhausen syndrome

From Kaliner MA. Anaphylaxis. In: Frieri M, Kettelhut B, eds. *Food Hypersensitivity and Adverse Reactions.* New York: Marcel Dekker; 1999:257.

Table 30–4. Differential diagnosis of food hypersensitivity.

Enzyme deficiencies
Transient fructose/sorbitol malabsorption
Lactase; sucrose deficiency
Phenylketonuria

Gastrointestinal disease
Postinfectious malabsorption
Viral, bacterial, parasitic
Hiatal hernia
Peptic ulcer
Gallbladder disease
Postsurgical dumping syndrome
Neoplasia
Inflammatory bowel disease
Pancreatic insufficiency

Additives and contaminants
Dyes
Tartrazine
Exogenous chemicals
Nitrates and nitrites
Monosodium glutamate
Sulfiting agents
Antibiotics

Endogenous chemicals
Caffeine
Tyramine
Phenylethylamine
Alcohol
Theobromine
Tryptamine

Toxins
Bacterial toxins
Aflatoxin
Botulism
Ergot
Fungi
Staphylococcal toxin
Toxigenic *Escherichia coli*
Vibrio cholerae
Endogenous toxins
Certain mushrooms (*Amanita muscaria*)
Shellfish (saxitoxin)
Psychological reactions
Bulimia
Anorexia nervosa

From Kaliner MA. Anaphylaxis. In: Frieri M, Kettelhut B, eds. *Food Hypersensitivity and Adverse Reactions.* New York: Marcel Dekker; 1999:257.

Many retired elderly play golf and can be exposed to insect allergy, and up to 3% of the population are at risk for anaphylaxis to insect stings with approximately 40 deaths per year. In addition, fire ants, biting insects, and mosquitoes can cause systemic reactions.

A recent review by Simons on long-term management of anaphylaxis in the community suggests specialists play a pivotal role. Comorbidities and concurrent medications in the elderly might interfere with recognition of triggers or symptoms, such as impairment of vision or hearing, neurology disease, or depression that might affect treatment of asthma, cardiovascular disease, or the inability to self-inject epinephrine. Concurrent administration of sedatives or hypnotics might affect treatment with β-adrenergic blockers or α-adrenergic blockers that decrease epinephrine efficacy by blocking effects at the adrenergic receptors.

Although food allergy is more common in children, most IgE-mediated reactions to foods in adults are caused by peanuts, tree nuts, fish, and shellfish. Many retired elderly travel and can have adverse food reactions. Foods may be contaminated by a wide variety of hidden substances that can be confused with food allergy, and other disorders in the elderly, such as hiatal hernia, peptic ulcer disease, malignancy, toxins or pharmacologic agents, can mimic food allergy. Table 30–4 reviews the differential diagnosis of food hypersensitivity.

Drug allergic reactions can be predictable or unpredictable due to an idiosyncratic reaction or intolerance, or they may be IgE mediated. Many elderly patients taking antibiotics, aspirin, nonselective nonsteroidal antiinflammatory medications or immunomodulators for arthritis, cancer, and other immune diseases can develop adverse drug reactions Such reactions could involve anaphylaxis or pseudoallergic reactions, angioedema, urticaria, maculopapular rashes, Stevens–Johnson syndrome or toxic epidermal necrolysis. Rigors, dyspnea, or hypotension can also occur with immunomodulators used to treat elderly patients with rheumatoid arthritis or Crohn disease, psoriasis, and other inflammatory disorders.

EVIDENCE-BASED MEDICINE

According to Sackett (*BMJ*; 1996:312:71), "evidence based medicine is conscientious, explicit and judicious use of current best evidence in making decisions about care of individual patients. The practice of evidence based medicine means integrity, individual clinical experience with the best available clinical evidence from systematic research." This chapter has provided several references from the literature in terms of review articles and sections from textbooks that critically explain mechanisms and can also be applied to patient care, intervention, and outcome.

BIBLIOGRAPHY

Georgitis JW. Differential diagnosis of chronic rhinitis at various ages. In: *Current Review of Rhinitis*. Philadelphia: Current Medicine; 2002:78.

Frieri M. Allergen and environmental triggers. *Emergency Med.* 1999;31:73.

Montanaro A. Allergic disease in the elderly: A wakeup call for the allergy community. *Ann Asthma Allergy Immunol.* 2000;85:85.

Slavin RG, Haselkorn T, Lee JH, et al. Asthma in older adults: Observation from the epidemiology and natural history of asthma: Outcomes and treatment regimes (TENOR) study. *Ann Asthma Allergy Immunol.* 2006;96:406.

Enright L. The diagnosis and management of asthma is much tougher in older patients. *Curr Opin Allergy Clin Immunol.* 2002;2:175.

Enright PL, McClelland RL, Newman AB, et al. Cardiovascular Health Study Research Group. Underdiagnosis and treatment of asthma in the elderly. *Chest.* 1999;116:606.

Mishra A. Asthma in the elderly. *Emerg Med.* 1999;95.

Barbee RA. Asthma in the elderly. In: Middleton E, et al., eds. *Allergy Principles and Practice.* Vol. 1. 3rd ed. 2001:1.

Frieri M. Seniors and asthma. *Asthma Magazine*, 2000. Available at: www.aaaai.org.

Kaliner MA, et al. Medical management of rhino sinusitis. In: Kaliner M, ed. *Current Review of Rhinitis.* Philadelphia: Current Medicine; 2003:101.

Frieri M. Management of asthma in women. *Women's Health Prim Care.* 2004;7(8):408.

Frieri M. Asthma concepts in the new millennium—update in asthma pathophysiology. *Allergy Asthma Proc.* 2005;26:83.

Kaliner MA. Anaphylaxis. In: Frieri M, Kettelhut B, eds. *Food Hypersensitivity and Adverse Reactions.* New York: Marcel Dekker; 1999:257.

Lieberman P. Anaphylaxis and anaphylactoid reactions In: Adkinson NE, Yunginger JW, Busse WW, et al., eds. *Middleton's Allergy Principles and Practice.* Vol 2. 6th ed. Philadelphia: Mosby; 2003.

Frieri M. Anaphylaxis. In: *Expert Guide to Critical Care.* Philadelphia: American College of Physicians. In press.

Attenhofer C, Rudolf S, Solomon F, et al. Ventricular fibrillation in a patient with exercise-induced anaphylaxis, normal coronary arteries, and a positive ergonovine test. *Chest.* 1994;105:620.

Frieri M, Linn N, Schweitzer M, et al. Lymphadenopathic mastocytosis with eosinophilia and biclonal gammopathy. *J Allergy Clin Immunol.* 1990;86:126.

Simons FER. Anaphylaxis, killer allergy. Long term management in the community. *J Allergy Clin Immunol.* 2006;117;367.

Frieri M. Cross-reactive and hidden allergies. In: Frieri M, Kettelhut B, eds. *Food Hypersensitivity and Adverse Reactions: A Practical Guide for Diagnosis and Management.* New York: Marcel Dekker; 1999:125.

Frieri M. Food allergy. In: Kaliner MA, ed. *Current Review of Allergic Disease.* Philadelphia: Current Medicine; 1999:173.

Shearer WM, Leung DYM. Mini-primer on allergic and immunologic disease. *J Allergy Clin Immunol.* 2006;117(suppl):S429.

Horne NS, Narayan A, Frieri M. Toxic epidermal necrolysis in systemic lupus erythematosus *Autoimmunity Rev.* 2006;5:160.

Diagnostic Testing in Allergic Diseases

31

Paul Cheng, MD, PhD, FAAAAI

When a medical history is suggestive of an allergic cause, proper testing is performed to identify clinically relevant allergens. The discovery of IgE antibody, along with the recognition of its central role in the allergic reaction, has established the identification of allergen-specific IgE as the key to the diagnosis of allergic diseases. Both in vivo skin testing and laboratory allergy testing are designed to detect allergen-specific IgE, although the pathophysiology of allergy is far more complex than just an IgE-mediated condition. Diagnostic testing for non–IgE-mediated allergic reactions and for allergies with predominant late-phase reaction, as well as challenge testing with food or other allergens, are beyond the scope of this chapter.

PERCUTANEOUS ALLERGY TESTING

The abundance of cutaneous mast cells, predominantly the MCTC phenotype that contains both tryptase and chymase, makes skin an idea place for in vivo allergy testing. Mast cell degranulation with the release of histamine and other immediate mediators on introduction of allergen extract to the skin is the hallmark of allergy skin testing. With the presence of allergen-specific IgE bound to it receptors on mast cells, an immediate wheal-and-flare response is elicited when two IgE-receptor molecules are cross-linked by their relevant allergens introduced to the skin. This immediate response is mediated mainly by histamine and, to a lesser extent, by tryptase. Through axon reflex, histamine released from mast cells can also trigger the release of neurogenic mediators, such as substance P and neurokinin A, which can further activate mast cell granulation and histamine release to intensify the wheal-and-flare response.

Prick/Puncture Method

The most widely used skin testing technique for allergy diagnosis is the prick/puncture method (Figure 31–1).

The skin is pricked or gently punctured, without causing bleeding, to allow allergen extract to penetrate into the epidermal space. Allergen extracts are placed on the volar surface of the arm or the back, and the test always includes histamine (positive control) and allergen extract diluent (negative control). Test for each allergen extract and control solution should be positioned at least 2 to 2.5 cm apart. The reactions from each allergen are read one by one, usually in 15 to 20 minutes, by comparing to the size of wheal in the histamine and diluent control. It is generally accepted that a reaction is considered positive if its wheal diameter is at least 3 mm greater than the negative control, which should be completely nonreactive. Reaction can be further graded qualitatively (grade 0 to 4) by comparison to the size of the histamine control (Table 31–1) or semi-quantitatively by measuring and recording the diameters of the wheal-and-flare from each allergen tested.

Several skin testing devices are available commercially. Practicing allergists usually consider accuracy, consistency, convenience, and cost in selecting their preferred devices. In a recent study comparing eight devices, it was found that single-headed devices demonstrated a higher degree of sensitivity and reproducibility as compared to multiheaded devices. Regardless of the device chosen, allergy skin testing should be performed by a well-trained staff under the supervision of an allergist to ensure consistent and reproducible results.

Here are some of the common errors in allergy skin testing that should be avoided:

1. False-negative from insufficient penetration of allergen extract into the epidermal space or using extracts with insufficient potency.

2. False-negative from drugs blocking the immediate wheal-and-flare reactions, including all H1 antihistamines, some tricyclic antidepressants, and ketotifen (not available in the United States). Patients are usually told to stop first-generation H1 antihistamines

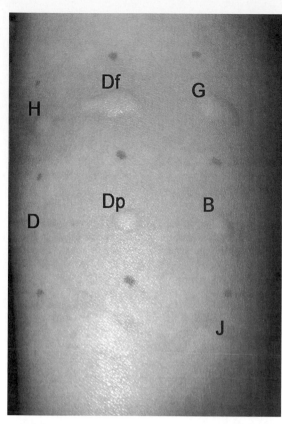

Figure 31–1. Prick allergy skin testing shows marked wheal-and-flare reactions to dust mites and grass allergens on a 4-year-old child with frequent sneezing and coughing for 2 months. H, histamine control; D, diluent; Dp, mite—major allergen from *Dermatophagoides pteronyssinus*; Df, *Dermatophagoides farinae*; G, mix of seven major grass allergens; B, Bermuda grass; J, Johnson grass.

Table 31–1. Grading criteria by wheal size for allergy skin testing.

Grade	Wheal reaction
0	No significant wheal reaction
1	Wheal size smaller than half of histamine control
2	Wheal size greater than half of histamine but smaller than histamine control
3	Wheal size about the same as histamine control
4	Wheal size greater than histamine control
4P	Pseudopod present

This grading system may be applied when the wheal reaction from histamine is at least 5 mm in diameter while negative control is completely nonreactive. Note that the histamine control reaction may often peak before the allergen reactions and may need to be read sooner.

for 2 days and second-generation H1 antihistamines for 5 days prior to skin testing. H2 antihistamines have minimal inhibitory effects on allergy skin testing. Likewise, leukotriene antagonist, now frequently prescribed for allergy patients, or oral steroid do not interfere with immediate reaction on skin testing. Intermittent use of topical corticosteroid or pimecrolimus does not appear to have a significant effect on skin testing either.

3. Applying allergy testing on patients with certain skin condition, such as eczema, may reduce skin reactivity. On the contrary, performing skin testing on patients with dermographism is very likely to get false-positive or nonspecific irritating reactions. The testing should always be performed on normal skin.

4. Skin testing should not be performed when the patient's history is suggestive of anaphylaxis or any severe systemic reactions from a particular allergen. This is more often in the case of food allergies. A thorough history should always be taken before carrying out skin testing to avoid unnecessary adverse reactions.

Intradermal Testing

When the history indicates allergy as a cause but prick testing is not revealing, further testing by the intradermal method may be used. A small volume (about 0.02 mL) of the allergen extract is injected intracutaneously (into the dermis) using a tuberculin syringe with a 26-gauge needle. The starting dose should be at least a 100-fold dilution of the extract used for prick/puncture testing to avoid large local reaction or potential systemic reactions. Intradermal testing has greater sensitivity but less specificity and should be interpreted cautiously with clinical history. It is not recommended for the diagnosis of food allergies because intradermal injection of food allergen extracts has a high false-positive rate and greater risks of systemic reactions. Intradermal testing is performed more often for the diagnosis of bee venoms or drug allergies (penicillin and local anesthetic agents). It is rarely indicated to perform intradermal testing with more than just a few selected allergens and would increase the unnecessary risks of systemic reactions to do so.

Diagnostic Value of Percutaneous Allergy Testing

It is critical that skin testing demonstrates high sensitivity and specificity in identifying allergens with clinical significance to make an effective allergen avoidance plan or formulate an allergen-specific immunotherapy program. Although allergy testing is conducted on the skin for the diagnosis of an allergy condition with symptoms often from different target organ systems, the diagnostic value of allergy skin testing is well established for conditions caused by inhalant allergens. The predictive value is over 95% for a positive skin test associated with an inhalant allergen when the history also suggests clinical sensitivity related to this allergen. With symptoms suggesting allergies, positive skin testing also correlates well with bronchial or nasal challenge. In the case of food allergy, correlation between positive prick testing and clinical symptoms or food challenge is not as significant. Although it has excellent negative predictive value, skin testing positive on food allergen has only about 30% predictive value of clinical sensitivity. Thus when performing allergy testing, it is critical to recognize that a positive reaction does not necessarily identify the allergens causing the symptoms. One should never make the diagnosis of allergy based on the results of the test alone.

IN VITRO MEASUREMENT OF ALLERGEN-SPECIFIC IMMUNOGLOBULIN E

In vitro testing is used when skin testing is not appropriate for patients under some circumstances previously mentioned, such as (1) those with a significant skin condition; (2) those who cannot discontinue antihistamines or other drugs that may interfere with a reaction to allergens on skin testing; or (3) those with a history of severe reaction to allergens and skin testing when these allergens may be of significant risk. Since it was introduced in the 1960s, radioallergosorbent test (RAST) has been the major form of in vitro measurement of allergen-specific serum IgE. In this assay, serum containing allergen-specific IgE from patients is incubated with allergens coupled to the sorbent. The bound IgE is further detected by ^{125}I-labeled anti-IgE antibodies. The level of specific IgE is measured by the percentage of total radioactivity bound to allergosorbent and reported in KU/L in which 1 KU/L equals 2.4 μg/L of IgE.

This widely used assay is gradually being replaced by a new fluorescence enzyme immunoassay (Pharmacia CAP system). In this system, the sensitivity level is greatly enhanced by using cellulose sponge to increase binding capacity to allergens and fluorescent-labeled anti-IgE antibodies for detection. Table 31–2 shows one of the commonly used score systems for this immunoassay.

Table 31–2. Scoring system of Pharmacia CAP System fluorescent immunoassay.

KU/L	Class	Interpretation
<0.10	0	Negative
0.10–0.34	0/1	Equivocal/borderline
0.35–0.69	1	Low positive
0.7–3.4	2	Moderate positive
3.5–17.4	3	High positive
17.5–49.9	4	Very high positive
50–99.9	5	Very high positive
>100	6	Very high positive

As in the case of skin testing, individuals with a positive in vitro test demonstrating the presence of allergen-specific IgE above normal range may show no clinical reactivity with no target organ symptoms to these allergens. However, the higher the level of IgE (class 3 or higher), the more likely one finds correlation to clinical symptoms, especially for inhalant allergens. A cutoff IgE level for selected food allergens, including egg, milk, peanut, tree nuts, fish, soy, and wheat, with greater than 95% correlation to clinical symptoms confirmed by a double-blind food challenge was established in recent studies.

Most commercial laboratories report total serum IgE along with individual allergen-specific IgE. Although total serum IgE is generally elevated in patients with an allergic condition, it has very limited value in the diagnosis of allergic diseases. In fact, when total IgE is very high (over 1000 IU/L), the results on individual allergens are more likely to be false-positive because of the presence of abundant IgE with no defined specificity competing with allergen-specific IgE in the assay. Total serum IgE is needed only in the diagnosis of certain conditions such as allergic bronchopulmonary allergic aspergillosis or hyper-IgE syndrome. It is also required when prescribing anti-IgE therapy because the initial dosage is calculated according to the body weight and total serum IgE level of the patients.

Allergists tend to advocate skin testing versus laboratory measurement of allergen-specific IgE. When properly performed, skin testing has the advantages of greater sensitivity, ease of performance, and immediate availability of the results.

With the improved sensitivity and specificity of the newer fluorescent enzyme immunoassay system, we may see a trend toward increasing usage of these tests, which are actively promoted by commercial laboratories to primary care physicians, allergists, and other specialists alike. It is critical that all ordering physicians have sufficient knowledge and clinical experience to interpret the results of these tests.

A related issue involves the selection of allergens to be tested. How many allergens should be included when ordering a test panel? Again, the decision is made after a thorough history is taken, and only clinically relevant allergens should be tested. Although the fluorescent enzyme immunoassay may be superior to other allergy tests, it is expensive. Ordering a large number of clinically irrelevant tests not only contributes to unnecessary cost, the information from these tests may be misleading, and the management plans based on the results from these tests may not be warranted. This principle of prudence in allergy testing applies to both inhalant and food allergens, either by skin testing or in vitro IgE measurement. When the history gives an impression of an allergic condition but does not suggest any allergen trigger, a screening test to cover large number of allergens hoping to find something positive is not how allergy should be practiced. Any screening panel should consist of limited tests according to the age and geographic location of the patients and the symptoms they present.

ALLERGY TESTING WITH NO PROVEN VALUE

Many allergy diagnostic tests are without scientific basis and have no proven diagnostic value. These are often promoted by the laboratories or by practitioners without formal allergy training. The following is a short list from the position paper published by the American Academy of Allergy, Asthma, and Immunology: measurement of serum IgG antibodies, mostly to food and mold allergens; food immune complex assay; kinesiology; end-point titration and provocation-neutralization, just to name a few. Many patients have received unwarranted or inappropriate treatments or have had unnecessary diet restriction based on the results of these tests. It is the responsibility of the entire medical community to be aware of and prevent the misuse of these scientifically unsound diagnostic tests and treatments.

EVIDENCE-BASED MEDICINE: NEWER TRENDS IN ALLERGY TESTING

As more standardized allergens become available, they should be used in both treatment and diagnostic testing for allergic diseases and research involving skin testing. The skin reaction can be better quantified and correlated to clinical symptoms when standardized reagents are used in the testing. Synthetic peptides with defined epitopes may offer higher specificity in allergy testing. Beyer et al have identified three immunodominant epitopes on peanut allergen Ara h 2 that preferentially bind to serum IgE from patients with symptomatic peanut allergies but not from those who are sensitized but asymptomatic or had "outgrown" their peanut allergies. Similarly, Ballmer-Weber and his group have shown higher specificity in the diagnosis of carrot allergies by using recombinant peptides.

Another new trend in the diagnosis of food allergies is to perform the so-called prick-to-prick skin testing. In this method, fresh allergens are used by first pricking raw fruits or vegetables and then pricking the skin immediately with the same needle. Again, the advantage of this approach is based on the assumption that clinically relevant epitopes from these foods have changed or been lost in the production of commercial food extracts used for conventional skin testing. This test has been applied more for the diagnosis of oral allergy syndrome. Bolhaar and her colleagues have shown the efficacy of prick-to-prick testing in assessing the allergenicity of apples confirmed by double-blind, placebo-controlled food challenge.

BIBLIOGRAPHY

AAAAI Work Group Report. Current approach to the diagnosis and management of adverse reactions to foods. Available at: www.aaaai.org/media/resources/academy_statements/practice_papers/adverse_reactions_to_foods.asp.

Bolhaar ST, van de Weg WE, van Ree R., et al. In vivo assessment with prick-to-prick testing and double-blind, placebo-controlled food challenge of allergenicity of apple cultivars. *J Allergy Clin Immunol.* 2005;116:1080.

Ballmer-Weber BK, Wangorsch A, Bohle B, et al. Component-resolved in vitro diagnosis in carrot allergy: Does the use of recombinant carrot allergens improve the reliability of the diagnostic procedure? *Clin Exp Allergy.* 2005;35:970.

Beyer K., Ellman-Grunther L, Jarvinen K-M, et al. Measurement of peptide-specific IgE as an additional tool in identifying patients with clinical reactivity to peanuts. *J Allergy Clin Immunol.* 2003:112:202.

Carr WW, Martin B, Howard RS, et al. Comparison of test devices for skin prick testing. *J Allergy Clin Immunol.* 2005;116:341.

European Academy of Allergology and Clinical Immunology. Allergen standardization and skin tests [position paper]. *Allergy.* 1993;48:48.

Sampson HA: Utility of food-specific IgE concentrations in predicting symptomatic food allergy. *J Allergy Clin Immunol.* 2001;107:891.

Sicherer SH, Bock SA. An expanding evidence base provides food for thought to avoid indigestion in managing difficult dilemmas in food allergy. *J Allergy Clin Immunol.* 2006;117:1419.

Primary Immunodeficiencies

Pedro C. Avila, MD

Deficiencies in the immune system increase susceptibility to infections, autoimmune disorders, and lymphoproliferative diseases. The characteristics of infections provide clues as to what functions of the immune system are defective. Infections in immunodeficient patients can be caused by common or opportunistic organisms and are frequent, severe, recurrent, and difficult to treat. Autoimmune diseases can be of any type, most commonly blood cytopenias, gastroenteropathies, and endocrinopathies. Malignancies are more often hematologic or gastrointestinal cancers.

The most common immunodeficiencies are those secondary to human immunodeficiency virus (see Chapter 33), to lymphoproliferative diseases, and to medical treatments (iatrogenic) resulting from radiation and chemotherapy for cancers as well as from immunosuppressant therapy for autoimmune diseases. Mild immunodeficiency defects also occur during certain infections (e.g., Epstein-Barr virus, malaria), chronic diseases (e.g., diabetes mellitus, chronic renal insufficiency), nutritional deficiencies (e.g., protein-energy malnutrition, zinc and vitamin deficiencies), protein-losing conditions (e.g., intestinal lymphangiectasis), and autoimmune leukocyte disorders (autoimmune neutropenia or lymphocytopenia). These acquired or secondary immunodeficiencies should always be considered in patients suspected of having an immunodeficiency.

In this chapter, we discuss the most common primary immunodeficiencies, which result from genetic defects or have unknown etiologies. This group of immunodeficiencies is rapidly expanding as new specific genetic defects are discovered in the immune system. Although more than 120 conditions have been characterized, for many only a few cases have been described.

WHEN TO SUSPECT IMMUNODEFICIENCY AND HOW TO WORK IT UP

The immune system is still developing in infants and children as they face their first antigenic challenges, mount specific adaptive responses, and build immunologic memory. Some immunologic parameters only achieve adult levels in adolescence. As a result, evaluation of the immune system needs to take into consideration the patient's age. If a local laboratory has not established its own age-specific normal ranges, consult appropriate references. For example, normal serum immunoglobulin concentration ranges are lower and lymphocyte count higher in newborns and infants compared with older children and adults (Table 32–1). Serum immunoglobulin concentrations are low in newborns and slowly rise until adolescence. A blood lymphocyte count of $1500/\text{mm}^3$ is low normal for adults but is a sign of severe combined immunodeficiency in neonates. Functional assays of adaptive immunity using antigens depend on previous exposure and sensitization to establish memory response and thus are not very helpful in infants. Therefore, the clinician needs to be aware of the patient's age and previous exposures and vaccinations when functionally assessing the immune system for memory adaptive immunity, particularly in neonates and infants.

The most common manifestations of immunodeficiencies are infections (Table 32–2). Because of the lack of previous exposures with development of memory adaptive immunity, healthy infants and children normally suffer infections more frequently than older children and adults. Infants attending child care can develop one acute upper respiratory infection (common cold) per month. Likewise, child care workers and teachers of young children develop respiratory infections more often than adults in jobs without much contact with the public or frequently ill people. Adults usually develop one to two common colds a year. Besides the frequency of infections, how a host handles common infections is important. Immunodeficient patients often have prolonged common colds lasting longer than 10 days, and they often develop postcold complications such as otitis media (in children), sinusitis (in adults), bronchitis, and even pneumonia. They may present with frequent prolonged infections that require antibiotic therapy, and infections may recur soon after the usual 7- to 10-day antibiotic courses,

Table 32–1. Normal characteristics of the developing immune system.

Test	Neonates		Infants		Children		Adults
Age	1–30d	1–6 mo	7–12 mo	13–24 mo	2–9y	10–17y	>18 y
Complete Blood Count							
White count (10^3/mm³)	9.1–34.0	6.0–14.0	6.0–14.0	6.0–14.0	4.0–12.0	4.0–10.5	4.0–10.5
Neutrophils (10^3/mm³)	6.0–23.5	1.1–6.6	1.1–6.6	1.1–6.6	1.4–6.6	1.5–6.6	1.5–6.6
• Segmented (10^3/mm³)	6.0–20.0	1.0–6.0	1.0–6.0	1.0–6.0	1.2–6.0	1.3–6.0	1.3–6.0
• Bands (10^3/mm³)	<3.5	<1.0	<1.0	<1.0	<1.0	<1.0	<1.0
Lymphocytes (10^3/mm³)	3.5–10.5	1.8–9.0	1.8–9.0	1.8–9.0	1.0–5.5	1.0–3.5	1.5–3.5
Eosinophils (10^3/mm³)	<2.0	<0.7	<0.7	<0.7	<0.7	<0.7	<0.7
Serum							
IgG (mg/dL)	140–930	250–1190	320–1250	400–1250	560–1380	680–1600	700–1500
IgA (mg/dL)	5–65	10–90	17–95	24–192	26–260	45–380	60–400
IgM (mg/dL)	14–140	14–170	14–170	24–170	35–250	35–250	35–250
IgE (IU/mL)*	0.0–6.6	0.0–6.6	0.0–6.6	0.0–20.0	0.0–60.0	3.6–100.0	3.6–100.0

*1.0 IU/mL of IgE = 2.4 ng/mL of IgE.

needing repeated and prolonged courses for what should be easily treatable common respiratory or mucocutaneous infections. Immunodeficient patients may also have opportunistic infections, deep-seated infections, and/or family history of immunodeficiency or of a relative who died young of an infection. Besides infections, a defective immune system may allow autoimmune and lymphoproliferative diseases to arise as already mentioned. Lastly, specific immunodeficiencies have characteristic accompanying disorders and physical signs that may hint at the diagnosis.

An initial workup for primary immunodeficiency can include (1) complete blood count and differential count; (2) quantitative serum immunoglobulins (IgG, IgA, IgM, and IgE); (3) flow cytometry typing of circulating T cells (CD3), T-cell subsets (CD4 and CD8 T cells), B cells (CD20 or CD19), and natural killer (NK) cells (CD16 and CD56 double positive); (4) complement hemolytic activity, CH50; (5) isohemagglutinin titers; (6) antibody titers to immunizations such as titers to pneumococcus serotypes and to diphtheria and tetanus toxoids. In addition, other tests can be obtained based on the history and types of infections, which can indicate what component of the immune system is defective, as shown in Table 32–2. Other tests may be appropriate to rule out other diseases. For example, the differential diagnosis for recurrent sinopulmonary infections includes HIV infection, aspiration (e.g., tracheoesophageal fistula, gastroesophageal reflux, impaired swallowing and gag reflex), anatomic obstruction (e.g.,

malformations, foreign body, cancer, polyps, scarring from recurrent nasosinus surgery), and mucociliary dysfunction (e.g., cystic fibrosis, ciliary dyskinesis). Low-serum IgG and IgA, but not usually the large pentameric IgM, occurs in (nephrotic syndrome) or in protein-losing enteropathy. The latter is caused by intestinal lymphangiectasis resulting in leak of lymph into intestinal lumen. It is diagnosed by measuring alpha-1 anti-trypsin in stools. In severe cases, patients may even lose lymphocytes and become lymphopenic.

ANTIBODY DEFICIENCIES

X-Linked Agammaglobulinemia

X-linked agammaglobulinemia (XLA) was the first reported primary immunodeficiency (by Ogden Bruton in 1952). It is caused by mutations in the Bruton tyrosine kinase (Btk, located in chromosome Xq22), which leads to an arrest in B cell development at the pre–B cell stage. As a result, patients have no B cells, and IgG is less than 200 mg/dL. The other immunoglobulins are also extremely low or absent (IgM, IgA, IgD, and IgE). Its prevalence is 1 in 100,000.

CLINICAL MANIFESTATIONS

Patients present with recurrent pyogenic infections starting at 5 to 6 months of age when passively placentally transferred maternal antibodies have waned. These

Table 32–2. Manifestations of immunodeficiency and laboratory investigation.

Manifestations	Immune Defects	Laboratory Investigation

Antibody Deficiencies
Recurrent sinopulmonary infections:[a]
• >2 sinusitis or bronchitis per year needing antibiotic therapy.
• Sinusitis needing antibiotics orally for >2 mo or intravenously.
• Repeated endoscopic sinus surgery for chronic sinusitis.
• >2 pneumonias per year.
• Bronchiectasis.
Enteroviral gastroenteritis or meningo-encephalitis (e.g., polio, echo)
	• X-linked agammaglobulinemia
	• Common variable immunodeficiency
	• Transient hypogammaglobulinemia of infancy.
	• Hyper-IgM immunodeficiency
	• IgA deficiency
	• IgM deficiency
	• IgG subclass deficiency
	• Immunodeficiency with thymoma
	• Transcobalamin deficiency
		Components:
		• Serum IgG, IgM, IgA.
		• Flow cytometry:
		  • B cell count (CD19 or CD20)
		  • CD40L (CD154) on T cells
		• Serum IgG subclasses
		Functional:[b]
		• Isohemagglutinins (IgM response)
		• Antibody response to vaccines (IgG response)

Complement Deficiencies Recurrent sinopulmonary infections with encapsulated microbes[c] Recurrent neisseria (gonococcal or meningococcal) invasive diseases.	• Deficiency of classic pathway proteins. • Deficiency of alternative pathway proteins.	*Components:* Serum complement proteins *Functional:* CH50, AH50

T-Cell Deficiencies
Recurrent opportunistic infections with:
• Herpesvirus infections (CMV, EBV, HSV)
• Vaccinia, adenovirus, measles
• Molluscum contagiosum
• Pyogenic bacteria[a]
• Mycobacterial infections
• Fungi: candida, aspergillus, *Pneumocystis carinii*
• Intracellular bacteria[d]
Growth failure in infants.
Persistent mucocutaneous candidiasis after 1 y of age.
Protracted diarrhea.
	Combined T- and B-cell deficiencies:
	• Severe combined immunodeficiencies
	• Wiskott-Aldrich syndrome
	• Ataxia-telangiectasis
	• Enzyme deficiencies
	• Bare lymphocyte syndrome
	• Omenn syndrome
	• X-linked lymphoproliferative disease
	• Reticular dysgenesis
	Isolated T-cell deficiencies:
	• DiGeorge and chromosome 22 anomaly
	• Idiopathic CD4 lymphopenia
	• Chronic mucocutaneous candidiasis
	Natural killer deficiency
		Components:
		• CBC lymphocyte count
		• Flow cytometry:
		  • T cells (CD3)
		  • T-cell subsets and ratio (CD4-to-CD8 ratio)
		  • Naive (CD45RA) and memory (CD45RO)
		  • B cells (CD20 or CD19)
		  • NK cells (CD16 + CD56 double stained)
		  • HLA-DR
		  • CD40L (CD154) on T cells
		• FISH of chromosome 22 (probe 22q11)
		Functional:
		• Delayed hypersensitivity testing[e]
		• Lymphocyte proliferation to mitogens[f]
		• Lymphocyte proliferation to antigens[g]
		• Mixed lymphocyte reaction[g]
		• NK cell cytolytic activity
		• Leukocyte enzyme assays: ADA, PNP

Phagocyte Deficiencies Recurrent infections with catalase-positive bacteria and fungi[h] Recurrent skin abscesses	Neutropenic syndromes Chronic granulomatous deficiency Myeloperoxidase deficiency Leukocyte adhesion molecule deficiencies	*Components:* • Serial CBC with neutrophil count • Flow cytometry: • CD18 on PMA stimulated granulocytes

(Continued)

Table 32–2. Manifestations of immunodeficiency and laboratory investigation. (Continued)

Manifestations	Immune Defects	Laboratory Investigation
Phagocyte Deficiencies		
Recurrent lymphadenitis Deep-seated abscesses (e.g., lung, liver) Mycobacterial infections Chronic periodontal disease, gingivitis	Leukocyte G6PD deficiency IFN-γ/IL12 axis deficiency	• Sialyl-Lewis^X on stimulated granulocytes • IFN-γ receptor • IL12p70 secretion from stimulated monocytes • Antineutrophil antibody *Functional:* • Neutrophil oxidative burst[i] • Leukocyte G6PD and MPO • Staphylococcal killing assay[j] • Neutrophil chemotaxis[j]

ADA, adenosine deaminase; AH50, alternative complement hemolytic activity 50%; CBC, complete blood count; CH50, classical complement hemolytic activity 50%; CMV, cytomegalovirus; EBV, Epstein-Barr virus; FISH, fluorescent in situ hybridization; G6PD, glucose-6-phosphate dehydrogenase; HLA, human leukocyte antigen; HSV, *Herpes simplex* virus; IFN, interferon; MPO, myeloperoxidase; NK, natural killer; PNP, purine nucleoside phosphorylase; PMA: phorbol myristate acetate.

[a]Recurrent sinopulmonary infections due to encapsulated organisms, such as pneumococci, streptococci, *Haemophilus influenzae*, and less often staphylococci. These and intestinal gram-negative bacteria are also known as pyogenic bacteria.

[b]Isohemagglutinins are IgM antibodies against ABO blood group antigens. Thus ABO blood typing needs to be performed simultaneously because AB blood type will not develop anti-A or anti-B antibodies. Titers become positive after 1 year of age (>1:4). Specific antibody titers to vaccines include titers to tetanus toxoid, diphtheria toxoid, *H. influenzae* type B (Hib), and hepatitis B surface antigen, which are all part of the regular immunization schedule in the first 6 months of life in the United States. Pneumovax is not very immunogenic in children younger than 2 years. Its immunogenicity improves slowly with age until adulthood. It contains capsular polysaccharides from 23 pneumococcus serotypes (1, 2, 3, 4, 5, 6B, 7F, 8, 9N, 9V, 10A, 11A, 12F, 14, 15B, 17F, 18C, 19F, 19A, 20, 22F, 23F, 33F). Prevnar contains aluminum adjuvant and polysaccharides from 7 pneumococcus serotypes (4, 6B, 9V, 14, 18C, 19F, 23F) conjugated with diphtheria CRM$_{197}$ protein, which makes it immunogenic in infants younger than 2 years. Toxoids and other protein vaccines generate a predominantly IgG$_1$ response, whereas polysaccharides generate a predominantly IgG$_2$ response. There is great controversy about what constitutes an adequate antibody response to rule out antibody deficiency. Comparing specific antibody levels before and 3 to 4 weeks after vaccination, many consider an adequate response either a fourfold increase in specific antibody levels or achieving immunity levels from previously nonimmune levels. In addition, for pneumococcus vaccines, an adequate response to only 30% to 50% of the serotypes for which antibodies were measured may be considered an adequate response.

[c]Both antibody and complement deficiency are associated with recurrent sinopulmonary infections with encapsulated organisms.

[d]Examples of intracellular bacteria are *Mycobacteria, Campylobacter,* and *Listeria.*

[e]Delayed hypersensitivity testing (DHT) assesses *in vivo* the specific lymphocyte memory response to antigens to which the patient should have been exposed and sensitized. Antigens are injected intradermically (0.1 mL) and an induration of more than 5 mm is expected in 48 to 72 hours. Antigens commonly used are *Candida,* tetanus toxoid, and mumps. Young children may not have yet acquired the appropriate immunity to respond normally to this test.

[f]Mitogens are lectins that bind to surface glycoproteins (e.g., receptors) activating leukocytes. They test lymphocyte proliferative capacity *in vitro*. Phytohemagglutinin (PHA) and concanavalin A (Con A) are T-cell mitogens. They bind to and crosslink T- cell receptors (TCR) inducing T-cell proliferation. Con A stimulation also requires a costimulatory signal to exert its effect. Pokeweed mitogen (PWM) induces proliferation of both T and B cells. To induce proliferation of B cells only, some laboratories use staphylococcal protein A, a B-cell superantigen, not a lectin.

[g]Specific lymphocyte proliferation to antigens *in vitro* depends on previous sensitization and memory cellular response to the relevant antigen. Thus young children may not have yet developed appropriate immunity to respond normally to this test. Antigens commonly used are tetanus toxoid and *Candida.* In mixed lymphocyte reaction, patient's lymphocytes are exposed to irradiated allogenic mononuclear cells and proliferate due to HLA incompatibility.

[h]Catalase-positive microbes include staphylococci, *Serratia marcescens, Klebsiella, Escherichia coli, Burkholderia cepacia, Candida, Aspergillus,* and *Nocardia.* Their catalases catabolize the abnormal small amount of hydrogen peroxide produced by defective neutrophils allowing their replication.

[i]Several tests to assess the ability of neutrophils to produce reactive oxygen species, particularly hydrogen peroxide, are available, including light microscopy (nitroblue tetrazolium [NBT] oxidation from a yellow to a dark blue color), flow cytometry, chemiluminescence, or superoxide production.

[j]Staphylococcal killing assay and neutrophil chemotaxis are very difficult to standardize and available in only a few laboratories.

infections include recurrent otitis media, bronchitis, pneumonia, and meningitis. Repeated pneumonias may lead to bronchiectasis. The most common microbes are pneumococci, *Haemophilus influenzae,* and other streptococci, but gram-negative bacteria may also be involved. Usually infections recur soon after antibiotic courses are finished with short periods of good health.

These patients are also more susceptible to a few virus infections even though they have normal T-cell function. These viruses include wild viruses or live attenuated vaccine viruses related to varicella, measles, paralytic poliomyelitis, and enteroviruses (e.g., echovirus, which can cause meningoencephalitis).

Other manifestations include abnormal dental decay, malabsorption, failure to thrive, chronic conjunctivitis, eczematoid skin infections, and rheumatoid arthritis–like disease. Malabsorption may be due to *Giardia lamblia* infestation. On physical examination, patients with XLA lack lymph nodes and tonsils but have a spleen.

Laboratory diagnosis is based on extremely low-serum IgG, IgA, and IgM and the absence of circulating B cells. Functional antibody responses are also greatly impaired to absent (isohemagglutinins and antibody response to vaccines), but they are not necessary when serum immunoglobulins are extremely low. CH50, T cells, and NK cells are all normal. Rarely, intestinal mucosal biopsy has been obtained to demonstrate lack of plasma cells in the lamina propria. In specialized genetic laboratories, analysis of the Btk gene for mutations can be performed to confirm the diagnosis. Diagnosis is particularly difficult in the first 6 to 9 months of age when maternal antibodies still circulate in the infant. Lack of circulating or tissue B cells can help diagnose XLA. Alternatively, serum immunoglobulins can be checked again in 3 months while infections are treated, antibiotic prophylaxis given, and live virus vaccines avoided. In XLA, the antibody levels progressively decline and never rise, whereas in transient hypogammaglobulinemia of infancy, the levels recover by 18 to 24 months of age. Normal T cells and the absence of circulating B cells, however, are characteristic of XLA and can help differentiate it from transient hypogammaglobulinemia of infancy, congenital HIV infection, early-onset common variable immunodeficiency, and severe combined immunodeficiency.

Treatment consists of immunoglobulin replacement, which leads to an excellent prognosis. In addition, clinicians should be vigilant for infections and the comorbidities just described that require specific workup and treatment.

Transient Hypogammaglobulinemia of Infancy

In transient hypogammaglobulinemia of infancy (THI), infants experience a delay in the maturation of their antibody synthesis ability. The cause is unknown, but it subsides by the end of infancy. Term infants naturally experience a decline in IgG concentrations with a nadir at 5 to 6 months, at which point maternally transferred IgG has been metabolized and the infant's own antibody production is developing. The lowest serum IgG levels reach about 350 mg/dL, and normal infants may begin to experience respiratory infections such as otitis media episodes. Premature infants may have less maternal IgG at birth and can experience a longer and deeper nadir in serum IgG levels until their own IgG synthesis reaches normal levels.

THI infants have persistent low IgG levels, whereas IgM and IgA levels are normal. They also have circulating B cells. If clinically significant, infants have poor antibody response to vaccines and experience unusually frequent respiratory infections requiring frequent antibiotic courses or continuous prophylactic antibiotics. They rarely need immunoglobulin replacement therapy, which may adversely impair the infant's own antibody production (e.g., response to vaccines). Most have normal serum IgG levels and antibody response by 18 to 24 months of age.

Common Variable Immunodeficiency

Patients with common variable immunodeficiency (CVID) usually have normal antibody production in their first years of life, but then, for unknown reasons, they have declining antibody production and start suffering frequent respiratory infections. Some patients have defects in the inducible T-cell costimulator (e.g., ICOS: inducible costimulator), and others in TACI (transmembrane activator and calcium modulator and cyclophilin ligand interactor), the receptor for the B-cell stimulating cytokines BAFF (B-cell activating factor of the tumor necrosis factor [TNF] family) and APRIL (a proliferation-inducing ligand). However, most patients have unknown immunologic defects, suggesting that many defects in the terminal B-cell differentiation into plasma cells can lead to similar clinical manifestations. CVID has rarely been reported following treatment with sulfasalazine, hydantoin, and carbamazepine. It occurs in 1 to 10,000 to 100,000 individuals.

CLINICAL MANIFESTATIONS

Although the onset of CVID can occur at any age, usually patients present between 15 and 35 years of age with recurrent sinopulmonary infections, particularly refractory chronic sinusitis. Infections are caused by common respiratory microbes such as pneumococcus, *Moraxella,* and *H. influenzae.* Other pyogenic bacteria may also be found. CVID patients may have recurrent bronchitis and pneumonia, and they may develop bronchiectasis.

Patients with CVID also have a high prevalence of gastrointestinal and autoimmune diseases, which may precede the onset of infections. These include achlorhydria, cholelithiasis, giardiasis, pernicious anemia, malabsorption, autoimmune blood cytopenias (usually thrombocytopenia and hemolytic anemia), rheumatoid arthritis, systemic lupus erythematosus (SLE), dermatomyositis, Graves disease, hypothyroidism, inflammatory bowel disease, autoimmune-induced diarrhea with malabsorption, and gastrointestinal bleeding.

Increased incidence of malignancies beyond 40 years of age is also observed. These include gastric carcinoma and a more than 100-fold increase in the incidence of lymphoma compared with the general population.

Noncaseating granulomas may affect liver and spleen, causing visceromegaly, abdominal lymphadenopathy, and obstructive symptoms. They may also affect the lungs. On examination, patients have mildly enlarged lymph nodes and may have splenomegaly.

Laboratory diagnosis is based on low immunoglobulin levels and poor antibody response. Serum IgA is low, usually absent, total IgG level is very low, and IgM is low in half of the patients. Frequently total immunoglobulin levels are very low, below 300 mg/dL, and IgG is below 250 mg/dL, which establishes the diagnosis. For patients with milder decreases in immunoglobulin levels, poor antibody response to vaccines establishes the diagnosis. Circulating B-cell number is normal, but plasma cells are decreased in lymph nodes and in lamina propria of the small intestine biopsies. Isohemagglutinins titers are usually low (less than 1:10). T-cell number and function are usually normal, but eventually many may have laboratory evidence of impaired T-cell number and function. However, opportunistic infections associated with T-cell deficiency do not occur, and if they do, the clinician should suspect other diseases such as hyper IgM syndrome or a combined T- and B-cell immunodeficiency. Examples of T-cell abnormalities in CVID include reduced CD4-to-CD8 ratio, impaired proliferative responses, and impaired delayed hypersensitivity testing. Differential diagnosis includes XLA (in which B cells are absent) and protein-losing enteropathy (low serum albumin and α1-trypsin in stools) or nephropathy (proteinuria).

TREATMENT

Patients with CVID are treated with immunoglobulin replacement, which leads to an excellent prognosis. Manifestations that often occur and need specific management are chronic sinus disease, chronic lung disease (e.g., bronchiectasis), and gastrointestinal diseases. Surveillance for malignancies is also important. Serology should not be relied on as a means to diagnose infectious diseases in patients with antibody deficiency and on immunoglobulin replacement. Instead, detection of the infectious agent should be sought (e.g., antigen, polymerase chain reaction [PCR], or culture).

Hyper IgM Syndrome

In hyper IgM syndrome (HIM) patients have an impaired immunoglobulin class switch from IgM to IgG, IgA, and IgE. As a result, serum IgM is normal or elevated, and levels of IgA and IgG are very low. Patients most commonly lack the CD40 ligand (CD40L or CD154, in chromosome Xq26.3–27), a surface molecule transiently expressed on activated T cells that provides the helper signal by binding to CD40 on B cells, inducing immunoglobulin class switching and triggering differentiation into plasma cells. CD40 is also expressed on monocytes, dendritic cells, and some myeloid progenitors.

CLINICAL MANIFESTATIONS

Male patients with X-linked HIM present early in the first or second year of life with recurrent pyogenic respiratory infections, particularly otitis media, pneumonia, and sepsis. They also have T-cell deficiency and develop *Pneumocystis carinii* pneumonia, which often is the presenting illness and a frequent cause of death. In addition, they have varying degree of neutropenia and may develop hemolytic or aplastic anemia. If patients survive beyond 20 years of age, they often develop chronic liver disease, sclerosing cholangitis, or hepatoma. Some may also develop cryptococcosis and protracted diarrhea due to *Cryptosporidium*.

LABORATORY DIAGNOSIS

HIM is suspected in a male patient with normal or elevated (150 to 1000 mg/dL) IgM and markedly reduced or absent IgG, IgA, and IgE. Half of the patients have normal serum IgM. Isohemagglutinin titers are normal or elevated, and antibody response to vaccines is poor. Diagnosis is confirmed by demonstrating lack of transient expression of CD40L (CD154) on stimulated T cells (mostly CD4 cells) using flow cytometry. However, some mutations in CD40L gene still allow surface expression of nonfunctional CD40L. Thus definitive diagnosis is made by identifying mutations in the CD40L gene. Several mutations have been identified in the extracellular transmembrane and intracytoplasmatic portions of the molecule. Circulating B- and T-cell numbers are normal. T cells proliferate normally to mitogens, but a third of patients have reduced proliferation to antigens. Neutropenia is present in two thirds of patients.

Treatment is based on immunoglobulin replacement therapy and on chronic prophylaxis for *Pneumocystis carinii* pneumonia (PCP) with sulfamethoxazole-trimethoprim. Granulocyte colony-stimulating factor (G-CSF) maybe needed to improve neutropenia. Mortality in early years is caused by infections, particularly PCP, and later due to the liver complications already mentioned. Liver disease tends to recur after liver transplantation. Because of poor prognosis, more aggressive therapy has been attempted. For example, matched bone marrow transplantation has been successful in a few patients.

Other Forms of Hyper-IgM Syndrome (Autosomal Recessive Forms)

Besides the X-linked form of HIM (*HIM type 1*), other autosomal recessive defects in molecules involved in immunoglobulin class switch can lead to similar diseases. CD40 (chromosome 20q12–q13.2. *HIM type 3*) deficiency causes disease very similar to CD40L deficiency.

Other forms lead to milder disease than CD40L and CD40 deficiencies. They include deficiencies of enzymes required for immunoglobulin class switch, such as activation-induced cytiditine deaminase (AID, chromosome 12q13. *HIM type 2*), and uracil N-glycosylase (UNG, chromosome 12q23–q24.1. *HIM type 5*). HIM types 2 and 5 have normal T-cell function (e.g., no susceptibility to PCP) and patients have lymphadenopathy. *HIM type 4* is caused by a defect downstream of AID, although the specific affected gene has not been identified. These enzyme deficiencies have better prognosis and may be diagnosed only in adulthood. Treatment is immunoglobulin replacement.

Another X-linked form of *HIM* is that *associated with ectodermal dysplasia*. In this disease, patients lack IKKγ (chromosome Xq28), also known as NF-κB essential modulator or NEMO. IKKγ binds to two kinases (IKKα and IKKβ) of the NF-κB inhibitor (IκB), a step required for NF-κB activation and translocation to the nucleus. NF-κB activation occurs after activation of CD40 by CD40L and in other cellular processes such as ectodermal formation in the fetus.

Selective IgA Deficiency

The exact cause of selective IgA deficiency (IgAD) and normal concentrations of other immunoglobulins is unknown despite this being the most common immune defect. It is encountered in about 1 in 600 whites, but it is 3 to 30 times less prevalent in Asians. Most patients do not have recurrent infections, but they may be predisposed to allergic and autoimmune diseases. B cells can switch from IgM to IgG but not to IgA, whereas T cells are normal and support IgA production in B cells from normal donors. Most cases are sporadic, although there are reports of it occurring in families with other IgAD and even CVID cases, suggesting shared etiopathogenesis between these deficiencies. IgAD is also associated with HLA-B8. Some cases of IgAD have been associated with drugs such as penicillamine, sulfasalazine, anticonvulsants, gold, chloroquine, captopril, and fenclofenac. It may also occur with chronic hepatitis C. It can occur in association with IgG2 deficiency, which increases susceptibility to infections.

In rare cases, patients have deficiency in the secretory component, and thus they can produce IgA but cannot secrete it in the mucosal lumen. In these cases, serum IgA is normal, but salivary IgA is decreased or absent.

CLINICAL MANIFESTATIONS

Patients with IgAD are usually asymptomatic, but they may have increased susceptibility to infections, allergies, autoimmune diseases, and cancer. If symptomatic, manifestations usually start in the first decade of life.

Infections are usually recurrent and refractory sinusitis, but not pneumonias or bronchiectasis as observed in patients with CVID. However, the combination with IgG2 deficiency increases infectious manifestations.

Allergic diseases are increased in patients with IgAD and are often difficult to treat. IgAD is twice as prevalent in atopic individuals than in the general population. It is postulated that mucosal IgA prevents absorption of allergens and immune sensitization, and that in IgAD this protective mechanism is absent. A unique allergy in patients with IgAD is mediated by antibodies to IgA, which are present in 20% to 40% of patients at the time of diagnosis. Many have not received any blood products, and it is unclear how they are sensitized. Sensitization may occur through ingestion of breast milk, transplacental maternal IgA transfer, cross-sensitization with cow's milk IgA, or exposure to mucosal IgA from normal individuals. Very rarely, patients with IgAD develop anaphylaxis to blood products.

Autoimmune diseases or autoantibodies are present in 37% of patients with IgAD. The mechanism for this high prevalence of autoimmunity is unknown. These patients are at risk for developing celiac disease, ulcerative colitis, Crohn disease, pernicious anemia, SLE, rheumatoid arthritis, dermatomyositis, Sjögren syndrome, Coombs-positive autoimmune hemolytic anemia, idiopathic thrombocytopenic purpura, autoimmune thyroiditis, Addison disease, and chronic autoimmune hepatitis.

Some cancers have been reported in association with IgAD, including thymoma, reticulum cell sarcoma, and squamous cell carcinoma of the lung and esophagus.

Laboratory diagnosis is made by detection of a low serum IgA (less than 15 mg/dL), although in most cases it is absent (less than 5 mg/dL). Other immunoglobulins are normal or elevated, and plasma cells are present in secondary lymphoid tissues and bone marrow. In infants, diagnosis may be delayed because serum IgA level is low in newborns, rises rapidly in the first 2 years of life, but only reaches adult levels by adolescence. Circulating B-cell numbers are normal, although the number of IgA-bearing B cells may be decreased. T-cell numbers and function are normal. Some patients may also have low IgG2. Rare patients may have deficiency in the secretory component leading to low mucosal IgA, which is diagnosed by detecting normal IgA in serum and its absence in saliva. On occasion, selective IgA deficiency may be the first manifestation of a more severe immunodeficiency such as ataxia-telangiectasia or chronic mucocutaneous candidiasis.

There is no specific *treatment* for IgAD. IgA is the antibody isotype most abundantly produced in the body, and a large proportion is secreted in mucosal lumen. Treatment, therefore, is limited to the associated conditions. In those with combined IgG2 deficiency, recurrent infections, and poor antibody response, immunoglobulin therapy to replace IgG can be considered. For patients reacting to blood products who need blood transfusion, washed (3X) packed red blood cells may minimize reactions. Prognosis for IgAD patients is excellent, and mostly determined by associated conditions.

Other Antibody Deficiencies

In *selective IgM deficiency*, patients have absent serum IgM but normal levels of other immunoglobulins. Circulating B-cell number is normal. T-cell number and function are also normal. They may or may not have poor antibody response. They may have recurrent respiratory infections with pneumococci and *H. influenzae*, and they may also have autoimmune diseases. Treatment focuses on antibiotics for infections. Immunoglobulin replacement therapy may also be beneficial.

In *selective IgG subclass deficiency*, total IgG may be normal or slightly decreased, but patients lack an individual IgG subclass, usually IgG1, IgG2, or IgG3 because they account for 65%, 20%, and 10%, respectively, of serum IgG. IgG4 is absent in many normal individuals, and it may make up to 5% of total IgG. Diagnosis of selective IgG deficiency is made if IgG1 is less than 250 mg/dL, IgG2 is less than 50 mg/dL, or IgG3 is less than 25 mg/dL. Like other antibody deficiencies, they may present with repeated pyogenic sinopulmonary infections and may also develop autoimmune diseases.

In patients with *functional antibody deficiency*, also known as *impaired polysaccharide responsiveness*, serum immunoglobulin levels are normal, IgG subclasses are normal, antibody responses to protein vaccines (e.g., toxoids) are normal, but they do not respond well to polysaccharide vaccines (e.g., pneumococcus and *H. influenzae* vaccines). They are usually young children with manifestations similar to those of other antibody deficiencies. Many improve their antibody response by 5 to 10 years of age, but others have persistent deficiency. For this deficiency and for selective IgG subclass deficiency, manifestations are mild and experts recommend antibiotic therapy and antibiotic prophylaxis. It is difficult to commit these patients to lifetime immunoglobulin replacement, but rare anecdotal refractory patients have benefited from such therapy.

In *immunodeficiency with thymoma (Good syndrome)*, elderly patients may initially present with recurrent sinopulmonary infections, chronic diarrhea, dermatitis, septicemia, stomatitis, and urinary infections, before a thymoma is discovered by chest radiograph. In 75% of cases, the thymoma is of the spindle cell type. They are susceptible to the development of myasthenia gravis, aplastic anemia, thrombocytopenia, amyloidosis, and chronic hepatitis. They have markedly reduced serum immunoglobulins, may lack circulating B cells, and may have impaired tests of T-cell function. Removal of thymoma does not improve immunodeficiency but can improve myasthenia gravis and aplastic anemia. Immunoglobulin replacement improves immunodeficiency and chronic diarrhea. Prognosis is poor, and death may occur from infection, aplastic anemia, or thrombocytopenia.

Immunoglobulin Replacement Therapy

Immunoglobulin preparations replace IgG only. The IgG is purified from serum of thousands of donors obtained by plasmapheresis. These are recurrent donors who are screened negative for blood-borne infectious diseases for at least 6 months before entering the donor pool. The IgG is purified by alcohol or Cohn fractionation and filtration steps, a process that by itself kills many viruses. Despite that, an outbreak of hepatitis C occurred in the early 1990s due to contaminated intravenous immunoglobulin (IVIG) preparations. As a result, immunoglobulin preparations now undergo additional processes to kill viruses such as solvent-detergent treatment to kill enveloped viruses (e.g., hepatitis B virus and HIV), pasteurization, low pH (pH = 4), together with pepsin treatment and nanofiltration. There has never been a case of transmissible spongiform encephalopathy (TSE) caused by a contaminated immunoglobulin preparation. Indeed, the alcohol fractionation steps partition prion proteins, which probably reduces the risk of transmission of prion disease by immunoglobulin products. Parvovirus B19 can survive the processing and virus inactivation steps and can be present in the final product. It is a cause of aplastic anemia, although parvovirus-induced disease caused by IVIG has not been reported.

The first immunoglobulin preparation was for intramuscular injection because IgG aggregates and causes complement activation leading to anaphylactoid reactions if injected intravenously. In the 1980s, intravenous immunoglobulin preparations became available through the addition of sugars—and later of amino acids—which solubilize IgG and prevent its aggregation (Table 32–3). A preparation is now also available for subcutaneous (SCIG) infusion. Besides precluding the need for intravenous access, subcutaneous infusions allow easier home self-administration than intravenous infusions, have similar efficacy, and are safer, causing less severe systemic side effects. A drawback is the need for weekly infusions with subcutaneous immunoglobulin instead of every 3 to 4 weeks with intravenous preparations.

The usual starting dose of intravenous immunoglobulins for primary immunodeficiencies is 400 to 600 mg/kg infused every 4 weeks. To minimize adverse events, the first infusion should start slowly at 1 mg/kg/min

Table 32–3. Preparations available for immunoglobulin replacement.

Product	Carimune NF	Flebogamma	Gammagard Liquid	Gammagard S/D	Gamunex	Octagam	Panglobulin NF	Vivaglobin
Manufacturer	ZLB Behring	Grifols	Baxter	Baxter	Telecris	Octa Pharma	American Red Cross	ZLB Behring
Form[a]	Lyophilized (3, 6, 9, or 12%)	5% liquid	10% liquid	Lyophilized (5% or 10%)	10% liquid	5% liquid	Lyophilized (3,6,9 or 12%)	16% liquid
Indications[b]	PID, ITP	PID	PID	PID, ITP, CLL, KS	PID	PID	PID, ITP	PID
Infusion Route	Intravenous	Intravenous	Intravenous	Intravenous	Intravenous	Intravenous	Intravenous	Subcutaneous
IgA Content	720 µg/mL	<50 µg/mL	37 µg/mL	<2.2 µg/mL	46 µg/mL	<50 µg/mL	720 µg/mL	Trace amounts
Stabilizer[c]	8.4 mg/mL sucrose	50 mg/mL D-sorbitol	18.8 mg/mL glycine	20 mg/mL glucose	18.0 mg/mL glycine	100 mg/mL maltose	100 mg/mL sucrose	22.5 mg/mL glycine
Sodium Content	Trace amounts	Trace amounts	Trace amounts	0.145 mEq/mL	Trace amounts	Trace amounts	Trace amounts	0.045 mEq/mL
Virus Inactivation[d]	Low pH Pepsin, NF	Pasteurization	S/D, low pH and NF	S/D	Low pH	S/D Low pH	NF	Pasteurization
TSE Removal Labeling	Yes	No	No	No	Yes	No	No	No
pH in Liquid Form	6.4–6.8	5.0–6.0	4.6–5.1	6.4–7.2	4.0–4.5	5.1–6.0	6.6	6.4–7.2
Osmolality (mOsm/kg)[e]	384 (at 6%) 768 (at 12%)	240–350	240–300	636 (at 5%) 1250 (at 10%)	258	310–380	384 (at 6%) 768 (at 12%)	Not specified
Storage (months)[f]	36 mo (at <30°C)	24 mo (at 2–25°C)	36 mo (at 2–8°C)	24 mo (at <25°C)	36 mo (at 2–8°C)	36 mo (at 2–8°C)	24 mo (at 2–25°C)	42 mo (at 2–8°C)

[a]Lyophilized preparations are best reconstituted in sterile water. Some may also be reconstituted in saline solution (NaCl 0.9%) or dextrose 5%, but these solutions will generate higher osmolality. Values in this table relate to reconstitution in sterile water at a final concentration of 5% or 6%.

[b]Indications: PID, primary immunodeficiency; ITP, idiopathic thrombocytopenic purpura; CLL, chronic lymphocytic leukemia; KS, Kawasaki syndrome.

[c]Stabilizer keeps IgG in solution, preventing formation of aggregates that may activate complement causing anaphylactoid reactions. Maltose in Octagam may cause spurious elevation of capillary blood glucose readings with certain strips and devices.

[d]Virus inactivation processes: The process of purifying IgG from plasma already inactivates many viruses such as HIV. This process involves protein fractionation, precipitation in alcohol, and filtration. In addition, specific steps are added to kill viruses. S/D: Solvent-detergent treatment kills enveloped viruses (e.g., HCV, HIV). NF: Nanofiltration eliminates viruses by removing any particles 35 nm or larger.

[e]Normal serum osmolality is 285 to 295 mOsm/kg. Values for lyophilized preparation reflect reconstitution in sterile water.

[f]Temperature conversion: 2°C = 36°F, 8°C = 46°F, 25°C = 77°F, 30°C = 86°F. Preparations cannot be frozen.

(or 0.01 mL/kg/min or, for adults, 1 mL/kg/h for a 5% IVIG preparation), and, if tolerated, doubled the infusion rate every 30 minutes to a maximum of 8 mg/kg/min (or 8 mL/kg/h for a 5% IVIG). In subsequent infusions, patients usually tolerate starting at faster initial rates, although the maximum rate should be maintained. Dose and interval are adjusted to improve clinical manifestations (e.g., infections and fatigue) and to maintain a trough serum IgG concentration of at least 500 mg/dL after 5 half-lives (3 to 4 months). Sometimes dosing at 3-week intervals or more often is necessary for patients who metabolize IgG rapidly.

Mild to moderate adverse events to infusion of immunoglobulin preparations are very common particularly with the first infusions, and include headache, nausea, rigors, and back pain. Less often patients experience fever, chest pain, abdominal pain, flushing, vomiting, arthralgia, myalgia, and hives. IVIG is better tolerated in subsequent infusions and eventually many patients tolerate them well without premedications (see below). However, they may recur with switching of immunoglobulin preparations. If adverse events occur during infusion, the infusion rate should be reduced or even temporarily stopped, depending on the severity of symptoms. Symptoms can be treated with oral acetaminophen, 500 to 650 mg (or 10 mg/kg for children), oral or parenteral diphenhydramine, 25 to 50 mg (1.25 mg/kg), and rarely systemic corticosteroids may be necessary (e.g., methylprednisolone 125 mg or 0.5 to 1 mg/kg IV). To prevent adverse events, one can (1) premedicate patient with acetaminophen and diphenhydramine 30 to 60 minutes before infusion, rarely oral corticosteroids may also be necessary; (2) infuse at a lower rate; (3) use a lower IVIG concentration (e.g., 3% or 5%); (4) use a preparation with low osmolality; (5) switch to a different immunoglobulin brand; (6) switch from intravenous to subcutaneous immunoglobulin. Extremely rarely anaphylactic reactions may be due to a patient's antibodies against IgA, in which case a preparation with low IgA content may help.

Immunoglobulin preparations can also cause severe adverse events. The IVIG preparations have a black box warning on the risk of renal dysfunction, acute renal failure, osmotic nephrosis, and death. The renal damage is caused by hyperosmotic insult. The risk increases in those with preexisting renal insufficiency, diabetes mellitus, age 65 years or older, with volume depletion, sepsis, paraproteinemia, and on concomitant nephrotoxic drugs. In addition, rapid infusion, high doses (e.g., 1 g/kg/day for 1 to 2 days used for autoimmune diseases), hyperosmolar preparations, and IVIG containing sucrose may also increase the risk for renal complications. Thromboembolic events have also been reported, particularly with high doses and rapid infusion and in those with preexisting cardiovascular diseases or a history of thromboembolic events. Other rare severe adverse events are aseptic meningitis, antibody-mediated (positive direct Coombs test) hemolysis, transfusion-related acute lung injury, cardiac arrest, bullous skin diseases, and anaphylactoid reactions.

Currently in the United States there is a single subcutaneous immunoglobulin (SCIG) preparation commercially available (Table 32–3). Subcutaneous infusion causes lower peak serum levels (minimizes dose-related adverse events) and higher trough serum levels (may minimize risk of infection). Indeed, serum IgG levels are very stable. In the clinical study that led to approval by the Food and Drug Administration, patients on IVIG were switched to SCIG 1 week after the last IVIG infusion at a dose 37% higher than the weekly IVIG dose. The recommended weekly dose is 100 to 200 mg/kg, 100 mg/kg/week if starting in immunoglobulin-therapy naïve patients. Systemic adverse events are similar to those of IVIG. In addition, local injection site adverse events occurred in 80% to 85% of patients, but they were mild to moderate and waned in intensity and frequency in subsequent infusions to 60% of patients by the 10th infusion, and stabilized at 30% to 40% by the 25th infusion. Local reactions included local edema, erythema, and pruritus, which usually disappear the day after the infusion. SCIG can be infused slowly into two to four sites simultaneously at 15 mL/site using bifurcated tubing. Sites need to be at least 2 in apart. It is infused in rotating sites in the lower abdomen—away from the navel and midline—upper thighs, upper arms, and lateral hips. The SCIG does not have a black box warning related to acute renal failure, nor has it been reported to cause thromboembolic events and the severe adverse events described earlier. However, only a few hundred patients have received SCIG and it has not been used in high doses (e.g., 1 g/kg) as an immunomodulatory drug for autoimmune diseases yet.

COMPLEMENT DEFICIENCIES

Defects in genes involved in the three major complement pathways have been described: classical pathway, alternative pathway, and mannose-binding lectin (MBL). All three pathways converge to activate C3, which then activates the late components that form the membrane attack complex (C5, C6, C7, C8, and C9). The complement system enhances phagocytosis by opsonization and directly kills bacteria and viruses (see Chapter 23).

Except for MBL deficiency, which may affect 5% of the population, all other complement deficiencies combined account for only 2% of all primary immunodeficiencies. Defects in all soluble complement components have been described. Most are autosomal recessive deficiencies. Exceptions are properdin deficiency (X-linked), and C1 esterase inhibitor deficiency (see Chapter 11), which is autosomal dominant. MBL deficiency is also autosomal dominant.

Deficiencies in the early components of the classical pathway (C1q, C1r, C1s, C4, and C2) manifest with pyogenic infections caused by encapsulated bacteria (pneumococcus and *H. influenzae*), but susceptibility to infections is attenuated by the ability to still activate C3 via alternative and MBL pathways. Deficiencies in these early components are also associated with autoimmune collagen vascular diseases (SLE) and glomerulonephritis.

C3 deficiency is associated with pyogenic infections, disseminated *Neisseria* infections, and vasculitis. Deficiencies in the late complement components C5, C6, C7, and C8 lead to recurrent disseminated or invasive neisserial infections (mainly *Neisseria meningitidis* and, to a much lesser extent, *Neisseria gonorrhea*). C9 deficiency is associated with pyogenic infections. These distinctions are not strict. Deficiency of early components can also be associated with neisserial infections, and late component deficiencies can occur with autoimmune diseases.

Deficiency in components of the alternative pathway can lead to recurrent disseminated or invasive neisserial infections (factor B and properdin deficiencies) or recurrent pyogenic infections (factor D and properdin deficiencies).

Deficiency in proteins that regulate the complement system also cause disease. Factor H and factor I deficiencies are associated with autoimmune collagen vascular diseases and recurrent pyogenic infections. C4bp deficiency is associated with angioedema and Behçet-like syndrome. These three deficiencies are autosomal recessive. C1 esterase inhibitor deficiency is autosomal dominant and causes hereditary angioedema (see Chapter 11) and is also associated with autoimmune diseases.

Mannan(or mannose)-binding lectin (or protein) (MBL or MBP, chromosome 10q11.2–q21) is a circulating lectin that binds to glycosylated surface components of microbes and activates complement via classical and alternative components leading to opsonization and killing of microbes. It is produced by the liver as part of the acute-phase response. MBP activates the complement pathways via its MBL-associated proteases 1 and 2 (MASP-1 and MASP-2). MBL is an important innate defense molecule in the first years of life when maternal antibodies wane and infants start to develop their repertoire of memory antibody responses. Thereafter, it becomes less clinically relevant. However, few cases of clinically significant MBL deficiency have been described in adults. Median normal plasma levels are 800 to 1000 μg/L. When deficient, its serum levels are more than 10-fold lower than normal (less than 50 μg/L). MBL-deficient infants present with recurrent respiratory tract infections, otitis media, and chronic diarrhea. This deficiency has been associated with increased susceptibility to HIV infection, SLE, arterial thrombosis, and increased morbidity in cystic fibrosis.

Deficiencies in *cell-bound complement proteins* also cause disease. *Complement receptor 1* (CR1) deficiency is probably an acquired disease due to autoimmune complex formation in SLE. CR1 is expressed on erythrocytes and is a cofactor for factor I, which cleaves C4b and C3b and inactivates C3 and C5 convertases. On erythrocytes, it binds and captures circulating immune complexes and facilitates their elimination via liver and splenic macrophages. Thus, excessive immune complex formation in SLE due to autoantibodies may consume CR1, causing an acquired, not inherited, deficiency. *Complement receptor 3* (CR3 or CD11b CD18) is an integrin beta 2 and its deficiency is described later (see leukocyte adhesion deficiency type 1). Mutations in the *phosphatidylinositol glucan A*, an enzyme that forms an anchor for three membrane-bound proteins, causes deficiency of three proteins that regulate complement activation: decay-accelerating factor (DAF), protectin (CD59), and homologous restriction factor (HRF). Other glycosyl phosphatidylinositol-linked proteins are also affected. CD59 deficiency is believed to result in intermittent hemolysis caused by uninhibited membrane attack complexes causing paroxysmal nocturnal hemoglobinuria (PNH).

Laboratory Evaluation of the Complement System

Complement hemolytic activity 50% (CH50) is a functional test of the complement system that determines the ability of the patient's serum complement to lyse 50% of antibody-sensitized sheep erythrocytes. It is a good screening test for complement deficiency. Patients with severe deficiency of a classical complement component will have a total complement CH50 of less than 5% of the normal (CH50 less than 5%). An exception is C9 deficiency where CH50 is 30% to 50% of normal because hemolysis is only partially impaired in this deficiency. Although CH50 is low in deficiencies of components of the classical pathway and of terminal components, deficiency in components of the alternative pathway can also cause low CH50. However, an alternative pathway hemolytic activity test (AH50) is also available in specialized laboratories and tests the ability of serum to lyse rabbit erythrocytes. The AH50 tests the function of alternative pathway components (factors B, H, I, and properdin), C3, and of the membrane attack complex (C5 to C9). If CH50 or AH50 is low, the specific complement deficiency may be pursued by quantification and functional assay for individual complement components, which is available in a few laboratories.

Two components need careful interpretation of results, C1 esterase inhibitor and C8, because they may be present but may not be functional. In the case of C1 inhibitor, certain mutations may allow production of nonfunctional molecules. In the case of C8, some of its three chains can be expressed in C8-deficient patients because C8 function is impaired in deficiency of either C8β alone, or both C8α and C8γ.

Treatment of Complement Deficiencies

There is no specific treatment for complement deficiencies, except for replacement of C1 esterase inhibitor (see below). Patients with deficiencies in complement components that increase susceptibility to infections should receive vaccines (meningococcal tetravalent vaccine, pneumococcal 23-valent vaccine, and conjugated *H. influenzae* vaccine). During severe infections, transfusion of fresh-frozen plasma to attempt replacement of the missing component may be beneficial, although in complete deficiencies patients may develop antibodies to nonself complement proteins after repeated transfusions reducing efficacy in the long term. Infections should be treated early and aggressively, and those with frequent infections may benefit from continuous antibiotic prophylaxis. Treatment of autoimmune diseases is not changed if a patient has concomitant complement deficiency.

Hereditary C1 esterase inhibitor deficiency can be treated with androgens, which increase its production in the liver, plasmin inhibitors, and replacement therapy (plasma purified or recombinant C1 esterase inhibitor, which were not available in the United States as of 2006). Acute angioedema may be treated with fresh-frozen plasma, although it may adversely worsen it by providing additional complement substrate (see also Chapter 11).

CELLULAR IMMUNODEFICIENCIES

These are immunodeficiencies affecting cellular immune response, which is mediated by lymphocytes and NK cells. These cells attach to the target cell to effect their function.

DiGeorge Syndrome

DiGeorge syndrome (DGS) is a triad of hypoparathyroidism, thymus hypoplasia, and congenital heart disease. However, this triad and many other manifestations are now recognized as part of a broader disorder called *chromosome 22q11.2 deletion syndrome*. It occurs in 13 per 100,000 live births, usually due to a sporadic deletion. This deletion leads to loss of many genes and abnormal embryonic migration of neural crest cells that form the third and fourth pharyngeal pouches (branchial arches). These branchial arches give rise to the thymus, parathyroid glands, cardiac outflow structures, skull, mesenchyme of face and palate, and neuronal structures of the head and neck. These structures are all formed in the embryo between weeks 4 and 8 of gestation. The clinical manifestations of this syndrome vary widely both in degree and number of tissues affected. It has also been named CATCH22 (Cardiac Abnormality/abnormal facies, T cell deficit due to thymic hypoplasia, Cleft palate, Hypocalcemia due to hypoparathyroidism resulting from 22q11 deletion), and Shprintzen (or velocardiofacial) syndrome.

Patients with DGS usually present with hypocalcemia and congenital heart disease, a combination that should lead to diagnostic investigation for chromosome 22q11.2 deletion and for other manifestations including lymphopenia and facial dysmorphism.

Hypoparathyroidism may manifest in the first day of life as hypocalcemia resistant to therapy. Serum phosphorus is high, and parathyroid hormone low. It is usually temporary but may persist into adulthood.

The congenital heart disease in DGS involves conotruncal defects affecting the outflow tract. These include tetralogy of Fallot, type B interrupted aortic arch, truncus arteriosus, right aortic arch, coarctation of aorta, and aberrant right subclavian artery. Ventricular septal defects are also common.

Facial dysmorphism affects face and palate including low-set ears with prominent overfolded helices, hypertelorism, narrow nasal alae with bulbous nasal tip, fish-shaped mouth (small mouth and prominent upper lip), malar flattening, and micrognathia. Palate may contain a submucosal cleft; that is, on palpation one notices a bone cleft in the distal portion of the hard (bony) palate, although the soft palate and uvula are present. Complete cleft palate or bifida uvula also occur. The facial features become more prominent as the child grows. They were first described by Shprintzen in 1981 and are called velocardiofacial syndrome (VCFS). Velopharyngeal insufficiency (short palate) may cause feeding difficulty, nasal regurgitation, and hypernasal and other speech problems.

Immunodeficiency results from hypoplastic and, rarely, aplastic thymus. Although thymus is not seen in lateral chest radiographs in newborns, usually there is a small thymus, or rests of thymus tissue scattered in submandibular and cervical areas so the immune defect is mild and transient in most patients.

Other less frequent clinical manifestations in DGS include microcephaly, inguinal and umbilical hernias, esophageal atresia, short stature, slender hands, scoliosis, and neuropsychiatric disorders (e.g., schizophrenia).

Laboratory diagnosis is confirmed by detecting the 22q11 deletion by fluorescent in situ hybridization (FISH), and decreased T-cell number. Absence of thymus shadow is noticed in chest radiographs of infants. The 22q11 deletion is detected in 90% of patients with the DGS triad, whereas the remaining DGS cases may be caused by other genetic defects, intrauterine exposure to retinoic acid or alcohol. CD3+ cells are low, in the range of 500 to 1500 cells/mm^3. Both CD4 and CD8 are affected, so the ratio of CD4 to CD8 is normal or high because CD8 depletion may be more severe than that of CD4. Lymphocyte proliferation to mitogens and allogenic cells is usually normal but is decreased in those with severe T-cell depletion. In severe cases, severe lymphopenia is persistent and can lead to opportunistic infections (Table 32–2). B cells are usually normal, but if CD4 helper function is markedly impaired, poor antibody production may be present. In most DGS patients, immunologic abnormalities correct in the first year of life.

Treatment of DGS often requires a multidisciplinary team because of the diverse manifestations. From the immunologic standpoint, it is important to monitor T-cell deficiency and institute prophylactic measures for T-cell deficiency. These measures include avoidance of live attenuated microbe vaccines (e.g., live virus and BCG vaccines), use of irradiated blood products to prevent graft-versus-host disease, and administration of PCP prophylaxis with sulfamethoxazole-trimethoprim. These measures should be started in those with persistent CD4 less than 500 cells/mm^3 at 2 months of age and should probably be continued until immunodeficiency resolves as determined by normalization of T-cell numbers and function: CD8 higher than 400/mm^3, CD4 higher than 1000/mm^3, normal T-cell proliferation to mitogens and antigens, and a normal antibody response. Because for most patients the T-cell deficiency is mild and transient, resolving in the first year of life, the prognosis of the immunologic defect in DGS is good. However, the immunodeficiency can be profound and persistent in a minority of DGS patients (less than 5%) and sometimes requires thymus or HLA-matched bone marrow transplants. In some of these cases, graft-versus-host disease develops due to transplacental transfer of maternal T cells or because of allogenic T cells from nonirradiated blood transfusions.

Hypocalcemia may require calcium supplements and 1,25-dihydrocholecalciferol therapy. Cardiac defects may require surgical repair, as may palate malformations. Some children may also need speech therapy.

Chronic Mucocutaneous Candidiasis

In this T-cell deficiency, patients suffer from impaired specific T-cell response to *Candida,* although the exact mechanism is not known. *Clinical manifestations* are mainly related to chronic candidal infections involving skin, nails, and oroesophageal and vaginal mucosa, but not usually sepsis of deep-seated infections. Skin infections may have a "stocking-glove" distribution. They may present in the first year of life or in teenage years. Some may have autoimmune disease, such as hypoparathyroidism, Addison disease, and, less often, diabetes mellitus, hypogonadism, and adrenocorticotropic hormone (ACTH) deficiency. Other manifestations include pernicious anemia, chronic hepatitis, vitiligo, alopecia, and pulmonary fibrosis. A form of this immunodeficiency is *autoimmune polyendocrinopathy, candidiasis, and ectodermal dystrophy (APECED),* an autosomal recessive disease caused by gene defects in the autoimmune regulator (AIRE) gene (21q22.3).

Laboratory diagnosis is based on evidence of deficient T-cell response to *Candida* antigens, such as the absence of delayed hypersensitivity skin response to candidin despite culture-proven chronic *Candida* infections. T-cell responses to mitogens, allogenic cells, and other antigens are normal. B cells are normal, including their ability to generate antibody response to *Candida.* *Treatment* often requires systemic rather than topical antifungal antibiotics and therapy for associated autoimmune disorders.

Immunodysregulation, Polyendocrinopathy, Enteropathy, X-Linked Syndrome

Immunodysregulation, polyendocrinopathy, enteropathy, X-linked (IPEX) syndrome is a rare X-linked deficiency of Foxp3 (chromosome Xp11.23), a member of the forkhead/winged-helix family of transcriptional regulators that is essential for generation of the CD4+CD25+ T regulatory (Treg) cells. These Treg cells inhibit effector T cells and cellular immune responses via both soluble factors (TGFβ and IL10) and via cell-to-cell contact (using inhibitory "costimulatory" molecules CTLA4 and GITR). Patients with IPEX lack Treg cells, which leads to exaggerated immune responses and autoimmune diseases.

CLINICAL MANIFESTATIONS

Patients present with various combinations of intractable diarrhea (autoimmune enteropathy with villous atrophy), eczema, hemolytic anemia, thrombocytopenia, diabetes mellitus type 1, chronic dermatitis, thyroid autoimmunity, and variable immunodeficiency. There are exaggerated responses to viral infections. Few survive the first decade of life, with death in infancy or early childhood occurring with infections or shortly after immunizations.

Laboratory diagnosis is made by lack of CD4+CD25+ T cells in the blood, and absence of Foxp3 expression. Total T- and B-cell numbers are normal at birth but seem to expand within weeks. Limited information exists on the natural history of immunologic markers.

Treatment of enteropathy with cyclosporine A has been temporarily successful, but prognosis is poor with death before the 10th birthday being common. Bone marrow transplantation once disease has manifested temporarily improves disease severity, but the few patients treated still died of complications.

Autoimmune Lymphoproliferative Syndrome

The defect in autoimmune lymphoproliferative syndrome (ALPS) is impaired FAS-induced apoptosis, a major pathway for lymphocyte homeostasis. Apoptosis eliminates harmful lymphocytes such as auto-reactive and proliferating effector lymphocytes, in the latter case as a means to terminate immune response once it is no longer necessary. Apoptosis also occurs in other immune cells. ALPS is both genetically and clinically heterogeneous. Both ALPS-0 and ALPS-1a are caused by a deficiency in CD95 (chromosome 10q24.1), but the former results from recessive mutations (homozygous), whereas the latter results from a dominant mutation. In ALPS-1b, patients lack FAS ligand (CD95L, chromosome 1q23), and in ALPS-2 they lack either caspase 8 or 10 (both in chromosome 2q33–q34). All these molecules participate in the FAS pathway. The defect in ALPS-3 has not been identified.

CLINICAL MANIFESTATIONS

Because of defective apoptosis, patients with ALPS have signs of excessive lymphoproliferation and autoimmune phenomena. Typically patients present around 24 months of age with a triad of lymphoproliferative disease, autoimmune cytopenias, and susceptibility to malignancies. However, many are diagnosed in adulthood.

Lymphoproliferative disease is characterized by chronic nonmalignant hepatosplenomegaly and lymphadenopathy. Lymph nodes can be normal in size or very prominent, forming very large distorting superficial lymph nodes and large thoracic and intraabdominal adenopathies that may cause obstructive disease. They may shrink with infections and improve in older patients. Autoimmune disorders affect 50% to 70% of patients. More often patients suffer from severe and difficult-to-treat blood cytopenias, including hemolytic anemia, thrombocytopenia, neutropenia, and Evan's syndrome, a combination of the first two cytopenias. Less often patients may develop glomerulonephritis, optic neuritis, Guillain–Barré syndrome, primary biliary cirrhosis/autoimmune hepatitis, arthritis, vasculitis, childhood linear IgA disease, and factor VIII coagulopathy. Risk of developing autoimmune diseases increases as patients age. Serum autoantibodies are found in up to 92% of cases.

Malignancies occur in 10% of patients with ALPS. Risk of developing Hodgkin and non–Hodgkin lymphomas is 51 times and 14 times higher than in the general population, respectively. Other malignancies may also occur.

LABORATORY FINDINGS

Patients have lymphocytosis and hypergammaglobulinemia. Diagnosis is made if patient has three features: nonmalignant lymphadenopathy plus splenomegaly, more than 1% double negative T cells, and impaired apoptosis of lymphocytes *in vitro*. Flow cytometry analysis of lymphocytes reveals more than 1% of CD3+CD4–CD8– (double-negative) T cells bearing $\alpha\beta$ T-cell receptors (range 1% to 75%), which are normally absent in the blood. However, some have reported normal subjects with up to 2.6% of double-negative

T cells. These double-negative CD3 cells also express CD45RA, CD57, CD27, CD28, perforin, and HLA-DR. Many tests can confirm impaired apoptosis of lymphocytes *in vitro*. An example of such a test is to isolate blood mononuclear cells, stimulate T cells with phytohemagglutinin (or anti-CD3 antibody), and incubate them with IL-2 for 1 week. Then expose cells to anti-FAS to induce apoptosis, which is assessed by surface expression of annexin using flow cytometry.

Besides these three required features already described, other characteristics that help diagnose ALPS are autoimmune disease, family history of ALPS, characteristic pathology of lymph node and spleen (see below), and identifying defective molecule in the apoptosis pathway at the protein and/or genetic level. At the protein level, missing molecules can be measured by flow cytometry or Western blot. At the DNA level, mutations can be identified by sequencing the affected gene.

Pathologic examination of lymph nodes reveals a prominent paracortical area T-cell zone with lymphoblasts. Immunohistochemistry shows that the majority of these cells is CD3+CD4–CD8–. CD4-to-CD8 ratio is markedly decreased, and a polyclonal plasma cell expansion may be present. In the spleen, there is follicular hyperplasia in an expanded white pulp and a massively expanded red pulp containing cells phenotypically identical to those seen in the lymph node paracortical regions.

Treatment with systemic corticosteroids or immunosuppressants improves lymphoproliferative manifestations, particularly if obstructive disease ensues. Patients should avoid contact sports to prevent splenic rupture. Autoimmune cytopenias also respond well to corticosteroids. If splenectomy becomes necessary, it should be followed by antibiotic prophylaxis until adulthood. Mycophenolate mofetil and rituximab with vincristine have been used with success for severe refractory immune thrombocytopenia. Neutropenia responds to G-CSF therapy. Few patients with severe and progressive disease have benefited from bone marrow transplantation.

Other Cellular Deficiencies

NATURAL KILLER CELL DEFICIENCY

NK cells are non–T (CD3-) non–B (CD19-) lymphocytes that express CD56 and FcγRIIIA (CD16). They attach to target cells and lyse them by contact. Attachment is via IgG and Fc-gamma receptor, or MHCI receptors. Target cell death occurs via perforin or by induction of apoptosis. The target cell is usually a virus-infected cell or a neoplastic cell. Few cases have been described of isolated NK cell deficiency that presented with Herpesviridae infections (e.g., herpes simplex, varicella, cytomegalovirus [CMV], and Epstein-Barr [EBV] viruses).

IDIOPATHIC CD4 LYMPHOCYTOPENIA

Several cases of low CD4 count in the absence of HIV infection (based on serology and PCR testing) have been described. Some cases may be a normal variant because their T-cell functional tests are normal. Others have impaired T-cell function and develop opportunistic infections that can be fatal. Most are adults from 17 to 70 years of age, and few have spontaneously recovered. In the case of T-cell impairment in functional assays and/or a history of opportunistic infections, chronic prophylaxis for PCP and avoidance of live virus vaccines may be considered.

COMBINED CELLULAR AND HUMORAL IMMUNODEFICIENCIES

In these deficiencies, patients have complete or partial defects in both T cells (cellular immunity) and in B cells (antibody response).

Severe Combined Immunodeficiencies

In severe combined immunodeficiencies (SCID), there is a marked impairment of T cells with a variable impairment of B cells, which may be primary or secondary to lack of T helper cell function. They are characterized by a common clinical presentation in the first months of life, and most require bone marrow transplantation therapy.

Despite the large number of genetic defects causing several types of SCIDs (Table 32–4), the *clinical manifestations* are similar and typically start within 3 months of age with persistent infections, failure to thrive, and diarrhea. Infections include persistent oral thrush and *Candida* diaper rash, PCP, bacterial pneumonias, protracted diarrhea, and severe virus infections with respiratory syncytial virus, EBV, and CMV. Live vaccines can also cause clinical infections, particularly oral polio vaccine and bacillus Calmette-Guérin (BCG), which are administered in the first months of life in some countries, but not in the United States. In addition, patients may have vomiting, fever, or rashes. On examination they have growth failure, absence of tonsils and of lymph nodes, and may have hepatosplenomegaly. Treatment of infections is difficult. Occasionally, patients may develop graft-versus-host disease (GVHD) from maternal or blood transfusion lymphocytes, which is fatal without immune reconstitution. Use of irradiated blood helps prevent GVHD, and live vaccines are contraindicated.

Laboratory diagnosis starts with identification of lymphopenia in neonates who should have more than 2500 lymphocytes/mm^3. In addition, they may have neutropenia (e.g., in X-linked SCID), thrombocytopenia,

Table 32–4. Phenotypes of combined T- and B-cell immunodeficiencies.

Lymphocyte Phenotype			Immune Defect	Chromosome and Inheritance
T	**B**	**NK**		
T–	B+	NK–	X-linked SCID (γ_c deficiency)	Xq13. X-linked
			Jak3 deficiency	19p13.1. Autosomal recessive
			CD45 deficiency	1q31–q32. Autosomal recessive
			IL-2R alpha chain deficiency	10p15.1.
T–	B+	NK+	IL7R alpha chain deficiency	5p13. Autosomal recessive
			CD3 delta chain deficiency	11q23. Autosomal recessive
			CD3 epsilon chain deficiency	11q23. Autosomal recessive
T–	B–	NK–	Adenosine deaminase deficiency	20q13.11. Autosomal recessive
T–	B–	NK+	RAG1 and RAG2 deficiency	11p13–p12. Autosomal recessive
			Artemis deficiency	10p13. Autosomal recessive
T4+ T8–	B+	NK+	Zap70 deficiency	2q12. Autosomal recessive
			HLA-I deficiency	6p21.3. Autosomal recessive
			CD3 zeta chain deficiency	1q22–q23. Autosomal recessive
T4– T8+	B+	NK+	HLA-II deficiency	Four genes in chromosomes 1, 13, 16, or 19. Autosomal recessive.

In T– deficiencies, total T cells (CD3 cells) are low and both of its subtypes are low (T4 = CD4 helper cells and T8 = CD8 suppressor cells). In T4+ T8– and T4– T8+ deficiencies, total T-cell number (CD3 cells) is usually normal.
RAG, recombination-activating gene (recombinase); γ_c, common gamma chain; Zap70, zeta-chain-associated protein kinase of 70 kd.

and hypogammaglobulinemia, although the latter can be masked by maternal IgG. Thymic shadow is absent in chest radiograph. As shown in Table 32–4, flow cytometry enumeration of blood T cells (and its subsets, CD4 and CD8 cells), B cells, and NK cells is very helpful to identify the type of SCID. CD4 count is usually very low (less than 200/mm^3), resulting in impaired lymphocyte proliferation to mitogens and to allogenic cells. However, if GVHD develops, the assessment of patient's lymphocytes is difficult. HLA typing and biopsy of rash can help diagnose GVHD. Once lymphocyte phenotyping is available, specific molecular defect can be pursued at the protein and genetic level. Definitive diagnosis is made by demonstrating deficiency of the affected protein and by identifying mutations in the affected gene.

The definitive *treatment* for SCIDs is bone marrow transplantation. In addition, patients receive supportive therapy with antibiotic treatment for infections, immunoglobulin replacement, PCP prophylaxis, avoidance of live microbe vaccines, and use of irradiated (2500 rads) blood products (to prevent GVHD). Ideally, an HLA-matched sibling is used for the bone marrow transplantation, but transplantation with HLA haploidential bone marrow depleted from T cells is more commonly available. Transplantation reconstitutes T-cell number and function in 3 to 4 months and B-cell function in 1 to 2 years or never. Pretransplant conditioning of the SCID recipient is not necessary because of the severe T-cell defect. Prophylaxis for GVHD with cyclosporine A is not needed for HLA-matched transplantation, but it is used for T-cell-depleted HLA-haploidential transplantation if T-cell depletion is not nearly complete. Use of CMV- and EBV-negative donors helps prevent fatal systemic virus infections immediately after transplantation.

FORMS OF SCIDs

The most common SCID is the *X-linked* form that accounts for 50% of cases and is due to lack of the common gamma chain (cγ), a cytokine receptor chain that transduces activation signal into the cytoplasma via phosphorylation of *Janus kinase 3* (Jak3). It is present in the receptors for IL-2, IL-4, IL-7, IL-9, IL-15, and IL-21. A similar phenotype ensues with deficiency in Jak3, the fourth most common SCID affecting 6% of cases. However, the lymphocyte counts in Jak3 deficiency are usually higher than in X-linked SCID.

The second most common SCID is *adenosine deaminase* (ADA) deficiency, which accounts for 17% of SCIDs. ADA participates in the catabolism of adenosine, as does purine nucleoside phosphorylase (PNP; Fig. 32–1), which participates in the catabolism of both purines (adenosine and guanosine). Deficiency in PNP also causes SCIDs. These enzymes similarly transform the deoxy forms of the nitrogen bases (Fig. 32–1).

ADA deficiency leads to accumulation of purine metabolites, which are toxic for thymocytes (thymic T lymphocyte precursors) and inhibit T-cell signaling. The high rate of apoptosis of the developing T cells in the thymus due to negative selection and consequent high rate of RNA/DNA catabolism renders this organ more susceptible to this enzymatic defect than other tissues. ADA deficiency leads to accumulation of adenosine (from RNA degradation), deoxyadenosine (from DNA degradation), and methyladenosine. Nucleotides also accumulate, one being 2'-deoxyadenosine triphosphate (dATP), which is toxic to lymphocytes, particularly T cells. Adenosine inhibits T-cell signaling. The dATP inhibits ribonucleotide reductase, which reduces purines and pyrimidines, a necessary step for DNA synthesis. The amount of dATP is increased in erythrocytes 100- to 2000-fold in this SCID. Adenosine and dATP also inhibit S-adenosyl-homocysteine hydrolase (SAHH), which is essential for methylation reactions and to maintain cell viability. Lastly, dATP initiates apoptosis by inducing cytochrome *c* release from mitochondria. ADA deficiency causes the most profound lymphopenia among all SCIDs with counts less than 500/mm^3. Diagnosis is confirmed by measuring ADA activity in cell lysates from erythrocytes as a screening tool (less than 1% of activity regardless of the age of onset of symptoms of ADA deficiency), and then confirmed in non–erythrocyte cells (blood lymphocytes, EBV-transformed B cells, or fibroblast). Depending on the activity of ADA in lymphocytes, the immunodeficiency may vary in onset. In 85% to 90% of ADA-deficient patients, lymphocyte ADA activity is less than 0.5%, and clinical manifestations of SCIDs with severe lymphopenia are noticed in the first months of life or may be delayed with onset by 1 to 2 years of life (delayed-onset form). When lymphocyte ADA activity is 0.5% to 3% (still will be less than 1% in erythrocytes), the onset of clinical disease is later (late-onset form) by 3 to 15 years of age, or even in adulthood, when patients present with recurrent sinopulmonary infections, lymphopenia, hyper-IgE, poor antibody response, and autoimmune diseases (thrombocytopenia, hemolysis, hypothyroidism). Partial ADA deficiency (5% to 80% of enzyme activity in nonerythrocyte cells) with normal immune function has been detected in population studies. Besides bone marrow transplantation, which is the first choice of therapy for ADA deficiency appearing in infancy, enzyme replacement and gene therapy have been partially successful and are used when an appropriate bone marrow donor is not available. Enzyme replacement with polyethylene glycol (reduces immunogenicity and prolongs half-life)-conjugated adenosine deaminase (PEG-ADA) derived from calf intestine (ADAGEN, pegademase bovine) is administered intramuscularly twice weekly at 15 to 30 U/kg of ideal body weight. Some patients need higher doses of 30 to

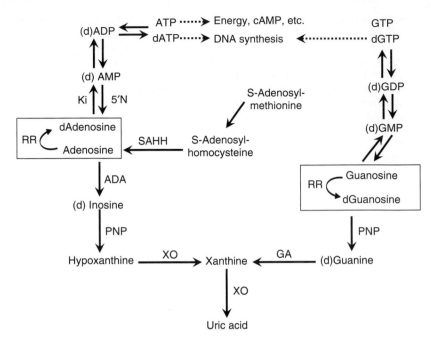

Figure 32–1. Function of adenosine deaminase (ADA) and of purine nucleoside phosphorylase (PNP) in the catabolism of purines. Other enzymes in this pathway are adenosine kinase (Ki), 5′ nucleotidase (5′N), ribonucleotide reductase (RR), s-adenosylhomocysteine hydrolase (SAHH), xanthine oxidase (XO), and guanase (GA). Note: d denotes deoxy; (d) denotes either nucleotide or deoxy-nucleotide forms. For example, (d)adenosine represents both adenosine and deoxy-adenosine.

60 U/kg at least initially. PEG-ADA response is monitored by measuring plasma ADA activity, erythrocyte levels of dATP accumulation, and the degree of inhibition of SAH hydrolase activity (less than 10% without therapy), which all improve dramatically. SAHH activity is the most sensitive marker to monitor therapy efficacy. Recovery of immune function is partial and delayed, taking 3 to 5 months for B- and T-cell numbers to start to increase and longer for antibody response to normalize, so that after 12 months 50% of patients may no longer need immunoglobulin replacement because they develop normal antibody response to bacteriophage. About 50% to 65% of patients develop antibodies to ADA, but it becomes a clinically significant problem in only a few patients, who because of faster elimination of PEG-ADA, experience decreasing plasma ADA levels and clinical deterioration. ADA deficiency was the first disease for which gene therapy was attempted. ADA cDNA was transfected *in vitro* using retrovirus vectors into expanding patient's own T cells, bone marrow cells, or cord blood CD34+ stem cells (in the few patients diagnosed prenatally) and administered back to patients, resulting in temporary replacement of ADA in immune cells. However, these patients continued to receive PEG-ADA, although sometimes at a

lower dose, so it is difficult to know how much clinical benefit gene therapy provided.

Purine nucleoside phosphorylase (PNP, chromosome 14q13.1) deficiency is a rare cause of SCID with similar manifestations as ADA deficiency, including severe lymphopenia (less than 500/mm³) and infantile and late-onset forms, but usually T cells are more affected than B cells. In PNP deficiency, uric acid is low in the serum (less than 1 mg/dL) and in the urine. A distinct feature is that half of the patients have neurologic symptoms, including spastic diplegia or tetraparesis, ataxia, tremor, reduced motor development, hyper- or hypotonia, behavioral difficulties, and varying degrees of mental retardation. Diagnosis is made by measuring enzyme activity in erythrocyte or other cell lysates similarly to ADA deficiency. There is no enzyme replacement available, and prognosis is poor even with bone marrow transplantation.

Less common forms of SCIDs involve molecules involved in the activation or development of lymphocytes. Lack of the *alpha chain receptor of IL-7* (9% of SCIDs) impairs development of memory lymphocytes. Deficiency in *recombinase proteins* (RAG1 and RAG2; 2.5% of SCIDs) impair V-D-J gene rearrangement of both immunoglobulins and T-cell receptors, thus affecting B and T cells, but sparing NK cells.

Rare SCIDs forms have been reported in a few patients. Deficiencies in the *subunits of CD3* impair transduction of activation signal between the T-cell receptor and cytoplasm blocking T-cell activation. Deficiency in CD3 zeta chain and in the transduction signaling molecule that binds to it, *zeta chain associated protein kinase 70* (Zap70), both lead to SCIDs characterized by depletion of CD8 cells (Table 32–4).

In *Artemis* deficiency, also known as Athabaskan SCID, the defect is in the gene encoding for the DNA-cross-link repair protein 1C, a nuclease involved in V(D)J gene rearrangement and in DNA repair. Besides defective rearrangement of immunoglobulin and T-cell receptor genes, this deficiency also increases susceptibility to DNA damage from radiation exposure, including X ray, which should be minimized.

In *reticular dysgenesis*, a very rare form of SCID, patients are born without leukocytes but with normal erythrocytes and platelets. The genetic defect is not known. Most die of overwhelming sepsis in the first days of life, or in weeks if kept in isolation in a sterile environment. Bone marrow shows no myeloid cells, and the thymus and spleen have no lymphocytes. One patient was successfully transplanted with the sibling's HLA-identical bone marrow.

OTHER FORMS OF COMBINED CELLULAR AND HUMORAL DEFICIENCIES

In nonsevere combined immunodeficiencies, the T-cell defect is milder than in SCIDs. Most are also treated with bone marrow transplantation, but because of the partial function of the patient's T cells, these patients require conditioning for ablation of their bone marrow prior to transplantation.

Bare Lymphocyte Syndromes Class I and II

Deficiencies in HLA class I and II lead to impaired stimulation of CD8 and CD4 lymphocytes, respectively. In HLA class I deficiency, or *bare lymphocyte syndrome type I*, HLA class I molecules are not expressed on the cell surface due to the lack of the peptide transporter that is composed of subunits TAP1 and TAP2 (Table 32–4). These patients can not be typed for HLA class I at the protein level. They may be asymptomatic or may present in late childhood with chronic lung disease.

HLA class II deficiency, or *bare lymphocyte syndrome type II,* is more frequent than the HLA class I deficiency. It frequently presents in infancy as SCIDs. It results from defects in factors essential for transcription of MHC class II genes. There are four genetic groups (A, B, C, and D), reflecting defects in four regulators of MHC class II expression. The factor defective in group A is MHC class II transactivator (CIITA, chromosome 16p13); in group B, regulatory factor-X ankyrin repeat-containing (RFXANK, chromosome 19p12); in group C, regulatory factor-5 (RFX5, chromosome 1q21.1–q21.3); and in group D, regulatory factor X-associated protein (RFXAP, chromosome 13q14).

Omenn Syndrome

In Omenn syndrome there is a partial deficiency in RAG1 or RAG2 leading to SCID. In addition to the immunodeficiency manifestations, these patients present with seborrheic erythrodermia, edema, alopecia, eosinophilia (usually more than 1000/mm^3), hepatosplenomegaly, lymphadenopathy, and elevated serum IgE. These additional signs resemble those of GVHD, and, indeed, patients with SCID who have been engrafted with maternal or blood transfusion–derived lymphocytes may develop overt GVHD and a similar clinical presentation, which is called by some the Omenn-like syndrome. In such a clinical presentation, Omenn syndrome due to deficiency of RAG1, RAG2, and GVHD must be evaluated with blood lymphocyte phenotyping, HLA typing, and skin biopsy. In Omenn syndrome, myeloablative conditioning prior to transplantation improves outcome of bone marrow transplantation because the recipient's T cells can jeopardize engraftment.

Wiskott-Aldrich Syndrome

The genetic defect in Wiskott-Aldrich syndrome (WAS) is in the WAS protein (WASP, Xp11.22), which participates in signal transduction that regulates cytoskeleton reorganization in hematopoietic cells. It is characterized by the triad of immunodeficiency, thrombocytopenia, and eczema. The first manifestation is bleeding due to thrombocytopenia with low platelet volume in the first year of life. It tends to improve in subsequent years. After 6 months of age, when maternal antibodies wane, patients develop recurrent respiratory infections with common bacterial microbes. Eczema ensues by 1 year of age and typically affects the lower face. Immunologic defects include low IgM, high IgA and high IgE, poor antibody response to polysaccharides, decreased T-cell function, and a predisposition to develop autoimmune diseases and cancer. Platelet count ranges from 5000 to 100,000/mm^3, platelets are small, and megakaryocytes are present in the bone marrow. Autoimmune-associated conditions include Coombs-positive autoimmune hemolytic anemia, vasculitis, renal disease, Henoch-Schönlein purpura, and inflammatory bowel disease. Malignancies occur in adolescence or adulthood, most commonly lymphoproliferative cancers, which worsen the prognosis even after bone marrow transplant. The best treatment for thrombocytopenia is intravenous immunoglobulin because prednisone and splenectomy increase the risk of life-threatening infections. Subcutaneous immunoglobulin is relatively contraindicated if thrombocytopenia is very severe due to the risk of bleeding. Diagnosis is made in boys with thrombocytopenic purpura and small platelets, together with eczema and the immune defects just mentioned. Identification of WASP gene mutations confirms that diagnosis. Prognosis is poor without bone marrow transplantation, which is curative.

Ataxia Telangiectasia

The multisystem disease of ataxia telangiectasia is caused by mutations in the ataxia-telangiectasia mutated gene (ATM, chromosome 22q22–q23), which encodes a phosphatidyl inositol-3 (PI-3) kinase. This is one of the kinases that responds to DNA damage by phosphorylating key substrates involved in DNA repair and in cell cycle control. This defect makes patients very sensitive to radiation, including x-ray, which leads to chromosome breakage. Eventually, the impaired ability to repair damaged DNA leads to lymphoproliferative and epithelial malignancies. Patients usually present with cerebellar ataxia in the first year of life, followed by telangiectasia in the second, and later, recurrent sinopulmonary infections. However, some present with delayed onset at 4 to 6 years of age. With time, neurologic status deteriorates with choreoathetosis, dysconjugated gaze, and extrapyramidal and posterior column signs. Telangiectasia appears first on the inner scleral conjunctiva (bulbar region) and then affects the nasal bridge, ears, and antecubital fossae. Immunodeficiency is manifested by recurrent sinopulmonary virus and bacterial infections. In puberty, secondary sexual characteristics do not develop, and mental retardation may ensue and progress. Laboratory findings include normal or low T- and B-cell functions. Patients may have lymphopenia (low CD4 cells, normal B and NK cells), low proliferation to mitogens and allogenic cells, no response to delayed hypersensitivity testing, IgA deficiency (present in 50% to 80%), or IgG2 and IgG4 subclass deficiency with poor antibody response. IgE may be absent as well. Patients have elevated α-fetoprotein. Definitive diagnosis is made by finding mutations in the ATM gene. No specific therapy exists. Patients may need aggressive antibiotic therapy for infections, antibiotic prophylaxis, immunoglobulin replacement, avoidance of live microbe vaccines, and be careful to receive only irradiated blood products. Bone marrow transplantation has not been performed, and thymus transplantation was not successful. Such approach will likely not reverse neurologic changes. Prognosis is poor because immunologic and neurologic functions deteriorate together with chronic lung disease, but some have lived to the fifth decade. Death results from infections or from malignancies such as non–Hodgkin lymphoma (45%), lymphocytic leukemias (14%), and carcinoma of the stomach, liver, and ovaries.

X-Linked Lymphoproliferative Disease or Duncan Syndrome

Males with this X-linked lymphoproliferative disease (XLPD), or Duncan syndrome, lack a gene encoding the SH2 domain protein-1A (chromosome Xq25), which leads to a lack of NKT cells. They are typically asymptomatic until they develop EBV infection, to which they are extremely sensitive. EBV causes a severe infectious mononucleosis around 2.5 years of age and is fatal in 50% of patients (death from liver failure). If patients survive the acute infection, they evolve with newly acquired hypogammaglobulinemia (approximately 30%) or Burkitt-type lymphoma (approximately 20%), usually in the ileocecal region. Some may develop aplastic anemia. Bone marrow transplantation is curative, but prognosis is poor, with 75% mortality by 10 years of age and longevity of less than 40 years of age.

PHAGOCYTE DEFICIENCIES

Neutropenic Syndromes

Neutropenia (less than 1000; severe if less than 500/mm^3) increases the risk of pyogenic infections, fever, and sepsis due to bacteria and fungi (Table 32–2). It may correct with administration of G-CSF.

Neutropenia can be secondary to chemotherapeutic agents, glycogen storage disease type 1b, myelokathexis (inability to release neutrophils from the marrow), autoimmune antibodies against neutrophils as in Felty syndrome with rheumatoid arthritis, bone marrow cancer invasion, myelofibrosis, infections, and deficiency of vitamin B$_{12}$ or folate. It also occurs in Shwachman-Bodian-Diamond syndrome, which involves exocrine pancreatic insufficiency, cytopenias, and hematologic malignancies caused by a defective SBDS gene (chromosome 7q11).

In primary immunodeficiencies, neutropenia can occur as part of other immunologic defects, such as in X-linked hyper IgM syndrome, X-linked agammaglobulinemia, and Wiskott-Aldrich syndrome (also X-linked), as mentioned earlier. In addition, as discussed later, neutropenia can be the principal defect in other primary immunodeficiencies, such as in congenital and cyclic neutropenia and Chédiak-Higashi syndrome.

Congenital Neutropenia or Kostmann Syndrome

Mutations in two genes can cause congenital neutropenia. Mutations in neutrophil elastase (ELA2 gene, chromosome 19p13.3) cause sporadic and autosomal dominant cases. Sporadic cases can also result from mutations in the growth factor-independent 1 (GFI1, chromosome 1p22), a repressor of ELA2 expression and also a transcriptional repressor protooncogene that inhibits hematopoieses. Some patients with GFI1 defects have also developed acute myeloid leukemia.

Mutations in neutrophil elastase gene have also been found in patients with *cyclic neutropenia*. These patients have cyclic inhibition of hematopoiesis and every 21 days develop cyclic fluctuations in the numbers of blood neutrophils, monocytes, eosinophils, lymphocytes, platelets, and reticulocytes. Patients with the disease typically have regularly recurring symptoms of fever, malaise, mucosal ulcers, and, occasionally, life-threatening infections during periods of neutropenia.

Chédiak-Higashi Syndrome

Chédiak-Higashi syndrome (CHS) is caused by a mutation in the lysosomal trafficking regulator gene (LYST, chromosome 1q42.1–q42.2), which impairs movement of lysosomes in the cytosol. As a result, giant lysosomal granules form in many cells including neutrophils (which allows diagnosis by analysis of blood smear), melanocytes, neural Schwann cells, renal tubular cells, gastric mucosa, pneumonocytes, hepatocytes, Langerhans cells, and adrenal cells. Large eosinophilic inclusion bodies (peroxidase positive) also form in myeloblasts and promyeloblasts in bone marrow. Clinical manifestations include partial albinism, photophobia, nystagmus, and neutropenia. Neutrophils have impaired chemotaxis and bactericidal activity. Death usually occurs by 7 years of age from severe infections or lymphoma. About 85% to 90% of patients develop a unique lymphoproliferative syndrome called the "accelerated phase" of CHS. This disorder is characterized by generalized lymphohistiocytic infiltrates, fever, jaundice, hepatosplenomegaly, lymphadenopathy, pancytopenia, and bleeding. The prognosis of the accelerated phase is poor, with death within 3 years from infection or bleeding unless bone marrow transplantation is performed successfully. Bone marrow transplantation corrects hematologic problems, but progressive neurologic symptoms ensue in the third decade of life (cerebellar ataxia, peripheral neuropathy, and cognitive abnormalities).

Chronic Granulomatous Disease

Patients with chronic granulomatous disease (CGD) have defective nicotinamide adenine dinucleotide phosphate (NADPH) oxidase, which produces superoxide, a precursor for other oxygen radicals produced during phagocyte respiratory burst to kill phagocytized bacteria. NADPH oxidase activity is tightly regulated. It becomes active when its four subunits come together. At rest, two subunits of the enzyme are bound to the plasma membrane and form the cytochrome b_{588}: a 91 kd glycoprotein (gp91^{phox}, CYBB gene or beta subunit, chromosome Xp21.2) and a 22 kd protein (p22^{phox}, CYBA or alpha subunit, chromosome 16q24). Upon NADPH oxidase activation, two other cytosolic subunits join these two membrane subunits to form the four-subunit functional enzyme. The cytosolic subunits are the p47^{phox} protein (neutrophil cytosol factor 1, NCF1, chromosome

7q11.23) and the p67^{phox} protein (neutrophil cytosol factor 2, NCF2, chromosome 1q25).

Deficiency of either CYBB or CYAA prevents expression of the cytochrome b_{588}, and causes the cytochrome-b negative CGD forms, whereas a deficiency of NCFs allows expression of cytochrome b_{588}, and causes the cytochrome-b positive CGD forms (type I due to NCF1/p47^{phox} deficiency and type II due to NCF2/p67-phox deficiency). The most common deficiency is lack of gp91^{phox}, an X-linked defect that accounts for 65% of all CGD cases. Deficiency in any of the other three subunits causes autosomal recessive disease (p22^{phox} deficiency in 5% of cases, p47^{phox} deficiency in 25%, and p67^{phox} deficiency in 5%).

Clinical manifestations are heterogeneous. They vary even between identical twins with the same mutations. Two thirds of CGD patients present in the first year of life with infections (recurrent suppurative lymphadenitis, pneumonia, impetigo), chronic dermatitis (sometimes since birth), and gastrointestinal symptoms (gastric antrum obstruction due to granulomas, bloody diarrhea from CGD colitis, perirectal abscesses with fistulas), and osteomyelitis. Other less common infections are otitis media, conjunctivitis, urinary tract infections, sinusitis, and abscesses in the liver, kidney, and brain. Many have a history of chronic diarrhea, gingivitis, and ulcerative stomatitis. On examination, most CGD patients have generalized lymphadenopathy and hepatosplenomegaly, which are enlarged because of noncaseating granulomatosis. Patients also have poor growth (underweight and short stature). Granulomatous disease can lead to obstruction of the gastric antrum, ileocolic junction, and to hydronephrosis. Some patients manifest the disease in adulthood.

Most organisms causing infections in CGD patients produce catalase, an enzyme that catabolizes hydrogen peroxide into water and oxygen. This enzyme eliminates bacterial peroxide, which cannot be used by neutrophils to produce other reactive oxygen species (Fig. 32–2). As a result, they escape phagocytosis and continue to multiply. The microbes—most catalase positive—that cause infections in CGD patients are *Staphylococcal aureus, Aspergillus* spp., enteric gram-negative bacilli (*Escherichia coli, Salmonella* spp., *Klebsiella* spp., *Enterobacter* spp., *Proteus* spp.), *Burkholderia cepacia, Serratia marcescens, Staphylococcus epidermidis, Streptococcus* spp., *Candida albicans,* and *Nocardia* spp.

Laboratory diagnosis is based on the inability of neutrophils to produce reactive oxygen species (ROS) when stimulated with zymosan or phorbol-myristate acetate because NADPH oxidase is inactive in resting phagocytes. In the past, nitroblue tetrazolium (NBT) was used as a substrate. When oxidized by ROS, NBT changes from yellow to dark brown-purple color inside the neutrophil granules, which is visualized by light microscopy in leukocyte smears. This has been replaced by newer tests using flow cytometry or chemiluminescence. In one

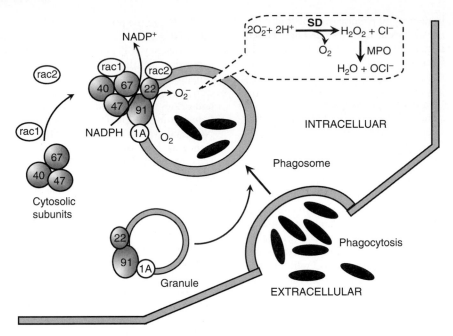

$$2O_2^- + 2H^+ \xrightarrow{\text{SD}} H_2O_2 + Cl^-$$

Figure 32–2. In the respiratory burst of phagocytes, nicotinamide adenine dinucleotide phosphate (NADPH) oxidase initiates formation of reactive oxygen species (ROS) in phagosomes, a process that consumes oxygen (O_2). NADPH is inactive at rest because its subunits are disassembled. In granules, two membrane-bound subunits (91^{phox} and 22^{phox}) form the cytochrome b_{588} next to the GTP binding protein rap1A (1A). Upon phagocytosis of microbes, granules fuse with the phagosome, and the cytoplasmic subunits (67^{phox}, 47^{phox}, and 40^{phox}) translocate and bind to cytochrome b_{588} to assemble the active NADPH oxidase. Small cytosolic GTP binding proteins rac1 and rac2 regulate translocation of 67^{phox} and electron transport in the cytochrome b_{588}, respectively. A case of rac2 deficiency causing chronic granulomatous disease (CGD) has been described. In the phagosome, superoxide (O_2^-) produced by NADPH oxidase is transformed by superoxide dismutase (SD) into hydrogen peroxide (H_2O_2), which is then transformed by myeloperoxidase (MPO) into hypochlorite (OCl^-). These three ROS kill bacteria.

flow cytometry assay, normal neutrophils become fluorescent when their hydrogen peroxide reacts with dihydrorhodamine. This is a highly reliable and sensitive assay to detect both disease and maternal X-linked carrier status. Additional tests include flow cytometry or Western blot to identify which of the four subunits is missing and detection of mutations in the gene alleles of the missing subunit. *In vitro* assays using patient's neutrophils and bacteria can also show that CGD neutrophils have impaired bacterial killing and impaired oxygen consumption.

Other laboratory abnormalities include hypergammaglobulinemia and anemia of chronic disease. Blood leukocytes and sedimentation rate are normal but increase with infections. Granulomatosis in the lungs, liver, and spleen can cause obstructive symptoms and are visualized in computerized tomography scan or magnetic resonance imaging studies.

Prognosis improves with aggressive *treatment* of infections, aspirating infected lymph nodes, draining

abscesses, and identifying infectious etiology by early biopsy of involved organs. Duration of antibiotic therapy is prolonged to 5 to 6 weeks instead of the usual duration of 1 to 2 weeks prescribed for immunocompetent hosts. Prophylactic treatment with trimethoprim-sulfamethoxazole reduces mortality due to bacterial infections, and recently, addition of prophylaxis for fungal infections using itraconazole was also beneficial. In addition, CGD patients treated continuously with subcutaneous interferon gamma (IFN-γ) at 60 μg/m², three times a week, have reduced mortality and morbidity. IFN-γ does not increase activity of NADPH oxidase, and it is unclear how it benefits CGD patients.

OTHER ENZYME DEFICIENCIES

Glucose-6-Phosphatase Dehydrogenase Deficiency

In glucose-6-phosphatase dehydrogenase (G6PD) deficiency, patients lack G6PD (chromosome Xq28) in leukocytes, which participates in the formation of NADH and NADPH. As a result, they have impaired production of hydrogen peroxide, but to a lesser extent than that in CGD. They are predisposed to infections with *S. aureus* and *E. coli,* but clinical manifestations are milder than those in CGD. This deficiency maybe related to G6PD deficiency in red cells, which predisposes to hemolysis with certain drugs such as sulfonamides.

Myeloperoxidase Deficiency

Patients with complete myeloperoxidase (MPO) (chromosome 17q23.1) deficiency in leukocytes cannot produce hypochlorite from hydrogen peroxide (Fig. 32–2) but have normal production of superoxide and hydrogen peroxide, and they have normal oxygen consumption. Bacterial killing assay shows delayed, but eventually even complete bacterial killing. Many patients are asymptomatic, but some may have increased susceptibility to infections with *Candida* and staphylococcus. Diagnosis is made by lack of peroxidase staining in blood neutrophils.

Hyper-IgE Syndrome or Job Syndrome

The specific defect in Hyper-IgE (HIE) syndrome is unknown. Lymphocytes produce excessive amounts of TH2 cytokines (IL4 and IL13), which explains increased IgE and eosinophilia. Patients also have recurrent pyogenic infections, intermittent defects in phagocyte chemotaxis, and facial dysmorphism.

Typically *clinical manifestations* start in childhood with recurrent skin abscesses and deep-seated abscesses caused by staphylococci including pneumonia (often with pneumatocele formation) and mastoiditis. The deep-seated infections differentiate HIE from atopic eczema, which can also cause high IgE and staphylococcal impetigo. Less commonly abscesses can affect bones, joints, and viscera. Dermatitis is prominent, but unlike atopic eczema, pruritus is uncommon. In HIE, staphylococcal infections with abscesses stand out, and rash is not related to food allergies. Other abnormalities include a characteristic facies (see below), osteopenia with fractures (osteoporosis) secondary to minor or unrecognized trauma, scoliosis, and hyperextensible joints. Dental abnormalities include the retention of primary teeth, the failure of secondary teeth to erupt, and delayed resorption of the roots of the primary teeth. On examination patients have coarse facial features, including frontal bossing, a broad nasal bridge, a wide, fleshy nasal tip, and deep-set eyes.

There is no specific *laboratory* test that establishes the diagnosis. Patients have very elevated IgE levels, usually more than 2000 IU/mL and often between 50,000 and 100,000 IU/mL, but levels fluctuate. IgD is also elevated, whereas IgA, IgM, and IgG are normal. Blood lymphocyte numbers and proliferative responses are normal. Eosinophils are elevated in blood, sputum, and tissues including in abscesses. Neutrophil respiratory burst and bacterial killing are normal, but they have a chemotactic deficiency probably mediated by T-cell soluble factors and/or IgE immunocomplexes.

There is no specific treatment. Treatment aims at controlling disease manifestations. Infections are treated with intravenous antibiotics to cover staphylococcus. Deep-seated abscesses need drainage or excision. Early treatment of sinusitis and bronchitis can help prevent pneumonias and the onset of chronic lung disease. Prophylaxis with trimethoprim-sulfamethoxazole may be beneficial. Topical cutaneous corticosteroids are used for dermatitis, and topical mupirocin for skin infections. Osteopenia and dental problems need early surveillance and treatment to avoid long-term complications. INF-γ and intravenous immunoglobulin have been attempted without clinical benefit.

Leukocyte Adhesion Deficiency Type 1

In leukocyte adhesion deficiency type 1 (LAD-1), an autosomal recessive disease, patients have mutations in the gene encoding CD18 (or integrin β-2, chromosome 21q22.3), which forms heterodimers with integrins α-L (CD11a), α-M (CD11b) or α-X to form, respectively, lymphocyte function-associated antigen 1 (LFA-1, CD11aCD18), complement receptor type 3 (Mac-1, CD11bCD18), and leukocyte surface antigen p150,95 (Leu5, CD11cCD18). LFA-1 is expressed on T, B, and NK cells; and Mac-1 on phagocytes and NK cells.

An initial *clinical manifestation* is the delayed separation of the umbilical cord (beyond 3 weeks). In the first weeks of life patients also develop pyogenic infections caused by *S. aureus, Pseudomonas aeruginosa, Klebsiella, Proteus,* and enterococci. Infections are omphalitis and other skin infections, pneumonia, ileocolitis, peritonitis, perineal abscesses, periodontitis, tracheobronchitis, and sepsis. Mortality is high in the first years of life. A milder protracted form with the same genetic defect also exists.

Laboratory findings include leukocytosis, which markedly increases during infections reaching 50,000 to 100,000 cells/mm^3, but infection sites (e.g., cellulitis) do not accumulate pus. LFA-1 deficiency impairs cellular cytotoxicity from NK and CD8 cells and interaction between antigen-presenting cells and lymphocytes. CR3 deficiency can impair binding to C3b, phagocyte adhesion, chemotaxis, respiratory burst with phagocytosis, and antibody-dependent cellular cytotoxicity. Diagnosis is made by demonstrating lack of expression of CD18 on blood leukocytes stimulated with phorbol myristate acetate.

Treatment is directed toward infections. Prophylactic antibiotic therapy may be beneficial as well (e.g., for dental procedures). Some have been successfully treated with bone marrow transplantation.

Leukocyte Adhesion Deficiency Type 2

In leukocyte adhesion deficiency type 2 (LAD-2), patients lack the GDP-fucose transporter-1 (chromosome 11p11.2) resulting in lack of expression of sialyl-Lewis^X (CD15s) on the surface of leukocytes. Sialyl-Lewis^X is the ligand for E-selectin, and its deficiency on neutrophils impairs their attachment and rolling on activated endothelial cells. As in LAD-1, neutrophils also have a chemotactic defect, and patients suffer recurrent pyogenic bacterial infections, periodontitis, and marked neutrophilia with poor pus formation at the infection site. However, unlike LAD-1, LAD-2 patients have mental retardation.

Deficiency in the IL12/IFN-γ Pathway

Macrophages stimulated by microorganisms produce IL12 that binds to the IL12 receptor on NK and T cells, inducing their production of IFN-γ, which, in turn, acts on macrophages via the IFN-γ receptor and increases their phagocytic and killing activity. This macrophage–lymphocyte interaction is important in the defense against mycobacteria because several deficiencies in this pathway increase susceptibility to mycobacterial infections.

The active form of IL12 is IL12p70, a heterodimer of IL12p40 (IL12B) and IL12p35 (IL12A). The IL12 receptor (IL12R) is also a heterodimer composed of IL12Rβ1 and IL12Rβ2. Similarly, the IFN-γ receptor (IFN-γR) is a heterodimer of IFN-γR1 and IFN-γR2. Stimulation via IFN-γR results in activation of the transcription factor STAT1.

Deficiencies in IL12p40, IL12Rβ1, IFN-γ-R1, IFN-γ-R2 and STAT1 have been described where patients *manifest clinically* with increased susceptibility to mycobacterial infections caused by usually nonpathogenic Bacille Calmette-Guérin (BCG) and environmental mycobacteria, including osteomyelitis, pneumonia, skin infections, and disseminated infection. Deficiencies in IL12p40 and IL12R also increase susceptibility to salmonella and nocardia infections.

Based on the frequency of the IFN-γ and IL12 axis defects, *laboratory evaluation* of patients with non–tuberculous mycobacterial infection and without other obvious cellular immunodeficiencies should be performed by flow cytometry as follows. First, expression of IFN-γR1 on monocytes should be examined, next phosphorylation of STAT1 (shows normal function of IFN-γR), and then, IFN-γR2 expression. If all normal, secretion of IL12p40 (or IL12p70) by monocytes stimulated with INF-γ and endotoxin [LPS]) should be undertaken, followed by examination of expression of IL12Rβ1 on stimulated and proliferating lymphocytes, and of phosphorylation of STAT4 (demonstrating functioning IL12R).

Besides acute antibiotic *treatment* for mycobacterial infections, many patients respond well to chronic INF-γ therapy and may need chronic mycobacterial antibiotic prophylaxis. BCG vaccine should be avoided.

EVIDENCE-BASED MEDICINE

Prenatal Diagnosis

Because the genetic defects for most primary immunodeficiencies are known, prenatal diagnosis is becoming widely available for the inherited diseases. Amniotic fluid cells or fetal blood are used to study leukocytes. In addition, there is ongoing research on developing molecular diagnostic tests to detect primary immunodeficiencies, particularly SCIDs, as part of newborn screening tests.

Gene Therapy for Immunodeficiencies

Gene therapy was first attempted in adenosine deaminase deficiency in 1990 resulting is temporary success as mentioned earlier. More recently, in 1999, gene therapy was performed for X-linked SCID where the common gamma chain (γc) was transfected into autologous bone marrow CD34+ stem cells *ex vivo* using a retrovirus vector. The transfected cells were then transferred back to the patients. Nine out of ten patients had excellent results, including reconstitution of specific antibody response, which is difficult to achieve with bone marrow transplantation. However, 3 years later, the two youngest patients developed clonal expansion of T cells because the gene transfection integrated the γc gene next to the proto-oncogene LM02, resulting in premalignant disorders. Future gene therapy technology will need to better control the site where new genes are integrated into the genome.

BIBLIOGRAPHY

Hacein-Bey-Abina S, Von Kalle C, Schmidt M, et al. LM02-associated clonal T cell proliferation in two patients after gene therapy for SCID-X1. *Science.* 2003;302(5644):415. Erratum in *Science.* 2003;302(5645):568.

Notarangelo L, Casanova JL, Conley ME, et al. International Union of Immunological Societies Primary Immunodeficiency Diseases Classification Committee. Primary immunodeficiency diseases: an update from the International Union of Immunological Societies Primary Immunodeficiency Diseases Classification Committee Meeting in Budapest, 2005. *J Allergy Clin Immunol.* 2006;117:883.

Ochs HD, Smith CIE, Puck JM. *Primary Immunodeficiency Diseases. A Molecular and Genetic Approach.* New York: Oxford University Press; 1999.

Online Mendelian Inheritance in Man (OMIM). Available at: http://www.ncbi.nlm.nih.gov/entrez/query.fcgi?db=OMIM.

Orange JS, Hossny EM, Weiler CR, et al. Primary Immunodeficiency Committee of the American Academy of Allergy, Asthma and Immunology. Use of intravenous immunoglobulin in human disease: a review of evidence by members of the Primary Immunodeficiency Committee of the American Academy of

Allergy, Asthma and Immunology. *J Allergy Clin Immunol.* 2006;117:S525. Erratum in *J Allergy Clin Immunol.* 2006;117:1483.

Parslow TG, Stites DP, Terr AI, et al. *Medical Immunology.* New York: McGraw-Hill; 2001.

Shearer WT, Buckley RH, Engler RJ, et al. Practice parameters for the diagnosis and management of immunodeficiency. The Clinical and Laboratory Immunology Committee of the American Academy of Allergy, Asthma, and Immunology (CLIC-AAAAI). *Ann Allergy Asthma Immunol.* 1996;76:282. Erratum in *Ann Allergy Asthma Immunol.* 1996;77:262.

Stiehm ER, Ochs HD, Winklestein JA. *Immunologic Disorders in Infants and Children.* London: Elsevier; 2004.

Wildin RS, Freitas A. IPEX and FOXP3: Clinical and research perspectives. *J Autoimmunol.* 2005;25(suppl):56.

Worth A, Thrasher AJ, Gaspar HB. Autoimmune lymphoproliferative syndrome: molecular basis of disease and clinical phenotype. *Br J Haematol.* 2006;133:124.

WEB-BASED RESOURCES

1. Jeffrey Modell Foundation. Available at: http://www.jmfworld.com/.

2. Immune Deficiency Foundation. Available at: http://www.primaryimmune.org/idf.htm.

3. National Institute of Allergy and Infectious Diseases resources on primary immunodeficiencies. Available at: http://www.niaid.nih.gov/publications/pid.htm.

HIV Infection

33

Mitchell H. Katz, MD and Andrew R. Zolopa, MD

Infection with the human immunodeficiency virus (HIV) causes progressive immunodeficiency, resulting in serious infections and cancers. Treatment focuses on inhibiting viral replication and, for those patients with immune dysfunction, administering prophylactic treatment to prevent serious infections. In this chapter we review the pathophysiology of HIV, the immunologic consequences of HIV infection, the treatment of HIV, and the management of two common allergic conditions associated with HIV/AIDS: hypersensitivity reactions and immune reconstitution inflammatory syndrome (IRIS).

PATHOPHYSIOLOGY OF HIV

HIV-1 is a single-stranded RNA retrovirus that infects humans. The virus envelope attaches itself to the human cell. The HIV virus has a high affinity for the CD4 receptors of the T lymphocytes and monocytes. Once attached to the receptor, the virus enters the cell. Replication of the virus depends on a reverse transcriptase (RNA-dependent DNA polymerase) to make a DNA copy of the viral RNA. Next, a second strand of DNA is synthesized making a double-stranded DNA replica of the viral RNA. The DNA strand becomes integrated into the host cellular DNA. The viral building blocks (HIV-1 RNA, gag proteins, and various enzymes) are synthesized and assembled inside the cell, and then they bud through the plasma membrane of the cell, creating mature viral particles that can infect other cells.

IMMUNOLOGIC CONSEQUENCES OF HIV INFECTION

Because HIV has a high affinity for CD4 receptor, the helper T lymphocyte cell is the major target of HIV. For this reason, measurement of the number of CD4 helper cells is the major laboratory parameter used for assessing the severity of immunodeficiency and response to treatment. Viral replication results in progressive killing and depletion of the CD4 cells. There is preferential loss of naive CD4 cells over memory CD4 cells early in infection. Besides loss of CD4 cells, HIV infection impairs the function of the remaining CD4 cells.

Although HIV causes CD4 cell loss, it simultaneously causes a state of immune activation of CD4 cells, CD8 cells, and monocytes. Activation enhances the ability of HIV to infect CD4 cells. Monocyte activation results in elevated production of the cytokines tumor necrosis factor alpha and interleukin 6. Overall, immune activation likely contributes to the dysfunction of the immune response against opportunistic infections. Although circulating CD8 cells expand initially with infection, with progressive infection there is loss of CD8 cells, B lymphocytes, and natural killer cells.

In the absence of treatment, HIV infection results in susceptibility to serious opportunistic infections and cancers. The average time between infection and serious immunodeficiency characterized by a CD4 count below 200 cells or an opportunistic infection or malignancy is about 10 years, with both rapid progressors (1 to 2 years from infection to serious immune deficiency) and slow progressors (persons who have been infected for longer than 15 years with intact immune systems.)

With potent antiretroviral treatment of HIV infection, there is a rapid increase (first few months after starting therapy) in circulating naive and memory CD4 and CD8 cells. This is followed by a slower increase (first year and beyond) in circulating naive CD4 and CD8 cells and a decrease in circulating memory cells. It is thought that the ability of T cells to respond to a variety of antigens improves during this second phase. Immune activation also decreases. It appears that these improvements in the immune system can continue for many years on effective antiretroviral treatment. With these immunologic improvements, marked reductions in the appearance of opportunistic infections and malignancies have occurred, including the successful eradication of some infections that were previously untreatable (e.g., cryptosporidial diarrhea).

TREATMENT OF HIV INFECTION

Antiretroviral Treatment

HIV replication (also commonly referred to as "viral load") is measured by either PCR tests that measure plasma RNA levels or branch chain test that measures DNA levels.

The best time to initiate antiretroviral treatment requires weighing the benefits of viral suppression against the side effects of the drugs for each patient. In general, treatment for asymptomatic HIV disease should be initiated when the CD4 cell count drops below 350 cells/mcL or when the patients develops symptoms of HIV disease (e.g., fever, weight loss). Patients with rapidly dropping CD4 counts or very high viral loads (above 100,000/mcL) should be considered for earlier treatment.

Once a decision to initiate therapy has been made, several important principles should guide therapy. First, because HIV patients develop drug resistance to antiretroviral agents, a major goal of therapy should be total suppression of viral replication as measured by the serum viral load. Therapy that achieves a plasma viral load below 50 or below 75 copies/mL (depending on the test used) correlates with antiviral effect in other compartments. To achieve this and maintain virologic control over time, aggressive combination therapy is essential. Partially suppressive combinations such as dual nucleoside therapy should be avoided, and caution should be exercised in starting treatment in patients who are not likely to adhere to this regimen (e.g., active substance users).

Similarly, if toxicity develops, it is preferable to either interrupt the entire regimen or change the offending drug rather than reduce individual doses. The current standard is to use at least three agents simultaneously. Because the number of drugs and potential combinations is finite and the development of drug resistance may severely compromise the efficacy of treatment, patients must be able to adhere to these regimens. Patients who may miss many doses of treatment should be counseled to defer starting therapy until they are able to adhere to the regimen. Adherence can be promoted through the use of medication boxes with compartments (e.g., MediSets), supportive counseling, or daily supervision of therapy.

Monitoring of antiretroviral therapy has two goals. Laboratory evaluation for toxicity depends on the specific drugs in the combination but generally should be done approximately every 3 months once a patient is on a stable regimen. Monitoring for efficacy is done with the CD4 cell count and HIV viral load tests. They should be repeated 1 to 2 months after the initiation or change of antiretroviral regimen and every 3 to 4 months thereafter in clinically stable patients. Reasons for changing antiretroviral regimens include intolerable adverse reactions, rising or persistently detectable viral loads, the clinical progression of disease, and continued immunologic deterioration as reflected by a declining CD4 cell count. Although a rebound in HIV viral load is cited as an indication to change therapy, exact parameters have not been established, and many patients appear to have continued clinical benefit in the face of rising viral load measurements. When therapy is modified, clinicians should attempt to start at least two agents to which an individual has not been exposed or to which there is minimal or no resistance at the same time. Conversely, there is a risk to stopping a single medication because of the possibility of its causing a side effect if the remaining regimen contains too few medications to prevent rapid development of resistance. Drug resistance testing is recommended for patients who are experiencing treatment failure (persistent or rising viral load despite adherence to an efficacious regimen).

Although the ideal combination of drugs has not yet been defined for all possible clinical situations, possible choices can be better understood after a review of the four major categories of medications: nucleoside and nucleotide reverse transcriptase inhibitors (NRTIs), nonnucleoside reverse transcriptase inhibitors (NNRTIs), protease inhibitors (PIs), and entry inhibitors. Table 33–1 shows the doses and side effects of these treatments.

NUCLEOSIDE AND NUCLEOTIDE REVERSE TRANSCRIPTASE INHIBITORS

There are currently seven approved NRTIs: zidovudine, lamivudine, emtricitabine, tenofovir, abacavir, didanosine, stavudine, and zalcitabine. Of these, lamivudine and emtricitabine are essentially interchangeable. Stavudine should be avoided because it causes significantly more side effects than the others. Zalcitabine is rarely used due to limited efficacy. Several combination medications of these medications have been formulated, including Combivir (zidovudine and lamivudine), Truvada (emtricitabine and tenofovir), Epzicom (lamivudine and abacavir), and Trizivir (zidovudine, lamivudine, and abacavir). These combinations decrease drug burden and increase compliance with regimens. Lamivudine, emtricitabine, and tenofovir all have activity against hepatitis B and are therefore often used in patients coinfected with HIV and hepatitis B. Coinfected patients who stop these medications may experience a flare of their hepatitis B infection characterized by liver function test abnormalities, right upper quadrant pain, fevers, and potentially fatal hepatic failure. Therefore, these agents should probably be continued as part of the patient's regimen even if the HIV infection has developed resistance to them.

NONNUCLEOSIDE REVERSE TRANSCRIPTASE INHIBITORS

There are three approved NNRTIs: efavirenz, nevirapine, and delavirdine. Of these three, efavirenz is the

Table 33–1. Antiretroviral therapy.

Drug	Dose	Side Effects	Monitoring
Nucleoside/Nucleotide Reverse Transcriptase Inhibitors			
Zidovudine (AZT) (Retrovir)	600 mg orally daily in two divided doses	Anemia, neutropenia, nausea, malaise, headache, insomnia, myopathy	Complete blood count (CBC) and differential (every 3 months once stable)
Lamivudine (3TC) (Epivir)	150 mg orally twice daily	Rash, peripheral neuropathy	No additional monitoring
Emtricitabine (Emtriva)	300 mg orally once daily	Skin discoloration of palms/soles (mild)	No additional monitoring
Tenofovir (Viread)	300 mg orally once daily	Gastrointestinal distress	Renal function
Abacavir (Ziagen)	300 mg orally twice daily	Rash, fever—if occur, rechallenge may be fatal	No special monitoring
Didanosine (ddI) (Videx)	400 mg orally daily (enteric-coated capsule) for persons ≥60 kg	Peripheral neuropathy, pancreatitis, dry mouth, hepatitis	CBC and differential, aminotransferases, K$^+$, amylase, triglycerides, bimonthly neurologic questionnaire for neuropathy
Stavudine (d4T) (Zerit)	40 mg orally twice daily for persons ≥60 kg	Peripheral neuropathy, hepatitis, pancreatitis	Monthly neurologic questionnaire for neuropathy, aminotransferases, amylase
Zalcitabine (ddC) (Hivid)	0.375–0.75 mg orally three times daily	Peripheral neuropathy, aphthous ulcers, hepatitis	Monthly neurologic questionnaire for neuropathy, aminotransferases
Nonnucleoside Reverse Transcriptase Inhibitors (NNRTIs)			
Efavirenz (Sustiva)	600 mg orally daily	Neurologic disturbances	No additional monitoring
Nevirapine (Viramune)	200 mg orally daily for 2 weeks, then 200 mg orally twice daily	Rash	No additional monitoring
Delavirdine (Rescriptor)	400 mg orally three times daily	Rash	No additional monitoring
Protease Inhibitors (PIs)			
Indinavir (Crixivan)	800 mg orally three times daily	Kidney stones	Trimonthly aminotransferases, bilirubin level, cholesterol, triglycerides
Nelfinavir (Viracept)	750 mg orally three times daily	Diarrhea	Cholesterol, triglycerides

Drug	Dose	Adverse Effects	Monitoring
Ritonavir (Norvir)	600 mg orally twice daily or in lower doses (e.g., 100 mg orally once or twice daily) for boosting other PIs	Gastrointestinal distress, peripheral paresthesias	Trimonthly aminotransferases, creatine kinase, uric acid, triglycerides
Saquinavir hard gel (Invirase)	1000 mg twice daily with 100 mg ritonavir orally twice daily	Gastrointestinal distress	Trimonthly aminotransferases, cholesterol, triglycerides
Fosamprenavir (Lexiva)	1400 mg orally twice daily or 1400 mg orally once daily with ritonavir 200 mg orally once daily	Same as amprenavir	Same as amprenavir
Lopinavir/ritonavir (Kaletra)	400 mg/100 mg orally twice daily	Diarrhea	Cholesterol, triglycerides, every other month aminotransferases
Atazanavir (Reyataz)	400 mg orally once daily	Hyperbilirubinemia	Bilirubin level
Darunavir (Prezista)	600 mg orally twice daily with ritonavir 100 mg twice daily with food	Diarrhea, intracranial hemorrhage, headache, rash	Cholesterol, triglycerides
Entry Inhibitors			
Enfuvirtide (Fuzeon)	90 mg subcutaneously twice daily	Injection site pain and allergic reaction	No additional monitoring

most frequently used because it is as effective as protease inhibitors with fewer side effects. Also, it can be administered once a day. Delavirdine is rarely used because of a large pill burden and no particular advantages over the other two drugs in this class.

NNRTIs inhibit reverse transcriptase at a site different from that of the nucleoside and nucleotide agents just described. The resistance patterns of the NNRTIs are distinct from those of the PIs, so their use still leaves open the option for future PI use.

Resistance to one drug in this class uniformly predicts resistance to other drugs in the class, although second-generation drugs are in development. There is no therapeutic reason for using more than one NNRTI at the same time or for sequential use once resistance had developed to one of these drugs.

PROTEASE INHIBITORS

Nine PIs—indinavir, nelfinavir, ritonavir, saquinavir, fosamprenavir, lopinavir (in combination with ritonavir), atazanavir, tipranavir, and darunavir are currently available. Of these, indinavir, ritonavir, and saquinavir are rarely used by themselves. Ritonavir is commonly used to boost the drug levels of indinavir, saquinavir, fosamprenavir, lopinavir, atazanavir, tipranavir, and darunavir, allowing use of lower doses and simpler dosing schedules of these PIs. Lopinavir is formulated with ritonavir (Kaletra). Tipranavir is the first approved nonpeptidic PI. Because of its unique structure it is active against some strains of the virus that are resistant to other available PIs. Tipranavir may be associated with intracranial hemorrhage.

All the PIs—to differing degrees—are metabolized by the cytochrome P-450 system, and each can inhibit and induce various P-450 isoenzymes. Therefore, drug interactions are common and difficult to predict. Clinicians should consult the product inserts before prescribing PIs with other medications. Drugs such as rifampin that are known to induce the P-450 system should be avoided.

All of the PIs, except atazanavir, have been linked to a constellation of metabolic abnormalities, including elevated cholesterol levels, elevated triglyceride levels, insulin resistance, diabetes mellitus, and changes in body fat composition (e.g., buffalo hump, abdominal obesity). These changes can also occur with NRTIs and NNRTIs, but with the exception of stavudine the metabolic consequences with these other agents are not as severe as seen with PIs). The lipid abnormalities and body habitus changes are referred to collectively as lipodystrophy. Of the different manifestations of lipodystrophy, the dyslipidemias that occur are of particular concern because of the likelihood that increased levels of cholesterol and triglycerides will result in increased prevalence of heart disease. All patients taking PIs should have a fasting cholesterol, low-density lipoprotein cholesterol, and triglyceride level performed

every 3 to 6 months. Elevated cholesterol and triglyceride levels that do not respond to dietary intervention require treatment with statins and or gemfibrozil.

ENTRY INHIBITORS

Peptide T-20 (enfuvirtide) is the first drug in the new class of fusion inhibitors, which block the entry of HIV into cells. Unfortunately it must be administered subcutaneously.

CONSTRUCTING COMBINATION REGIMENS

Only combinations of three or more drugs have been able to decrease HIV viral load by 2 to 3 logs and allow suppression of HIV RNA to below the threshold of detection for longer than 10 years in some individuals. Current evidence supports the use of Truvada (tenofovir and emtricitabine) as the "nucleoside/nucleotide backbone" combined with efavirenz as the initial regimen of choice. It has the advantage of being formulated in a single once-daily pill (Atripla). Because 8% to 10% of newly infected persons in some urban areas of the United States have NNRTI resistance, resistance testing should be performed prior to initiating efavirenz in this population.

Increasing data suggest the virologic and clinical inferiority of regimens that include only nucleoside and nucleotide analogs without nonnucleoside agents or PIs. Thus triple nucleoside/nucleotide regimens should be avoided when other options exist.

In the absence of head-to-head comparisons of different regimens in different situations, several general principles should guide the choice of combinations. The most important determinant of treatment efficacy is adherence to the regimen. Therefore, it is vitally important that the regimen chosen be one to which the patient can easily adhere. In general, patients are more compliant with medication regimens that are once or twice a day only, do not require special timing with regard to meals, can be taken at the same time as other medications, do not require refrigeration or special preparation, and do not have bothersome side effects. Second, it is desirable to prescribe combinations that have demonstrated clinical benefit; because these data do not exist for many combinations, it is reassuring to know that the combination under consideration has shown beneficial effects on HIV viral load levels in short-term studies. To the extent possible, agents to which the patient has not been exposed are preferable to drugs for which resistance mutations may have already occurred. Toxicities should ideally be nonoverlapping. Interactions between drugs that result in potentially toxic levels should be avoided. For example, didanosine levels are increased when it is administered with tenofovir, potentially resulting in increased side effects. Therefore, this combination should be used very cautiously, and the didanosine dose should be reduced. An individual's relative contraindications to a given drug or drugs should be considered. The regimen should not include agents that are either virologically antagonistic or incompatible in terms of drug–drug interactions. Compatible dosing schedules—prescribing medications that can be taken at the same time—improve adherence to treatment. Finally, highly complex therapeutic regimens should be reserved for individuals who are capable of adhering to the rigorous demands of taking multiple medications and having this therapy closely monitored. Conversely, simplified regimens that deliver the lowest number of pills given at the longest possible dosing intervals are desirable for patients who have difficulty taking multiple medications.

A number of points about the "nucleoside/nucleotide backbone" of regimens have become clearer. The combination of stavudine plus didanosine should be avoided because there is increased risk of toxicities, in particular in pregnant women because of the increased risk of lactic acidosis. Also notable is the fact that the addition of lamivudine to didanosine does not appear to result in the same level of viral suppression as when lamivudine is combined with zidovudine or stavudine. Moreover, the nucleoside pair of zidovudine and stavudine should be avoided because of increased toxicity and the potential for antagonism that results from intracellular competition for phosphorylation. Finally, the combination of didanosine with tenofovir can cause declines in CD4 counts despite excellent virologic response and appropriate dose reduction of didanosine; the reason for this is unknown.

For some patients, it is impossible to construct a tolerable regimen that fully suppresses HIV. In such cases, clinicians and patients should consider their goals, and expert advice should be sought. Patients maintained on effective antiretroviral agents often benefit from these regimens (e.g., higher CD4 counts, fewer opportunistic infections) even if their virus is detectable. In some cases, patients may request a drug holiday during which they are taken off all medications. Patients often immediately feel better because of the absence of drug side effects. Unfortunately, structured treatment interruptions generally result in viral rebound and rapid CD4 decline, and patients who interrupt their treatment fare poorly compared to patients who continue their regimens without interruption.

DRUG RESISTANCE

HIV-1 drug resistance limits the ability to fully control HIV replication and is a leading cause for antiretroviral regimen failure. Resistance has been documented for all currently available antiretrovirals including the new class of fusion inhibitors. The problem of drug resistance is widespread in HIV-infected patients undergoing treatment in countries where antiretroviral therapy is widely available. A recent prevalence study of a representative sample of patients being treated in U.S. clinics revealed that nearly 80% of patients with detectable

viremia had at least some degree of drug resistance. Drug resistance is particularly a problem because of cross-resistance between drugs within a class. For example, the resistance patterns of lopinavir/ritonavir and indinavir are overlapping, and patients with virus resistant to these agents are unlikely to respond to nelfinavir or saquinavir even though they have never received treatment with these agents. Similarly, the resistance patterns of nevirapine and efavirenz are overlapping.

However, the issue of resistant virus does not just concern the treatment-experienced patient. Resistance is now also documented in patients who are treatment naive but who have been infected with a drug-resistant strain—"primary resistance." Cohort studies of treatment-naive patients entering care in North America and Western Europe show that roughly 10% to 12% of recently infected individuals have been infected with a drug-resistant strain of HIV-1.

Current expert guidelines recommend resistance testing for patients who are recently infected and for pregnant women. Resistance testing is also recommended for patients who are on an antiretroviral regimen and have suboptimal viral suppression (i.e., viral loads above 1000 copies/mL). Both genotypic and phenotypic tests are commercially available, and in randomized controlled studies their use resulted in improved short-term virologic outcomes compared to making treatment choices without resistance testing. Furthermore, multiple retrospective studies have conclusively demonstrated that resistance tests provide prognostic information about virologic response to newly initiated therapy that cannot be gleaned from standard clinical information (i.e., treatment history, examination, CD4 count, and viral load tests).

Because of the complexity of resistance tests, many clinicians require expert interpretation of results. In the case of genotypic assays, results may show that the mutations selected for during antiretroviral therapy are drug specific or contribute to broad cross-resistance to multiple drugs within a therapeutic class. An example of a drug-specific mutation for the reverse transcriptase inhibitors would be the M184V mutation that is selected for by lamivudine or emtricitabine therapy—this mutation causes resistance only to those two drugs. Conversely, the thymidine analog mutations ("TAMs") of M41L, D67N, K70R, L210W, T215Y/F, and T219Q/K/E are selected for by either zidovudine or stavudine therapy but cause resistance to all the drugs in the class and often extend to the nucleotide inhibitor tenofovir when three or more of these TAMs are present. Further complicating the interpretation of genotypic tests is the fact that some mutations that cause resistance to one drug can actually make the virus that contains this mutation more sensitive to another drug. The M184V mutation, for example, is associated with increased sensitivity to zidovudine, stavudine, and tenofovir. Phenotypic tests also require interpretation in that the distinction between a resistant virus and a sensitive one is not fully defined for all available drugs.

Both methods of resistance testing are limited by the fact that they may measure resistance in only some of the viral strains present in an individual. Resistance tests are only valid with reference to the antiretroviral medications patients are taking at the time of the test. Thus resistance results must be viewed cumulatively; that is, if resistance is reported to an agent on one test, it should be presumed to be present thereafter even if subsequent tests do not give the same result.

Prophylaxis of Opportunistic Infections

All HIV-infected patients with positive purified protein derivative (PPD) reactions (defined for HIV-infected patients as more than 5 mm of induration) should receive prophylaxis against *Myobacterium tuberculosis* infection. A chest radiograph should be performed first to exclude active tuberculosis.

For patients with severe immune suppression, prophylaxis of opportunistic infections is needed. In the era prior to highly active antiretroviral therapy (HAART), patients started on prophylactic regimens were maintained on them indefinitely. However, studies have shown that in patients with robust improvements in immune function—as measured by increases in CD4 counts above the levels that are used to initiate treatment—prophylactic regimens can safely be discontinued.

Primary prophylaxis for *Pneumocystis carinii* pneumonia (PCP) should be prescribed to patients with CD4 counts below 200 cells/mcL, a CD4 lymphocyte percentage below 14%, or weight loss or oral candidiasis

(Table 33–2). Patients with a history of PCP should receive secondary prophylaxis until they have had an optimal virologic response (i.e., <50 copies/mL) to HAART for at least 3 to 6 months and maintain a CD4 count of above 250 cells/mcL.

Four regimens for prophylaxis of PCP are trimethoprim-sulfamethoxazole, dapsone, atovaquone, and aerosolized pentamidine. Trimethoprim-sulfamethoxazole is inexpensive, widely available, and the most effective agent for prophylaxis. However, hypersensitivity reactions are common (see later). Dapsone is a second-line prophylactic agent with minimal side effects. Before prescribing dapsone, clinicians should make certain that the patient is not glucose-6-phosphate dehydrogenase deficient because such patients are at high risk of developing hemolytic anemia with dapsone therapy. For patients unable to take trimethoprim-sulfamethoxazole or dapsone, and aerosolized pentamidine are third- and fourth-line treatment options, respectively.

Prophylaxis against *Myobacterium avium complex* (MAC) infection should be given to patients whose CD4 counts fall below 75 cells/mcL. The preferred regimen is azithromycin (1200 mg orally weekly). Before initiating prophylaxis, clinicians should establish with a blood culture that the patient does not have disseminated MAC infection. Prophylaxis against MAC infection may be discontinued among patients whose CD4 counts go above 100 cells/mcL in response to HAART and whose plasma viral load has been optimally suppressed to below 50 to 75 copies/mL.

Toxoplasmosis prophylaxis is desirable in patients with positive IgG toxoplasma serology and CD4 counts below 100 cells/mcL.

Table 33–2. Infection prophylaxis for HIV-infected persons.

Infection	Indication	Treatment
Tuberculosis	+PPD >75-mm induration and normal chest radiograph	Isoniazid, 300 mg daily, with pyridoxine, 50 mg daily, for 9 mo
Pneumocystis jiroveci	CD4 cells <200 cells or CD4 lymphocyte percentage below 14% or weight loss or oral candidiasis	Trimethoprim-sulfamethoxazole, one double-strength tablet three times a week to one tablet daily, or dapsone, 50–100 mg daily or 100 mg two or three times per week
Toxoplasmosis	CD4 cells <100 cells and positive IgG for *Toxoplasmosis gondii*	Trimethoprim-sulfamethoxazole, one double-strength tablet daily, or pyramethathine, 50 mg orally once a week, with dapsone, 50 mg orally daily, with leucovorin, 25 mg/wk
Mycobacterium avium complex	CD4 cells <75 cells	Azithromycin, 1200 mg weekly

PPD, purified protein derivative.

Cytomegalovirus (CMV) infection is also common in late HIV disease. Oral ganciclovir (1000 mg orally three times daily with food) is approved for CMV prophylaxis among HIV-infected persons with advanced disease (e.g., CD4 counts below 50 cells/mcL). However, because the drug causes neutropenia, it is not widely used.

Cryptococcosis, candidiasis, and endemic fungal diseases are also candidates for prophylaxis. One prophylactic trial showed a decreased incidence of cryptococcal disease with the use of fluconazole, 200 mg orally daily, but the treated group had no benefit in terms of mortality. Fluconazole (200 mg orally once a week) was found to prevent oral and vaginal candidiasis in women with CD4 counts below 300 cells/mcL. In areas of the world where histoplasmosis and coccidioidomycosis are endemic and frequent complications of HIV infection, prophylactic use of fluconazole or itraconazole may prove to be useful strategies. However, the problem of identifying individuals at highest risk makes the targeting of prophylaxis difficult.

Because individuals with advanced HIV infection are susceptible to a number of opportunistic pathogens, the use of agents with activity against more than one pathogen is preferable. It has been shown, for example, that trimethoprim-sulfamethoxazole confers protection against PCP and toxoplasmosis.

Treatment of HIV Manifestations

HIV can affect every organ system in the body. For references on the diagnosis and treatment of HIV-related infections and malignancies, see the evidence-based medicine section and the reference list at the end of the chapter.

HYPERSENSITIVITY REACTIONS

Hypersensitivity reactions are drug-specific immune responses (production of a specific antibody or reaction of sensitized T cells) that are independent of drug dose. Patients with HIV are more likely to develop hypersensitivity reactions.

Severity of the reaction can vary from mild to life threatening with a wide variety of manifestations, including rash, fever, hepatitis, Stevens-Johnson syndrome, toxic epidermal necrolysis (TEN), hypotension, anaphylaxis, and death. Typically symptoms occur within a few weeks of starting the medication. They can begin much sooner in the case of rechallenge.

Among drugs used in the treatment of HIV, hypersensitivity reactions are particularly common with abacavir, the nonnucleoside reverse transcriptase inhibitors, and trimethoprim-sulfamethoxazole, which commonly is used in both the treatment and the prophylaxis of PCP.

With mild hypersensitivity reactions (e.g., a morbilliform rash not involving mucosal structures occurring 7 to 14 days after starting trimethoprim-sulfamethoxazole), it is sometimes possible to continue treatment with supportive care (e.g., antihistamines). Severe reactions should prompt immediate discontinuation of treatment.

For patients in whom treatment is stopped due to hypersensitivity, it is best to switch them to an alternative agent. Sometimes, however, this is not possible. In such cases, patients can sometimes be successfully desensitized to a particular drug. Experiences with desensitization protocols have been published for sulfonamides, efavirenz, nevirapine, and enfuvirtide. Rechallenge should never be attempted with abacavir because of life-threatening reactions to this medication.

Because reliable skin testing for hypersensitivity only exists for penicillin allergy, clinicians should take a good mediation history prior to the start of new treatments, noting regimens that the patient previously took and the cause of termination.

IMMUNE RECONSTITUTION INFLAMMATORY SYNDROME

Immune reconstitution inflammatory syndrome (IRIS) is a local or systemic inflammatory response to a specific preexisting organism that occurs following rapid immune recovery due to antiretroviral therapy. These inflammatory reactions may present with generalized signs of fevers, sweats, and malaise with or without more localized manifestations that usually represent unusual presentations of opportunistic infections. For example, patients with CMV retinitis have developed vitreitis after being treated with highly active antiretroviral treatment. MAC can present as focal lymphadenitis or granulomatous masses in patients receiving highly active antiretroviral treatment. Tuberculosis may paradoxically worsen with new or evolving pulmonary infiltrates and lymphadenopathy. Progressive multifocal leukoencephalopathy (PML) and cryptococcal meningitis may also behave atypically. The diagnosis of IRIS is one of exclusion and can be made only after recurrence or new opportunistic infection has been ruled out as the cause of the clinical deterioration.

A prospective study of 180 HIV-infected patients with preexisting *M. tuberculosis*, MAC, or *Cryptococcus neoformans* begun on highly active antiretroviral therapy found that 32% developed IRIS. The median time between start of therapy and diagnosing IRIS was 46 days. Individuals with a more rapid initial fall in HIV-1 RNA level in response to therapy were more likely to develop IRIS.

Management of IRIS is conservative and supportive with use of steroids only for severe reactions. Most authorities recommend that antiretroviral therapy be continued unless the reaction is life threatening.

EVIDENCE-BASED MEDICINE

A central question facing clinicians is choosing the best available antiretroviral regimen. Robbins et al used a factorial design to randomize antiretroviral naive patients to a variety of different regimens. The initial use of zidovudine, lamivudine, and efavirenz was superior to the other regimens, including a PI-containing regimen of zidovudine, lamivudine, and nelfinavir. This study had a major impact on practice because previously most clinicians thought that PI-containing regimens would be more efficacious than regimens that had a NNRTI but no PI.

The best choice for initial treatment of HIV was further refined by a study by Gallant et al that randomized antiretroviral naive patients to tenofovir, emtricitabine, and efavirenz versus zidovudine, lamivudine, and efavirenz. The patients treated with tenofovir, emtricitabine, and efavirenz had greater viral suppression. Taken together these two studies have made tenofovir, emtricitabine, and efavirenz the leading treatment for HIV-infected persons. This has been furthered by the availability of these three medications in a single once-daily pill formulation. Unfortunately, the best regimen for retroviral experienced patient has not been determined and needs to be individualized based on history of response and side effects to prior medications and resistance patterns.

The known side effects and high cost of antiretroviral treatments have led some to question whether treatment can be delayed or interrupted for patients who are doing well. The Strategies for Management of Antiretroviral Therapy (SMART) trial compared continuous viral suppressive treatment to a drug conservation strategy (stopping or deferring antiretroviral treatment until the CD4 count is below 250 cells and using episodic antiretroviral therapy to increase counts to above 350 cells). Almost all persons enrolled in the study had been previously treated (95%). Patients in the drug conservation arm were significantly more likely to suffer HIV progression or death. Surprisingly, severe complications (cardiac, hepatic, or renal) were higher in the drug conservation arm. The impact of this trial is to encourage earlier treatment and discourage treatment interruptions for HIV.

RESOURCES

HIV treatment guidelines are still changing rapidly. Therefore, the best sources of information are regularly updated websites. Johns Hopkins AIDS Service has a number of useful features including expert question and answer, publications, treatment guidelines and links to other websites (www.hopkins-aids.edu). From the website, copies of the most current edition of: Bartlett and Gallant's *Medical Management of HIV Infection* can be ordered for a minimal fee. This book represents the standard of care for both Johns Hopkins University AIDS Service and the quality assurance program of Maryland Medicaid. A second useful website is AIDSinfo (www.aidsinfo.nih.gov). This site, provided as a service of the U.S. Department of Health and Human Services, has a database of drugs and clinical trials, as well as information for providers, researchers, and patients.

BIBLIOGRAPHY

Bartlett JG, Gallant JE. *2005–2006 Medical Management of HIV Infection.* Baltimore, Md: John Hopkins Medicine Health Publishing Group; 2005.

Benson CA, Kaplan JE, Masur H, et al. Treating opportunistic infections among HIV-infected adults and adolescents: recommendations from CDC, the National Institutes of Health, and the HIV Medicine Association/Infectious Diseases Society of America. *MMWR Recomm Rep.* 2004;53(RR15):1.

Clavel F, Hance AJ. HIV drug resistance. *N Engl J Med.* 2004;350:1023.

DeSimone JA, Pomerantz RJ, Babinchak TJ. Inflammatory reactions in HIV-1-infected persons after initiation of highly active antiretroviral therapy. *Ann Intern Med.* 2000;133:447.

El-Sadr W, Neaton J, for the SMART Study Team. Strategies for management of antiretroviral therapy study. http://www.smart-trial.org. Accessed July 10, 2006.

Gallant JE, DeJesus E, Arribas JR, et al. Tenofovir DF, emtricitabine, and efavirenz vs. zidovudine, lamivudine, and efavirenz for HIV. *N Engl J Med.* 2006;354:251.

Greene WC. Molecular insights into HIV. In: Sande MA, Volberding PA, eds. *The Medical Management of AIDS.* 4th ed. Philadelphia: Saunders; 1995:22.

Hetherington S, McGuirk S, Powell G, et al. Hypersensitivity reactions during therapy with the nucleoside reverse transcriptase inhibitor abacavir. *Clin Ther.* 2001;23:1603.

Hirsch MS, Brun-Vézinet F, Clotet B, et al. Antiretroviral drug resistance testing in adults infected with human immunodeficiency virus type 1: 2003 recommendations of an International AIDS Society-USA Panel. *Clin Infect Dis.* 2003;37:113.

Powderly WG, Landay A, Lederman MM. Recovery of the immune system with antiretroviral therapy: the end of opportunism? *JAMA.* 1998;280:72.

Shelburne SA, Visnegarwala F, Darcourt J, et al. Incidence and risk factors for immune reconstitution inflammatory syndrome during highly active antiretroviral therapy. *AIDS.* 2005;19:399.

Shepherd GM. Hypersensitivity reactions to drugs: evaluation and management. *Mt Sinai J Med.* 2003;70:113.

Zolopa AR, Katz MH. HIV Infection. In: Tierney LH, McPhee SJ, Papadakis MA, eds. *Current Medical Diagnosis and Treatment.* 46th ed. New York: Lange Medical Books, 2007;1346.

Complementary and Alternative Medicine in the Treatment of Allergic and Asthmatic Disease

34

Jennifer Heimall, MD and Leonard Bielory, MD

The field of complementary and alternative medicine (CAM) in allergic disease is a constantly growing one; in the sections that follow we provide recent evidence-based examples of its use in the treatment of asthma and allergic disease. In this chapter, the current literature discussing CAM interventions, the prevalence and pattern of use, discussion of CAM use with patients, and examples of specific modalities are discussed. The specific risks of CAM interventions associated with the use of these modalities, omission of traditional therapeutic modalities, and the liability risk for physicians who either provide or counsel their patients regarding CAM interventions are also reviewed.

WHAT IS COMPLEMENTARY AND ALTERNATIVE MEDICINE?

CAM, as defined by the National Center for Complementary and Alternative Medicine (NCCAM), is a group of diverse medical and health care systems, practices, and products that are not presently considered part of conventional medicine. "Conventional medicine" is medicine as practiced by holders of MD (medical doctor) or DO (doctor of osteopathy) degrees and by their allied health professionals, such as physical therapists, psychologists, and registered nurses. Other terms for conventional medicine include *allopathy, Western, mainstream, orthodox and regular medicine,* and *biomedicine.* Some conventional medical practitioners are also practitioners of CAM (e.g., osteopathic manipulation). Other terms for complementary and alternative medicine include *unconventional, nonconventional, unproven,* and *irregular medicine* or *health care.*

CAM involves of the use of various modalities in a variety of domains (Fig. 34–1) to relieve symptoms and treat various diseases. Some of the most commonly used CAM modalities include herbal therapy, homeopathy, acupuncture, Ayurveda, and behavior modification techniques. CAM has its roots in many different cultures, Western and

Eastern. It should be remembered that many medications used today in traditional medicine for allergic, asthmatic, and immunologic disorders found their origin in herbs and other alternative medicines of the past. For example, corticosteroids, which are prominently used in the treatment of both asthma and atopic disease, have their origin in ground placenta and the urine of pubescent boys, and the mast cell stabilizer cromolyn is historically derived from the Middle Eastern khella plant.

DEFINITIONS AND DESCRIPTIONS OF COMMONLY USED MODALITIES

Herbal Therapies

Several herbal remedies are noted in the literature to have efficacy in the treatment of allergies. A diverse sampling of various antiinflammatory plants has been described, as have a variety of plants and herbals that provide solely symptomatic relief.

Homeopathy

Homeopathy works on the principle of treatment with "similars." The remedies prescribed by homeopathic practitioners are essentially very dilute solutions of drugs known to cause the very symptoms that are to be treated. According to the literature reviewed, 3% to 4% of CAM users use homeopathy, and about 75% of patients seen by a homeopathic practitioners report symptomatic improvement. Homeopathic remedies are determined by "provings" and are listed in the *Homeopathic Materia Medica.*

Acupuncture

Acupuncture is a form of traditional Chinese medicine that was originally thought to work on the principle of redistribution of *qi,* the life energy. In traditional Chinese

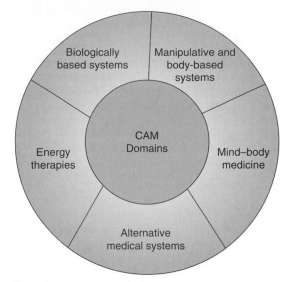

Figure 34–1. CAM domains. The five CAM domains (alternative medical systems), which include Traditional Chinese Medicine/acupuncture, homeopathy, naturopathy medicine, and Ayurvedic medicine; energy therapies, including bioelectromagnetic applications, Reiki, and Qi gong; biologically based systems, including diet, nutrition, lifestyle changes, herbal agents, and pharmacologic and biologic treatments; manipulative and body-based systems, including chiropractic and massage; and mind–body medicine, including meditation, yoga, imagery, prayer, hypnosis, music therapy, and biofeedback.

medicine, it is believed that an imbalance of qi or poor flow of qi is the origin of disease. By placing needles at specific points along meridians, qi can be redirected into better balance. The National Institutes of Health Consensus Development Panel (NIHCDP) within the Office of Alternative Medicine (now the NIH National Center for Complementary and Alternative Medicine) has already been working to prove the efficacy of acupuncture in the treatment of specific conditions, most notably nausea, pain, and addictions.

Ayurveda

Very little disease-specific research appears to have been completed in Ayurveda, a medical tradition originating from India. Ayurvedic medicine is derived from the teachings of ancient Hindu healers and first appeared in texts between 1500 and 1000 BC. Ayurvedic therapeutic interventions include yoga, meditation, breathing exercises, and herbal preparations. In its truest form, Ayurveda exists for the "*promotion of health*" rather than the prevention of specific disease states that have already begun to affect the body.

Behavior Modification Techniques

Behavior modification techniques include yoga and breathing retraining used by some asthmatic patients and teaching patients to respond differently or avoid allergic stimuli.

HOW MODALITIES HAVE BEEN STUDIED TO DATE

The integration of CAM interventions into the conventional day-to-day care of patients recommended by health care providers is limited by the lack of acceptance due to inadequate randomized placebo-controlled studies used to prove their efficacy. Although there is a paucity of data detailing the mechanisms or even the efficacy of many modalities, one must start to carefully review the literature for CAM interventions that have undergone randomized clinical studies with scientific scrutiny. The design of randomized placebo-controlled studies in CAM is complicated by difficulties in blinding, difficulties in creating an appropriate placebo (particularly for acupuncture), and difficulties in designing a control treatment when the mechanisms of actions of the modality to be tested are poorly delineated. Additionally, the difference in philosophy of CAM interventions from conventional health care allows for significant variation in the way CAM modalities are practiced. Therapies are often individualized for a particular patient and their particular disease state. Results can vary with patient's perception of their interaction with the CAM provider, which is often more personal than the interaction between patients and traditional health care providers. Study results may easily vary between CAM providers. Although one recent study showed no link between a patient's positive or negative attitude regarding a homeopathy remedy and outcomes in the treatment versus placebo groups, in studying the efficacy of CAM interventions, one must also appreciate and assess the importance of placebo effect because of the relationship that patients have with CAM providers.

As difficult as the design will be, the effort needs to be made to ensure patient safety and to prove the efficacy of these modalities. By establishing the mechanisms and efficacy of CAM modalities currently in use, new options for traditional intervention may be discovered and currently used medications may be improved.

IDENTIFYING PATIENTS MOST LIKELY TO USE CAM

Epidemiology of CAM use

The use of CAM has increased markedly in the worldwide population and specifically in the U.S. population (Fig. 34–2). Recent research continues to reflect that a majority of people worldwide use CAM interventions in some form for either the prevention and/or the treatment of disease with estimates of 80% noted by the World Health Organization. In the United States, a third of the population has tried some form of CAM. It is thought that perhaps two thirds (40% to 67%) of the population with chronic disorders imparting devastating mortality, such as the immunodeficiency associated with HIV, have used CAM interventions Other studies have shown that between 20% and 55% of pediatric patients have used some form of CAM interventions in the past year. This is particularly important for allergists because children suffer disproportionately from atopic disease.

Why Patients May Use CAM

CAM interventions are most commonly used for chronic conditions. Although the most common conditions associated with CAM interventions are either neuropsychiatric or musculoskeletal, atopic and immunologic disorders such as asthma, allergies, or immunodeficiencies are also common problems for which people use CAM. Asthma and atopic disease are frustrating to patients because of the lack of a permanent and reliable cure or even a predictable remission. Patients generally understand that CAM intervention is not curative, but in some instances, it provides some form of benefit in terms of symptom relief and improvement in quality of life. In regard to CAM interventions for the treatment of allergic disorders, most have concentrated on the use of herbal remedies derived from medicinal plants, homeopathy, acupuncture, and Ayurvedic interventions. In recent data published, 55% of adults said they were most likely to use CAM because they believed it would help them when combined with conventional medical treatments. Additionally, 28% of adults used CAM because they believed conventional medical treatments would not help them with their health problem. Thirteen percent used CAM because they felt that conventional medicine was too expensive.

Identifying Populations Likely to Use CAM

One study in California focusing on patients with the diagnosis of asthma or rhinosinusitis revealed that 42% of all patients surveyed had used CAM interventions; 24% of all patients had used herbs. Forty-two percent of the herb users used ephedra-containing products. The majority (more than 75%) of all patients were college educated. Although earlier studies have shown education to be a factor in herbal use, no statistically significant link was found between level of education and the use of CAM interventions. Considering issues of health disparities, Hispanic patients and those with incomes less than $20,000 annually were less likely to have used CAM interventions. Women were found more likely to

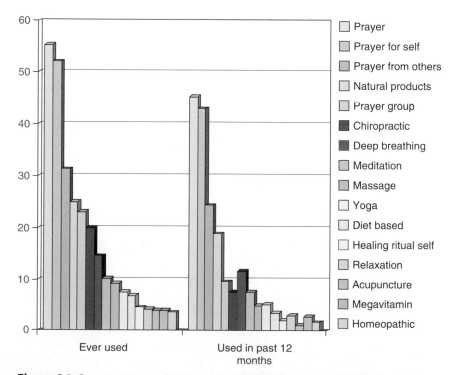

Figure 34–2. Prevelance of CAM use in the U.S. population as of 2002.

have used homeopathy, acupuncture, and massage; younger age was associated with medicinal caffeine use. Finally, self-assessed disease severity did not have an impact on herb use, but patients who felt they had more severe disease used homeopathy. These data reemphasize the importance of discussing CAM interventions with all patients.

Screening for CAM Use by Patients

Many patients and patients' parents are reluctant to discuss their use of CAM interventions with their physician, so it is important that the physicians ask their patients about CAM intervention use. To better assist their patients, physicians should be prepared to discuss some of the benefits and risks associated with various CAM modalities so patients will feel open to share their CAM experiences with the physician. The importance of inquiring about CAM intervention is exemplified in a survey of 142 pediatric patients seen in the emergency department, in which 45% of parents reported giving their child an herbal supplement. The most commonly used supplements were aloe, echinacea, sweet oil, eucalyptus, gingko, ginseng, and goldenseal. One parent reported the concomitant administration of albuterol and ephedra. Many of these patients did not share their use of these therapies with their physicians. This lack of open communication puts the patient at risk of drug interactions leading to therapeutic toxicity or inefficacy of traditional therapies.

MODALITIES COMMONLY USED IN THE TREATMENT OF ASTHMA

Herbals

A wide variety of herbs are used in the treatment of asthma. Particularly common is the use of Ma Huang, a traditional Chinese medicine whose main active ingredient is ephedrine. Although theophylline, an established asthma treatment, is found in tea leaves, regular black tea and coffee have also been used for the therapeutic effects of their methylxanthine component, caffeine, in the treatment of asthma. In a study of 601 adult asthmatics comparing the use of CAM agents, 8% reported the use of herbal remedies, and 37% of herb users used ephedrine-containing products. Six percent of all patients used ephedrine alone, and 6% used coffee or black tea. This study found that whereas coffee, black tea, or other herb use was associated with an increased risk of visits to the emergency department and hospitalization related to asthma, the ephedrine-containing herbs and ephedrine supplementation were not. These agents did have cardiac and neurologic adverse effects.

Traditional Chinese Medicine (TCM) remedies often involve the use of several herbs, but they most commonly include Ma Huang (ephedra). Gingko biloba has been used, and although the mechanism of efficacy is often questioned, several platelet-activating factor antagonist effects have been identified. Licorice has been used for its antiinflammatory properties, and various other herbs have anticholinergic actions, such as the smoke of henbane leaves and stramonium cigarettes.

Herbal combinations used in Traditional Japanese Medicine are similar to those in TCM, and these agents are commonly known as *saibuko-to/sho-saiko-to*. Some of these agents have a downregulating effect on lipoxygenase and cyclooxygenase activity. There have been numerous citations of the adverse effects, including hepatotoxicity and pneumonitis, regarding these agents. Other common plants known to have active ingredients include the Ayurvedic datura plants, as a source of atropine, and *Coleus forskohlii* plants, which produce a β-sympathomimetic effect.

Mucokinetic drugs used in Europe include mustard and horseradish. The North American–derived echinacea has been used for the prevention and treatment of the common cold for hundreds of years. However, recent evidence using various echinacea preparations showed no effect over that of a placebo. There may be an effect when *Echinacea purpurea* is used for the treatment of colds, but no definitive evidence was found for this. There have been recent reports of complications of the use of echinacea, including anaphylaxis, bronchospasm, urticaria, and angioedema that are more commonly reported in individuals with atopy.

Acupuncture

Acupuncture's common use for asthma treatment may stem from its nonpharmacologic nature, low cost, and ready accessibility in many urban centers. There is a paucity of reliable data to support its use. Even in studies with sham acupuncture used as a control, the data have not been reliable in supporting the efficacy of acupuncture. In studies where acupuncture and β-agonists were compared, the β-agonists have proven superior therapeutic benefits for patients. There are case reports of mechanical side effects from the needles, including contact dermatitis and pneumothorax. As in any practice involving sharp metal piercing of the skin, there is a risk for infectious disease transmission (hepatitis B and C, HIV) with this modality.

Homeopathy

There have been several reviews of the use of homeopathy in the treatment of both adult and pediatric patients with chronic stable asthma. This modality is tailored to the individual needs of each patient, which leads to difficulties in standardization of the studies. In all cases, however, the studies were placebo controlled. However, none of the studies were able to demonstrate an objective improvement in patient's disease status, pulmonary function, or quality of life scores. A Cochrane Database review concluded that there is not enough evidence to assess reliably the possible role of homeopathy in asthma.

Behavioral Techniques and Behavior Modification

Many patients have reported benefits from disciplined breathing exercises, including yoga and relaxation exercises, for control of their asthmatic symptoms. There have been some studies that demonstrate superior benefits when compared to traditional pharmacologic therapy alone. When yoga is compared to a control of a stretching program, these benefits are lost. However, there are many different forms of yoga, and these differences will need to be carefully studied before it will be possible to recommend for or against yoga in the treatment of asthma.

MODALITIES COMMONLY USED IN THE TREATMENT OF ALLERGIC RHINOCONJUNCTIVITIS

Herbals

Many studies of herbs in the treatment of allergic disease can be found; the following are examples of herbal remedies for rhinitis, dermatitis, and conjunctivitis. Butterbur, a petasine (*Petasites hybridus)*, is an herbaceous plant native to Europe, North Africa, and Southwest Asia in the Petasine family. The petasines have been shown in vitro to cause their effects by the inhibition of leukotriene synthesis, inhibition of histamine binding to H1 receptors, and blockage of degranulation of inflammatory cells. In a randomized, double-blind parallel group comparison study, the effects of butterbur were compared with the effects of the commonly used oral antihistamine cetirizine. The 125 study participants scored their allergic symptoms; global functioning was assessed by questionnaire. The "overall" outcome was that butterbur's effects compared to cetirizine were similar. Symptom specific outcomes were not individually evaluated. It was noted that there was no pattern of side effects noted with butterbur, whereas drowsiness was noted with cetirizine. Honey has been anecdotally been reported to modulate the allergic response of seasonal allergy sufferers. In a randomized double-blind, placebo-controlled study comparing the effects of pasteurized honey, unpasteurized honey, and placebo, 36 subjects ingested 1 tablespoon of honey per day for 195 days during peak allergy seasons (May through August). The patients rated the severity of the following symptoms: sore eyes, swollen eyes, watery eyes, itchy eyes, headache, runny nose, sneezing, itchy nose, postnasal drip, and stuffy blocked nose. No change in symptoms was noted consistently when honey users were compared to the placebo-controlled group. Eight weeks of daily treatment with a Chinese herbal remedy (extract of 18 herbs) reduced the severity of nasal symptoms and non-nasal symptoms and improved measures of quality of life in a randomized, double-blind, placebo-controlled study of 55 patients with seasonal allergic rhinitis seen in a Chinese medicine clinic in Australia.

One of the first studies of herbal therapy in atopic dermatitis involved 47 children with severe eczema treated with Zymophyte (active ingredients, Ledebouriella *seseloides, Potentilla chinensis, Anebia clematidis, Rehmannia glutinosa, Paeonia lactiflora, Lophatherum gracile, Dictamnua dasycarpus, Tribulus terrestris, Glycyrrhiza uralensis,* and *Schizonepta tenuifoua).* After an 8-week treatment period, the study group demonstrated a 91% decrease in erythema compared to a 10% decrease observed in the placebo group. A similar study was conducted in adults with similar results. These herbs have been theorized to work by several mechanisms, including stimulation of the adrenal cortex leading to increased endogenous cortisone and cortisol release; potentiation of endogenous corticosteroids by slowing metabolic degradation; corticosteroid activity of the plants themselves; decreased production of inflammatory compounds (leukotrienes, prostaglandins, and arachidonic acid); antipruritic effects (possibly via vasoconstriction); and antibacterial action. More recently, 2 weeks of topical treatment with a licorice extract gel (made with 2% licorice extract; 19.6% glycyrrhizinic acid in gel) reduced erythema, edema, and itching in a double-blind study of 60 patients with atopic dermatitis.

Euphrasia drops (from the *Euphrasia rostkovianaofficinalis)* were studied in a prospective cohort trial for their efficacy in the symptomatic treatment of conjunctivitis of any etiology (allergic, irritative, or infectious). Eighty patients were enrolled in the study, and 65 patients completed the study in which patients used were permitted to use 1 drop of Euphrasia eye drops up to five times daily as needed for symptoms: reddening, burning, and veiling of vision. At the conclusion of the study it was reported that more than 95% of patients experienced a complete disappearance of their symptoms within 3 to 17 days of starting the Euphrasia drops, with optimal results from the administration of 1 drop thee times a day.

Flavonoids have inhibitory activity on mast cells and thus can decrease allergic symptoms. This activity appears be enhanced by combining these compounds with sulfated proteoglycans.

Acupuncture

Acupuncture has also been studied in the treatment of allergic rhinitis. In a small randomized and controlled study (n = 30) of patients suffering from seasonal allergic rhinitis, the efficacy of treatment with acupuncture was assessed. The group was divided into two and treated with acupuncture or a sham control, each performed three times a week for 4 weeks. After the initial 4 weeks the groups were crossed so the original placebo group became the treatment group and vice versa. In both cases, the subjects treated with acupuncture, when compared to a control group receiving sham acupuncture, had a 70% relief of their non-nasal (itching eyes and eye watering) and nasal seasonal allergy symptoms. The sham control group had a 30% relief of their symptoms. The participants used no antihistamines, although they were available if the individual was to deem them necessary. Acupuncture has also been noted to have a limited but appreciable effect in the treatment of severely dry eyes.

Homeopathy

In a study designed to determine if homeopathy was primarily a placebo response, a 30 mL (1 part in 10^{60}) solution of grass pollen extract was given to 70 patients and a placebo remedy was given to an additional 70 patients. When patients' symptoms scores (based on symptoms of sneezing, blocked and runny nose, and watery, red, irritated eyes) were compared between the two groups, there was a significant improvement in the homeopathically treated group. However, some members of this group also suffered from exacerbation of their symptoms, leaving the author of the study to recommend that homeopathy may be more useful as a preventative measure than for acute symptomatic relief. In a retrospective study assessing systemic medication use in allergy sufferers, those patients who had used homeopathy in addition to traditional medication for allergy had an average reduction of their use of antihistamines by 70% due to symptomatic relief from homeopathy treatment.

Nontraditional Immunotherapy

Also important in the prevention of allergic response is immunotherapy. There has been some interesting research into the feasibility of sublingual and direct conjunctival immunotherapy for the prevention of allergic rhinitis. In a double-blind, placebo-controlled study, an accelerated course of sublingual immunotherapy (SLIT) was used in the prevention of seasonal rhinoconjunctivitis due to grass pollen. A statistically significant change was found in the study group, who received two sublingual grass pollen extracts daily for 15 days. The dose was scaled upward in the induction period and readministered three times a week during the allergy season. A similarly efficacious use of sublingual immunotherapy was demonstrated in a double-blind, placebo-controlled study of children allergic to *Parietaria juadacia*. This study also noted that children who used this modality tolerated it well and demonstrated good compliance with the administration schedule. Finally, in a double-blind

study comparing efficacy of SLIT to traditional injection therapy, the subjective efficacy noted by patient in daily symptom diaries was equitable. When IgG levels and skin reactivity were analyzed, only the injective therapy was of benefit. Overall, the subjective patient response to SLIT seems to be comparable to more traditional injection therapy, and it has been recognized by World Health Organization as a reasonable alternative means of administrating immunotherapy in the prevention of allergic rhinoconjunctivitis.

Local conjunctival immunotherapy entails instilling antigen drops in the eyes of patients known to suffer from allergic conjunctivitis. In a double-blind, placebo-controlled study, 24 subjects were divided into two groups. An increasingly concentrated dose of antigen was administered to each eye daily. At the conclusion of the 6-month trial, the antigen-specific conjunctival provocation test score was significantly lower in the study than placebo populations. This may represent, in addition to the previously described SLIT, a viable alternative to injected immunotherapy.

Behavioral Techniques and Behavior Modification

Eye rubbing worsens the symptoms of ocular allergies. In a study of 33 patients with cat allergy exposed to cat dander for 75 minutes and 15 minutes after exposure, one of their eyes was rubbed for 15 to 20 seconds. Rubbed eyes experienced increased itching and hyperemia when compared with the nonrubbed eye. Teaching patients to modify their response to allergic symptoms (i.e., avoiding rubbing itchy eyes) may effectively decrease the severity of symptoms experienced.

ETHICAL AND LEGAL ISSUES RAISED BY PATIENT'S USE OF CAM

Risks associated with CAM interventions include direct toxicities of the therapies themselves, the lack of conventionally tested medical interventions, and the liability risk for physicians who provide or counsel patients in the use of CAM.

Side Effects of CAM

The majority of adverse effects reported have been associated with herbal formulations similar to the risks associated with conventional pharmaceutical agents and have included hepatic and renal toxicities and hypersensitivity reactions (Table 34–1). Hepatotoxicity has previously been reported with Kinshi-gan and Sho-saiko-to. Both formulations contain Ginseng Radix, Scutellariae Radix, and Glycyrrhizae Radix. Liver injuries generally peaked within 3 to 4 days of challenge and resolved within 2 weeks; challenge testing may induce severe allergic reactions in addition to hepatic injury, particularly in

Table 34–1. Herbs in allergy and asthma: mechanisms of action/symptoms treated and observed adverse effects.

Herb	Mechanism of Action/ Symptom Treated	Adverse Effect
Allium cepa (onion)	Inhibits mast cell degranulation	Strong odor
Aloe arborescens	Bronchodilation	Electrolyte imbalances, abdominal cramps, pseudomelanosis coli
Atropa belladonna	Anticholinergic and bronchodilating properties	Ataxia, hallucinations, extrapyramidal reactions, decreased bowel sounds, photophobia, sinus tachycardia, thirst and urinary retention
Bu-zhong-yi-qi-tang (Traditional Chinese Medicine)	Decreased capillary permeability; decreased eosinophils, CD4 cells, IL-4 and IL-5; inhibited TH2 cell responses	None reported
Caffeine	Bronchodilator	Insomnia, gastroesophageal reflux, hypertension
Coleus forskohlii	Bronchodilator; possibly due to intracellular stimulation of adenylate cyclase to produce cAMP; high doses required to produce effect	Tremor and hypokalemia, although proportionally less than effect of β-agonist in study
Datura stramonium (Jimsonweed)	Tropane alkaloids (atropine, hyoscyamine, hyoscine, scopolamine); bronchodilator	Ataxia, hallucinations, extrapyramidal reactions, decreased bowel sounds, photophobia, sinus tachycardia, thirst and urinary retention
Echinacea	In vitro antiviral effects vs. influenza; limited effect in recent studies	Anaphylaxis, bronchospasm, urticaria, angioedema, hepatitis, hypertension, atrial fibrillation, acute renal failure, vasculitis
Eucalyptus	Cold/Influenza remedy; mucokinetic/decongestant; cockroach repellant	Allergic reactions
Chamazulene (chamomile)	Leukotriene inhibitor	Rarely, anaphylaxis in patients allergic to ragweed/chrysanthemum; botulism
Golden seal (hydrazine)	Treatment of urinary tract infection, diarrhea, conjunctivitis, acute otitis media, eczema	Peripheral vasoconstriction/hypertension; irritation of the oropharynx; nausea, vomiting, diarrhea
Hi Chun (Korean)	Stabilizes mast cell membrane; inhibits histamine release	None reported
Jisil (Korean)	Stabilizes mast cell membrane; inhibits cAMP and decreased IgE production	None reported
Kutki/Kurro (Indian Ayurvedic)	Stabilizes mast cell membrane	None reported
Licorice	Slows the change of cortisol to cortisone, blocks histamine-induced capillary permeability, inhibits platelet-activating factor and has antitussive activities	Hypokalemia; hyperaldosteronism
Ma Huang (ephedra) Wu-Hu-Tang	Oral adrenergic agonist; inhibits mast cell degranulation and has sympathomimetic activity; for treatment of asthma/allergic rhinitis, doses are usually 15, 25, or 30 mg three times a day	Concern of safety when used in high doses, particularly for weight loss (100 mg two times a day); common side effects include hypertension, tachycardia, palpitations, nervousness, headache, insomnia, dizziness, euphoria, nephrolithiasis, seizure, stroke, and myocardial infarction; has caused sudden death

(Continued)

Table 34–1. Herbs in allergy and asthma: mechanisms of action/symptoms treated and observed adverse effects. (continued)

Herb	Mechanism of Action/ Symptom Treated	Adverse Effect
Menthol (mint)	Decongestant action	Ingestion may be fatal (mechanism of death not reported)
Minor Blue Dragon	Stabilizes mast cell membranes	None reported
Peppermint oil (mint)	Decongestant action/stabilizes mast cell membranes	Cardiac arrhythmias
Sho-seiry-to (Japanese)	Decreased IgE-mediated cutaneous reactions; complement inhibition; anticholinergic effect leads to drying of secretions and decreased inflammation	None reported
Urticaria dioica (Nettle)	Stem nettles contain histamine, serotonin, choline; used in the treatment of allergic rhinitis	Contact urticaria with natural plant leaves; diarrhea; gastric irritation; edema; decreased urinary volume
Tylophora indica (India)	Alkaloid derivative plant that acts as a bronchodilator; induced peak expiratory flow improvement in one study	Nausea, vomiting, and sore mouth; worse when plant is chewed
Saiboku-to (Japanese) Chaipo-tang (Chinese)	Inhibition of 11-β-dehydrogenase leads to increased endogenous cortisol levels; in studies patients dropped their steroid doses. Did not induce downregulation of glucocorticoid or β-2-adrenergic receptors	Pneumonia/pneumonitis
Sho-seiry-to (Japanese)	Decreased IgE-mediated cutaneous reactions; complement inhibition; anticholinergic effect leads to drying of secretions and decreased inflammation	None reported

patients with known allergic disease. However, more serious adverse effects have also been reported, such as fatal cases of liver failure associated with restarting Kinshi-gan and Sho-saiko-to and acute pneumonitis with Sho-saiko-to.

Renotoxicity examples include hypokalemia, water retention, and sodium retention associated with licorice ingestion and nephrolithiasis associated with ephedra. The widely used ephedra has also been linked with severe cardiovascular and neurologic side effects, including 10 fatalities. Ephedra has recently come under even more scrutiny for its use in diet and performance enhancement. In the doses required to effect weight loss, side effects are commonly observed. California banned the distribution and sale of ephedra alkaloid-containing products effective January 1, 2004. Under the law, licensed health care practitioners may prescribe or dispense ephedra-containing products only for purposes other than weight loss, bodybuilding, or athletic performance enhancement.

As with any unregulated substance, one must also be concerned about the amounts of the pharmacologically active drug in any given preparation and about any contaminants. TCM has been linked with both dosage toxicities and contamination. Many of the remedies may be safe at low doses but at higher doses become markedly toxic. However, without studies to establish the therapeutic index, it is difficult if not impossible to advise patients on the use of CAM interventions. Contaminants that have been found range from nonsteroidal antiinflammatory drugs (NSAIDs), steroids, and benzodiazepines to heavy metals (e.g., lead) (Table 34–2). The wealth of misleading anecdotal and poorly obtained scientific evidence is dangerous for patients who expect so-called natural complementary/alternative medications to be safe.

There have also been adverse effects reported with acupuncture (Table 34–3). Side effects reported include vasovagal effects, earaches, gastrointestinal complaints, five reports of pneumothorax, one case of cardiac tamponade, and one documented case of hepatitis B, among others.

Table 34–2. Adverse effects reported from contaminants of herbs and homeopathic remedies.

Contaminant	Number of Reports	Adverse Effect Noted
Mercury	4	Motor and vocal tics
Lead	111	Anemia/ encephalopathy
Steroids	2	None
Arsenic	75	

Significant Interactions with Western Therapies

Aside from CAM modalities taken for the control of asthma or allergic disease, physicians must also remember to ask about remedies taken for other conditions. As noted earlier, echinacea is often taken as prophylaxis for the common cold. It has been associated with anaphylaxis, bronchospasm, urticaria, angioedema, hepatitis, hypertension, atrial fibrillation, acute renal failure, and vasculitis. One case report describes a middle-aged woman who developed anaphylaxis within a few minutes of ingesting a solution of echinacea. She had been taking the supplement for several years prior to the event without incident; she had a history of atopy; oral

Table 34–3. Acupuncture and other physical modalities: observed adverse effects.

Modality	Sample Size	Adverse Effect
Acupuncture	Unknown	Hepatitis B
Acupuncture	1	Cardiac tamponade
Acupuncture	1	Septic sacroiliitis
Acupuncture	1	Septic arthritis
Acupuncture	1	HIV
Acupuncture	1	Pneumothorax
Spinal manipulation	Unknown	Cerebrovascular accident
Spinal manipulation	1	Holocord astrocytoma
Massage	1	Large hematoma
Cupping	1	Sepsis

allergy syndrome, and urticaria/angioedema associated with bananas. After the incident, allergy was confirmed with skin prick and intradermal testing to the same solution the patient had ingested. Findings were further confirmed by radioallergosorbent test (RAST). Further investigation of other patients in the practice found that even among those who had not been using echinacea but were sensitive to grass pollen, 94% had positive immediate skin tests to echinacea. As such, patients with atopy may be at higher risk than the general population of developing serious adverse reactions to herbal modalities. Green tea has antioxidant, antibacterial, and antiviral activity, and it is taken by many patients as a preventative measure. In one case report, 11 patients developed occupational asthma associated with the inhalation of green tea dust; 5 of the 11 had symptoms after drinking green tea as well. The allergen association was confirmed with intradermal tests and challenge inhalation. Another commonly used herb, ginseng, has also been associated with adverse effects. Ginseng is often used for weakness and fatigue; additionally it is thought to have efficacy in boosting immune system function. Adverse effects reported include nausea, diarrhea, euphoria, insomnia, headaches, hypertension, hypotension, mastalgia, and vaginal bleeding. Due to liver effects it may lower blood alcohol concentration and decrease warfarin efficacy. Interactions with caffeine may lead to hypertension. Ginseng may lead to hypoglycemic episodes in patients taking insulin or oral hypoglycemic agents. It is contraindicated in hypertension, acute asthma, acute nosebleeds, acute infections, or menorrhagia. Garlic has been used for its cardiovascular benefits and for relief of cold, colds, and rhinitis. But it has been associated with gastrointestinal disturbances, change in body odor, hypoglycemia, and allergic reactions. St. John's wort is commonly used for treatment of depression. It has been found to induce cytochrome 3A4. This action can decrease levels of conventional medications, including cyclosporine (commonly used as an immunomodulator in transplantation), indinavir (commonly used in the treatment of HIV), and oral contraceptive pills. Decreased levels and the resultant diminished therapeutic effect of any of these medications can lead to significant complications.

Risks Associated with Lack of Western Therapeutic Involvement

Traditional physicians are not needed to refer patients for complementary/alternative modalities. As such, traditional therapies may be delayed or omitted for these patients. In one study of adherence to allopathic treatment among asthmatics in India, CAM intervention, particularly yoga, Ayurveda, and homeopathy, were seen as barriers to achieving adherence with β-agonists or other traditional interventions. Twenty-six percent of individuals using CAM interventions were not concomitantly using traditional treatment for asthma/rhinitis, and there is concern that use of CAM interventions may delay the use of specific antiinflammatory therapy, leading to increased visits to the emergency department or to hospitalizations. Additionally, some patients may be swayed by CAM practitioners regarding immunization. Only 30% of chiropractors, homeopaths, and naturopaths recommend immunization; 7% of American naturopaths actively oppose immunization.

Liability Risks for Physicians

Some patients may seek the advice or referral from their physician before seeing the care of a CAM provider. This discussion is more likely when CAM use has been discussed in the past, so the patient feels comfortable discussing alternative treatment options with the primary physician. In this role, it must be remembered that the physician is still responsible for the coordination of the patient's overall care. Physician liability may stem from recommendations to pursue CAM interventions or from failing actively to discourage the use of certain CAM interventions.

There are essentially four categories under which the risks fall (from low to high):

1. Evidence supports both efficacy and safety (e.g., acupuncture for chemotherapy-induced nausea)
2. Evidence supports safety, but evidence regarding efficacy is inconclusive (e.g., homeopathy for rhinitis)
3. Evidence supports efficacy, but evidence regarding safety is inconclusive (e.g., gingko for dementia)
4. Evidence indicates serious risk or inefficacy (e.g., injections of unapproved substances; inattention to known herb–drug interactions)

The liability risk associated with a particular modality increases as less is known about positive efficacy or safety. In determining the category of a particular CAM intervention, the physician must document the literature supporting a particular therapeutic choice, document that the risks and benefits of a given CAM intervention were discussed with a patient, and, if possible, patients should sign documentation of their assumption of risk. This is particularly advisable if the patient will be replacing traditional treatment with CAM interventions. One method of dividing modalities into risk groups for patients uses three categories: sufficient evidence to view the therapy as reasonable and sometimes recommend, reasonable with caveats, and clearly unwise. These categories were originally developed for the use of oncologists to use when discussing treatment options with their patients, but they can be used effectively for any patient considering CAM

interventions. When referring a patient, it is also prudent to confirm the competency or certification of the practitioner to whom your patient is referred.

CONCLUSION

CAM interventions are continuing to grow in popularity among patients in the United States and abroad for the treatment of a myriad of conditions. Asthma and allergic disease are among the conditions most commonly treated with CAM. These modalities may offer exciting opportunities for patients who respond poorly to or have difficulty tolerating traditional treatment, but it is advisable to discourage patients from abandoning conventional therapy completely.

Herbs are among the CAM modalities most commonly used and unfortunately also appear to cause adverse effects most commonly. Adverse effects associated with CAM use may be due to toxicity of the intervention itself or to contaminants of the intervention. For these reasons, and because atopic patients may be more susceptible to adverse reactions from these modalities, allergists and clinical immunologists should be well versed in the benefits and risk associated with CAM use. Because patients may not volunteer their experiences with CAM interventions, physicians must screen all patients routinely. Furthermore, well-designed randomized and placebo-controlled studies are needed to clearly establish the efficacy and safety of these modalities so patients and physicians can reasonably establish the risk-to-benefit ratio associated with various modalities

EVIDENCE-BASED MEDICINE

CAM in the Prevention of Allergic and Asthmatic Disease

Most CAM treatment of allergic disease aims at prevention or alleviation of symptoms. The mechanism of allergy development has been fodder for medical science for many years. Hygiene hypothesis is one of the popular theories of how allergic disease develops in some individuals and basically relates that as the developing immune system has had to fend off fewer pathologic antigens, it has become reactive to benign and common environmental allergens. Recently, there has been increased interest in the use of newer modalities, including CAM, in decreasing the so-called atopic march. Some of the modalities currently being considered as a means of primary prevention are: probiotics, prebiotics, and helminths. These agents are thought to have their effects via improved immunoregulation of TH1 and TH2 cell subclass activity. Recently, evidence has indicated that intestinal dendritic cells absorb dietary proteins and then act in the mesenteric lymph nodes to induce regulatory T-cell differentiation of both the TH1 and TH2 subclasses. As evidence is discovered about new dietary protein uptake is affected by probiotics, prebiotics, and helminths, an expanded therapeutic or preventative role may be established for these agents.

In probiotics, *Lactobacillus* is purposely given to infants and young children with the intention of reducing their development of allergic disease. *Lactobacillus* taken orally can lead to late induction of IL-10. This response has been found to vary with the immunologic status of the patient. When IL-4 is absent or at low levels, IL-10 diminishes eosinophilic inflammation and IgE responses. A recent study demonstrated that probiotics given to atopic pregnant mothers and their infants for 6 months led to a decreased incidence of atopic dermatitis. This protective effect was shown to persist to age 4 years. However, no benefit has been noted for atopic adults given *Lactobacillus*. It is thought that by increasing the antigenic stimulation in the intestinal tract of newborns, it may be possible to decrease the development of an atopic responder phenotype. Further study is warranted to determine more clearly whether lasting effects on the prevention of atopic disease can be achieved by the use of probiotics, prebiotics, and helminths.

BIBLIOGRAPHY

Barnes PM, Powell-Griner E, McFann K, et al. Complementary and alternative medicine use among adults: United States, 2002. Advance data from vital and health statistics #343. Hyattsville, Md: HCHS; 2004.

Bielory L, Russin J, Zuckerman G. Clinical efficacy, mechanisms of action, and adverse effects of complementary and alternative medicine therapies for asthma. *Allergy Asthma Proc.* 2004; 25(5):281.

Chan-Yeung M, Becker A. Primary prevention of childhood asthma and allergic disorders. *Curr Opin Allergy Clin Immunol.* 2006;6:146.

Furrie E. Probiotics and allergy. *Proc Nutr Soc.* 2005;64(4):465.

Heimall J, Bielory L. Defining complementary and alternative medicine in allergies and asthma: benefits and risks. *Clin Rev Allergy Immunol.* 2004;27(2):93.

Linde K, Barrett B, Wolkart K, et al. Echinacea for preventing and treating the common cold. *Cochrane Database Syst Rev.* 2006;(1):CD000530.

Mantani N, Kogure T, Tamura J. Challenge tests and kampo medicines: case report and review of the literature. *Am J Chinese Med.* 2003;31(4):643.

McCarney RW, Linde K, Lasserson TJ. Homeopathy for chronic asthma. *Cochrane Database Syst Rev.* 2004;(1):CD000353.

Ogden NS, Bielory L. Probiotics: a complementary approach in the treatment and prevention of pediatric atopic disease. *Curr Opin Allergy Clin Immunol.* 2005;5(2):179.

Rautava S, Kalliomaki M, Isolauri E. New therapeutic strategy for combating the increasing burden of allergic disease: Probiotics-A Nutrition, Allergy, Mucosal Immunology and Intestinal Microbiota (NAMI) Research Group report. *J Allergy Clin Immunol.* 2005;116:31.

Sabina A, Williams A. Yoga intervention for adults with mild-to-moderate asthma: a pilot study. *Ann Allergy Asthma Immunol.* 2005;94(5):543.

Strobel S, Mowat AM. Oral tolerance and allergic responses to food proteins. *Curr Opin Allergy Clin Immunol.* 2006;6(3):207.

Turner R, Bauer R, Woelkart K, et al. An evaluation of Echinacea angustifolia in experimental rhinovirus infections. *N Engl J Med.* 2005;353(4):341.

Theoharides TC, Bielory L. Mast cells and mast cell mediators as targets of dietary supplements. *Ann Allergy Asthma Immunol.* 2004;93(2 suppl 1):S24.

Xue CC, Thien FC, Zhang JJ, et al. Treatment for seasonal allergic rhinitis by Chinese herbal medicine: a randomized placebo controlled trial. *Altern Ther Health Med.* 2003;9(5):80.

Nutrition, Diet, and Allergic Diseases 35

Avraham Giannini, MD

Patients have always wanted to control their own lives, which is positive. A physician works best in an environment where—in addition to the list of prescription medications—individuals present histories that include all their disciplines: nutrition, dietary supplements and restrictions, over-the-counter pharmaceuticals, including homeopathic and naturopathic remedies, and even their belief systems regarding illness. Whether patients perceive disease as a punishment, a consequence of behavior, or a random deviation of nature, these perceptions may affect outcomes. Many diseases remain out of anyone's control.

This chapter addresses the areas of allergy where patients most definitely can take control of their disease by what they eat or drink every day. First I look at the concept of control and nutrition from infancy on. A historical perspective frames the picture. Then simple dietary guidelines lead to an overview of the effects of nutrition on allergy and asthma. Finally, I present the world of supplements—vitamins, minerals, and herbs, with a perspective on allergy and asthma.

CONTROLLING ONE'S DESTINY

Infants spit out their food. This is often their only way of controlling their lives. The one thing a child can do to get the attention of Mom and Dad as well as grandparents is to refuse to eat certain foods and spit them out when the foods are "force-fed" into their mouths. This "control" continues into the toddler and grammar school years. And the response is always the same: constant nagging and attention from everyone in the family, even the pediatrician. What power! This is something that the infant discovers in the first year of life. Why give up that control and power, with the family, the nanny, and the doctor all making such a fuss? Later in high school, there are even more options, including special dietary requirements—vegetarian, vegan, raw foods, partial fasts (including detox diets), and even the very dangerous behavioral disorder bulimia.

A series of wonderful books by Mollie Katzen are guides that allow very young children to self-select and

enjoy foods with important nutrients. By their natural attraction to the foods' color, shape, and smell, very young children are able to indeed control in a positive manner—instead of resistance and rebellion. My favorite titles are *Pretend Soup, Honest Pretzels,* and *The Enchanted Broccoli Forest.* I keep Katzen's books in my allergy office waiting room.

HISTORICAL PERSPECTIVE

The desire to control our destiny motivates every new "health food fad." Americans really drank snake oil sold from the back of trucks and out of the tents of messianic health care providers in the 19th and 20th centuries. These providers were often referred to as "quacks"; nevertheless, they traveled from city to city with their message of self-improvement, and their products sold like hotcakes!

The general public was never really fooled: people just wanted some way to control their health and their destiny. During this same period, Dale Carnegie was selling self-improvement through self-confidence, and Charles Atlas was doing the same thing by touting bigger muscles. Atlas did it from the inside of matchbooks. Incidentally, cigarette companies used photos of physicians to sell their product.

We now are certainly aware of the dangers of cigarettes; unfortunately, many are unaware of the similar dangers with marijuana. There were reports in the 1960s that marijuana actually was beneficial for asthma. This, together with other myths about marijuana, is dangerous misinformation. Marijuana is second to alcohol among the most common drugs associated with fatal auto accidents. Paternal as well as maternal use of marijuana in pregnancy is risky. Now we are told that cigarette smoking can possibly avert Alzheimer's disease and even benefit schizophrenia. Again, beware of myths. Throughout all the various fads, the trained physician remained a beacon in care. When an illness requires a prescription medication or an operation, everyone still calls the doctor. Physicians continue to be very well trained in anatomy and physiology, the function of organ systems, then the diagnosis, the treatment of disease/pathology, and, in recent years, evidence-based medicine. Nutrition is still only allotted very few hours in the curriculum. Medical training generally does not offer an adequate wellness approach.

This catch-all term *wellness* enters our vocabulary at a time when Americans are no longer battling serious disease. With polio paralyzing and killing, and tuberculosis sending family members to sanitariums, there was not a great deal of energy focused on staying well. Now that these scourges have generally come under control, everyone (in developed countries) wants to stay well and live to an old age with the greatest quality and energy of life, thus the desire for wellness. Starvation does not lend itself to a focus on good nutrition; nevertheless, the populations of Northern Europe actually had fewer problems with cardiovascular disease during World War II when milk products and other animal fats were in short supply. And these cardiovascular problems again reappeared after the war was over. "You can dig your own grave with a knife and fork."

From ancient times to the 21st century, attempts continue by a variety of authors to address the need for dietary guidance. Maimonides taught about medicinal plants, and he really did recommend chicken soup over a thousand years ago. Soybeans were championed by the cereal tycoon John Kellogg and also by Henry Ford. After the devastation of the Second World War, soyprotein became America's favorite "health food." Now French and Israeli health agencies warn that dietary soybean products especially soymilk must be limited because of the side effects of genistein the major soy isoflavone on the thyroid as well as the estrogenic side effects of soy isoflavones. Adele Davis had a following in the 1950s: some of her nutritional advice was appropriate and helpful. Dr. Seuss's appeal came with wonderful illustrations and titles such as *Green Eggs and Ham*. The brilliant pediatrician Benjamin Spock gave mothers a guide for raising children. Cardiologist Dean Ornish continues to advise patients from a cardiovascular metabolic focus. Naturopaths run limited detoxification programs, and some physicians guide patients on the master-cleanse-detox regimen. Finally, many of us still recall drinking cod liver oil every morning before school from that greasy bottle. The cod liver oil regimen of the 1940s and 1950s was left over from the English. During World War II, every English child was provided with daily cod liver oil with its vitamin D content to protect against rickets.

DIETARY GUIDELINES

Daily requirements (based on 2500 calories: 55% carbohydrates, 30% fats, 15% protein) are as follows:

- *Protein:* 80 g (a very small hamburger has about 15 g, and a McDonald's quarter pounder weighs a little more than 100 g)
- *Carbohydrate:* 350 g
- *Fat:* 80 g

A diet high in fruits and vegetables has been cited as protective against asthma. Additionally, obesity is repeatedly cited as a contributing factor in asthma. Again, the desire to control our destiny continues. Somehow, if we did things differently, then we would not have asthma. Conversely, if we change what we are doing (eating less fat and more fruits and vegetables and losing weight) then our asthma will go away. I don't dispute the research articles. Nevertheless, in my own experience in my private practice as well as in clinics, most severe asthmatics are not obese, and the most important factor is always the family history of asthma linked with a viral illness. Research into the role of bacteria and viruses as a factor in obesity is very compelling. Could these microbial factors also have a role in allergy and asthma?

Trained registered nurses with diet specializations are currently important sources of knowledge and instruction. They have a practical approach to food requirements. For example, their patients learn that the total protein requirement for a meal may look like a deck of cards. American beef and poultry industries do not want to hear this. Yet our neighbors across the pond in France and Italy know this. Restaurants there do not serve the enormous portions we see here. Perhaps we thought this was economic: *We in America had more so we ate more.* I hope the wisdom of these nurse/dietitians will trickle down to culinary academies and then school cafeterias, as well as the kitchens of Moms, Dads, and nannies.

SUPPLEMENTS WITH AN EYE ON ALLERGY

In the 21st century, the word *supplement* dominates the world of nutrition and wellness. A supplement can refer to vitamins, minerals, enzymes, essential components of our cellular and intracellular structures, and herbs (often with acupuncture). These include the following:

- Glucosamine (may be derived from shellfish so beware).
- Methylsulfonylmethane (MSM) (may be helpful for hayfever).
- Antioxidants/vitamins: the word *vitamin* was coined by Polish biochemist Casimir Funk in 1912. Remember vitamin C and vitamin D eradicated scurvy and rickets, respectively. (Cod liver oil has vitamin D, although halibut has higher amounts and is used now instead of cod.)
- Probiotics/orally administered live microorganisms (e.g., *Lactobacilli* and *Bifidobacteria*). These may help in a regulatory role, fitting into the hygiene hypothesis of atopic disease.
- Wheat grass juice (be careful if you are allergic to grass or wheat).

- Sorbitol (a sweetener; beware because it can cause diarrhea).
- Omega-3 fish oil (here goes the cod liver oil again!).
- Homeopathic remedies.
- Bee pollen (beware if you have pollen allergy).
- Herbs (phytotherapy)

Vitamins are necessary for health: see Table 35-1. They are found in minute quantities in our food staples like milk, bread, and fruit juices. It is commonplace to see "vitamin enriched" on a food label. We never even question whether vitamins are really necessary and if they can instead be harmful. One study found that *multivitamins in infancy actually increase the incidence of asthma and allergy.* Another study cites antioxidant vitamin E as beneficial for an infant if taken during pregnancy. Go figure! In addition to immune regulation, probiotic *Lactobacillus* may alter the intestinal flora and protect an eczema patient from the damaging effect of certain foods that flare atopic dermatitis.

Here are some herbal names I encounter in my practice:

- Calendula
- Chamomile
- Cohosh
- Colophony
- Comfrey

Table 35–1. Table of vitamins (daily requirements).

Fat-Soluble Vitamins	
Vitamin A	900 µg
Vitamin D	5–10 µg
Vitamin E	10 µg
Vitamin K	100 µg
Water-Soluble Vitamins	
Vitamin B$_1$ Thiamine	1.1 mg
Vitamin B$_2$ Riboflavin	1.5 mg
Vitamin B$_{12}$	3 µg
Vitamin B$_9$ Folic acid	400 µg
Vitamin B Biotin	150 µg
Vitamin B Pantothenic acid	5 mg
Vitamin B$_6$	2 mg
Vitamin B Niacin	15 mg
Vitamin C	60 mg

- Cottonseed oil
- Dandelion
- Echinacea
- Edelberry
- Ephedra
- Eucalyptus
- Evening primrose
- Fenugreek (a favorite in Egypt, especially in Port Said)
- Feverfew
- Flax
- Garlic
- Ginger
- Ginkgo biloba
- Ginseng
- Goldenseal
- Guar
- Kombucha
- Nettle
- Poison oak
- Propolis
- Quercetin
- Saint John's wort
- Saw palmetto
- Star anise
- Valerian

Be very careful with all herbs, including those just listed. I do not recommend that you use these. Some have toxic side effects. Other herbs are prepared as combinations, such as AirBorne and Windbreaker.

Here are some warnings:

- Calendula can cause contact dermatitis (be careful especially if you work with flowers).
- Chamomile (used by my grandmother to sleep; beware because it is related to ragweed, a very potent cause of hayfever and asthma).
- Ephedra (used for decades; called "Ma Huang" or "Mormon tea.") It is a very potent adrenaline-like herb that can cause irritability, difficulty sleeping, elevation of blood pressure, and in males difficulty with urination.
- Glucosamine may have shrimp/crab (read the label and be careful if you have shellfish allergy).
- Kombucha is made from a fermenting mushroom soaking in black tea. It should not be taken by people allergic to mold spores!
- Poison oak has been used by some Native Americans since birth, so that they will not become sensitized at a later date. This can have serious side effects, and this method of inducing tolerance to poison oak should not be used by anyone.

Table 35–2. Table of minerals (daily requirements).

Sodium	2300 mg
Calcium	1000 mg
Magnesium	400 mg
Zinc	15 mg
Selenium	70 µg

- Saw palmetto may help with prostate hypertrophy and the repeated need to urinate, but patients should check with their physician to rule out prostate cancer.

The following minerals may play a role in allergy and asthma (see Table 35-2):

- Magnesium and selenium may play a beneficial role in bronchial inflammation.
- Calcium may be beneficial or possibly dangerous (regarding kidney stones).
- Zinc in infant vitamins/formulas may benefit immune function and asthma treatment.
- Sodium: A low-salt diet benefits exercise-induced asthma.

EVIDENCE-BASED MEDICINE

Evidence-based medicine has documented significant improvement of exercise-induced asthma with higher spirometry values when asthma patients took fish oil for 3 weeks. Salt restriction has also been demonstrated to improve exercise-induced asthma. Antioxidant vitamins E and C have benefited asthmatics exposed to air pollution ozone. These and other citations for evidence-based medicine support supplements such as the probiotic *Lactobacillus* for atopic dermatitis and weight loss for asthma.

Evidence-based medicine does not support treatment of asthma with acupuncture, herbs, or homeopathic remedies. Even though there are reports of improvement with these disciplines; it could really be dangerous to depend on them alone for asthma care. Patients should be seen by their Primary Care Physicians then possibly have Allergy or Pulmonary Consultation. There have been some studies that appear to improve hayfever: nevertheless there are no clear evidence-based recommendations for treatment of rhinitis or asthma with alternative medicine regimens. Again, beware of the potential dangerous side effects of some herbs. Remember, hayfever puts patients at a greater risk for asthma: treat the hayfever properly and asthma may be prevented.

CONCLUSION

Physicians must always try to guide their patients carefully and guard against any harmful treatments. At the same time, 21st century medicine incorporates the assistance of other professionals: physician assistants and nurse practitioners together with the caring LVN's and RN's who closely attend out-patients. Unfortunately, the highly trained nutritionists are still underutilized. Homeopathy, Chinese medicine, holistic, homeopathic, and naturopathic disciplines continue to offer patients something their physicians do not always provide. We can continue to provide the best medicine only if we listen to the needs and desires of our patients. Not everything they desire is what they need. But if we listen actively, perhaps we can help and guide their quest for healing.

Physicians as well as patients must keep their minds open to new ideas. Many diseases have been found to be related to nutritional factors. Mental institutions were filled with phenylketonuria (PKU) patients before special low phenylalanine diets were instituted in infancy. Scurvy was taught as a disease by the medical community even decades after nutritionists suspected and later confirmed a dietary deficiency, and lemons, in fact, were the cure. Listen to your patients and to anyone who is trying to cure them: do not be afraid that the brush will tarnish the painter. Always be ready to learn: from the Mom who just has a hunch of what may be going on, as well as the University Professor who sometimes bases very sophisticated research on a hunch. Two leading 20th-century allergists—Dr. William Deamer and Dr. Benjamin Finegold—were ahead of their time, unfolding the various manifestations of food allergy; while Professor O. Lee Frick, M.D. Ph.D. continues into the 21st Century guiding physicians onto paths that will lead to clear scientific understanding. They remain role models for all physicians, continuing the quest for knowledge with compassion and understanding.

BIBLIOGRAPHY

Baker JC, Ayres JG. Diet and asthma. *Respir Med.* 2000;94(10):925.

Bauer J. *The Complete Idiot's Guide to Total Nutrition.* New York: Alpha Books/Penguin Group; 2005.

De Smet P. *Adverse Effects of Herbal Drugs.* Berlin: Springer-Verlag; 1993.

Fligiel SE, Roth MD, Kleerup EC, et al. Tracheobronchial histopathology in habitual smokers of cocaine, marijuana, and/or tobacco. *Chest.* 1997;112(2):319.

Fugh-Berman A. Herb-Drug interactions. *Lancet.* 2000;355:134.

Gotshall RW, Mickleborough TD, Cordian L. Dietary salt restriction improves pulmonary function in exercise-induced asthma. *Med Sci Sports Exerc.* 2000;32(11):1815.

Gratzer W. *Terrors of the Table: The Curious History of Nutrition.* New York: Oxford University Press; 2005.

Katzen M. *The Enchanted Broccoli Forest.* Berkeley: Ten Speed Press; 2000.

Knonoff-Cohen H, Lam-Kruglick P. Maternal and paternal recreational drug use and sudden infant death syndrome. *Arch Pediatr Adolesc Med.* 2001;155(7):765.

Martindale S. Antioxidant intake in pregnancy in relation to wheeze and eczema in the first two years of life. *Am J Respir Crit Care Med.* 2005;171(2):121.

Mickleborough TD, Lindley MR, Lonescu AA, et al. Protective effect of fish oil supplementation on exercise induced bronchoconstriction in asthma. *Chest.* 2006;129(1):39.

Milner JD, Stein DM, McCarter R. Early infant multivitamin supplementation is associated with increased risk for food allergy and asthma. *Pediatrics.* 2004;114(1):27.

Passalacqua G, Bousquet PJ, Carlsen KH, et al. ARIA update: 1—Systematic review of complementary and alternative medicine for rhinitis and asthma. *J Allergy Clin Immunol.* 2006;117(5): 1054.

Shore SA. Obesity, smooth muscle, and airway hyperresponsiveness. *J Allergy Clin Immunol.* 2005;115(5):925.

Spector SL, Surette ME. Diet and asthma: has the role of dietary lipids been overlooked in the management of asthma? *Ann Allergy Asthma Immunol.* 2003;90(4):371.

Stenius-Aarniala B, Poussa T, Kvarnstrom J. Immediate and long term effects of weight reduction in obese people with asthma: randomized controlled study. *BMJ.* 2000;320(7238):827.

Trenga CA, Koenig JQ, Williams PV. Dietary antioxidants and ozone induced bronchial hyper responsiveness in adults with asthma. *Arch Environ Health.* 2001;56(3):242.

Weston S, Halbert A, Richmond P. Effects of probiotics on atopic dermatitis: a randomized controlled trial. *Arch Dis Child.* 2005;90(9):892.

Prevention and Control Measures in the Management of Allergic Diseases

36

Shuba Rajashri Iyengar, MD, MPH and Massoud Mahmoudi, DO, PhD

The causal relationship between allergic disease and allergen exposure has been well documented throughout the literature. Therefore, measures to reduce allergen exposure have been fundamental in the treatment of all types of allergic disease, including asthma and allergic rhinitis. The significance of this can be seen in studies conducted over 80 years ago, in which patients with asthma and atopic dermatitis were successfully treated by living in a climate chamber. Comparable studies have been performed more recently, demonstrating that changing asthmatic patients from their domestic environment to a hospital room for several months resulted in significantly decreased airway hyperresponsiveness from bronchial provocation studies.

Although these measures are impractical in outpatient medicine, they demonstrate the importance of allergen exposure and sensitization in the pathogenesis of allergic disease. Sensitization to one or more of the major indoor allergens has been consistently found to be the strongest risk factor for asthma. In addition, studies examining the reunification of East Germany with the more industrialized West Germany demonstrated the effects of environmental exposure on the development of asthma and allergic disease in two genetically similar populations. The prevalence of asthma (and bronchial hyperresponsiveness) as well as atopy was greater in West German than East German children shortly after reunification. West German children also had significantly greater rates of sensitization to mite, cat, and pollen allergens during this time period. However, follow-up studies performed years later (after greater spread of industrialization) demonstrated increasing rates of hay fever and atopic sensitization, but not of asthma and bronchial hyperresponsiveness, among a cohort of East German schoolchildren. This suggests that the development of different atopic disorders may depend on when during childhood development the allergen exposure has occurred.

Therefore, identifying pertinent indoor and outdoor allergens (through skin and serum IgE testing) is essential in the management of asthma and atopic disease. Further steps include determining and reducing allergen reservoirs (through barrier methods, air filtration, etc.), ambient environmental changes, and long-term strategies to maintain allergen reduction and control.

INDOOR ALLERGENS

Dust Mite

BACKGROUND

Household dust can contain many different species of mites, but in most countries the pyroglyphid mites are the majority. This includes *Dermatophagoides pteronyssinus* and *Dermatophagoides farinae*. These mites are eight-legged microscopic creatures that are invisible to the naked eye. They live on skin scales and other debris. In addition, mites are not capable of drinking liquids and so must absorb water through a substance extruded from their leg joints. This makes them entirely dependent on the humidity of the ambient environment. In addition to humidity, they have strict temperature requirements and can only grow between temperatures of 65°F and 80°F (18°C and 27°C).

Ideal areas for mites to live include carpets, mattresses, pillows, sofas, and clothing because these can be very humid environments. However, even with reductions in the ambient humidity, it may take several months for mites to die and even longer for allergen levels to decrease in carpets, pillows, mattresses, and sofas. This is because as the moisture level drops, mites withdraw from the surface to the deeper layers of carpet and upholstery, making them difficult to eradicate.

The largest quantity of the mite allergen is found in its fecal particles. This is the major particulate source of dust allergen in house dust. Many of these allergens have now been characterized and are referred to as *group 1* (Der p 1 and Der f 1) and *group 2* (Der p 2 and Der f 2).

Control Strategies

Key principles behind reducing dust mite exposure include identifying and reducing dust mite reservoirs. Reservoirs are objects that harbor large amounts of a specific allergen. For example, dust mite reservoirs include bedding, carpets, furniture, and other upholstered items (Table 36–1). Measures to reduce reservoir carriage of dust mite include obtaining dust mite impermeable covers, washing bedding in hot water, and carpet removal. The next step in reducing dust mite exposure involves strategies to change the ambient

Table 36–1. Dust mite avoidance measures.

Reservoir Reduction
1. Bedding
   a. Impermeable zippered covers for pillows and mattresses (on all beds that patient sleeps on).
   b. Washing all bedding (pillowcases, sheets, blankets) at 130°F (54°C) weekly.
   c. Removing blankets/comforters that are not washable or using them with an impermeable zippered cover.
   d. Removing all upholstered toys on bed (unless washed at 130°F [54°C] or placed in freezer overnight weekly).
2. Carpets
   a. Vacuum weekly with a filtration system (i.e., high-efficiency particulate air [HEPA] filter) or cleaner.
   b. If possible, replace carpets with linoleum or wood flooring in the bedroom (first priority) and other living spaces.
   c. Remove carpets on concrete slabs.
   d. Clean and wash area rugs.
3. Furniture (sofa, draperies, throw pillows, and other upholstered items)
   a. Reduce upholstered items, especially old sofas and draperies. If necessary, consider plastic covers for old sofas/chairs.
   b. Clean and dust items often, especially those in the bedroom (household member rather than patient should do this).

Ambient Environmental Changes
1. Humidity: Reduce humidity to <50% of the relative humidity.
   a. If possible, avoid living in the basement or overly humid environments.
   b. Consider second-floor bedroom of house or apartment.
2. Air Filtration Systems: They are generally not very effective for mite control.

---

environment. This includes measures to decrease humidity (like a dehumidifier) as well as changing the bedroom or entire home. Most strategies target the former because these measures are relatively simple, inexpensive, and have a greater impact (Table 36–1).

Reservoir reduction Reservoir reduction methods are aimed at finding those items that harbor dust mites and eliminating or reducing the amount of mites and mite antigen in them (see examples in Table 36–1).

Impermeable zippered covers to reduce dust mite and mite allergen exposure are widely used. Traditionally used items were entirely plastic, but now tightly woven synthetic fibers or nonwoven synthetics that allow vapor to pass through (but not allergen) are available. Dust mite allergens (Der f 1 and Der p 1) were blocked below detectable limits by fabrics less than 10 μm in pore size. Fabrics with an average pore size of 6 μm or less blocked cat allergen (Fel d 1). The effect of dust mite–impermeable covers on reducing clinical symptoms is under debate, but most studies show that these measures should not be performed in isolation. Most practitioners recommend these methods be performed in combination with the washing of bedding, the avoidance of stuffed animals, and the frequent vacuuming/removal of carpets (Table 36–1).

Many investigators have studied the use of chemicals to kill mites or denature allergens, but there is modest data favoring this approach. Only benzyl benzoate and tannic acid have been marketed in the United States and have resulted in minimal mite reduction when applied to carpets.

Lastly, those studies that have been successful in demonstrating a clinical benefit from allergen avoidance measures have ensured sustained use for greater than 6 months. Therefore, patient education and follow-up to ensure compliance is extremely important.

Ambient environmental changes Because dust mites thrive in humidity, decreasing the humidity to below 50% of the relative humidity can decrease mite growth. However, this can be difficult to accomplish in humid geographical areas (e.g., southeastern states, areas along the Pacific Coast). General recommendations include not living in basement areas and, if living in an apartment, to live on the second floor or above. Air filtration units are not helpful for dust mite reduction because most of the airborne mite allergen is carried on large particles (larger than 10 μm) that fall rapidly after disturbance. Therefore, after several minutes, little airborne mite allergen is detectable.

Animal Dander

BACKGROUND

The domestic animals most commonly encountered in the United States include cats and dogs.

Cats The main cat allergen is Fel d 1, although other characterized proteins produced by cats are allergenic for patients (i.e., Fel d 2, Fel d 3). The most important sources of the allergen are the sebaceous, salivary, and perianal glands, with the skin and fur being the principal reservoirs. Several properties of the Fel d 1 protein contribute to its high allergenicity. First, it is very heat stable. For example, exposure at 284°F (140°C) for 60 minutes resulted in only a 30% denaturation of the molecule. Next, it is easily airborne. Both Fel d 1 and Can f 1 (main dog antigen) are carried by small particles (5 to 10 μm in diameter) that are light and readily airborne for long periods of time after minimal disturbance. Lastly, cat dander particles can stick to all available surfaces, such as furniture, clothing, and walls. Therefore, they frequently travel to indoor environments that theoretically should be cat free (like houses without cats, schools, and other types of public buildings). Many studies have shown that the clothes of cat owners represent the main source for the dispersal of cat allergens in cat-free environments. Because of these properties of the Fel d 1 antigen, the allergen can persist for many months even when cats are removed from the house.

Cat allergen is a major risk factor for asthma. Asthma was found to be strongly associated with sensitization (assessed by skin testing) to cat allergens in a cross-sectional study conducted in New Mexico. In addition, a Dutch cohort study found that cat allergen exposure was associated with both sensitization and persistent wheezing at 4 years of age.

Dogs Can f 1 is the major allergen found in dogs. Similar to Fel d 1, it can accumulate in house dust and is easily airborne. In addition, it can also collect in public areas like schools. However, Can f 1 allergy is less common than Fel d 1 allergy as a cause of asthma. Like Fel d 1, it was associated with both sensitization and persistent wheezing at 4 years of age but only in a subgroup of patients with maternal atopy.

CONTROL STRATEGIES

Source and reservoir reduction The same principles that have been applied to dust mite exposure reduction can be applied to animal dander. This includes reservoir identification and reduction as well as long-term strategies to maintain allergen reduction (Table 36–2). Most practitioners agree that an atopic patient who is sensitized to cat or dog allergen should not live with a pet in their home. However, because most families are reluctant to part with the pet, eliminating the source of allergen in sensitized individuals becomes difficult. Because pets are quite mobile and pet allergen particles are very sticky, these antigens become widely distributed in a home, as discussed previously.

Table 36–2. Animal dander avoidance measures.

Reservoir Reduction
1. Pet Removal
   a. The most effective strategy is to remove the pet from the house.
   b. After removal, vacuum clean and wash all surfaces (including walls) on which Fel d 1 or Can f 1 may have accumulated. Carpets and upholstery must be cleaned. Bedding and clothing must be washed.
   c. Restricting animals to areas of the house is not effective.
   d. Cats should be washed twice weekly to obtain a significant reduction of Fel d 1 shedding; however, protein reaccumulates quickly.
2. Clothing (especially important for cat owners)
   a. Washing (water superior to dry cleaning) the clothes and avoiding use of allergen-contaminated clothes outdoors.
3. Carpet
   a. Remove carpeting from all environments and replace with linoleum or wood flooring, if possible. Alternatively, use vacuum cleaner with a high-efficiency particulate air HEPA (or polyethylene) filter and double-thickness bags.
4. Bedding
   a. Wash bedding in water weekly. Using detergent solutions at 25°C (77°F) for at least 5 minutes is recommended.
5. Furniture
   a. Remove or limit all upholstered furniture (sofas, draperies, chairs, etc.).
   b. Clean and dust items often.

Ambient Environment
Air filtration systems: Recommended in combination with methods cited earlier, HEPA, or electrostatic units.

Like dust mite allergen, pet allergen reservoirs in the home include all upholstered items (bedding, sofas, carpet, chairs, draperies, etc.). Measures to reduce allergen are similar to those already discussed, but these measures are frequently ineffective if the source (i.e., the pet) is not removed from the home. Pet allergen concentrations are 10 to 1000 times higher in homes with a pet than without.

Cockroach

BACKGROUND

Although several species of cockroaches are found in North American homes, the best known are the German cockroach (*Blattella germanica*) as well as the American cockroach (*Periplaneta americana*). These insects are common in inner-city apartments in the United States. Aerosolized proteins from secretions, fecal material, saliva, debris, and the dead bodies of cockroaches induce IgE-mediated hypersensitivity. The characterization of allergens derived from German and American cockroaches (Bla g 1–5) has been reported.

Cockroach allergy is an important risk factor for emergency department visits for asthma and hospital admissions. This association is restricted to urban areas, where cockroach allergens have been found in houses.

Control Strategies

Reservoir reduction Attempts at reducing exposure to cockroach allergen with the goal of improving clinical outcome in inner-city patients with asthma have been generally unsuccessful. One of the most well known attempts was the National Cooperative Inner City Asthma Study in which 265 inner-city families with asthmatic children underwent several different interventions, including insecticide application and directed education. Approximately 20% of the families were randomly selected to have Bla g 1 measured in settled dust from the kitchen, bedroom, and TV/living room. After 1 year, no significant changes were seen from preextermination levels, and only 50% of families had been compliant with cleaning instructions.

Major reservoirs for cockroaches are areas where food waste is available. These are typically areas of the kitchen/dining room and are commonly used dishes and cooking utensils, garbage, and open food containers. Therefore, recommendations include the following:

- Using multiple baited traps or poisons. This ranges from boric acid, which can kill roaches by destroying their foregut, to a range of chemicals, including hydramethylnon, abamectin, and fipronil.
- Washing dishes and cooking utensils immediately after use.
- Disposing of domestic garbage and food waste quickly.
- Removing cockroach debris promptly.

OUTDOOR ALLERGENS

Background

The most widely recognized and abundant sources for outdoor allergens are pollen grains and fungal spores. However, insect stings should always be included in the discussion of outdoor allergic triggers. See Chapter 25 for information regarding this topic.

Pollen allergens were believed to play a role in allergic rhinitis, but the particle size of pollen was considered too large to penetrate the lower airways, and therefore too large to lead to asthma. However, increasing evidence indicates a relationship between exposure to pollen, fungal, and other airborne allergens and the exacerbation of asthma and other forms of allergic disease. For example, studies examining data from the second National Health and Nutrition Surveys have demonstrated an association between increased skin test reactivity to several different outdoor pollens and significant decrements in forced expiratory volume in 1 second (FEV_1) in symptomatic asthmatic children. In addition, asthma and allergic rhinitis were associated with skin test reactivity to specific outdoor allergens, like Alternaria. In addition, allergic rhinitis alone (without the presence of asthma) was associated with skin test reactivity to rye grass and ragweed.

PLANT POLLENS

Pollen allergen exposure depends on the pollination process occurring in wind-pollinated (anemophilous) plants, including trees, grasses, and weeds, rather than insect-pollinated plants. This is because in wind-pollinated plants, pollen grains are released into the atmosphere and must passively find their way onto an appropriate receptive female. This process is very inefficient, so these plants produce large amounts of pollen to ensure successful fertilizations. Therefore, pollen from these types of plants is the most abundant and significant in regard to human exposure.

Pollen grains are usually spherical with a rigid cell wall formed of a complex polysaccharide-based substance. They are identified using light microscopy by the size and shape of the grain as well as wall structure. Most airborne pollen grains are 15 to 50 µm in diameter, although the overall range is broad (10 to 100 µm).

The potency of pollen allergens is not just a matter of protein abundance. Comparable amounts of two allergens in rye grass pollen, for instance, can produce widely different allergenicities based on radioallergosorbent test (RAST) inhibition. Therefore, there are differences in structure and composition that confer allergenicity.

Up to this point, most attention has been directed at allergens contained within pollens as the primary sources of allergen. However, attention is now being focused on small particle fractions and their association with pollen allergens. For example, grass allergens measured in fine-particle aerosols have been found joined to diesel exhaust particles and starch grains. The role of pollen-derived allergens associated with these small particle fractions is still unclear. However, because of the microscopic size of these particles, they could easily enter the lower airways. Therefore, they may play a role in asthma exacerbations. In addition, there is a potential increased risk of exposure because of longer amounts of time spent airborne.

FUNGAL SPORES

Fungal spores are either actively released from the plant source or dispersed passively, with the aid of wind or

Table 36–3. Outdoor allergen avoidance measures.

1. Keep windows and doors closed to prevent outdoor allergens from coming into the home.
2. Remove indoor sources that can collect pollen, support fungal growth.
   a. Dust all surfaces frequently.
   b. Eliminate/reduce the number of indoor plants.
   c. Clean moldy surfaces.
   d. Keep the house well ventilated and free of dampness.
   e. Avoid basements.
   f. Do not use window fans.
3. Stay indoors during the times when the allergen is abundant outdoors.
   a. Learn about the prevalence patterns of for each relevant allergen, including seasonal, geographic, and daily variation patterns (see Chapter 5).

rain. The active mechanisms all depend on changes in moisture conditions. For instance, Ascospores and basidiospores are released as the spore-bearing cell absorbs water, either during rainfall or as humidity increases. Some dry-weather spores (e.g., *Cladosporium*) are shaken loose as the spore-bearing cell twists as it dries. During instances where passive mechanisms are used, air movements alone are sufficient to cause release of spores. Rainfall is also well known to cause release of spores. Because rainfall both disperses and removes spores, it is difficult to predict airborne spore concentrations during rainfall. However, during long gentle rains, there is thought to be much higher spore concentrations than on sunny days without rain.

Control Strategies

Control strategies include keeping windows and doors closed to minimize outdoor allergens in the home, removing indoor reservoirs, and avoiding high pollen environments (Table 36–3).

EVIDENCE-BASED HOME INTERVENTION METHODS

Because children with asthma who live in the inner city are exposed to multiple indoor allergens, several recent studies have looked at the impact of different home-based environmental intervention methods on asthma symptomatology and morbidity. Morgan et al from the Inner-City Asthma Study Group performed a randomized, controlled trial looking at the efficacy of an environmental intervention that lasted 1 year and included education for exposure to allergens and environmental tobacco smoke as well as allergen reduction interventions

(encasements, high efficiency particulate air filters, cockroach extermination). The study group consisted of 937 children with atopic asthma (5 to 11 years of age) living in seven major U.S. cities. Home environmental exposures were assessed every 6 months, and asthma-related complications were assessed every 2 months during the intervention and for 1 year after the intervention. There were greater declines in the levels of indoor allergens, such as *D. farinae* and *D. pteronyssinus*, in the bed and cockroach allergen on the bedroom floor. In addition, the intervention group had fewer days with symptoms than the control group during both the intervention year and the year afterward. However, there was no significant effect of the environmental intervention on lung function during the intervention year as measured by either spirometry or peak flow monitoring.

More recently, Eggleston et al conducted a randomized controlled trial also involving a 1 year home-based environmental intervention. This included education, cockroach and rodent extermination, mattress and pillow encasings, and high-efficiency particulate air cleaner. The study group consisted of 100 asthmatic children age 6 to 12 years. Outcomes were assessed by home evaluations at 6 and 12 months, a clinic evaluation at 12 months, and multiple telephone interviews. Levels of particulate matter (10 μm or smaller) declined by up to 39% in the treatment group but increased in the control group. In addition, cockroach allergen levels decreased by 51% in the treatment group. Daytime symptoms decreased in the treatment group and increased in the control group. However, other measures of morbidity, such as spirometry findings, nighttime symptoms, and emergency department use, were not significantly changed.

Therefore, both studies demonstrate that a tailored, multifaceted environmental treatment reduced indoor allergen levels in inner-city homes, as well as symptomatology, but had no effect on spirometry measurements. It is possible that longer intervention and/or follow-up periods are needed to demonstrate a significant effect on lung function measurements.

BIBLIOGRAPHY

Almqvist C, Larrson PH, Egmar A-C, et al. School as a risk environment for children allergic to cats and a site for transfer of cat allergen to homes. *J Allergy Clin Immunol.* 1999;103:1012.

Brussee JE, Smit HA, van Strien RT, et al. Allergen exposure in infancy and the development of sensitization, wheeze, and asthma at 4 years. *J Allergy Clin Immunol.* 2005;115(5):946.

Burge HA, Rogers CA. Outdoor allergens. *Environ Health Perspect.* 2000;108(suppl 4):653.

Carter MC, Perzanowski MS, Raymond A, et al. Home intervention in the treatment of asthma among inner-city children. *J Allergy Clin Immunol.* 2001;108(5):732.

Chapman RS, Hadden WC, Perlin SA. Influences of asthma and household environment on lung function in children and adolescents: the third national health and nutrition examination survey. *Am J Epidemiol.* 2003;158(2):175.

Eggleston PA, Butz A, Rand C, et al. Home environmental intervention in inner-city asthma: a randomized controlled clinical trial. *Ann Allergy Asthma Immunol.* 2005;95(6):518.

Gergen PJ, Mortimer KM, Eggleston PA, et al. Results of the National Cooperative Inner-City Asthma Study (NCICAS) environmental intervention to reduce cockroach allergen exposure in inner-city homes. *J Allergy Clin Immunol.* 1999;103(3 Pt 1):501.

Luczynska C, Tredwell E, Smeeton N, et al. A randomized controlled trial of mite allergen-impermeable bed covers in adult mite-sensitized asthmatics. *Clin Exp Allergy.* 2003;33(12):1648.

Morgan WJ, Crain EF, Gruchalla RS, et al. Results of a home-based environmental intervention among urban children with asthma. *N Engl J Med.* 2004;9;351(11):1068.

Rosenstreich DL, Eggleston P, Kattan M, et al. The role of cockroach allergy and exposure to cockroach allergen in causing morbidity among inner-city children with asthma. *N Engl J Med.* 1997;336(19):1356.

Tovey ER, Taylor DJ, Mitakakis TZ, et al. Effectiveness of laundry washing agents and conditions in the removal of cat and dust mite allergen from bedding dust. *J Allergy Clin Immunol.* 2001;108:369.

von Mutius E, Martinez FD, Fritzsch C, et al. Prevalence of asthma and atopy in two areas of West and East Germany. *Am J Respir Crit Care Med.* 1994;149(2 Pt 1):358.

Wood RA, Eggleston PA, Rand C, et al. Cockroach allergen abatement with extermination and sodium hypochlorite cleaning in inner-city homes. *Ann Allergy Asthma Immunol.* 2001;187:60.

Woodcock A, Forster L, Matthews E, et al. Control of exposure to mite allergen and allergen-impermeable bed covers for adults with asthma. *N Engl J Med.* 2003;17;349(3):225.

Antihistamines and Mast Cell Stabilizers

Giselle S. Mosnaim, MD, MS and Timothy J. Craig, DO

MECHANISM OF ALLERGIC DISEASE

The allergic response is comprised of an early phase and a late phase. The early phase, which occurs within minutes of allergen exposure in sensitized individuals, is characterized by the release of preformed mediators including histamine and proteases. The late phase, which tends to occur within 3 to 12 hours after antigen exposure, involves the recruitment of additional cells to augment the inflammation. These cells may include eosinophils, basophils, monocytes, and lymphocytes (Fig. 37–1).

Histamine is a key mediator in allergic disease and primarily produced in mast cells and circulating basophils. In response to antigen exposure in an appropriately sensitized atopic individual, IgE antibodies are produced and bind to high-affinity receptors for the Fc portion of the IgE antibody on these mast cells and basophils. This binding, and subsequent cross-linking of bound IgE antibodies by antigen, begins a series of events that leads to the extracellular release of histamine. Histamine may cause a variety of physiologic effects depending on its target cell. Binding to smooth muscle may cause bronchoconstriction and vasodilation, binding to endothelial cells can lead to increased vascular permeability, and binding to sensory nerves may lead to a burning sensation as well as itching. These physiologic effects may translate clinically into symptoms of sneezing, rhinorrhea, pruritus, and urticaria.

ANTIHISTAMINE MECHANISM OF ACTION

Four distinct histamine receptor subtypes have been identified, designated as H_1, H_2, H_3, and H_4. In allergic disease, the focus is on the H_1 receptor. H_1 antihistamines function as inverse agonists at the histamine H_1 receptor, stabilizing the receptor in the inactive conformational state (Fig. 37–2).

The clinical efficacy of H_1 antihistamines is mainly due to this inverse agonist activity at the H_1 histamine receptor. Independent of their histamine-blocking action, antihistamines also exert antiinflammatory effects, including downregulation of mediator release, intracellular adhesion molecule expression, superoxide generation, chemotaxis, and cytokine expression; and upregulation of neutrophil and epithelial cell immunoreactivity, and number and function of β-adrenergic receptors. The clinical significance of these antiinflammatory effects still requires further investigation, and this research is leading to a new understanding of the mechanisms for allergic disease and the development of new drugs to treat the clinical symptoms.

ANTIHISTAMINES

Antihistamines currently available on the market in the United States include: oral first-generation, oral second-generation, topical intranasal, topical skin, and topical intraocular formulations.

Oral First-Generation Antihistamines

Oral first-generation antihistamines include diphenhydramine, clemastine, tripelennamine, pyrilamine, brompheniramine, chlorpheniramine, triprolidine, hydroxyzine, promethazine, and cyproheptadine. Hydroxyzine is available by prescription, and some of the other agents, such as diphenhydramine and chlorpheniramine, are available over the counter. They are nonselective receptor antagonists and exert antiserotonergic, anticholinergic, antidopaminergic, and anti-α-adrenergic effects. Due to their blockage of muscarinic receptors, they may cause significant anticholinergic effects, including dry mouth, constipation, urinary retention, and sinus tachycardia. The lipophilic properties of oral first-generation antihistamines allow them to cross the blood-brain barrier and interact with central nervous system H_1 receptors. Because histamine controls vigilance during the waking

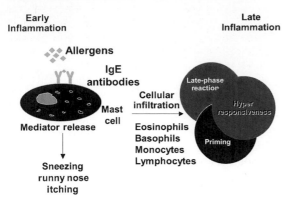

Figure 37–1. Early-and late-phase response of allergic inflammation. The early-phase response (early inflammation) is characterized by the cross linking of IgE antibodies on the surface of the mast cell by the allergen, releasing preformed mediators such as histamine. The late-phase response (late inflammation) occurs several hours later due to cellular infiltration by eosinophils, basophils, monocytes, and lymphocytes. (Reproduced, with permission, from Naclerio, RM. Allergic rhinitis. *N Engl J Med.* 1991;325:861.)

state, this blockade of the effects of endogenous histamine in the central nervous system may lead to sedative effects. As a class, they are also often referred to as *sedating* antihistamines, a term that has been operationalized to indicate both drowsiness and impairment in motor and cognitive abilities. Studies have

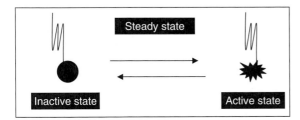

Figure 37–2. The H_1 histamine receptor. This figure shows the histamine H_1 receptor active state in equilibrium with the inactive state. A histamine H_1 receptor agonist, histamine, as it preferentially binds the active state, stabilizes the receptor in the active conformation, and thus causes a shift in the equilibrium toward the active state. A histamine H_1 receptor inverse agonist, an H_1 antihistamine, preferentially binds the inactive state, stabilizing the receptor in the inactive conformation, and thus causes a shift in the equilibrium toward the inactive state.

also demonstrated discrepancies between patient self-reported and objective measures of drowsiness and impairment due to these medications. Further corroborating these findings, oral first-generation antihistamines cause significant loss of productivity at school and at work and impair driving performance. Dosing for oral first-generation antihistamines is several times a day. Because the terminal elimination half-life of these drugs varies from 9.2 to 27.9 hours, even if taken only at bedtime, there may be potential sedation the following day. In general, their rate of sedation is twice that of placebo, and 25% to 50% of patients are affected.

Oral Second-Generation Antihistamines

Oral second-generation antihistamines currently available in the United States include cetirizine, desloratadine, fexofenadine, and loratadine. These drugs are referred to by a variety of different names, including *nonsedating, low-sedating, new-generation, next-generation,* and *third-generation antihistamines,* for which there are no universally accepted definitions. This terminology should be avoided because it may cause confusion among clinicians and patients.

In contrast to the oral first-generation antihistamines, the oral second-generation antihistamines have more specific peripheral H_1 receptor selectivity and are thus less likely to cause antiserotonergic, anticholinergic, antidopaminergic, anti-α-adrenergic effects. Furthermore, they are lipophobic, and therefore the possibility of their penetration of the blood-brain barrier to act on central H_1 receptors to cause sedative effects is diminished. Overall, they also have a quicker onset of action, longer duration of action, increased potency, or reduced adverse events. The second-generation antihistamines have been well studied in clinical trials, and their clinical efficacy, safety profiles, significant drug interactions, use during pregnancy and lactation, clinical indications, dosage and administration, as well as comparative efficacy with respect to other agents used to treat allergic diseases, are clearly established.

CLINICAL EFFICACY

All four oral second-generation antihistamines have shown efficacy in controlling symptoms of allergic rhinitis, 24-hour symptom control, and antiinflammatory potential. Pollen challenge studies conducted in an environmental exposure unit (EEU) are often used to characterize the time to onset of clinically important relief with oral second-generation antihistamines.

SAFETY PROFILE

Central nervous system effects Undesirable effects of antihistamines are related to their ability to cross the blood-brain barrier and function as inverse agonists at

H_1 receptors in the brain, causing sedation. The oral second-generation antihistamines, due to their lipophobic properties, are less likely than their liphophilic first-generation counterparts to exert these effects. Cetirizine has demonstrated sedative properties even at recommended doses in patients 12 years of age or older (11% to 14%, vs. 6% receiving placebo). Sedative properties have been observed with desloratadine and loratadine at two to four times higher than recommended doses, but not at therapeutic doses. At clinically indicated doses, or higher than therapeutic doses, fexofenadine does not cause sedation.

Cardiotoxicity Antihistamines are more likely to cause cardiotoxicity when plasma concentrations are elevated. Thus it is important to consider overdose and drug–drug interactions when discussing cardiotoxicity.

The first oral second-generation antihistamines approved for use in the United States, terfenadine and astemizole, were removed from the market in the late 1990s because of their association with rare but serious adverse cardiac events, including ventricular arrhythmias, cardiac arrest, and death. In 20 of the first 25 cases of proarrhythmic effects related to terfenadine reported to the U.S. Food and Drug Administration (FDA), patients had at least one documented risk factor causing elevation of blood concentrations of terfenadine and predisposing them to these adverse reactions: 11 patients were taking concomitant drugs known to inhibit hepatic terfenadine metabolism, 3 had taken an intentional overdose, and 6 likely had hepatic cirrhosis.

In summary, first-generation oral antihistamines, including diphenhydramine and hydroxyzine, have demonstrated QT_c prolongation at higher-than-recommended doses. Terfenadine and astemizole were withdrawn from the market due to their cardiotoxicity. Even at higher than therapeutic doses, cetirizine, desloratadine, fexofenadine, and loratadine have not demonstrated clinically significant cardiac effects. It is important to underscore that fexofenadine, although it is the primary metabolite of terfenadine, does not exhibit cardiotoxicity.

DRUG INTERACTIONS

Terfenadine, astemizole, and loratadine are substrates of the hepatic cytochrome P-450 isoenzymes, which can be found in the liver and small intestine. Specifically, loratadine is a substrate for cytochrome P-450 isoenzymes 3A4 and 2D6. Other drugs that inhibit the cytochrome P-450 isoenzymes 3A4 and/or 2D6, including ketoconazole, erythromycin, cimetidine, and clarithromycin, may elevate the plasma concentrations of loratadine. The clinical significance of this elevation is unknown. Cetirizine, fexofenadine, and desloratadine do not undergo cytochrome P-450 metabolism.

Fexofenadine and desloratadine interact with the efflux transporter P-glycoprotein, and fexofenadine interacts with the uptake transporter organic anion transporting peptide (OATP). Due to P-glycoprotein, ketoconazole taken concomitantly with desloratadine and fexofenadine may increase the plasma concentration of these antihistamines by 40% and 135%, respectively. However, adverse effects associated with this elevation have not been reported. Coadministration of 1.2 L of grapefruit juice decreased plasma levels of fexofenadine likely due to the saturation of OATP carrier proteins with grapefruit juice. The effectiveness of fexofenadine should also be monitored when taken concurrently with antacids. Antacids may bind fexofenadine and thus decrease its absorption.

Sedation and driving impairment due to cetirizine may be augmented by the concomitant use of alcohol (Table 37–1). Cetirizine, desloratadine, fexofenadine, and loratadine all accumulate with renal impairment, and the dose should be adjusted accordingly. Cetirizine, desloratadine, and loratadine undergo significant liver metabolism to varying degrees, 30%, more than 90%, and more than 98%, respectively. These three drugs require dose reduction in patients with hepatic impairment. Fexofenadine undergoes less than 4% liver metabolism. It does not accumulate in patients with hepatic dysfunction, nor does it require dose adjustment.

PREGNANCY AND LACTATION

Because they have been out on the market longer and thus more data are available in pregnancy, oral first-generation antihistamines are considered first-line therapy for allergic rhinitis in pregnancy. Specifically, chlorpheniramine, tripelennamine, and diphenhydramine are category B. Brompheniramine should be avoided during pregnancy. Second-generation antihistamines are reasonable alternatives, especially for women who have not responded to or had significant side effects on taking oral first-generation antihistamines. Testing in animal models has led the FDA to label cetirizine and loratadine as Pregnancy Category B, and fexofenadine and desloratadine as Pregnancy Category C.

Based on animal and human studies in nursing mothers taking oral second-generation antihistamines that examine the amount of drug secreted into breast milk, cetirizine and desloratadine are not recommended for nursing mothers. Caution should be exercised when prescribing fexofenadine and loratadine to a nursing mother.

CLINICAL INDICATIONS

Oral second-generation antihistamines are indicated for the treatment of seasonal and perennial allergic rhinitis, as well as chronic idiopathic urticaria.

Allergic rhinitis Allergic rhinitis is a chronic condition affecting 10% to more than 40% of the population worldwide. It is one of the top ten reasons for patients to visit their primary care physicians. Clinical symptoms

Table 37–1. Comparison of second-generation oral antihistamines.[*]

	Cetirizine	Desloratadine	Fexofenadine	Loratadine
Age Indication	≥6 mo	≥6 mo	≥6 mo	≥2 y
Pregnancy Category	B	C	C	B
Sedation	Yes	No	No	No
Performance Impairment	Yes	No	No	No
QT$_c$ Prolongation with Increased Drug Levels	No	No	No	No
Substantial Effect of Macrolides on Bioavailability	No	No	Yes	Yes
Accumulation in Renal or Hepatic Dysfunction	Both hepatic and renal	Both hepatic and renal	Renal only	Both hepatic and renal

[*]Cetirizine, desloratadine, and fexofenadine are indicated down to ≥6 months of age. Loratadine is indicated down to ≥2 years of age. Cetirizine and loratadine are Pregnancy Category B, whereas desloratadine and fexofenadine are category C. Cetirizine may cause sedation and performance impairment at recommended doses. Clinical trials do not show sedation or performance impairment with the use of recommended doses of desloratadine, fexofenadine, and loratadine. None of these agents cause clinically significant QT$_c$ prolongation with increased drug levels. Macrolides may have a substantial effect on the bioavailability of fexofenadine and loratadine but not on the bioavailability of cetirizine or desloratadine. Whereas cetirizine, desloratadine, and loratadine may accumulate in both renal and hepatic impairment, fexofenadine accumulates only with renal impairment.

include pruritus, sneezing, rhinorrhea, and nasal congestion. Allergic rhinitis is part of a systemic inflammatory process and often associated with other inflammatory conditions such as asthma, rhinosinusitis, allergic conjunctivitis, and otitis media with effusion. It has traditionally been classified as either seasonal or perennial, depending on whether the patient is sensitized to cyclical pollens or year-round allergens such as mold, pets, dust mites, and cockroaches. More recently a new classification system, the Allergic Rhinitis and Its Impact on Asthma (ARIA) guidelines, were developed by the World Health Organization. Under this new system, allergic rhinitis is defined as intermittent or persistent, and mild or moderate-severe. Intermittent symptoms are present less than 4 days per week or less than 4 weeks per year. Persistent symptoms are present more than 4 days per week and more than 4 weeks per year. Mild symptoms do not interfere with sleep; do not impair daily activities; do not affect work and school; and do not cause troublesome symptoms. A patient is considered to have moderate-severe disease if one or more of the following symptoms are present:

abnormal sleep; impairment of daily activities, impairment of work and school activities, and troublesome symptoms.

The ARIA guidelines outline a stepwise approach to the treatment of allergic rhinitis. Initial pharmacotherapy for mild intermittent allergic rhinitis consists of an oral antihistamine, an intranasal antihistamine, or an oral decongestant. For persistent and moderate-severe symptoms, intranasal steroids are the first-line recommended treatment. Appropriate follow-up care accompanied by step-up or step-down therapy is the cornerstone for long-term management of this chronic disease.

Oral second-generation antihistamines, including cetirizine, desloratadine, loratadine, and fexofenadine, have been studied in patients with allergic rhinitis and concomitant asthma. These studies have led to several clinical findings regarding oral second-generation antihistamines, including the following: Whereas the oral first-generation antihistamines had the potential to exacerbate asthma because of their anticholinergic effects, the oral second-generation antihistamines, with their lack of anticholinergic effects, do not pose this problem; by ameliorating allergic rhinitis, they may

Table 37–2. Therapeutic options in the treatment of allergic rhinitis.*

	Sneezing	Rhinorrhea	Nasal Congestion	Nasal Pruritus	Ocular Symptoms
Intranasal Steroids	3+	3+	3+	2+	2+
Intranasal Chromones	1+	1+	1+	1+	Ø
Oral Decongestants	Ø	Ø	3+	Ø	Ø
Intranasal Anticholinergics	Ø	2+	Ø	Ø	Ø
Antileukotrienes	Ø	1+	2+	Ø	2+

*Medications used in the treatment of allergic rhinitis have different degrees of effectiveness in targeting specific symptoms.

indirectly improve symptoms of asthma; and they may serve as a useful adjunctive therapy in patients with allergic rhinitis and concomitant asthma.

Other treatment options for allergic rhinitis in addition to antihistamines There are a variety of other options for the treatment of allergic rhinitis in addition to oral and intranasal antihistamines (Table 37–2.) These medications include intranasal steroids, intranasal chromones/mast cell stabilizers, oral and topical decongestants, oral decongestant-antihistamine combinations, topical anticholinergics, and antileukotrienes.

Intranasal steroids Intranasal steroids are currently the most effective class of medications for the treatment of allergic rhinitis and improve all nasal symptoms, including rhinorrhea, pruritus, congestion, and sneezing. They are first-line treatment for patients with persistent moderate-severe symptoms or whose main complaint is nasal congestion. Nasal steroids are superior to antihistamines for nasal congestion. In contrast, antihistamines appear to be superior for ocular symptoms. Intranasal steroids are superior to intranasal chromones for overall symptom reduction.

Oral decongestants and oral decongestant/antihistamine combinations Antihistamines are frequently combined with oral decongestants to offer better symptom control of nasal congestion. Oral decongestants such as pseudoephedrine are currently available in the United States. These medications produce vasoconstriction in the nasal mucosa via stimulation of β-adrenergic receptors and can ameliorate nasal congestion. They do not improve any of the other symptoms of allergic rhinitis. Side effects of oral decongestants include insomnia, irritability, palpitations, and tachycardia. Oral decongestants are contraindicated in patients with severe hypertension; severe cardiovascular disease; narrow-angle glaucoma; urinary retention; and during or within

14 days of use of monoamine oxidase inhibitors. Pseudoephedrine is available in 30-mg tablets, 120-mg sustained-release tablets, 15-mg chewable tablets, and 15-mg/5-mL liquid. Multiple over-the-counter first-generation antihistamine plus decongestant combination products are available. The second-generation antihistamine plus decongestant products include loratadine, 10 mg, and pseudoephedrine, 240 mg combination; loratadine, 5 mg, and pseudoephedrine, 120 mg, combination; desloratadine, 5 mg, and pseudoephedrine, 240 mg, combination; cetirizine, 5 mg, and pseudoephedrine, 120 mg, combination; fexofenadine, 60 mg, and pseudoephedrine, 120 mg, combination; and fexofenadine, 180 mg, and pseudoephedrine, 240 mg, combination.

Urticaria Chronic idiopathic urticaria is characterized by the appearance of transient pruritic erythematous wheals. Individual lesions resolve within 24 hours, and then new ones appear. Chronic urticaria is defined as recurring episodes of hives lasting more than 6 weeks. Oral second-generation antihistamines are first-line therapy as well as the mainstay of treatment. Both first- and second-generation antihistamines are used for acute urticaria, although neither are FDA approved for this indication.

Allergic conjunctivitis Ocular allergy symptoms may present alone, and this condition is termed *allergic conjunctivitis*. The symptoms often present in combination with allergic rhinitis, and this is then termed *allergic rhinoconjunctivitis*. Topical intraocular antihistamines and oral antihistamines are the cornerstone of treatment for allergic conjunctivitis and allergic rhinoconjunctivitis, respectively.

Atopic dermatitis It is controversial whether antihistamines are effective for the relief of pruritus associated with atopic dermatitis. Although not FDA indicated, in practice, antihistamines are often used to treat itching associated with these conditions. Sedative effects of first-generation antihistamines are frequently used to induce sleep at night in those with sleep disturbance from pruritus.

Other uses of antihistamines in nonallergic diseases
Meclizine is an antihistamine used for the treatment of motion sickness prophylaxis as well as vertigo of vestibular origin. A combination tablet, acetaminophen plus diphenhydramine, is available over the counter as a pain reliever/sleep aid.

DOSAGE, ADMINISTRATION, FDA INDICATIONS, AND DOSAGE ADJUSTMENT IN HEPATIC OR RENAL IMPAIRMENT

The second-generation oral antihistamines come in a variety of formulations and dosages appropriate for children and adults. Cetirizine, desloratadine, and fexofenadine are available by prescription only. Loratadine is available over the counter. All four are also available as antihistamine/decongestant combination tablets.

Cetirizine   Cetirizine is available as 5-mg and 10-mg tablets, 5-mg and 10-mg chewable tablets, and 1 mg/mL syrup. It is indicated for seasonal allergic rhinitis in patients older than 2 years, perennial allergic rhinitis in patients older than 6 months, and chronic idiopathic urticaria in patients older than 6 months. For patients 6 to 23 months of age, the recommended dose is 2.5 mg daily; for patients 12 to 23 months of age, the recommended starting dose is 2.5 mg daily, and the maximum recommended dose is 2.5 mg every 12 hours; for patients 2 to 5 years of age, the recommended starting dose is 2.5 mg daily, and the maximum recommended dose is 2.5 mg every 12 hours to 5 mg daily; for patients older than 6 years, the recommended dose is 5 to 10 mg daily. For patients with renal or hepatic impairment older than 6 years or the elderly (older than 77 years), the recommended dose is 5 mg daily. Cetirizine is not recommended in patients with renal or hepatic impairment who are younger than 6 years.

Desloratadine   Desloratadine is available as 5-mg tablets, 5-mg orally disintegrating tablets, and 0.5 mg/mL syrup. It is indicated for seasonal allergic rhinitis in patients older than 2 years, perennial allergic rhinitis in patients older than 6 months, and chronic idiopathic urticaria in patients older than 6 months. For patients 6 to 11 months of age, the recommended dose is 2 mL; for patients 1 to 5 years of age, the recommended dose is 2.5 mL; for patients 6 to 11 years of age, the recommended dose is 2.5 mg daily; and for patients older than 12 years, the recommended dose is 5 mg daily. For patients older than 12 years with renal or hepatic impairment, the recommended starting dose is 5 mg every other day.

Fexofenadine   Fexofenadine is available as 30 mg, 60 mg, and 180 mg tablets, as well as a 6 mg/1 ml oral suspension. It is indicated for seasonal allergic rhinitis in patients

≥2 years of age and for chronic idiopathic urticaria in patients ≥6 months of age. For patients 6–24 months of age, the recommended dose is 15 mg twice daily; for patients 2–11 years of age, the recommended dose is 30 mg twice daily; for patients ≥12 years of age, the recommended dose is 180 mg daily or 60 mg twice daily. For patients 6–24 months of age with renal impairment, the recommended starting dose is 15 mg once daily; For patients 2–11 years of age with renal impairment, the recommended starting dose is 30 mg once daily. For patients ≥12 years of age with renal impairment, the recommended starting dose is 60 mg once daily.

Loratadine   Loratadine is available as 10-mg tablets, 10-mg orally disintegrating tablets, and 1 mg/1 mL syrup. It is indicated for seasonal allergic rhinitis in patients older than 2 years, and chronic idiopathic urticaria in patients older than 2 years. For patients 2 to 5 years of age, the recommended dose is 5 mL daily; for patients older than 6 years, the recommended dose is 10 mg daily. For patients 2 to 5 years of age with renal or hepatic impairment, the recommended starting dose is 5 mL every other day. For patients older than 6 years with renal or hepatic impairment, the recommended starting dose is 10 mg every other day.

Topical Nasal Antihistamines

With respect to intranasal antihistamines, the only agent available in the United States is azelastine. It is available by prescription only and approved for use in adults as well as children down to 5 years of age. Azelastine is indicated for perennial allergic rhinitis, seasonal allergic rhinitis, and vasomotor rhinitis at the recommended dose of two sprays per nostril twice daily. Studies have shown an onset of action within 3 hours after initial dosing and sustained efficacy over the following 12-hour interval. The most common side effects reported are bitter taste (19.7% vs. 0.6% placebo) and sedation (11.5% vs. 5.4% placebo). Azelastine is labeled Pregnancy Category C.

Topical Skin Antihistamines

The topical skin antihistamines include over-the-counter diphenhydramine, but its use is associated with a high rate of contact dermatitis. For this reason, allergy specialists generally recommend oral antihistamines over topical skin agents.

Ocular Antihistamines and Antihistamine/Mast Cell Stabilizer Combination Products

A variety of topical intraocular antihistamine and antihistamine/mast cell stabilizer combination products are available on the market in the United States. Three ophthalmic H_1 antihistamines and their dosages include emedastine difumarate 0.05%, one drop in each eye up to four times daily; levocabastine hydrochloride, 0.05% one drop in each eye four times daily; and azelastine hydrochloride, 0.05% one drop in each eye twice daily. Emedastine difumarate and azelastine hydrochloride are indicated for the treatment of patients older than 3 years with allergic conjunctivitis, and levocabastine hydrochloride is indicated for the treatment of seasonal allergic rhinitis in patients older than 12 years. Mast cell stabilizer plus antihistamine intraocular combination products include olopatadine hydrochloride 0.1% and ketotifen fumarate 0.025%. Both are indicated for the treatment of allergic conjunctivitis in patients older than 3 years. Olopatadine hydrochloride 0.1% is dosed at one drop in each affected eye twice daily at 6- to 8-hour intervals, and ketotifen fumarate 0.025% is dosed at one drop to each affected eye every 8 to 12 hours.

MAST CELL STABILIZERS

Intranasal Chromones/Mast Cell Stabilizers

Intranasal mast cell stabilizers currently available include cromolyn sodium and nedocromil sodium. By inhibiting the degranulation of sensitized mast cells, cromolyn sodium blocks the release of inflammatory mediators involved in causing the symptoms of allergic disease. Clinical trials have shown cromolyn sodium to be effective in ameliorating both the early- and late-phase reaction in participants with allergic rhinitis. The drug is indicated for use in both seasonal and perennial allergic rhinitis. Patients usually get symptom relief within the first week of treatment, and there is enhanced symptom improvement over the following weeks with continued use. The four times daily dosing may impede adherence initially. Once desired symptom control has been achieved, a less frequent dosing schedule may suffice to maintain control. Because local adverse effects are uncommon, and they have poor systemic absorption, mast cell stabilizers have an excellent safety profile. The 4% intranasal solution is indicated for adults as well as children down to 2 years of age.

Intraocular Mast Cell Stabilizers

Some examples of intraocular mast cell stabilizers and their dosage indications include pemirolast potassium, 0.1% 1 to 2 drops in each eye four times daily; nedocromil sodium, 2% 1 to 2 drops in each eye twice daily; cromolyn sodium 4%, 1 to 2 drops in each eye four to six times daily at regular intervals; and lodoxamide tromethamine 0.1%, 1 to 2 drops in each eye four times daily. Cromolyn sodium is indicated for allergic conjunctivitis for patients older than 4 years, pemirolast potassium and nedocromil sodium are indicated for allergic conjunctivitis for patients older than 3 years, and lodoxamide tromethamine is indicated for the

treatment of vernal keratoconjunctivitis, vernal conjunctivitis, and vernal keratitis in patients older than 2 years.

The adverse effect profile of this class of medications is minimal, and it is unlikely that adverse effects will interfere with adherence to therapy; however, the need for frequent dosing may interfere with compliance to therapy.

CONCLUSION

Oral second-generation antihistamines are the cornerstone of treatment for allergic rhinitis and chronic idiopathic urticaria. Extensive clinical studies attest to their safety and efficacy in both adult and pediatric populations. The variety of formulations, including tablet, chewable tablet, rapidly disintegrating tablet, and liquid preparations, once-a-day dosing, and onset of action within a few hours and 24-hour duration of action, enhance their widespread use.

EVIDENCE-BASED MEDICINE

Two new agents have completed Phase III clinical trials in the United States: oral levocetirizine and olopatadine nasal spray. Levocetirizine is the active enantiomer of cetirizine. The olopatadine nasal spray contains the same active ingredients as that found in the currently available olopatadine eye drops. In one double-blind, placebo-controlled randomized clinical trial that examined the efficacy and safety of levocetirizine in 306 participants 6 to 12 years of age with perennial allergic rhinitis, the investigators found that the levocetirizine group had a significant improvement in Total 4 Symptoms Score (e.g., sneezing, rhinorrhea, as well as nasal and ocular pruritus) and Health-Related Quality of Life scores compared with placebo. In a multicenter, randomized, double-blind, placebo-controlled study of 677 participants ranging from 12 to 81 years of age who were dosed with olopatadine nasal spray (0.6% or 0.4%) or placebo twice daily for 2 weeks, the investigators reported improvements in nasal allergy symptom scores and well as Rhinoconjunctivitis Quality of Life scores.

BIBLIOGRAPHY

Blaiss, MS. Antihistamines: treatment selection criteria for pediatric seasonal allergic rhinitis. *Allergy and Asthma Proc.* 2005;26:95.

Biospace Beat. Alcon releases clinical results on new nasal allergy spray. http://www.biospace.com/news_story.aspx?StoryID=15504020&full=1. Accessed on June 21, 2006.

Bloebaum RM, Grant JA. Levocetirizine, the allergist's arsenal grows larger. *Expert Opin Pharmacother.* 2004;5:1581.

Bousquet J, van Cauwenberge P, Khaltaev N. World Health Organization. Allergic rhinitis and its impact on asthma. In collaboration with the World Health Organization. Executive summary of the workshop report. Geneva, Switzerland, December 7–10, 1999. *Allergy.* 2002:57:841.

Golightly LK, Greos LS. Second-generation antihistamines: actions and efficacy in the management of allergic disorders. *Drugs.* 2005;65:341.

Greiner AN. Allergic rhinitis: impact of the disease and considerations for management. *Med Clin North Am.* 2006;90:17.

Lai L, Casale TB, Stokes J. Pediatric allergic rhinitis: treatment. *Immunol Allergy Clin North Am.* 2005;25:283.

Leurs R, Church MK, Taglialatela M. H1-antihistamines: inverse agonism, anti-inflammatory actions and cardiac effects. *Clin Exp Allergy.* 2002;32:489.

Meltzer EO. Evaluation of the optimal oral antihistamines for patients with allergic rhinitis. *Mayo Clin Proc.* 2005;80:1170.

Naclerio RM. Allergic rhinitis. *N Engl J Med.* 1991;325:860.

Ohmori K, Hayashi K, Kaise T, et al. Pharmacological, pharmacokinetic and clinical properties of olopatadine hydrochloride, a new antiallergic drug. *Jpn J Pharmacol.* 2002;88:379.

Physicians' Desk Reference. 59th ed. Montvale, NJ: Thomson PDR; 2005.

Potter PC, Paediatric Levocetirizine Study Group. Efficacy and safety of levocetirizine on symptoms and health related quality of life of children with perennial allergic rhinitis: a double-blind, placebo-controlled randomized clinical trial. *Ann Allergy Asthma Immunol.* 2005;95:175.

Simons FER. Advances in H_1-antihistamines. *N Engl J Med.* 2004;351:2203.

van Cauwenberge P, Bachert C, Passalacqua G, et al. Consensus statement on the treatment of allergic rhinitis. EAACI Position paper. *Allergy.* 2000;55:116.

Bronchodilators

38

Jennifer S. Kim, MD and Rachel E. Story, MD, MPH

Bronchodilators are an essential component of asthma treatment, especially in acute exacerbations. In this chapter, we review pharmacology, methods of delivery, and clinical indications for the use of various bronchodilators.

PHARMACOLOGY OF BRONCHODILATORS

β-Agonists

β-Agonists are the most effective agents to produce bronchodilation.

β-Adrenoreceptors

β-Adrenergic agonists exert their effects through transmembrane G protein–coupled receptors. There are three types of β-adrenergic receptors: β_1, β_2, and β_3: β_1 receptors exist predominantly in the heart, whereas β_3 receptors are found in adipose tissue; β_2 receptors, however, are ubiquitous and can be found in the lung, liver, kidney, and gastrointestinal smooth muscle. In the lung, they are widely distributed in smooth muscle, submucosal glands, epithelium, alveoli, and the arterial system. They also are found on inflammatory cells that are associated with asthma. These include macrophages, mast cells, neutrophils, eosinophils, and lymphocytes.

Mechanism of Action and Cellular Effects

The active site of the β_2 receptor is located within the transmembrane region consisting of seven β helices. Once the β-agonist attaches to its receptor, signal transduction occurs. Adenylate cyclase is activated, increasing cyclic adenosine monophosphate (cAMP). cAMP then is believed to activate protein kinase A, which causes phosphylation, thereby leading to cellular effects, such as relaxation of bronchial smooth muscle.

Important nonbronchodilator actions of β-agonists include increased mucociliary clearance, protection of respiratory epithelium against bacteria, inhibition of cholinergic neurotransmission, and priming of the glucocorticoid receptor.

Structure and Development of β-Adrenergic Agents

EPINEPHRINE

The first catecholamine introduced for the treatment of asthma was epinephrine by injection in 1903. Epinephrine has both α- and β-adrenergic effects. It acts rapidly but for a short time. Epinephrine remains the drug of choice for anaphylaxis but has diminished importance for asthma.

EPHEDRINE

In the late 1930s, another catecholamine, ephedrine, became widely used as the first effective oral adrenergic bronchodilator. Although employed for several decades, ephedrine is a relatively weak bronchodilator that is no longer used for asthma.

ISOPROTERENOL

Introduced in 1941, isoproterenol was the first β-specific (but non-β_2 selective) adrenergic agonist developed. It has a very short duration of action and is not useful as an oral medication because of gastrointestinal inactivation. For decades, however, it was the preferred drug for aerosol administration. Modifications made to isoproterenol have produced improved medications so the progenitor is no longer recommended for use.

Short-Acting Nonselective β-Agonists

METAPROTERENOL

Metaproterenol is a noncatecholamine bronchodilator that can be administered by aerosol and is also active orally due to its resistance to gastrointestinal activation. Its structure and clinical activity is otherwise similar to isoproterenol. At high doses, it loses β_2-adrenergic specificity and is no longer useful clinically.

FENOTEROL

Fenoterol has never been approved for use in the United States. Its unique characteristic is that is a complete agonist for the β-adrenergic receptor. At high doses, therefore, its potency induces more cardiac stimulation and extra-pulmonary side effects compared to other β_2-agonists.

Short-Acting Selective β_2-Agonists

Once the differentiation between β_1 and β_2 adrenergic receptors was made, efforts were directed toward the development of β_2 selective agonists. More selectivity for the β_2 receptor can be achieved structurally by increasing the bulk of the side chain (Fig. 38–1.)

ALBUTEROL, PIRBUTEROL, AND TERBUTALINE

The selective β-agonists albuterol (also called salbutamol) and terbutaline both produce bronchodilation but with decreased cardiac stimulation. Pirbuterol, which is very similar in structure to albuterol, has comparable effects. These are currently in wide use for a variety of respiratory diseases such as asthma.

Long-Acting Selective β_2-Agonists

Two β_2-agonists were developed in the early 1990s that provide more than 12 hours of bronchodilation: salmeterol and formoterol.

Structurally, increasing the size of the terminal amino group protects against monoamine oxidase (MAO) degradation, thereby prolonging the duration of action.

SALMETEROL

Salmeterol has a long lipophilic side chain that interacts with the "exosite" (an auxiliary binding site) of the receptor. This interaction prevents dissociation from the β_2 receptor and results in repeated stimulation of the active site of the receptor, thereby producing prolonged bronchodilation.

FORMOTEROL

Formoterol, due to its more moderate lipophilicity, penetrates the plasma membrane and gradually escapes out to interact with the β_2 receptor. Formoterol has a faster onset of action compared to salmeterol. However, they are equally β_2 selective.

Enantiomers

LEVALBUTEROL

More recently, in 1999, levalbuterol, a preservative-free formulation of R-albuterol, was made available. The rationale for isolating the R-isomer was that this enantiomer induced bronchodilation. In contrast, the S-isomer does not produce bronchodilatory effects. Furthermore, the S-isomer enhances contractile responses in bronchial tissue and has proinflammatory effects in in vitro studies. In vivo, S-albuterol is metabolized 10 times more slowly than R-albuterol. However, clinical studies in patients with asthma have failed to illustrate that significant toxicity is associated with S-albuterol.

Xanthines

Theophylline is a methylxanthine similar in structure to caffeine. It has been in clinical use for over 60 years, but the mechanisms of action on a molecular level are not entirely clear. It is a bronchodilator that may have additional antiinflammatory and immunomodulatory effects.

Magnesium Sulfate

The mechanism of action of magnesium sulfate is not clearly defined. Magnesium ion decreases the uptake of

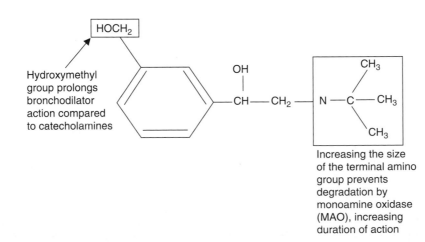

Figure 38–1. Albuterol structure.

calcium by bronchial smooth muscle cells, which in turn leads to bronchodilation. Magnesium may also have a role in inhibiting mast cell degranulation, thus reducing inflammatory mediators. In addition, magnesium inhibits the release of acetylcholine from motor nerve terminals and depresses the excitability of muscle fibers.

ROUTES OF ADMINISTRATION FOR β-AGONISTS

Inhalation of aerosolized medication is the preferred route of administration for short-acting β-agonists. Seventy-five percent of maximum bronchodilation is noted after 5 minutes with a peak in 30 to 90 minutes. Significant bronchodilation is maintained for 4 hours after a single treatment. The same degree of bronchodilation is achieved with systemic administration of β-agonists, but there are far fewer side effects with aerosolized administration. There is no role for oral β-agonists in the treatment of asthma because side effects are dose limiting and there is an equivalent degree of bronchodilation in both oral and inhaled formulations.

DEVICES FOR AEROSOLIZED ADMINISTRATION OF β-AGONISTS

Metered-Dose Inhalers

Metered-dose-inhalers (MDIs) are pressurized canisters that use propellants to generate aerosolized particles. Chlorofluorocarbons (CFCs) have traditionally been used as the propellant, but they deplete the ozone layer and there is a December 31, 2008 deadline beyond which CFCs cannot be used. Therefore,

a newer propellant containing hydrofluoroalkanes (HFAs) is increasingly being used. CFC-MDIs have 80% oral deposition and a higher proportion of large particles that cannot reach the lower airways. In contrast, HFA-MDIs have decreased oral deposition and a higher proportion of fine particles that can penetrate the lower respiratory tract. Even with HFA-MDIs, coordination between actuation of the device and inhalation is required. This is the limiting factor in the efficacy of most MDIs, particularly in children. Thus valved holding chambers or spacers are recommended for use with MDIs. For children 4 years and younger, a spacer with a mask is recommended. Table 38–1 has details of available devices with description of the proper technique and patient ages.

Nebulizers

Nebulizers do not require coordination and therefore are preferred for use in young children (2 years and younger) and during moderate to severe exacerbations in all age groups.

Dry Powder Inhalers

Dry powder inhalers (DPIs) do not use propellants and are the only delivery system currently available for long-acting β-agonists (LABAs). The LABAs in DPIs are inhaled in a dry form, requiring a rapid, deep inhalation. Children younger than 4 years are not able to produce an inspiratory flow capable of delivering the medication. Thus they are not appropriate for children younger than 4 to 6 years. Depending on the specific device, DPIs require an inspiratory flow rate of 30 to 50 L per minute.

Table 38–1. Devices for aerosolized administration of B$_2$-agonists.

Device	Age	Technique
Nebulizer	<2 y or any age if patient is unable to use a MDI with spacer/mask	Tidal breathing with tight fitting mask or mouthpiece
CFC or HFA-MDI and spacer with face mask	>2y[*]	Tidal breathing for 6 respiratory cycles per actuation
with mouthpiece	>4y[*]	Slow inhalation (3–5 sec) with 10-sec breath hold
HFA-MDI (no spacer)	>5 y[*] Even over the age of 5, most patients will benefit from the use of a spacer	Slow inhalation (3–5 sec) with 10-sec breath hold
DPIs	>4 y[*]	Rapid (1–2 sec) deep inhalation

[*]Proper inhalation and coordination may be difficult and should be assessed on an individual basis. CFC, chlorofluorocarbon; DPI, dry powder inhaler; HFA, hydrofluoroalkane; MDI, metered-dose inhaler.

CLINICAL USE OF BRONCHODILATORS FOR ACUTE SEVERE ASTHMA

Selective Short-Acting β-Agonists

Selective short-acting β-agonists are the mainstay of treatment in acute severe asthma. Less β_2-selective medications, such as isoproterenol, metaproterenol, and epinephrine, are not recommended because of increased cardiac stimulation.

In most cases airway obstruction is secondary to both inflammation and smooth muscle contraction. Thus therapy with bronchodilators does not completely reverse obstruction, and treatment with systemic steroids is usually required in moderate to severe exacerbations. Because systemic steroids require at least 4 hours to improve asthma symptoms, they should be given promptly. However, acute therapy focuses on inhaled β-agonists.

Inhaled preparations of β-agonists are strongly preferred over oral preparations because side effects are dose limiting in the oral preparations. For moderate to severe exacerbations, continuous or repetitive administration of inhaled β-agonists is recommended. Racemic albuterol (R- and S-albuterol) is the most commonly used β-agonist in the United States. The pure (R)-enantiomer of albuterol, called levalbuterol, produces comparable bronchodilation to racemic albuterol. When given in equivalent dose with proper technique administered via nebulizer or MDI, racemic albuterol and the pure (R)-enantiomer produce equal results.

Second-Line Agents for Acute Severe Asthma

Bronchodilators other than the short-acting β-selective agonists, such as methylxanthines, anticholinergics, epinephrine, and magnesium, can be used as adjuvant therapy in acute asthma.

EPINEPHRINE

The use of subcutaneous epinephrine is beneficial in some patients who fail to improve with inhaled therapy with short-acting β-agonists; however, there is no proven benefit of systemic therapy with epinephrine over aerosolized albuterol.

ANTICHOLINERGICS

The anticholinergic medication ipratropium bromide may increase the degree of bronchodilation when used in conjunction with β-agonists, especially in children. In addition, anticholinergics are the recommended treatment for β-blocker–induced bronchospasm.

METHYLXANTHINES

Studies show no additional benefit to treatment with methylxanthines (aminophylline, theophylline) in acute asthma if a patient has optimal treatment with inhaled β-agonists. Furthermore, the short-acting β-agonists produce three to four times more bronchodilation than methylxanthines.

MAGNESIUM

Several clinical prospective trials failed to show a benefit to the use of intravenous magnesium sulfate in acute asthmatics in emergency departments. Others have demonstrated benefit. Several meta-analyses have been performed on the subject and conclude that no evidence supports routine use of magnesium in acute asthma. Additional data are needed to establish a clear role for magnesium in the management of acute asthma.

Long-Acting β_2-Agonists

There is no role for the use of long-acting β_2-agonists in the treatment of acute asthma.

LONG-TERM CONTROL MEDICATION USE IN ASTHMA

Short-Acting β-Agonists

National Heart, Lung, and Blood Institute (NHLBI) guidelines recommend the use of short-acting β-agonists as "quick relief" medications. Daily scheduled use of β-agonists is not recommended because it shows no benefit in mild asthma and may cause worsening of asthma symptoms in moderate asthma. There are genetic polymorphisms in the β receptor such that some genotypes will have improved lung function with daily β-agonist administration, whereas others will have significant deterioration in lung function with regular use. Use of more than one canister of a short-acting β_2-agonist per month or increase in use is associated with life-threatening asthma, and daily anti-inflammatory treatment should be instituted or increased in these situations.

Long-Acting β-Agonists

Long-acting β-agonists (LABAs) can be used as adjuvant therapy with inhaled corticosteroids in moderate and severe persistent asthma. Because LABAs are not antiinflammatory, the NHBLI recommends their use only as an adjunct to inhaled corticosteroids and not for use as monotherapy. Studies suggest that the addition of a LABA is superior to increasing the dose of inhaled corticosteroids in asthma control, and the addition of a LABA is superior to the addition of theophylline or a leukotriene pathway modifying agent in improving asthma. LABAs should not be used for quick relief for acute symptoms. LABAs have a black box warning because some studies report an increase in asthma-related deaths in patients on LABAs. This is discussed further in the evidence-based medicine section of this chapter.

Methylxanthines

Sustained-release theophylline is primarily a bronchodilator and is not a NHLBI preferred medication for persistent asthma because its antiinflammatory activity is modest. Its use may benefit a subset of severe persistent asthmatics when used as an adjunctive controller medication. Common side effects include headache, nausea, vomiting, abdominal discomfort, and restlessness. Serum concentrations of 10 to 15 µg/mL indicate therapeutic levels for asthma. Regular monitoring of serum levels is recommended to prevent toxic side effects, which include seizure and cardiac arrhythmias. There is a narrow therapeutic index, and many commonly used medications, such as erythromycin and cimetidine, affect theophylline blood levels.

Exercised-Induced Bronchospasm

Exercised-induced bronchospasm (EIB) occurs secondary to loss of heat and water from the lung during exercise. Use of short-acting β-agonists prior to exercise prevent EIB in more than 80% of patients and is effective for 2 to 3 hours. A single dose of a LABA prevents EIB for up to 12 hours but, as discussed earlier, should only be used in conjunction with daily antiinflammatory therapy, primarily inhaled corticosteroids.

ADVERSE EFFECTS AND SAFETY OF β-AGONISTS

Adverse Effects of β-Agonists

Because β_2 receptors are found in many organ systems, including skeletal muscle, lung, liver, kidney, and gastrointestinal smooth muscle, there is a wide variety of adverse effects. Tolerance to nonbronchodilatory effects of β-agonists often occurs within 2 weeks. Use of short-acting β-selective agonists decreases side effects. Administration via inhalation also decreases side effects.

The most common side effect of β-agonists is tremor caused by activation of β_2 receptors in skeletal muscle. Tolerance to tremor often develops in 2 weeks. Palpitations and tachycardia occur less often with use of selective β-agonists but is still present. Myocardial ischemia can occur, and isoproterenol is particularly noted for altering coronary blood flow with resultant subendocardial ischemia. Prolonged QTc occurs with both selective and nonselective β-agonists and can lead to arrhythmia. Metabolic effects of β-agonists include hyperglycemia, hypokalemia, and hypomagnesemia. Table 38–2 offers a more complete list of potential side effects.

Safety of β-Agonists

The safety of both short- and long-acting β-agonists has been debated since the introduction of MDI β-agonists.

Table 38–2. Adverse effects of inhaled β-agonists.

Tremor
Restlessness
Hyperactivity
Insomnia
Palpitations
Prolonged QTc
Arrhythmia
Myocardial ischemia
Seizures
Transient decrease in PaO_2
Abdominal discomfort
Nausea
Hyperglycemia
Hypokalemia
Hypomagnesemia
Paradoxical bronchospasm

In the 1960s, a significant increase in asthma mortality occurred in the United Kingdom and six other countries, coinciding with the introduction of MDI β-agonists. The increased mortality occurred only in countries using high-dose inhaled isoproterenol, and many deaths were attributed to the medication. In the 1970s, a similar epidemic occurred in New Zealand that some studies attributed to the use of fenoterol. Fenoterol produces a significant decrease in pulmonary function and asthma control when used regularly in moderate asthma. However, a subsequent study in New Zealand found that fenoterol was used more often in patients with severe asthma. After adjusting for asthma severity, the use of fenoterol did not increase the risk of life-threatening asthma.

Studies do not agree on whether an increased risk of life-threatening asthma is associated only with specific β-agonists such as fenoterol and high-dose isoproterenol or whether increased risk for life-threatening asthma is a class effect of β-agonists. In a study that reviewed the health insurance database of more than 12,301 patients who were prescribed asthma medication in Saskatchewan Canada, increased asthma mortality occurred only when β-agonists were used in excess of 1.4 canisters per month. The investigators argued that increased use of β-agonists was not responsible for increased mortality but was simply a marker of increased asthma severity, which is itself a risk factor for fatal asthma.

Safety questions around the use of long-acting β-agonists are discussed in detail in the next section.

EVIDENCE-BASED MEDICINE

On March 2, 2006, the Food and Drug Administration (FDA) approved labeling changes with new black box safety warnings for asthma LABAs, namely medications containing salmeterol xinafoate. These warnings were issued due to evidence that regular treatment with LABAs may be associated with an increased risk of severe exacerbations and even death from asthma in a small subset of patients.

Because of early safety concerns after the introduction of LABAs, the manufacturer of salmeterol, GlaxoSmithKline, on the FDA's request, designed a study called the Salmeterol Multicenter Asthma Research Trial (SMART), which was initiated in June 1996. The outcomes measured included respiratory-related deaths and life-threatening experiences (intubation or mechanical ventilation). Approximately 26,000 patients were enrolled and randomized to receive either salmeterol or placebo for 28 weeks in addition to their usual therapy. Compliance was not reinforced, and the use of inhaled corticosteroid (ICS) was not a prerequisite to participation in the study. The study was stopped due to findings of a small but significant increase in combined respiratory-related deaths or life-threatening experiences in subjects receiving salmeterol as opposed to placebo. This was more pronounced in the African American population. In contrast, multiple well-designed clinical studies have confirmed the superiority of combination therapy (LABA + ICS) over monotherapy with a higher dose of ICS.

How can we reconcile these findings? Certainly, combination therapy of a LABA with an ICS has benefited many patients with asthma. However, in a small subset of patients, regular use of LABAs may have the potential to increase the risk of exacerbations and death. Further studies are necessary to reach definite conclusions, but reserving combination therapy for more severe disease (as per the NHLBI guidelines) seems prudent. Prior to the addition of LABAs, consider lack of patient adherence or the presence of other concomitant medical conditions when a patient fails to respond appropriately to ICS therapy. Patients, once prescribed LABAs, would benefit from close medical monitoring, particularly if symptoms become difficult to control.

BIBLIOGRAPHY

Barnes PJ. Theophylline and phosphodiesterase inhibitors. In: Adkinson NF, Yunginger JW, Busse WW, et al., eds. *Middleton's Allergy Principles and Practice.* 6th ed. Philadelphia: Mosby; 2003:823.

Castle W, Fuller R, Hall J, et al. Serevent nationwide surveillance study: comparison of salmeterol with salbutamol in asthmatic patients who require regular bronchodilator treatment. *BMJ.* 1993;306:1034.

Corbridge T, Mokhlesi B. Management of acute severe asthma. In: Grammer LC, Greenberger PA, eds. *Patterson's Allergic Diseases.* 6th ed. Philadelphia: Lippincott Williams & Wilkins; 2002:595.

Johnson M. Molecular mechanisms of beta(2)-adrenergic receptor function, response, and regulation. *J Allergy Clin Immunol.* 2006;117:18.

McFadden ER. Acute severe asthma. *Am J Respir Crit Care Med.* 2003;168:740.

National Heart, Lung, and Blood Institute. *Expert Panel Report 2: Guidelines for the Diagnosis and Management of Asthma.* Bethesda, Md: National Institutes of Health; 1997.

Nelson HS. Beta-adrenergic agonists. In Adkinson NF, Yunginger JW, Busse WW, et al., eds. *Middleton's Allergy Principles and Practice.* 6th ed. Philadelphia: Mosby; 2003:803.

Nelson HS. Is there a problem with inhaled long-acting β-adrenergic agonists? *J Allergy Clin Immunol.* 2006;117:3.

Nelson HS, Weiss ST, Bleecker ER, et al. The salmeterol multicenter asthma research trial: a comparison of usual pharmacotherapy for asthma or usual pharmacotherapy plus salmeterol. *Chest.* 2006;129:15.

Pongracic JA. β agonists. In: Grammer LC, Greenberger PA, eds. *Patterson's Allergic Diseases.* 6th ed. Philadelphia: Lippincott Williams & Wilkins; 2002:717.

Glucocorticoids

Joseph D. Spahn, MD

Glucocorticoid (GC) therapy remains one of the most valuable treatment modalities in the management of asthma and allergic rhinitis. GCs have been used in the treatment of allergic diseases for more than 50 years. Pioneering studies performed in the 1950s found cortisone, the first synthetic GC, to result in significant improvements in asthma symptoms and pulmonary function. Unfortunately, reports describing the multitude of adverse effects associated with chronic cortisone began to appear and much of the early enthusiasm of chronic oral GC treatment for asthma waned. Over the next couple decades, attempts to deliver GCs topically were a major focus of research and development. By the mid-1970s, the first inhaled GC was approved for use in the treatment of asthma. The development of highly effective inhaled GC preparations has revolutionized how we care for patients with asthma. By virtue of their high topical to systemic potency, inhaled GC therapy has proven to be both safe and effective in the treatment of asthma. This chapter provides a broad overview of the structure, mechanisms of action, pharmacokinetics, efficacy, adverse effects, and current issues associated with both systemic and inhaled GC therapy in asthma, in addition to a brief discussion of intranasal GC therapy for the treatment of allergic rhinitis.

CHEMISTRY

Synthetic GCs are cortisone-based molecules that have undergone structural modifications designed to enhance their potencies and prolong their durations of action. Antiinflammatory GCs have a 17-hydroxyl group and methyl groups at carbons 18 and 19 (Fig. 39–1). Further modifications to the basic steroid structure have increased the antiinflammatory while decreasing mineralocorticoid effects. Unfortunately, it has not been possible to separate the unwanted metabolic effects from the desired antiinflammatory properties of GCs.

MECHANISMS OF ACTION

Both asthma and allergic rhinitis are immune mediated-diseases in which a specific inflammatory reaction involving TH2 lymphocytes, eosinophils, and IgE

occurs. Given that GCs have broad and potent antiinflammatory effects, it should come as no surprise that GCs are among the most effective classes of medications available for use in allergic disease. GCs act at several levels of the inflammatory response (Table 39–1), with their primary effect coming mainly from their ability to inhibit the expression and/or production of molecules involved in the initiation and maintenance of the inflammatory response. Specifically, they inhibit the upregulation of adhesion molecules on endothelial cells that are required for the adhesion and subsequent migration of inflammatory cells to sites of inflammation. They also inhibit the production of cytokines involved in inflammatory cell recruitment, activation, and proliferation. GCs also have potent vasoconstrictive properties. By decreasing capillary permeability at sites of inflammation, plasma exudation is inhibited, which results in a reduction of tissue edema, as well as reductions in the concentration of inflammatory and chemotactic factors and ultimately in a decrease in the inflammatory response. Lastly, GC upregulate β-adrenergic receptors on airway smooth muscle cells thereby rendering these cells more responsive to β-agonist therapy.

SYSTEMIC GLUCOCORTICOID THERAPY

Pharmacokinetics

The pharmacokinetics of GCs can influence dosing strategies; however, in general GC dosing regimens do not depend on pharmacokinetic parameters. Rather, dosing is either empirical or based on the patient's history of prior response. Exceptions to this are when gross abnormalities of absorption or elimination result in a clinically significant reduction of systemic GC exposure. In this scenario, clinical response to treatment would be expected to diminish. Prednisone, prednisolone, and methylprednisolone are all rapidly and nearly completely absorbed following oral administration, with peak plasma concentrations occurring within 1 to 2 hours. Of interest, prednisone is an inactive prodrug that requires biotransformation of the 11-ketone group to an 11-hydroxyl group (Fig. 39–1A). This conversion to

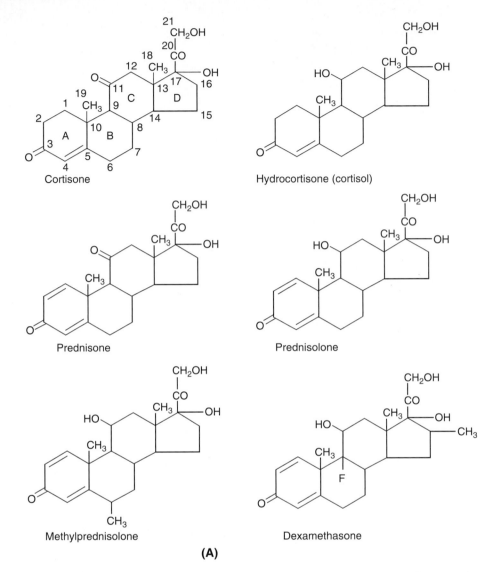

(A)

Figure 39–1. **(A)** Systemically administered glucocorticoids (GCs). Molecular structures of commonly administered systemic GCs used in the treatment of asthma. Carbon and ring nomenclature is noted for cortisone. **(B)** Inhaled and intranasal GCs. Molecular structures of the available inhaled GCs used in the treatment of asthma. All of the currently available inhaled GCs (beclomethasone dipropionate [BDP], triamcinolone acetonide [TAA], flunisolide [FN], budesonide [BUD], fluticasone propionate [FP]), and mometasone furoate [MF]) have further alterations at the 17 and/or 21 carbon positions that result in further increases in antiinflammatory effects and subsequent metabolism to inactive or nearly inactive metabolites. All of the inhaled GC preparations are halogenated except for budesonide.

prednisolone (its active form) occurs via first-pass hepatic metabolism.

Once absorbed, GCs bind to serum proteins and are metabolized in the liver by the cytochrome P-450 isoform 3A4 (CYP3A4) into inactive compounds. The rate of

metabolism or clearance of GCs can be altered by drug interactions and disease states. Cystic fibrosis and hyperthyroidism are diseases where higher GC doses may be required due to intrinsically enhanced clearance and metabolism. GC elimination may also be altered by

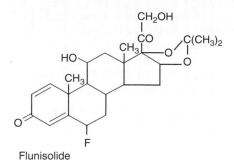

Flunisolide

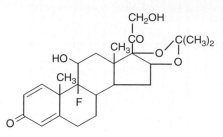

Triamcinolone acetonide

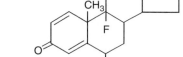

Beclomethasone dipropionate

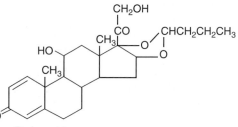

Budesonide

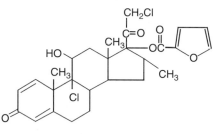

Fluticasone propionate

Mometasone furoate

(B)

Figure 39–1. (Continued)

numerous concomitant medications (Table 39–2). Drug interactions may result in either reduced or enhanced clearance and consequently an increased risk for adverse effects or a diminished therapeutic response, respectively. The anticonvulsants phenytoin, phenobarbital, and carbamazepine are potent inducers of CYP3A4, and when used concurrently with systemic glucocorticoids can significantly enhance the metabolism of all of the systemic GCs, with methylprednisolone especially vulnerable to enhanced clearance. Rifampin is another inducer of CYP3A4 and will substantially enhance the clearance of GCs. Several case reports have described breakthrough symptoms and worsening asthma control in steroid-dependent asthmatics who were placed subsequently on rifampin. In this scenario, one may require higher doses of prednisone or more frequently administered doses to maintain adequate asthma control.

Other medications can delay GC elimination by inhibiting CYP3A4. Significant reductions of GC clearance have been noted with concomitant ketoconazole administration. The macrolide antibiotics erythromycin, troleandomycin, and clarithromycin can also delay GC clearance; however, this effect is limited to methylprednisolone. Methylprednisolone elimination can be reduced from 50% to 70% with the macrolides just cited. In addition, oral contraceptives and estrogen replacement therapy can significantly delay prednisolone metabolism.

If a drug interaction that increases clearance is identified, one can simply increase the GC dose. Alternatively, a split dosing regimen may be considered

Table 39–1. Mechanisms of glucocorticoid action in asthma.

I. Inhibitory Effects
  A. Inhibition of leukocyte activation, function, and survival
    1. T lymphocytes
    2. Eosinophils
    3. Monocyte/macrophages
  B. Inhibition of leukocyte adhesion/migration
  C. Inhibition of the production of cytokines important in the differentiation, proliferation, and activation of inflammatory cells
    1. IL-2, IL-3, IL-4, IL-5, IL-13, granulocyte-macrophage colony-stimulating factor (GM-CSF)
  D. Inhibition of the production and/or release of inflammatory mediators
    1. Lipid mediators (platelet-activating factor, leukotrienes, prostaglandins)
    2. Cytokines (IL-1, IL-6, tumor necrosis factor alpha [TNF-α])
    3. Eosinophil-derived cytotoxic proteins (eosinophil cationic protein [ECP], major basic protein [MBP])
  E. Inhibition of transcription factor function
II. Positive Effects
  A. Vasoconstrictive properties
  B. Potentiation of β-adrenergic receptor
  C. Stimulation of lipocortin expression

---

with two-thirds of the total daily GC dose administered in the morning and the remaining third administered in the afternoon. This strategy may provide for a more normal plasma concentration versus time curve and could result in better responsiveness. If these changes offer no benefit, a change to a GC with a longer half-life, such as dexamethasone, could be another option.

Efficacy of Oral Glucocorticoid Therapy in Asthma

GLUCOCORTICOID THERAPY FOR ACUTE ASTHMA IN ADULTS

Systemic GC therapy is considered first-line therapy for the treatment of acute severe asthma. Over the past 50 years, numerous studies have demonstrated the efficacy of systemic GC therapy in the outpatient clinic, the emergency department and in hospitalized patients. Short courses of GC administered in the outpatient department decrease the rate of asthma relapse, and intravenous (IV) methylprednisolone administered in the emergency room can decrease the need for subsequent hospitalization. In studies evaluating the effectiveness of IV GC therapy in hospitalized patients, GC therapy is superior to placebo with respect to multiple clinical outcomes. Despite their widespread use, the optimal dose of GC in the acute setting has not been firmly established. In one of the few studies that have attempted to determine a dose response, 40 mg of methylprednisolone was found to be as effective as 125 mg administered every 6 hours in patients admitted with status asthmaticus. In contrast, a study that evaluated three doses of prednisolone (0.2, 0.4, and 0.6 mg/kg/day) for 2 weeks in asthmatics requiring a prednisolone burst due to worsening asthma symptoms found the highest dose to be the most effective. There is also no consensus regarding the duration of GC treatment for acute asthma. Because duration of treatment is in part related

Table 39–2. Potential drug interactions with systemic glucocorticoids.

Glucocorticoid	Drugs That Increase Clearance	Drugs That Decrease Clearance
Methylprednisolone	Carbamazepine	Ketoconazole
	Phenobarbital	Troleandomycin
	Phenytoin	Erythromycin
	Rifampin	Clarithromycin
		Oral contraceptives
Prednisolone	Antacids (decrease absorption)	Ketoconazole
	Carbamazepine	Oral contraceptives
	Phenobarbital	
	Phenytoin	
	Rifampin	

to the severity of the initial episode, recommendations for the length of treatment must be tailored to the individual case. With that in mind, it has recently been recommended to treat patients admitted in status asthmaticus with at least 36 to 48 hours of IV therapy with a transition to oral GC therapy when tolerated. The duration of the oral GC taper will depend on the individual's response but should span 4 to 12 days.

In summary, systemically administered GCs are highly effective for acute asthma. With that said, a clear consensus on the optimal type, dose, route of administration (oral vs. intravenous), and duration of treatment does not exist. A number of protocols outlining systemic GC therapy in acute asthma have been published, but therapy should always be tailored to the individual patient's condition. The National Heart, Lung, and Blood Institute (NHLBI) Guidelines on the Diagnosis and Management of Asthma recommends either prednisolone, prednisone, or methylprednisolone, 120 to 180 mg/day in 3 or 4 doses for 48 hours, then 60 to 80 mg/day until peak expiratory flow (PEF) reaches 70% of predicted or personal best for adults.

GLUCOCORTICOID THERAPY FOR ACUTE ASTHMA IN CHILDREN

Systemic GC therapy improves multiple outcomes in children with acute asthma. Studies performed over the past several decades have shown improvements in peak expiratory flow rate (PEFR), forced expiratory volume in 1 second (FEV_1), PaO_2, and reductions in the rate of asthma relapse. In addition, studies evaluating a single dose of GC administered either parenterally or orally in the emergency department setting have demonstrated a reduction in subsequent hospitalization. Lastly, studies comparing the effectiveness of oral prednisone to IV methylprednisolone in treatment of acute asthma have shown both modalities to be equally effective. This is important information because placing an IV line in an agitated toddler in respiratory distress is no small feat. Liquid formulations of prednisone (i.e., Prelone, Pediapred, or Orapred) can be administered to infants and young children who cannot swallow pills. Liquid preparations are more completely and more rapidly absorbed, with peak serum levels occurring within 1 hour compared to 2 hours with tablets.

A study published nearly two decades ago demonstrates how early oral GC use during an acute asthma exacerbation can significantly reduce the progression of asthma symptoms. In this placebo-controlled study of 41 children presenting to the clinic with acute asthma, all 22 patients randomized to prednisone improved during treatment, with only one relapse noted following discontinuation of therapy. In contrast, 42% of those who received placebo developed worsening asthma symptoms requiring rescue intervention. Because continued asthma symptoms often lead to emergency care

and/or hospitalization, this classic study was the basis for the recommendation of the early institution of prednisone during acute exacerbations.

Issues such as the optimal dose, duration of treatment, and the route of administration remain largely empirical and depend largely on the severity of the acute exacerbation. A recent study in children with acute asthma found no difference in efficacy when prednisolone was administered in doses of 0.5, 1, or 2 mg/kg/day. As mentioned previously, oral GCs can be used in many cases, although hospitalized children requiring high flow rates of oxygen to treat hypoxemia adequately are obvious candidates for IV GC therapy. In this situation, methylprednisolone sodium succinate (Solu-Medrol), 1 to 2 mg/kg as a loading dose followed by 0.5 to 1 mg/kg every 6 hours, is administered. Once oral medications are tolerated, a switch to oral prednisone can be made at a dose of 2 mg/kg/day (maximum dose, 60 mg/day) in two divided dose for an additional 2 to 4 days followed by a taper to 1 mg/kg/day administered in a single morning dose for an additional 2 to 4 days prior to stopping. For outpatient management of acute exacerbations, a short course of prednisone is administered with a starting dose of 2 mg/kg/day (maximum, 60 mg/day) in two divided doses for 2 to 3 days followed by a reduction to 1 mg/kg in a single morning dose for an additional 2 to 3 days. The NHLBI guidelines recommend administering prednisone, prednisolone, or methylprednisolone, 1 mg/kg/dose every 6 hours for 48 hours, then 1 to 2 mg/kg/day (maximum dose, 60 mg/day) in two divided doses until PEF is 70% of predicted or personal best.

ORAL GLUCOCORTICOID THERAPY IN THE MANAGEMENT OF CHRONIC SEVERE ASTHMA

Since the advent of inhaled GC therapy, the number of patients with so-called steroid-dependent asthma has substantially declined. Unfortunately, a small number of patients continue to require regular use of oral GC despite optimal therapy consisting of combination high-dose inhaled GCs and long-acting β-agonist therapy. In these patients, chronically administered oral GCs are required to maintain adequate asthma control. Studies performed three decades ago found that the therapeutic effects of steroids persisted longer than their metabolic effects. Consequently, investigators began to evaluate several dosage schedules and found that morning dosing of prednisone on alternate days resulted in the greatest improvement in asthma control while minimizing adverse effects. As a result of these pioneering studies, all patients who require chronic oral GCs should be on alternate-day dosing schedules if at all possible.

There are several management issues to consider when caring for patients with possible steroid-dependent asthma. First, all other asthma therapy should be optimized, including inhaled GC, long-acting β-agonists and leukotriene-modifying agents, in addition to judicious use of short-acting β-agonists. Second, the diagnosis of asthma should be firmly established. Third, factors such as inappropriate inhalation technique and poor compliance with asthma medications should be considered and remedied. Fourth, environmental control measures (especially in atopic patients) should be undertaken, and concomitant disorders such as gastroesophageal reflux, and sinusitis, which can contribute to poor asthma control, should be considered and, if present, adequately treated. Lastly, given the inevitable development of potentially severe steroid-associated adverse effects, every attempt should be made to determine the lowest possible oral steroid dose administered and, if at all possible, administered on alternate days.

Adverse Effects of Chronically Administered Systemic Glucocorticoids

Because all nucleated cells in the body have a common GC receptor, all are potentially affected and thus susceptible to the development of untoward effects. These effects can occur immediately (i.e., metabolic effects) or can develop insidiously over several months to years (i.e., osteoporosis and cataracts). In addition, some adverse effects are limited to children (growth suppression), whereas others appear to require interaction with other drugs (nonsteroidal antiinflammatory agents and peptic ulcer disease). Most adverse effects occur in a dose-dependent and duration of treatment manner, although this has not been uniformly noted. Table 39–3 lists many of the common adverse effects associated with chronic GC use.

OSTEOPOROSIS

Osteoporosis, a significant and common adverse effect, is often overlooked secondary to its insidious onset. All patients who have received more than 7.5 mg of prednisone (or the equivalent) daily for at least 6 months are at risk for developing osteoporosis. Risk factors for steroid-induced osteoporosis include inactivity, sex hormone deficiency, a diet deficient in calcium, and concurrent use of drugs such as furosemide, anticonvulsants, and excessive thyroid hormone replacement. Because demineralization of bone is not detectable on conventional radiographs until a significant degree of bone mineral density is lost, the diagnosis of osteoporosis is best made using bone mineral densitometry.

Treatment of osteoporosis consists of attempting to decrease the oral GC dose and/or frequency of dosing, increasing calcium intake to 1000 to 1500 mg of elemental calcium per day supplemented with at least 400 IU/day of vitamin D (Table 39–4), and increasing weight-bearing physical activities such as walking. Avoidance of activities such as heavy lifting, high-impact

Table 39–3. Adverse effects associated with systemic glucocorticoid use.

1. Dermatologic Effects
   - Dermal thinning/increased skin fragility
   - Acne
   - Striae
   - Hirsutism
2. Endocrinologic Effects
   - Adrenal suppression
   - Growth suppression
   - Delayed sexual maturation in children
   - Weight gain
   - Cushingoid habitus
   - Diabetes mellitus
3. Musculoskeletal Effects
   - Osteoporosis/vertebral compression fractures
   - Aseptic necrosis of bone (hips, shoulders, knees)
   - Myopathy (acute and chronic forms)
4. Metabolic Effects
   - Hypokalemia
   - Hyperglycemia
   - Hyperlipidemia
5. Ophthalmologic Effects
   - Cataracts (posterior subcapsular)
   - Glaucoma
6. Immunologic Effects
   - Diminished immunoglobulin G (IgG) levels
   - Loss of delayed-type hypersensitivity (DTH)
   - Potential for increased risk of opportunistic infection/severe varicella infection
7. Psychological/Neurologic Effects
   - Mood swings, depression, psychosis
   - Steroid withdrawal syndrome
   - Pseudotumor cerebri
8. Hematologic Effects
   - Lymphopenia
   - Eosinopenia
   - Neutrophilia
9. Cardiovascular Effects
   - Hypertension
   - Atherosclerosis

aerobics, and contact sports is recommended because these activities can result in compression fractures of the vertebral bodies in addition to fractures of the long bones. Patients with severe osteoporosis may require treatment with a remittive medication (e.g., bisphosphonate therapy) and a referral to an endocrinologist.

MYOPATHY

Two distinct types of myopathy can occur with systemic GC therapy. An acute, severe myopathy has been reported in patients hospitalized with severe asthma exacerbations. Affected patients often have markedly

Table 39–4. Management of glucocorticoid-induced osteoporosis.

I. Taper oral GC dose to ≤20 mg in adults and ≤10 mg in children on alternate days if at all possible.
II. Increase calcium intake to 1000–1500 mg elemental calcium/d.
  A. Increase dietary calcium intake by eating foods high in calcium: milk (1 cup) (300 mg calcium); cheddar cheese (1 oz) (204 mg calcium).
  B. Consider additional calcium in the form of a calcium supplement* such as:
    1. Calcium carbonate (40% elemental calcium)
      • Os-Cal 500, Os-Cal 500 + D (400 IU vitamin D)
      • Tums (500 mg)
      • Viactiv (500 mg; chewable)
    2. Calcium citrate (21% elemental calcium)
      • Citracal (200 mg elemental calcium)
      • Citracal-D (265 mg elemental calcium + 200 IU vitamin D)
    3. Calcium gluconate (9% elemental Ca^{2+})
  C. Vitamin D supplementation (400 IU/d)
    1. Increase physical activity:
      • Gravity-dependent activities such as walking/low-impact aerobics are most effective
    2. Avoid heavy lifting, contact sports, and high-impact aerobics
    3. Other agents used for severe osteoporosis (often with consultation from endocrinologist):
      • Bisphosphonate (alendronate [Fosamax]; risedronate [Actonel])
      • Calcitonin
      • Calcitriol
      • Sodium fluoride
      • Estrogen (indicated for postmenopausal osteoporosis)

---

*Note that Ca^{2+} is in the form of a salt; thus the amount of elemental Ca^{2+} is a percentage of the total weight of the tablet unless the label specifies the amount of elemental Ca^{2+} per tablet.

elevated serum creatine phosphokinase (CPK) levels and diffuse necrosis of skeletal muscle on biopsy. This rare form occurs primarily in patients who were intubated and received paralytic agents in addition to high-dose parenteral GC therapy. Recovery begins after GC withdrawal, but more than 6 months may be required for complete recovery. The more commonly encountered form is the insidious development of proximal muscle atrophy in patients receiving chronically administered GCs for prolonged periods of time. Isokinetic muscle testing (Cybex) of hip flexor strength appears to be the most sensitive and objective measure of proximal muscle weakness. Enzymes of muscle origin, such as CPK, aldolase, and lactate dehydrogenase (LDH), are not typically elevated, and biopsy of affected muscle reveals atrophy rather than necrosis. To correct and/or prevent GC-induced myopathy, every attempt should be made to taper the GC dose, and a program designed to improve muscle strength should be initiated.

CATARACTS

Posterior subcapsular cataracts (PSCs) are a well-described complication of chronic GC use with a prevalence rate of up to 29%. GC-induced cataracts are often small but can at times significantly affect visual acuity, requiring surgical intervention. Although the development

of cataracts appears to be related to the daily dose, cumulative dose, and the duration of treatment, there is a significant degree of variability with respect to individual susceptibility to cataract formation. It is unknown whether GC dose reduction will result in regression or disappearance of the cataract, although some studies suggest that if recognized early, regression can occur. A yearly ophthalmologic exam to evaluate for the presence of cataracts and glaucoma is recommended for all patients receiving maintenance oral GC therapy.

GROWTH SUPPRESSION

Growth suppression is the GC-associated adverse effect that causes the most concern for clinicians caring for children. Regular daily therapy, frequent short courses, or high-dose alternate-day GC therapy often results in the suppression of linear growth. Doses of prednisone as small as 0.1 mg/kg administered daily for as short a period as 3 months have resulted in significant suppression of linear growth. When a GC is administered on alternate days, the degree of suppression may be less, but significant growth suppression can still occur. Complicating the issue of GC-induced growth suppression is the finding that asthma itself can impair growth. This is a significant issue, especially as it pertains to whether chronic inhaled GC therapy is associated with growth suppression (see later). Because daily or high-dose alternate-day GC therapy for extended periods of time can result in permanent growth retardation, every effort should be made to decrease the amount of oral GC to less than 20 mg on alternate days. If the child's oral GC dose cannot be tapered to 20 mg or less on alternate days, treatment with recombinant growth hormone can be considered. Growth hormone therapy can increase linear growth in children on chronic GC therapy, but the response depends on the dose of GC administered; the higher the daily dose of prednisone, the less effective the GH therapy.

ADRENAL INSUFFICIENCY

Patients who are adrenally suppressed as a consequence of oral chronic GC therapy are at risk of developing acute adrenal insufficiency at times of stress, such as surgical procedures, gastroenteritis resulting in dehydration, or trauma. Patients who develop acute adrenal insufficiency can present with dehydration, shock, electrolyte abnormalities, severe abdominal pain, and lethargy out of proportion to the severity of the presenting illness. This is a medical emergency requiring prompt diagnosis and rapid treatment with IV hydrocortisone (2 mg/kg initially followed by 1.5 mg/kg every 6 hours until stabilization is achieved and oral therapy is tolerated) and vigorous fluid replacement if dehydration and hypotension are present. All patients on chronic oral GC therapy should be considered adrenally suppressed and wear a MedicAlert bracelet that identifies them as being at risk for acute adrenal insufficiency. All adrenally suppressed individuals should be given hydrocortisone at the time of any surgical procedure (1 to 2 mg/kg) and every 6 hours thereafter for the next 24 to 48 hours with a switch to their usual oral GC dose when oral medications are tolerated. The same recommendations are to be followed at other times of acute stress. Complete recovery from adrenal suppression can take from 6 months to 1 year after cessation of long-term GC use. Thus all patients with a history of chronic GC use should be considered adrenally suppressed and be managed as such for up to 1 year following cessation or significant reduction of oral GC therapy.

OTHER ADVERSE EFFECTS

Other common adverse effects of chronic GC therapy include increased appetite with weight gain and the development of a cushingoid habitus consisting of a moon facies, buffalo hump, central obesity with wasting of the extremities, atrophy of the skin with the development of striae, and hirsutism. Psychological disturbances from increased emotional lability to frank psychosis can occur, as well as hypertension, peptic ulcer disease, atherosclerosis, aseptic necrosis of bone, and diabetes mellitus. Chronic GC use can also result in immunologic attenuation with loss of delayed-type hypersensitivity, diminished IgG levels without change in functional antibody response, the potential for reactivation of latent tuberculosis infection, and possible increased risk for infection, especially the development of severe varicella.

INHALED GLUCOCORTICOID THERAPY

The first inhaled GC available for use in the treatment of asthma was approved in the mid-1970s. By effectively delivering small quantities of a potent GC directly into the airway, inhaled GC therapy maximizes the beneficial effects while minimizing the systemic effects. As a result these preparations have a superior therapeutic index compared to oral GCs. Although inhaled GCs have been available for more than 30 years, their use, especially in pediatric patients, until recently had been limited to those patients with severe asthma. As our understanding of asthma has changed, with increasing emphasis on airway inflammation even in mild asthma, inhaled GCs are now considered first-line therapy in all patients including children with persistent asthma.

Efficacy of Inhaled Glucocorticoid Therapy

Bronchial hyperreactivity (BHR) describes the enhanced twitchiness of the airway that characterizes asthma. No other class of asthma controller medications has as big an effect on attenuating BHR as inhaled GC therapy. Reductions in BHR from two- to sevenfold have been reported within 6 weeks of instituting inhaled GC therapy. Associated with improvements in BHR come reductions in asthma symptoms, need for rescue short-acting β-agonist use, and improved pulmonary function, in addition to reductions in acute exacerbations. Scores of publications over the past two decades have demonstrated that inhaled GCs significantly reduce airway inflammation. In addition, inhaled GCs, administered for as little as 6 weeks, can result in modest reductions in thickness of the basement membrane in the airways of asthmatics. Basement membrane thickening is a characteristic finding in chronic asthma, and although its role in asthma is unclear, thickening of the basement membrane may contribute to the development of chronic and potentially irreversible airflow obstruction. In summary, chronic administration of inhaled GC therapy results in improvement in lung function, reduction in BHR, asthma symptoms, and need for supplemental β-agonist use, in addition to suppression of airway inflammation and reduction in basement membrane thickening.

Several studies have also demonstrated that inhaled GCs protect against asthma morbidity and even mortality. Inhaled GC therapy can decrease the need for prednisone, visits to the emergency department, and hospitalizations by up to 50%. In patients with severe and/or poorly controlled asthma, the reduction in hospitalization can approach 70%! In an important epidemiologic study from Canada, Suissa et al found inhaled GCs, in a dose-dependent manner, to reduce the risk of death from asthma significantly. Specifically, they found low-dose beclomethasone dipropionate (200 µg/day) therapy to reduce the risk of a fatal asthma attack by 50% compared to age- and severity-matched asthmatics not on regular inhaled GC therapy. No other class of asthma medication reduces the morbidity and mortality associated with acute asthma to the same extent as inhaled GCs.

Inhaled Glucocorticoids as First-Line Therapy

Inhaled GCs are now recommended as the preferred controller agent in all patients with persistent asthma, including children. This recommendation was made in the 2002 Update to the NHLBI Guidelines, based on a comprehensive review of both the efficacy and safety of long-term inhaled GC use in both adults and children with asthma. This review found inhaled GCs not only the most extensively studied but also the most effective controller class of medications. Lastly, and most important, two recently published landmark studies demonstrated the long-term safety of inhaled GC therapy in children with mild to moderate asthma.

Further support of using inhaled GCs earlier in the course of the disease come from studies that suggest inhaled GC therapy is most effective if begun within the first couple of years of diagnosis. As expected, these studies found inhaled GC therapy to be effective in decreasing asthma symptoms, supplemental β-agonist use and improving pulmonary function. Of greater importance, they found that the longer one delayed instituting inhaled GC therapy after the diagnosis was made, the less effective it was in improving lung function and BHR. Although speculative, the loss of response may be due to the development of some degree of irreversible airflow obstruction secondary to airway remodeling.

Available Inhaled Glucocorticoids

Currently six inhaled GCs are available for use in the United States (Fig. 39–1B): beclomethasone dipropionate (BDP), marketed as Qvar, which is available in 40 and 80 µg per actuation; triamcinolone acetonide (TAA), marketed as Azmacort, which delivers 200 µg from the canister but only 100 µg per inhalation from the built-in spacer device; flunisolide (FLN), marketed as AeroBid, which delivers 250 µg per actuation; fluticasone propionate (FP), marketed as Flovent, which is available in three doses: 44, 110, and 220 µg/actuation;

budesonide (BUD), marketed as Pulmicort Turbuhaler (200 µg/actuation) and Pulmicort Respules (0.5 and 1.0 mg); and mometasone furoate (MF), marketed as Asmanex (220 µg/actuation). Table 39–5 lists the recommended dosages for both adults and children for all of the inhaled GCs. BUD, FP, and MF are often called second-generation inhaled GCs in that they have greater topical-to-systemic potencies. In addition, BUD, FP, and MF all have oral GC-sparing effects in adults with steroid-dependent asthma. Few studies have attempted to compare the clinical efficacy of the available inhaled GCs. FP and MF are thought to be roughly twice as potent as the other available inhaled GCs. In addition, high-dose FP therapy (1000 µg/day or more) results in two to four times greater suppression of adrenal function than equivalent doses of BUD. Thus it appears as if FP may be more potent than the other inhaled GC products on the market, both in terms of efficacy and the potential for systemic effects at high doses.

Qvar is unique, in that although the BDP has been available for decades, its delivery is novel. It is the first inhaled GC preparation that uses the ozone-friendly propellant hydrofluoroalkane-134a (HFA) as opposed to chlorofluorocarbon (CFC). Because BDP dissolves in HFA, smaller particles are generated, resulting in a mean diameter size of 1.1 µm compared to particle sizes of 3.5 to 4.0 µm for most inhaled GCs that remain in suspension with CFC. The smaller particle size, in turn, results in enhanced lung deposition and greater drug delivery to the distal portions of the lung. As a result, lower doses of Qvar provide equivalent to superior efficacy compared to BDP delivered using the traditional CFC propellants.

Dose/Frequency of Use

Asmanex is recommended as a once-daily agent. Pulmicort can also be used once daily, once asthma control is achieved. The remaining products recommend twice-daily administration. With respect to dosage, the more severe or poorly controlled the asthma, the higher the initial dose (Table 39–5 lists recommended doses). High-dose inhaled GC therapy is often used in an attempt to rapidly optimize pulmonary function and clinical symptoms. Once asthma control is optimized, the dose is tapered, following clinical symptoms and pulmonary function closely. Whether starting with high-dose inhaled GC results in more rapid or greater initial improvement in asthma control remains debatable. At least two studies have shown low-dose to be as effective as high-dose therapy as initial treatment. In any case, the ideal inhaled steroid dose should be large enough to control asthma symptoms yet small enough to avoid the potential for adverse systemic effects.

Table 39–5. Dosage guidelines for inhaled glucocorticoids.*

Glucocorticoid	Low Daily Dose	Medium Daily Dose	High Daily Dose
ADULTS			
Beclomethasone HFA 40 or 80 µg/puff	80–240 µg	240–480 µg	>480
Budesonide Turbuhaler 200 µg/dose	200–400 µg (1–2 inhalations)	400–600 µg (2–3 inhalations)	>600 µg (>3 inhalations)
Flur.isolide 250 µg/puff	500–1000 µg (2–4 puffs)	1000–2000 µg (4–8 puffs)	>2000 µg (>8 puffs)
Fluticasone propionate MDI: 44, 110, 220 µg/puff	88–264 µg (2–6 puffs; 44 µg) or (2 puffs; 110 µg)	264–660 µg (2–6 puffs; 110 µg)	>660 µg (>6 puffs; 110 µg) or (>3 puffs; 220 µg)
Triamcinolone acetonide 100 µg/puff	400–1000 µg (4–10 puffs)	1000–2000 µg (10–20 puffs)	>2000 µg (>20 puffs)
Mometasone furoate 220 µg/inhalation	220 (1 puff)	220–440* (1–2 puffs)* may be delivered twice daily	440–880* (2–4 puffs)* may be delivered twice daily
CHILDREN			
Beclomethasone HFA 40 or 80 µg/puff (approved for children ≥5 y)	80–160 µg	160–320 µg	>320
Budesonide Turbuhaler 200 µg/dose (approved for children ≥6 y)	200 µg	200–400 µg	>400 µg
Budesonide suspension for nebulization 0.5 mg, 1 mg/2 mL (approved for children 12 mo–8 y)	0.5 mg	1 mg	2.0 mg
Flunisolide 250 µg/puff (approved for children ≥6 y)	500–750 µg (2–3 puffs)	1000–1250 µg (4–5 puffs)	>1250 µg (>5 puffs)
Fluticasone propionate MDI: 44, 110, 220 µg/puff (approved for children ≥12 y)	88–176 µg (2–4 puffs; 44 µg)	176–440 µg (4–10 puffs; 44 µg) or (2–4 puffs; 110 µg)	>440 µg (>4 puffs; 110 µg)
Triamcinolone acetonide 100 µg/puff (approved for children ≥6 y)	400–800 µg (4–8 puffs)	800–1200 µg (8–12 puffs)	>1200 µg (>12 puffs)
Mometasone furoate 220 µg/inhalation (approved for children≥12 y)	220 µg (1 puff)	220 µg (1 puff)	440* µg (2 puffs) may be delivered twice daily

*Adapted from National Asthma Education and Prevention Program Report. Guidelines for the diagnosis and management of asthma. Update on selected topics—2002. *J Allergy Clin Immunol.* 2002;110:S141.

Adverse Effects of Inhaled GC Therapy

ADRENAL SUPPRESSION

Inhaled GC therapy can result in suppression of the hypothalamic-pituitary-adrenal (HPA) axis. The degree of suppression depends largely on the dose and frequency of the inhaled GC delivered, the duration of treatment, route of administration, and the time of day the drug is administered. The preponderance of data would suggest that doses of 400 μg/day or less of budesonide (or equivalent) are not associated with changes in the HPA axis, but as the inhaled dose is increased to more than 1000 μg/day, significant suppression of the HPA axis can occur. Although FP is thought to have comparable systemic effects to the other inhaled GCs at doses recommended for the treatment of mild and moderate asthma (176 to 440 μg/day), the same cannot be said regarding high-dose FP therapy (1000 μg/day or more). A number of studies have demonstrated significantly greater HPA axis suppression with FP compared to equivalent doses of BUD. In addition, there have been a few case reports of children who developed acute adrenal insufficiency while on high-dose FP therapy (1000 μg/day or more). Because FP is twice as potent as the other inhaled GCs, one should only use high-dose FP in patients with severe poorly controlled asthma or in patients with steroid-dependent asthma.

GROWTH SUPPRESSION

Growth suppression is the steroid-associated adverse effect that causes the most concern for parents and clinicians who care for children. In the late 1990s, several studies suggested that BDP, in doses as little as 400 μg/day, could result in suppression of linear growth. Unfortunately, these studies were limited by the short duration of the study (1 year or less). In addition, in many of the studies, the pubertal status of the children was not ascertained, baseline growth velocity data were lacking, or there were significant differences in baseline height and/or age between the different treatment groups at entry into the study. Complicating this issue further was the long known but often overlooked observation that asthma, especially poorly controlled asthma, can adversely affect growth.

Two long-term studies published in 2000 helped clarify the effect of inhaled GCs on growth. In the largest and longest placebo-controlled trial performed to date in children with asthma, the Childhood Asthma Management Program (CAMP) study found children who had received a mean of 4.3 years of BUD (200 μg twice daily) to be 1.1 cm shorter than those who received placebo. Of significance, the loss of growth velocity occurred primarily in the first year of therapy, and using the Tanner equation to calculate anticipated adult height, the adult was calculated to be 174.8 cm for both the BUD and placebo-treated groups. The CAMP study strongly supports the contention that inhaled GC therapy can result in a modest but transient effect on growth that is unlikely to have any adverse effect on adult-attained height.

This point was strengthened by Agertoft and Pedersen, who followed and evaluated the growth of 211 asthmatic children until they attained adult height. They studied 142 children who had been treated with a mean daily dose of 412 μg of BUD for a mean of 9.2 years and 18 asthmatics who were not treated with inhaled GCs. Fifty-two healthy nonasthmatic siblings of the BUD-treated patients served as controls. The investigators found no difference in the measured versus the expected adult heights in any of the groups studied. In addition, no correlations were found between duration of treatment and cumulative dose of BUD. Of interest, they too noted a transient suppression of growth during the first few years of therapy, but it did not adversely impact adult-attained height.

OSTEOPOROSIS

Despite the fact that osteoporosis can be a debilitating complication of oral GC therapy, whether inhaled GC therapy can adversely affect bone mineral density (BMD) is less clear. Some studies have found significant reductions in BMD of the femoral neck of asthmatics treated with inhaled GCs compared to age-matched controls, with significant inverse correlations found between BMD and the dose duration (product of the average daily dose of inhaled GC in grams and the duration of therapy in months). In contrast, other studies have failed to demonstrate any deleterious effect on BMD.

Given the discrepancy in results among these studies, Toogood et al sought to differentiate between the effect of inhaled GCs compared to the effect of other important variables, including past or current oral GC use, age, physical activity level, and postmenopausal state. They found inhaled GC therapy to result in a dose-dependent reduction of BMD with a decrease of approximately 0.5 standard deviations for each increment of inhaled GC dose of 1000 μg/day. Of surprise, a larger lifetime exposure to inhaled GCs was associated with a more normal BMD. The authors speculated that this so-called protective effect was due to reconstitution of BMD following conversion from oral to inhaled GC therapy.

The CAMP study remains the best study performed to evaluate the effect of inhaled GCs on BMD in children with asthma. Every child underwent yearly BMD determinations, and at no point during the study did the BMD differ in those children treated with budesonide (400 μg/day) versus children treated with nedocromil or placebo. In addition, there was no difference in the bone age among the three groups studied at the end of the 5-year study. The CAMP study strongly suggests that long-term inhaled GC therapy, when given in pediatric-size doses, has no adverse effect on bone growth or BMD in children with mild to moderate asthma. In summary, many factors appear to contribute to the development of osteoporosis, including dose, frequency of administration, and duration of inhaled GC use.

CATARACTS/GLAUCOMA

Recent reports have suggested that chronic inhaled GC therapy can be associated with the development of these cataracts and/or glaucoma. These large epidemiologic studies found weak but statistically significant associations between inhaled GC therapy and either cataracts or glaucoma. Of note, these studies evaluated elderly individuals with mean ages of 65 or older. In addition, the studies failed to provide any indication of clinical significance or visual impairment. Agertoft and Pedersen performed slit-lamp evaluations on 157 asthmatic children on BUD for an average of 4.5 years and in 111 age-matched asthmatic controls with only one posterior subcapsular cataract identified. This was in a child receiving BUD, but this was a known cataract with the diagnosis made 2 years before the child was placed on BUD therapy. On completion of the CAMP study, all children underwent eye exams for cataracts with one possible cataract identified. Thus long-term treatment with inhaled GCs in children is unlikely to cause cataracts, and ophthalmologic surveillance is probably not warranted.

OTHER ADVERSE EFFECTS

A number of other adverse effects are associated with inhaled GC therapy, including hypoglycemia, the development of cushingoid features, opportunistic infections, dermal thinning, and psychosis. Most of these adverse effects have been reported as case reports, with few controlled studies performed to evaluate objectively the potential for and significance of these complications.

INTRANASAL GLUCOCORTICOIDS FOR THE TREATMENT OF ALLERGIC RHINITIS

Antiinflammatory Effects

Intranasal GCs are first-line therapy for patients with moderate to severe seasonal allergic rhinitis (SAR) and perennial allergic rhinitis (PAR). Allergic inflammation plays a prominent role in the pathogenesis of allergic rhinitis with activation of TH2 cells and the subsequent influx of eosinophils into the nasal mucosa following inhalation of allergen. No other therapy is as effective as GC therapy in terms of reducing nasal inflammation. Nasal GCs inhibit the influx and activation of inflammatory cells, inhibit the expression of proinflammatory cytokines, inhibit the production of nasal nitric oxide, and can attenuate the production of allergen-specific IgE.

In addition, nasal GCs, when chronically administered, can block the development of both the immediate- and late-phase allergic responses.

Clinical Efficacy

Presently six nasal GC products are available, including beclomethasone dipropionate, triamcinolone, flunisolide, budesonide, fluticasone propionate, and mometasone furoate. These products are available in aqueous suspensions. Multiple studies over the past couple of decades have demonstrated this class of medications to result in reduced nasal secretions, sneezing, and decreased nasal congestion. For this reason they are the most effective therapy for patients with allergic rhinitis. As noted, with oral and inhaled GC therapy for the treatment of asthma, clear dose–response relationships are difficult to demonstrate with intranasal GC therapy. Low-dose (32 µg/day) aqueous budesonide therapy is as effective as a dose eightfold larger (256 µg/day) in reducing nasal blockage, runny nose, and sneezing while significantly improving in quality of life in patients with PAR. These findings suggest that the lowest dose studied was already at the plateau of the dose–response curve. Studies evaluating the onset of effect of intranasal glucocorticoids in PAR found improvements in runny nose and nasal congestion within 36 to 60 hours. Nasal GCs are also effective in patients with SAR. Intranasal GCs have been compared to oral and intranasal antihistamines and result in a greater reduction in nasal symptoms scores in addition to significant reductions in nasal inflammation.

Adverse Effects of Nasal Glucocorticoid Therapy

LOCAL EFFECTS

Reported adverse effects of nasal GC therapy from controlled clinical trials in seasonal and perennial rhinitis include headache, nasal dryness, nasal irritation or burning sensation, epistaxis, nausea/vomiting, cough, asthma symptoms, viral infection, upper respiratory infection, pharyngitis, otitis, sinusitis, conjunctivitis, tinnitus, dyspepsia, and, rarely, septal perforation. More constitutional complaints, such as abdominal pain, diarrhea, fever, aches and pains, dysmenorrhea, dizziness, flulike symptoms, and bronchitis have also been reported. Whether intranasal GC results in atrophy of the epithelium has been evaluated in patients with perennial allergic rhinitis compared to healthy control subjects before and after long-term mometasone therapy. No significant changes in the nasal mucosa were noted the in pre- and posttreatment specimens in both normal subjects and subjects with perennial rhinitis. In addition, complete resolution of inflammatory changes were seen in about a third of the mometasone-treated patients.

ADRENAL SUPPRESSION

Although the potential for systemic absorption through the nasal route is far less than that via the systemic route, recent studies indicate that intranasal GC can have effects on HPA axis and growth. Wilson et al evaluated the systemic HPA-axis activity of triamcinolone acetonide (220 μg/day), beclomethasone dipropionate (336 μg/day), and fluticasone propionate (200 μg/day), using overnight urinary cortisol excretion and low-dose adrenocorticotropic hormone (ACTH) stimulation test in a single-blind, randomized, four-way, crossover, placebo-controlled study of 16 healthy subjects. Suppression of overnight urinary cortisol was found with fluticasone (43%), triamcinolone (23%), and beclomethasone (21%), although compared to placebo, the only statistically significant difference was seen with fluticasone. In addition, no significant differences between placebo and the three active drugs were seen with regard to suppression of morning serum cortisol and ACTH-stimulated response.

The same group of investigators using a single-blind, randomized, four-way, crossover, placebo-controlled design separated by a 7-day washout period compared the systemic activity of triamcinolone acetonide (220 μg/day), budesonide (200 μg/day), and mometasone (200 μg/day) given for 5 days in patients with allergic rhinitis. No significant difference between the placebo and any of the active treatments was found for fractionated or 24-hour plasma cortisol levels, fractionated and 24-hour uncorrected urinary-free cortisol or cortisol/creatinine levels, osteocalcin, and blood eosinophil count. These findings are suggestive of the lack of significant bioactivity in markers of adrenal function, bone metabolism, and blood eosinophils from currently available nasal GCs at the specified doses.

GROWTH SUPPRESSION

Few studies have investigated the long-term effects of nasal GC therapy on linear growth in children. In a double-blind, randomized, parallel group study by Skoner et al, prepubertal children with perennial allergic rhinitis age 6 to 9 years were treated for 1 year with either aqueous beclomethasone dipropionate, 168 μg twice daily, or placebo. The growth velocity in the beclomethasone-treated group (0.013 cm/day) was significantly slower than the placebo-treated children (0.017 cm/day, $p < 0.01$). After 1 year, the change in standing height was 5.0 cm for the beclomethasone-treated patients and 5.9 cm for the placebo-treated patients ($p < 0.01$), with significant differences in mean height change between the two groups detected as early as 1 month into the study that persisted throughout the

study. There were no significant differences between treatment groups in baseline morning plasma cortisol or response to 0.25 mg cosyntropin stimulation at baseline, 6 months, and 12 months into the study.

In contrast, a study that evaluated the linear growth of children who received intranasal mometasone furoate (100 μg once daily) versus placebo showed no differences in heights at all time points for both mometasone- and placebo-treated groups. In addition, at weeks 8 and 52, the mean increase in height from baseline in the group treated with nasal GCs was actually higher than the placebo group (at week 52, 6.95 vs. 6.35 cm, $p = 0.02$). However, no significant difference in the rate of growth was found between the two treatment groups (mean growth, 0.018 cm/day for both groups). As in the case of oral inhaled GC, whether short-term effects of nasal GC therapy on growth suppression reflect long-term changes and ultimately final adult height is not yet be determined.

CONCLUSION

GCs are an important pharmacologic modality in the treatment of the two most common allergic diseases: asthma and allergic rhinitis. Systemically administered GCs are first-line agents for acute severe asthma; inhaled GCs are first-line agents for the long-term management of all patients with persistent asthma, and intranasal GCs are first-line agents for the treatment of moderate to severe SAR and PAR. It is a well established fact that long-term systemic GC therapy can result in serious adverse effects. Fortunately, topically applied GC preparations have been developed that greatly minimize the systemic adverse effects while retaining beneficial airway effects. Many previously steroid-dependent asthmatics have been tapered off oral GC following institution of inhaled GC therapy. As with oral GC therapy, high-dose inhaled GC therapy can result in systemic adverse effects. Of importance, recent studies suggest that low-dose inhaled GC therapy even when administered long term is unlikely to result in any clinically meaningful adverse effects. By using the lowest possible effective GC doses, as well as maximizing other therapeutic modalities, adverse systemic effects from GCs can be greatly minimized.

EVIDENCE-BASED MEDICINE

Two recent studies published in the *New England Journal of Medicine* provide much needed information regarding the recommendation for long-term controller therapy in young children with recurrent wheezing. The current guidelines recommended institution of inhaled GCs in children 5 years or younger who have had three or more episodes of wheezing and who are at risk for developing persistent asthma (one of the following: a parent with asthma, presence of eczema, or allergic sensitization to an aeroallergen).

The purpose of the first study was to determine whether long-term inhaled steroid therapy in young children at risk for asthma would alter the natural course of the disease. Nearly 300 children (2 to 3 years of age) received either fluticasone (Flovent), 88 μg, or matching placebo for 2 years, followed by a 1-year observational period, with the primary outcome the proportion of episode-free days during the observation year. The investigators found that 2-year treatment with an inhaled GC had no effect on the natural course of the disease, but that it was associated with less asthma morbidity (fewer exacerbations and less need for supplemental controller therapy) while improving lung function. The results of this study mirror those seen in older children. Inhaled GCs are effective in improving asthma control and reducing exacerbations requiring prednisone, urgent care/emergent care, and hospitalizations, but they have no disease-modifying effects.

The second study sought to determine whether intermittent inhaled GC therapy begun at the first episode of wheezing is effective in treating acute wheezing episode as well as altering the subsequent course of the disease. More than 400 infants of mothers with asthma were enrolled at 1 month of age into the study, with 294 receiving at least one 2-week course of budesonide or matching placebo. The proportion of symptom-free days during the 3-year study was 83% for the budesonide group and 82% in the placebo group. There was no difference in the percentage of children with persistent wheezing in the budesonide (24%) versus placebo-treated (21%) groups, and the mean duration of each acute wheezing episode was 10 days in both groups. In summary, the investigators found intermittent inhaled corticosteroid therapy to have no effect on either the natural history of wheezing in at-risk infants or any short-term effect during acute episodes of wheezing.

These two studies provide important information for all who care for children with asthma. First, we should reconsider the common practice of using intermittent courses of inhaled corticosteroids in young children with recurrent episodes of wheezing because they have no effect on the duration of the acute episode, nor do they influence the natural history of the disease. Second, although long-term inhaled GC failed to prevent persistent asthma in young children with recurrent wheezing at risk for asthma, they were effective in reducing exacerbations and improving asthma control. These two studies clearly support the NHLBI Guidelines and strengthen the evidence behind what were, at the time, recommendations based on the extrapolation of findings in older children and adults.

BIBLIOGRAPHY

Agertoft L, Pedersen S. Bone mineral density in children with asthma receiving long-term treatment with budesonide. *Am J Respir Crit Care Med.* 1998;157:178.

Agertoft L, Pedersen S. Effect of long-term treatment with inhaled budesonide on adult height in children with asthma. *N Engl J Med.* 2000;343:10064.

Bisgaard H, Hermansen MN, Loland L, et al. Intermittent inhaled corticosteroids in infants with episodic wheezing. *N Engl J Med.* 2006;354:1998.

The Childhood Asthma Management Program Research Group. Long-term effects of budesonide or nedocromil in children with asthma. *N Engl J Med.* 2000;343:1054.

Fanta CH, Rossing TH, McFadden ER. Glucocorticoids in acute asthma: a critical controlled study. *Am J Med.* 1983;74:845.

Guilbert TW, Morgan WJ, Zeiger RS, et al. Long-term inhaled corticosteroids in preschool children at risk for asthma. *N Engl J Med.* 2006;354.

Harris JB, Weinberger MM, Nassif E, et al. Early intervention with short courses of prednisone to prevent progression of asthma in ambulatory patients incompletely responsive to bronchodilators. *J Pediatr.* 1987;110:627.

National Asthma Education and Prevention Program Report. Guidelines for the diagnosis and management of asthma. Update on selected topics—2002. *J Allergy Clin Immunol.* 2002;110:S141.

Schenkel EJ, Skoner DP, Bronsky EA, et al. Absence of growth retardation in children with perennial allergic rhinitis after one year of treatment with mometasone furoate aqueous nasal spray. *Pediatrics.* 2000;105(2). http://www.pediatrics.org/cgi/content/full/105/2/e22.

Skoner DP, Rachelefsky GS, Meltzer EO, et al. Detection of growth suppression in children during treatment with intranasal beclomethasone dipropionate. *Pediatrics.* 2000;105(2). http://www.pediatrics.org/cgi/content/full/105/2/e23.

Suissa S, Ernst P, Benayoun S, et al. Low dose inhaled corticosteroids and the prevention of death from asthma. *New Engl J Med.* 2000;343:332.

Toogood JH, Baskerville JC, Markov AE, et al. Bone mineral density and the risk of fracture in patients receiving long-term inhaled steroid therapy for asthma. *J Allergy Clin Immunol.* 1995;96:157.

Webb JR. Dose response of patients to oral corticosteroid treatment during exacerbations of asthma. *Br J Med.* 1986;292:1045.

Wilson AM, McFarlane LC, Lipworth BJ. Effects of repeated once daily dosing of three intranasal corticosteroids on basal and dynamic measures of hypothalamic-pituitary-adrenal-axis activity. *J Allergy Clin Immunol.* 1998;101:470.

Wilson AM, Sims EJ, McFarlane LC, et al. Effects of intranasal corticosteroids on adrenal, bone, and blood markers of systemic activity in allergic rhinitis. *J Allergy Clin Immunol.* 1998;102:598.

Anti–Immunoglobulin E Therapy 40

Kari C. Nadeau, MD, PhD

BACKGROUND
Immunoglobulin E and Inflammation

Immunoglobulin E (IgE) is an important mediator in allergic responses. Its discovery occurred approximately 40 years ago. Ishizaka, Johannson, and Bennich were some of the initial investigators who performed early immuno-chemical methods to identify IgE as the skin-sensitizing antibody. The World Health Organization (WHO) International Reference Center for Immunoglobulins in Lausanne, Switzerland, in February 1968, accepted the term *immunoglobulin E* as that component in serum that carries allergenic activity. IgE replaced other terminology such as *E-globulin, IgND*, and *reagin*, which were previously used in the literature to refer to skin-sensitizing antibodies present in the serum of individuals with allergy. IgE was shown to have antimmunoglobulin enic determinants in common with the other four human immunoglobulin classes (IgG, IgA, IgM, and IgD), and IgE from non-myeloma sources was shown to contain both light chains (κ and λ). Studies with two IgE myeloma proteins confirmed the molecular weights of the IgE heavy and light polypeptide chains as 75,500 and 22,500, respectively. IgE's overall molecular weight is 180,000. Knowledge of its role in allergy has led to improved diagnostic methods and enhanced clinical management. The discovery of IgE is a critical historical event that will have a lasting effect on the study of human allergic disease into the future.

IgE binds to high-affinity receptors (FcϵRI) on mast cells in the tissues as well as circulating basophils and triggers the cascade that leads to allergy symptoms involved in sinopulmonary, ocular, gastrointestinal, cardiovascular, and skin organs. Allergies are manifested by positive skin prick tests or measurable specific serum IgE following exposure to a sensitizing allergen and the release of interleukin-4 (IL-4), IL-5, and IL-13. Mast cells and basophils, upon IgE-mediated activation, release chymase, tryptase, and histamine. The reactions following an antimmunoglobulin E exposure of a sensitized individual have been categorized into two phases: early- and late (per Milgrom). IgE binds to its receptor on inflammatory cells in the airways, the gastrointestinal system, and the skin. Cross-linking by allergen molecules of a critical mass of IgE antibodies bound to the surface of mast cells initiates the first phase of the allergic reaction. Bronchoconstriction can occur, which clinically is diagnosed in asthma. It can be confirmed by a decrease in forced expiratory volume in 1 second (FEV$_1$) within 1 hour of allergen exposure. Typically, the early phase resolves within an hour of onset.

Mast cell survival and growth are promoted by the binding of monomeric IgE to its high-affinity receptor. The binding of IgE molecules to FcϵRI induces activation of mast cells and does not depend on specific IgE. Surface expression of FcϵRI can increase as a result of the allergic cascade; therefore, mast cells may be sensitized to more allergens, release mediators at lower allergen concentrations, and release larger amounts of chemokines and other products in response to an allergen. In summary, the mast cell amplifies both acute and prolonged IgE-mediated tissue responses, and IgE enhances the activity of the mast cell.

Research focusing on stopping these events has resulted in the development of a monoclonal antibody to human IgE that interferes with the initiation of the inflammatory cascade. Anti-IgE interferes with allergic responses in several ways. It attaches to the FcϵRI binding domain of free IgE, making it unavailable to mast cells. It also prevents IgE from interacting with FcϵRI on monocytes, eosinophils, dendritic cells, epithelial cells, and platelets, thus interfering with mediator/cytokine release. Also, it prevents IgE from interacting with the low-affinity receptor (FcϵRII) on antigen presenting cells and it downregulates FcϵRI on basophils, mast cells, and dendritic cells.

Anti-IgE therapy inhibits allergen-induced increases in sputum eosinophils and reduces peripheral blood eosinophilia. Similar inhibition of eosinophilia occurred in bronchial biopsy specimens obtained from patients with asthma after 16 weeks of therapy with anti-IgE. In early trials, anti-IgE reduced free-serum IgE levels by more than 90% (Fig. 40–1).

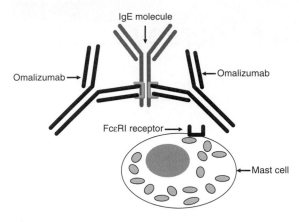

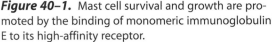

Figure 40–1. Mast cell survival and growth are promoted by the binding of monomeric immunoglobulin E to its high-affinity receptor.

Measurement of IgE for Diagnostic Purposes

After acceptance of IgE in 1968, a group of Swedish investigators moved rapidly to develop a clinically useful serologic assay for total and allergen-specific IgE antibody (RAST, or radioallergosorbent test). For the first time, the diagnosis of human allergic disease could be accomplished by an in vitro alternative to skin testing that involved detection of allergen-specific IgE in serum. The first commercially available RAST for clinical laboratories used a paper disk allergosorbent to bind specific IgE antibody, and radioiodinated antihuman IgE Fc was then used to detect bound IgE. Over the next 40 years, many versions of IgE antibody assays have been created. An alternative approach was adopted, the method of heterologous interpolation, in which allergen-specific IgE results were interpolated from a (heterologous) total serum IgE dose–response curve. The quantitative nature especially of the commercially available allergen-specific IgE assays has allowed the identification of IgE antibody 95% confidence limits for some food allergen specificities.

The competitive inhibition format of the RAST and its modern nonisotopic counterparts, such as the ImmunoCAP System (Pharmacia, Kalamazoo, MI) and Immulite 2000 (Diagnostic Products Corporation, Los Angeles, CA), have become important assays to allergen manufacturers and regulatory agencies for assessing allergenic potency of biologic extracts and to the food industry for detecting and quantifying residual allergenic proteins in food products for the purposes of labeling. More specifically, the power of IgE-based competitive inhibition immunoassays to quantify the presence and amount of allergens with immunoreactive epitopes has remained unsurpassed in comparison with total protein assays, IgE immunoassays, and polymerase chain reaction (PCR)-based DNA assays.

Anti-IgE Therapy

A number of studies are currently ongoing to evaluate the therapeutic potential of a variety of anti-IgE antibodies. Two different approaches have been proposed: (1) producing antibodies to the portion of IgE that is part of membrane but not secreted IgE, and (2) targeting the IgE binding site for the high-affinity IgE receptor (FcεRI). The latter relies on an analysis of IgE/FcεRI interactions, and on the generation of high-affinity humanized antibodies capable of preventing IgE binding to the receptor, such as rhuMAb-E25 (omalizumab). Clinical trials have demonstrated that omalizumab is effective in the suppression of allergen-induced symptoms of allergic asthma, such as reduced FEV_1 and reduced serum IgE levels. This is most likely due to lower densities of IgE on the surface of mast cells and basophils. This treatment appears to have some promise for patients with moderate to severe asthma because it has been reported to allow for tapering of glucocorticoid dosages. Omalizumab is the only anti-IgE therapy currently on the market. It binds to the portion of the IgE recognized by the FcεR1 (high-affinity) receptor. This reduces, in a dose-dependent manner, the amount of free IgE available to crosslink with an allergen. This minimizes effector cell activation and decreases the release of inflammatory mediators. The use of anti-IgE antibodies may represent a potentially promising approach to the treatment of allergic diseases.

ANTI-IGE THERAPY IN ASTHMA

Asthma currently affects an estimated 300 million people worldwide and is associated with significant mortality and morbidity. The mainstay of modern treatment has been the use of inhaled corticosteroid (ICS) and bronchodilator drugs. However, patients with severe asthma often require oral steroids and other immunosuppressive regimens that have deleterious side effects. Recent reports have confirmed the safety of omalizumab and have shown reductions in asthma symptoms and ICS requirement in asthmatic adults and children.

Studies Using Anti-IgE in Asthma

Fourteen trials (15 group comparisons) were included in a recent Cochrane meta-analysis (Walker), contributing a total of 3143 mild to severe allergic asthmatic participants with high levels of IgE. Treatment with intravenous and subcutaneous omalizumab significantly reduced free IgE compared with placebo. Omalizumab led to a significant reduction in ICS consumption compared with placebo (–119 μg/day [95% confidence interval (CI), –154 to –83; three trials]). There were significant increases in the number of participants who were able to reduce ICS by more than 50% (odds ratio [OR], 2.50; 95% CI, 2.02 to 3.10; four trials) or completely withdraw their daily ICS intake (OR, 2.50; 95% CI, 2.00 to 3.13; four trials). Participants treated with omalizumab were less likely to suffer an asthma exacerbation with treatment as an adjunct to ICS (OR, 0.52; 95% CI, 0.41 to 0.65; five trials) or as an ICS tapering agent (OR, 0.47, 95% CI, 0.37 to 0.60; four trials).

Route of Administration

Three routes of drug administration have been used as part of clinical trials: inhaled, intravenous, and subcutaneous injection. In all studies anti-IgE was compared with placebo, although doses of omalizumab differed. The study using intravenous omalizumab compared high (5.8 µg/kg/ng IgE/mL) and low (2.5 µg/kg/ng IgE/mL) doses with placebo. Inhaled omalizumab was given at doses of 1 mg or 10 mg, and subcutaneous omalizumab at doses of 0.016 mg/kg/IU/mL every 2 to 4 weeks.

Efficacy

OVERALL

Subcutaneous omalizumab reduced asthma exacerbations when used as either an adjunctive or steroid-sparing therapy. Omalizumab was better than placebo in allowing participants to withdraw their inhaled steroid treatment following subcutaneous or intravenous administration of the drug. There were significant improvements in health-related quality of life with omalizumab compared with placebo. There was no consistent effect of omalizumab on lung function.

PIVOTAL STUDIES FOR GOVERNMENT APPROVAL

The pivotal studies leading to Food and Drug Administration (FDA) approval found that omalizumab resulted in a reduction in exacerbations (33% to 75% vs. placebo in the steroid-stable phase and 33% to 50% in the steroid-reduction phase) as well as the ability to reduce the dose of inhaled corticosteroid (41.3% of patients receiving omalizumab were able to eliminate beclomethasone vs. 19.3% of patients receiving placebo) over the 28 weeks.

EXACERBATION REDUCTION

Omalizumab reduced exacerbations when assessed as both an adjunctive treatment and as a steroid-sparing agent in moderate to severe asthma. However, in the subgroup of patients requiring oral steroids, omalizumab had no significant effect on asthma exacerbations or reduction in daily oral steroid dose.

STEROID USE REDUCTION

The reduction in daily inhaled steroid dose following treatment with omalizumab was significant. Treatment with omalizumab increased the likelihood of steroid reduction. Not all participants across the studies benefited from omalizumab treatment. Approximately 16% of severe patients achieved less than 25% reduction in daily inhaled steroid use over the steroid reduction phase. Not all asthmatics at the severe end of the spectrum who may benefit most from steroid reduction respond to omalizumab treatment, which could reflect the heterogeneity of asthma.

LONG-TERM EFFICACY ASSESSMENT

The long-term clinical efficacy of omalizumab has been assessed in extension phases from some of the core studies reviewed in this analysis. Complete data from the extension phase (Soler) have now been published. It is possible that longer term use of omalizumab would enable patients to maintain reductions in steroid use and exacerbate less frequently than control. Discontinuation of omalizumab treatment is associated with increases in circulating free IgE to prebaseline values within 8 weeks. Therefore, it is possible that treatment would be needed long term to maximize its therapeutic effect.

SIDE EFFECTS

Side effects following treatment with omalizumab were mild to moderate and did not differ significantly from placebo with the exception of injection site reactions. The most common side effects observed in patients treated with omalizumab are headaches, viral infections, upper respiratory tract infections, and injection-site reactions (45%), such as pain, redness, swelling, itching, and bruising. Most injection-site reactions occur within 1 hour of dosing.

Omalizumab is a humanized monoclonal antibody with less than 5% of the molecule composed of murine complementarity-determining regions and over 95% as a IgG1κ human framework. It forms small biologically inert complexes with IgE and does not activate complement. Anti-IgE binds to free IgE either in the forms of trimers or hexamers and is cleared by the reticuloendothelial system (Fig. 40–2).

Anaphylactoid reactions have been observed in only three patients in the pivotal clinical trials representing less than 0.1% of patients. To date, more than 50,000 patients have been prescribed omalizumab in the United States. Most clinicians observe the patient for up to 2 hours following the first injection, and then for 1 hour or less thereafter. If a severe hypersensitivity reaction to omalizumab occurs, therapy should be discontinued.

Use of a humanized anti-IgE antibody has raised theoretical concerns about immune complex–mediated pathology and abnormal immune responses to parasitic infection. Administration of parenteral anti-IgE results in the formation of small immune complexes (less than 10 kd) that are cleared through the kidney. There were no reports of immune complex–mediated side effects in

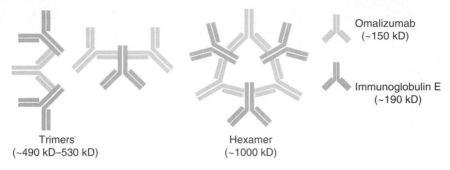

Omalizumab
(~150 kD)

Immunoglobulin E
(~190 kD)

Trimers
(~490 kD–530 kD)

Hexamer
(~1000 kD)

Figure 40–2. Anti–immunoglobulin E binds to free immunoglobulin E either in the forms of trimers or hexamers and is cleared by the reticuloendothelial system.

up to 16 weeks of administration. Aerosolized omalizumab showed no significant effects on allergen induced early and late asthmatic responses. Many of the observed side effects were similar in adults and children, although pruritus was reported only in children. Additionally, antibodies to omalizumab did not develop in participants treated with subcutaneous or intravenous omalizumab but did occur transiently in one participant who received inhaled anti-IgE therapy.

Pediatric Trials

Population-based studies that followed children into adulthood have clarified some aspects of the development of asthma. Three phenotypes have been identified in children: transient wheezing, nonatopic wheezing of the preschool-age child, and IgE-mediated wheezing. IgE-mediated wheezing associated with allergic sensitization is found in the cohort most likely to develop persistent asthma.

Studies Using Anti-IgE Therapy in Pediatric Subjects with Asthma

Anti-IgE treatment was evaluated in 334 children with moderate to severe allergic asthma who had been controlled on inhaled corticosteroids and as-needed bronchodilators. The patients, 6 to 12 years of age, were treated with subcutaneously administered placebo (n = 109) or anti-IgE (n = 225) at a dose based on body weight and initial serum IgE concentration (0.016 mg/kg/IgE per 4 weeks). Beclomethasone dipropionate (BDP) dose (initial range, 168 to 420 µg/day) was kept stable for 16 weeks (stable-steroid phase), reduced over 8 weeks to the minimum effective dose (steroid-reduction phase), and maintained constant for the final 4 weeks. More subjects in the anti-IgE group were able to reduce their BDP dose, compared with those treated with placebo (median reduction, 100% vs. 66.7%; $p = 0.001$). BDP was withdrawn completely in 55% of patients treated with anti-IgE versus

39% of patients treated with placebo ($p = 0.004$). The incidence and frequency of asthma exacerbations requiring treatment with doubling of BDP dose or systemic corticosteroids were lower in the anti-IgE group. The treatment differences were statistically significant during the steroid-reduction phase, when fewer subjects in the anti-IgE group had asthma exacerbation episodes (18.2% vs. 38.5%, $p < 0.001$), and the mean number of episodes per patient was smaller than with placebo (0.42 vs. 0.72; $p < 0.001$). Five asthma exacerbations requiring hospitalization all occurred in the placebo group. Over the entire treatment period, patients in the anti-IgE group missed a mean of 0.65 school days, compared with a mean of 1.21 days in the placebo group ($p = 0.040$). The mean number of unscheduled medical contacts due to asthma-related medical problems was significantly smaller in the anti-IgE than in the placebo group throughout the treatment period (0.15 vs. 0.35, $p = 0.001$). Median reduction in serum-free IgE was 95% to 99% among anti-IgE patients. Anti-IgE treatment was well tolerated.

There were no serious treatment-related adverse events. The frequency and types of all adverse events were similar in the anti-IgE and placebo groups. Treatment with anti-IgE inhibited airway inflammation measured by exhaled nitric oxide (FE_{NO}). The degree of inhibition of FE_{NO} was similar to that seen for ICS, consistent with evidence that anti-IgE inhibits eosinophilic inflammation in induced sputum and endobronchial tissue

Although results from the pediatric trial were generally similar to those reported for trials involving adult and adolescent participants, there were some differences, notably in exacerbation data during the stable steroid phase, suggesting the need for further evaluation of omalizumab in exclusively pediatric study populations.

Cost-Effectiveness Studies

Corren et al conducted a pooled analysis of three multicenter, randomized, double-blind, placebo-controlled, phase III trials investigating the effect of long-term treatment with omalizumab on the rate of serious asthma exacerbations. Patients in the omalizumab groups had fewer asthma exacerbations and asthma-related hospitalizations. Omalizumab was able to decrease hospitalizations by 92% and decrease the average hospital stay by up to 63%. This should substantially lower the cost of care for asthma patients. A retrospective study was conducted to determine the cost effectiveness of therapy and found benefits primarily for patients with multiple hospitalizations despite maximal asthma therapy. More economic studies are needed to determine the cost effectiveness of omalizumab in the treatment of asthma in the long term.

OMALIZUMAB INDICATED FOR TREATMENT OF ASTHMA

The FDA-approved indication is as follows: Xolair (omalizumab [Genentech, Inc; South San Francisco, CA]) is indicated for adults and adolescents (12 years and older) with moderate to severe persistent asthma who have a positive skin test or in vitro reactivity to a perennial aeroallergen and whose symptoms are inadequately controlled with inhaled corticosteroids. Xolair decreases the incidence of asthma exacerbations in these patients. Safety and efficacy have not been established in other allergic conditions.

Recommended Dosing

The dosing of omalizumab has been standardized, and many aids have been developed to allow the clinician to determine the correct dose. The dosage is determined by matching the IgE level drawn at baseline and matching it to the patient's weight (per product insert, Genentech).

IgE levels, once drawn, should not be repeated because no dosage adjustments occur thereafter. The dosage of omalizumab chosen should result in neutralization of free IgE to levels less than 5% at baseline and equates to 0.016 mg/kg of omalizumab per IU/mL per 4 weeks. However, total IgE may actually increase secondary to formation of omalizumab-IgE complexes. The decision to begin omalizumab therapy should be made with full understanding that this is a long-term therapy, administered subcutaneously every 2 or 4 weeks depending on body weight and baseline IgE level.

Indicated Patient Population

Several studies have tried to determine the ideal patient for omalizumab therapy. The FDA-approved indication for this agent is moderate-to-severe persistent asthma of an allergic nature, not controlled with the use of inhaled corticosteroids. In addition, the patient should have an IgE level between 30 IU and 700 IU and not weigh more than 150 kg. The patient should also demonstrate allergies either via skin testing or RAST testing. Rosenwasser and Nash proposed the therapy be used in patients with severe persistent asthma who are controlled with high doses of inhaled corticosteroids as well as those requiring bursts of oral steroids, and also be considered for patients with moderate persistent asthma not well controlled on inhaled corticosteroids and long-acting β-agonists or leukotriene modifiers. Lastly, they propose a role for omalizumab in patients poorly adherent to prescribed therapy and requiring frequent medical services.

OTHER INDICATIONS

Food Allergy

Like other atopic disorders, food allergy is a growing problem in prosperous countries. Recent estimates suggest that IgE-mediated food allergies affect 3.5% to 4% of Americans. Although effective treatment is available for other atopic disorders, the only proven countermeasure for food hypersensitivity is the elimination of the offending allergen. For these reasons the demonstration that anti-IgE increases the threshold of response to peanut challenge, an effect that should translate into protection against unintended ingestion of this intensely feared food allergen, is an important clinical development.

Omalizumab has been successfully used in patients with moderate to severe allergic asthma; however, TNX-901, another anti-IgE antibody, made by Tanox, was tested in 84 peanut-allergic patients in clinical trials. TNX-901 reduced serum IgE levels and successfully increased the sensitivity threshold to peanuts from an average of half a peanut to almost nine peanuts. Patients would still have to eliminate peanuts from the diet, but TNX-901 therapy would ensure protection from accidental ingestion or exposure, which is the cause of most fatalities. In addition, anti-IgE administered during specific immunotherapy for food may reduce the risk of anaphylaxis. Omalizumab is currently in phase I studies in atopic dermatitis in children and adults with severe eczema and food allergy. On other fronts, an inhibitor of the IgE receptor on mast cells, R112, is a possible candidate for food allergy. Preclinical experiments are being conducted on a human IgG-IgE Fc fusion protein that inhibits mast cells, basophils, and B cells. This potential drug may also have an application in food allergy.

Allergic Rhinitis

Clinical trials in allergic rhinitis have demonstrated that anti-IgE reduces both symptoms and the use of rescue medication and improves rhinitis-specific quality of life (RQoL). In the course of a 16-week trial, the mean daily nasal severity score was significantly lower in patients treated with anti-IgE than with placebo ($p < 0.001$). The improvement in symptoms of patients receiving anti-IgE occurred with a reduction in the use of rescue antihistamine and improvement in RQoL. In another 16-week study, treatment with anti-IgE inhibited nasal symptoms.

Atopic Dermatitis

The skin of patients with atopic dermatitis contains increased numbers of Langerhans cells and inflammatory dendritic epidermal cells expressing FcεRI. The highest FcεRI expression is observed in the lesional skin of patients with active atopic dermatitis. Researchers have proposed that elevated IgE levels enhance the expression of FcεRI on dendritic cells of atopic individuals, a process that might be impeded by the reduction of these levels with anti-IgE therapy. Unfortunately, the serum concentrations of IgE in patients with atopic dermatitis may be too high to achieve good results with the current generation of anti-IgE.

Immunotherapy

Combined treatment with anti-IgE and allergen-specific immunotherapy is superior to either treatment administered alone to children and adolescents with seasonal allergic rhinoconjunctivitis. In published trials, omalizumab pretreatment enhanced the safety of rush immunotherapy (RIT) for ragweed allergic rhinitis. Furthermore, combined therapy with omalizumab and allergen immunotherapy may be an effective strategy to permit more rapid and higher doses of allergen immunotherapy to be given more safely and with greater efficacy to patients with allergic diseases.

EVIDENCE-BASED MEDICINE

Randomized Controlled Study Using Anti-IgE In Rush Immunotherapy

RIT presents an attractive alternative to standard immunotherapy. However, RIT carries a much greater risk of acute allergic reactions, including anaphylaxis. Casale et al hypothesized that omalizumab, a humanized monoclonal anti-IgE antibody, would be effective in enhancing both the safety and efficacy of RIT. Adult patients with ragweed allergic rhinitis were enrolled in a three-center, four-arm, double-blind, parallel-group, placebo-controlled trial. Patients received either 9 weeks of omalizumab (0.016 mg/kg/IgE [IU/mL]/month) or placebo, followed by a 1-day rush (maximal dose, 1.2 to 4.0 mug Amb a 1) or placebo immunotherapy, then 12 weeks of omalizumab or placebo plus immunotherapy. Of the 159 patients enrolled, 123 completed all treatments. Ragweed-specific IgG levels increased more than 11-fold in immunotherapy patients, and free IgE levels declined more than 10-fold in omalizumab patients. Patients receiving omalizumab plus immunotherapy had fewer adverse events than those

receiving immunotherapy alone. Post hoc analysis of groups receiving immunotherapy demonstrated that the addition of omalizumab resulted in a fivefold decrease in risk of anaphylaxis caused by RIT (odds ratio, 0.17; $p = .026$). On an intent-to-treat basis, patients receiving both omalizumab and immunotherapy showed a significant improvement in severity scores during the ragweed season compared with those receiving immunotherapy alone (0.69 vs. 0.86; $p = .044$). Overall, omalizumab pretreatment enhances the safety of RIT for ragweed allergic rhinitis. Furthermore, combined therapy with omalizumab and allergen immunotherapy may be an effective strategy to permit more rapid and higher doses of allergen immunotherapy to be given more safely and with greater efficacy to patients with allergic diseases.

Use of Anti-IgE Therapy Reduces Leukotrienes in Children with Allergic Rhinitis

Binding of allergens with IgE to the IgE receptors on mast cells and basophils results in the release of inflammatory mediators as sulfidoleukotrienes (SLTs), triggering allergic cascades that result in allergic symptoms, such as asthma and rhinitis. Kopp et al sought to investigate whether omalizumab in addition to specific immunotherapy (SIT) affects the leukotriene pathway. Ninety-two children (age range, 6 to 17 years) with sensitization to birch and grass pollens and with seasonal allergic rhinitis were included in a phase III, placebo-controlled, multicenter clinical study. All subjects were randomized to one of four treatment groups. Two groups subcutaneously received birch SIT and two groups received grass SIT for at least 14 weeks before the start of the birch pollen season. After 12 weeks of SIT titration, placebo or anti-IgE was added for 24 weeks. The primary clinical efficacy variable was symptom load (i.e., the sum of daily symptom severity score and rescue medication score during pollen season). Blood samples taken at baseline and at the end of the study treatment after the grass pollen season were used for separation of leukocytes in this substudy. After in vitro stimulation of the blood cells with grass and birch pollen allergens, SLT release (LTC4, LTD4, and LTE4) was quantified by using the enzyme-linked immunosorbent assay (ELISA) technique. Before the study treatment, SLT release to birch and grass pollen exposure did not differ significantly among the four groups. Under treatment with anti-IgE + SIT grass (n = 23), a lower symptom load occurred during the pollen season compared to placebo + SIT grass (n = 24, $p = .012$). The same applied to both groups receiving birch SIT (n = 23 and n = 22, respectively; $p = .03$). At the end of treatment, the combination of anti-IgE plus grass SIT, as well as anti-IgE plus birch SIT, resulted in significantly lower SLT release after stimulation with the corresponding allergen

(416 ng/L [5th to 95th percentile; 1 to 1168] and 207 ng/L [1 to 860 ng/L], respectively) compared with placebo plus SIT (2490 ng/L [384 to 6587 ng/L], $p = .001$; 2489 ng/L [1 to 5670 ng/L], $p = .001$). In addition, treatment with anti-IgE was also followed by significantly lower SLT releases to the allergens unrelated to SIT (grass SIT: 300 ng/L [1 to 2432 ng/L] in response to birch allergen; birch SIT: 1478 ng/L [1 to 4593 ng/L] in response to grass pollen) in comparison with placebo (grass SIT: 1850 ng/L [1 to 5499 ng/L], $p = .001$; birch SIT: 2792 ng/L [154 to 5839 ng/L], $p = .04$). In summary, anti-IgE therapy reduced leukotriene release of peripheral leukocytes stimulated with allergen in children with allergic rhinitis undergoing allergen immunotherapy independent of the type of SIT allergen used.

FUTURE DIRECTIONS

There remains need for further information on the safety profile of the drug following long-term use and in different populations such as those with endemic parasitism. Finally, it is possible that omalizumab may have clinical efficacy in IgE-mediated diseases impacting other organ systems, such as eosinophilic esophagitis, dermatitis, allergic bronchopulmonary aspergillosis, and anaphylaxis. Anti-IgE in patients with hyper-IgE syndrome may help alleviate some of their symptoms.

Further investigations into the cost effectiveness of omalizumab will be required to identify its role in the management of IgE-mediated airways disease, and future studies should include comparisons with other available treatment options at step two of the asthma guidelines. Study design should try and overcome the confounding effect of improved adherence to ICS therapy due to the intensity of study monitoring.

CONCLUSION

In almost every situation, the decision to institute omalizumab therapy should be made on sound principles including the diagnosis of moderate or severe persistent IgE-mediated asthma with evidence for poor control despite the use of inhaled corticosteroids, and usually other controller medications as well; an IgE level between 30 and 700 IU/mL; and evidence of reactivity to one or more aeroallergens. The benefits of omalizumab therapy may take up to several weeks to months to manifest and frequent assessments of symptoms and quality of life are necessary.

Omalizumab should be considered a second-line therapy for patients with moderate-to-severe persistent allergic asthma not fully controlled with standard therapy. The use of this agent has resulted in improvements in quality of life for many patients, and in most settings it should not result in a significant increase in cost because of a reduction in emergency care including hospitalization, as well as indirect cost reductions such as productivity and absenteeism.

Anti-IgE therapy decreases free IgE, downregulates FcεRI, improves symptoms, and reduces the need for other medications. Anti-IgE provides a benefit in asthma, allergic rhinitis, and food allergy, and it may be effective in other conditions that involve IgE such as atopic dermatitis, anaphylaxis, occupational allergies, urticaria, eosinophilic esophagitis, hyperimmunoglobulin E syndrome, and allergic bronchopulmonary aspergillosis. Its place in the treatment of diseases other than asthma remains to be defined. New therapeutic approaches are still needed in asthma, and more indications for therapy with anti-IgE will emerge in the future.

BIBLIOGRAPHY

Busse W, Corren J, Lanier BQ, et al. Omalizumab, anti-immunoglobulin E recombinant humanized monoclonal antibody, for the treatment of severe allergic asthma. *J Allergy Clin Immunol.* 2001;108:184.

Casale TB, Busse WW, Kline JN, et al. Immune Tolerance Network Group. Omalizumab pretreatment decreases acute reactions after rush immunotherapy for ragweed-induced seasonal allergic rhinitis. *J Allergy Clin Immunol.* 2006;117:134.

Corren J, Casale T, Deniz Y, et al. Omalizumab, a recombinant humanized anti-immunoglobulin E antibody, reduces asthma-related emergency room visits and hospitalizations in patients with allergic asthma. *J Allergy Clin Immunol.* 2003;111:87.

Fahy JV. Anti-immunoglobulin E: Lessons learned from effects on airway inflammation and asthma exacerbation. *J Allergy Clin Immunol.* 2006;117:1230.

Hamilton RG. Science behind the discovery of immunoglobulin E. *J Allergy Clin Immunol.* 2005;115:120.

Kawakami T, Galli SJ. Regulation of mast-cell and basophile function and survival by immunoglobulin E. *Nature Rev Immunol.* 2002;2:773.

Kopp MV, Brauburger J, Riedinger F, et al. The effect of anti-immunoglobulin E treatment on in vitro leukotriene release in children with seasonal allergic rhinitis. *J Allergy Clin Immunol.* 2002;110:728.

Leung DY, Sampson HA, Yunginger JW, et al. Effect of anti-immunoglobulin E therapy in patients with peanut allergy. *N Engl J Med.* 2003;348:986.

Milgrom H. Anti-immunoglobulin E therapy in allergic disease. *Curr Opin Pediatr.* 2004;16:642.

Rosenwasser LJ, Nash DB. Incorporating omalizumab into asthma treatment guidelines: consensus panel recommendations. *P & T.* 2003;28:400.

Soler M, Matz J, Townley R, et al. The anti-immunoglobulin E antibody omalizumab reduces exacerbations and steroid requirement in allergic asthmatics. *Eur Respir J.* 2001;18:254.

Walker S, Monteil M, Phelan K, et al. Anti-immunoglobulin E for chronic asthma in adults and children. *Cochrane Database Syst Rev.* 2006;CD003559.

Xolair, Omalizumab for Subcutaneous Use [package insert]. San Francisco: Genentech; 2005.

Allergy Immunotherapy

41

Jeffrey R. Stokes, MD and Thomas B. Casale, MD

Allergic diseases have increased in prevalence over the last 20 years, affecting as many as 40 to 50 million people in the United States. Allergen immunotherapy has been a therapeutic option for more than 100 years, and its use is supported by multiple placebo-controlled trials. Allergen immunotherapy alters the course of allergic diseases through a series of injections of a mixture of extracts composed of clinically relevant allergens. The World Health Organization has replaced the term *allergen extract* with *allergen vaccine* to reflect that allergen vaccines are used in medicine as immune modifiers.

INDICATIONS

Allergen immunotherapy is used in the treatment of allergic rhinitis, allergic asthma, and stinging insect venom hypersensitivity. The diagnosis of these diseases is made by history and physical examination supported by testing to confirm IgE sensitization. Skin testing by prick or intradermal method is the preferred objective assessment, but in vitro tests such as the radioallergosorbent test (RAST) are an alternative, especially when skin testing is unable to be performed.

Candidates for venom or Hymenoptera immunotherapy include all patients who have experienced life-threatening allergic reactions or non–life-threatening systemic reactions to Hymenoptera stings. The risk of anaphylaxis for a venom-allergy patient from an insect sting is greater than the risk of anaphylaxis from immunotherapy. In patients younger than 16 years with only urticaria to Hymenoptera stings, immunotherapy is not generally recommended. However, in patients older than 16 years with only cutaneous reactions, immunotherapy is a recommended option. Venom immunotherapy is not indicated for patients who have only had local reactions at the stinging site, even large local reactions.

Immunotherapy is also effective for pollen, mold, animal dander, dust mite, and cockroach allergies. Symptomatic patients with allergic rhinitis and asthma despite allergen avoidance and pharmacotherapy are candidates for immunotherapy (Table 41–1). Other candidates include allergic rhinitis or asthma patients having undesirable adverse reactions to medications, or those wishing to reduce or eliminate long-term pharmacotherapy. In addition to reducing symptoms to current allergens, immunotherapy may prevent the development of sensitization to new allergens or progression of allergic rhinitis to asthma, especially in children.

MECHANISM

The exact mechanism of how immunotherapy works is not fully understood, but it involves shifting a patient's immune response to allergen from a predominantly allergic T-lymphocyte (TH2) response to a "nonallergic" T-lymphocyte (TH1) response. Lymphocytes of a TH2 phenotype typically produce IL-4 and IL-5, cytokines needed for IgE production and eosinophil survival. Findings of increased production of IFN-γ and a decreased production of IL-4 and IL-5 have not, however, been consistently demonstrated after immunotherapy. What has been consistent is the increased production of allergen-specific IL-10. IL-10 causes a shift in allergen-specific IgE to allergen-specific IgG4. This change may be orchestrated by regulatory T cells that downregulate allergic immune responses in part through the release of IL-10 and T-cell growth factor alpha (TGF-α). With allergen immunotherapy, the seasonal increase in allergen-specific IgE is blunted while protective allergen-specific IgG4 production is increased. However, these changes in IgE and IgG may not correlate with clinical efficacy, so periodic skin testing or in vitro IgE antibody measurements are not always useful in evaluating responses to immunotherapy.

CONTRAINDICATIONS

Relative contraindications for immunotherapy include medical conditions that reduce patients' ability to survive a serious systemic allergic reaction, such as coronary artery disease or the concurrent use of β-blockers (including eye drops) or angiotensin-converting enzyme

Table 41–1. Immunotherapy.

Currently Indicated	Allergic rhinitis Allergic asthma Venom allergy
Not Indicated	Atopic dermatitis Food allergy Chronic urticaria/angioedema
Relative Contraindications	Unstable asthma Concurrent use of β-blockers or angiotensin-converting enzyme inhibitors Severe coronary artery disease Malignancy Unable to communicate clearly (children <5 y)

inhibitors (Table 41–1). β-Adrenergic blocking agents may make the treatment of immunotherapy-related systemic reactions more difficult. Despite this, immunotherapy is indicated for patients with life-threatening stinging insect hypersensitivity receiving β-blockers. Allergen immunotherapy should not be initiated in asthmatic patients unless the patient's asthma is relatively stable with pharmacotherapy. Patients who are mentally or physically unable to communicate clearly, such as very young children, are not good candidates for immunotherapy because it may be difficult for them to report early symptoms of a systemic reaction. Pregnancy is not a contraindication for immunotherapy, but by custom immunotherapy is not initiated during pregnancy. If a patient becomes pregnant while already on immunotherapy, the dose is not increased during the pregnancy but maintained at the current level in an attempt to avoid anaphylactic reactions.

DOSING

Standard allergen immunotherapy is administered as a subcutaneous injection. The allergist selects the appropriate allergen extracts (vaccines) based on the patient's clinical history, allergen exposure history, and the results of tests for allergen-specific IgE antibodies. The immunotherapy vaccine should contain only clinically relevant allergens. When preparing mixtures of allergen vaccines, the prescribing physician must take into account the cross-reactivity of allergens, the optimal dose of each constituent, and the potential for allergen degradation caused by proteolytic enzymes in the mixture. The efficacy of immunotherapy depends on achieving an optimal therapeutic dose of each allergen in the vaccine.

Allergen immunotherapy dosing consists of two treatment phases: the buildup phase and the maintenance phase. The prescribing physician must specify the starting immunotherapy dose, the target maintenance dose, and the immunotherapy buildup schedule. The highest concentration of vaccine projected to provide the therapeutically effective dose is called the "maintenance" dose or concentrate. In general, the starting immunotherapy dose is 1000- to 10,000-fold less than the maintenance dose. For highly sensitive patients, the starting dose may be even lower. Dilute concentrations are more sensitive to degradation and lose potency more rapidly than the more concentrated preparations. Thus their expiration dates are much shorter and must be closely monitored.

The buildup phase involves injections with increasing amounts of allergens. The frequency of the injections can vary depending on the protocol. The most common or "conventional" protocol recommends dosing once to twice a week with at least 2 days between injections (Table 41–2). It is customary to repeat or reduce the dose if there has been a substantial time interval between injections. Patients with greater sensitivity may require a slower buildup phase to prevent systemic reactions. With this schedule, maintenance is usually achieved after 3 to 6 months (Table 41–3). Alternative schedules such as "rush" or "cluster" immunotherapy rapidly achieve maintenance dosing and should only be administered by an allergist/immunologist because of an increased risk for systemic reactions. Immunotherapy dosing schedules should be written by trained allergists/immunologists, and primary care physicians should seek their advice if questions or issues arise during administration.

The maintenance phase begins when the effective therapeutic dose is achieved. This final dose is based on several factors, including the specific allergen, the concentration of the extract, and how sensitive a patient is to the extract. Once maintenance is achieved, the intervals for injections range from every 2 to 6 weeks but are individualized for each patient. Clinical improvement can be demonstrated shortly after the patient reaches his or her maintenance dose. If no improvement is noted

Table 41–2. Conventional immunotherapy.

Buildup
- 1000–10,000-fold dilution starting dose (depending on sensitivity)
- Increase dose once to twice a week with at least 2 d in between injections
- Maintenance achieved after 4–6 mos

Maintenance
- Therapeutic dose administered q2–6wk
- Therapy continued for 3–5 y

Table 41–3. Typical buildup schedule for conventional immunotherapy.

1:1000 (v/v)	0.05
	0.10
	0.20
	0.40
1:100 (v/v)	0.05
	0.10
	0.20
	0.30
	0.40
	0.50
1:10 (v/v)	0.05
	0.07
	0.10
	0.15
	0.25
	0.35
	0.40
	0.45
	0.50
Maintenance Concentrate	0.05
	0.07
	0.10
	0.15
	0.20
	0.25
	0.30
	0.35
	0.40
	0.45
	0.50

after 1 year of maintenance therapy, a reassessment should be done. Possible reasons for lack of efficacy need to be evaluated, and if none are found, discontinuation of immunotherapy should be considered. Patients should be evaluated at least every 6 to 12 months while on immunotherapy by the prescribing allergist/immunologist. Duration of maintenance therapy is generally 3 to 5 years. Treatment may lead to prolonged clinical remission and persistent alterations in immunologic reactivity. The severity of disease, benefits from sustained treatment, and the convenience of treatment are all factors that are considered when deciding the length of therapy for each individual patient.

Many studies, especially from Europe, have shown that high-dose sublingual allergen immunotherapy is effective for certain patients, but this mode of therapy is not approved by the U.S. Food and Drug Administration and is considered investigational. Many questions still remain unanswered on sublingual immunotherapy including effective dose concentrations, schedule for buildup and maintenance therapy, and timing of dosing (i.e., seasonal or continuous throughout the year). Additionally, sublingual therapy requires much larger doses of allergen, anywhere from 10 to 300 times greater, making cost an issue. Finally, the utility of sublingual immunotherapy for polysensitized patients is not yet determined.

SAFETY

The greatest concern with immunotherapy is safety. Local reactions at the injection site, such as redness, swelling, and warmth, are common. These reactions can be lessened with H1 antagonists prior to injections. Local reactions can be managed with treatments such as cold compresses or topical corticosteroids. Large local, delayed reactions (25 mm or larger) do not appear to be predictors of developing severe systemic reactions, and generally they do not require adjustment of dosing schedules. However, some patients with a greater frequency of large local reactions (more than 10% of injections) may be at increased risk for future systemic reactions, and dosing adjustments may be necessary.

The incidence of systemic reactions, such as urticaria, angioedema, increased respiratory symptoms (nasal, pulmonary, ocular), or hypotension, ranges from 0.05% to 3.2% per injection, or 0.84% to 46.7% of patients. Risk factors for systemic reactions include errors in dosing, symptomatic asthma, a high degree of allergen hypersensitivity, concomitant use of β-blocker medications, injections from a new vial, and injections given during periods when allergic symptoms are active, especially during the allergy season. A recent survey of 1700 allergists reported that 58% of responders had an event in which a patient received an injection meant for another patient, and 74% reported that patients had received an incorrect amount of vaccine. These errors resulted in a multitude of adverse events, including local reactions, systemic reactions, and even one fatality. Thus it is extremely important to make sure patients are questioned about potential risk factors and the correct vials are used to administer immunotherapy injections.

It is unclear if premedication with antihistamines can reduce the frequency of systemic reactions in conventional immunotherapy, but in cluster or rush immunotherapy, premedication can reduce the rate of systemic reactions.

The incidence of fatalities due to immunotherapy has not changed much over the last 30 years in the United States. From 1990 to 2001, fatal reactions occurred at a rate of 1 per 2.5 million injections, with an average of 3.4 deaths per year. Most fatal reactions occurred with maintenance doses of immunotherapy. The patient population at greatest risk was poorly controlled asthmatics. In many of the fatalities, there was either a substantial delay in giving epinephrine or epinephrine was not administered at all. The incidence of near-fatal reactions (respiratory compromise, hypotension, or both, requiring epinephrine) is 2.5 times more frequent than fatal reactions.

TREATMENT OF ANAPHYLAXIS

Systemic allergic reactions can be life threatening and need to be treated rapidly. Most systemic reactions are limited to the skin, such as urticaria. Respiratory symptoms are seen alone or with skin manifestations in 42% of systemic reactions. Epinephrine is the standard of care for severe systemic or anaphylactic reactions. Treatment of anaphylactic reactions includes placing a tourniquet above the injection sites and immediately injecting epinephrine 1:1000 intramuscularly. For adults, the dose is typically 0.2 to 0.5 mL, and for children, 0.01 mL/kg (maximum, 0.3 mg dose) every 5 to 10 minutes as needed. For convenience, subcutaneous injection at the arm (deltoid) is frequently used, but intramuscular injection into the anterolateral thigh produces higher and more rapid peak levels of epinephrine.

IMMUNOTHERAPY IN GENERAL PRACTICE

Immunotherapy should be administered in a setting that permits the prompt recognition and management of adverse reactions. The preferred setting is the prescribing physician's office, especially for high-risk patients. However, patients may receive immunotherapy injections at another health care facility if the physician and staff at that location are equipped to recognize and manage systemic reactions, in particular anaphylaxis. Because of the potential for anaphylaxis, immunotherapy should not be administered at home. Informed consent should be obtained prior to administering immunotherapy. A full, clear, and detailed documentation of the patient's immunotherapy schedule must accompany the patient when receiving injections at another health care facility. Use of a constant uniform labeling system for dilutions may reduce errors in administration. The maintenance concentration and serial dilutions should be prepared and labeled for each individual patient. Table 41–4 shows the American Academy of Allergy, Asthma and Immunology's recommended nomenclature and color-coded system.

A brief review of a patient's current health status is recommended prior to dosing. It is important to assess any current asthma symptoms, increased allergic symptoms, any new medications, or any delayed reactions to the previous injection. In patients with asthma, peak expiratory flow rate measurements should be obtained prior to each injection. In general, immunotherapy

Table 41–4. Immunotherapy vaccine labeling.

Dilution from Maintenance	Dilution Designation in Volume per Volume (V/V)	Color	Number
Maintenance	1:1	Red	1
10-fold	1:10	Yellow	2
100-fold	1:100	Blue	3
1000-fold	1:1000	Green	4
10,000 fold	1:10,000	Silver	5

injections should be withheld if the patient presents with an acute asthma exacerbation or if peak flow measurements are below 20% of the patient's baseline values. Immunotherapy may need to be decreased or held if significant allergic symptoms are present prior to an injection.

Most severe reactions develop within 20 to 30 minutes after the immunotherapy injection, but reactions can occur after this time. Patients need to wait at the physician's office for at least 20 to 30 minutes after the immunotherapy injection. In some cases, the wait may need to be longer depending on the patient's history of previous reactions.

It is usual practice to reduce the dose of vaccine when the interval between injections is longer than prescribed. This reduction in dose should be clearly stated on the patient's immunotherapy schedule. Because of the potential of extract degradation over time, when new vials are started the initial dose is decreased and then built back up to maintenance. When a systemic reaction occurs, the physician needs to decide if immunotherapy should be continued. This should be done in consultation with the allergist/immunologist who prescribed the immunotherapy. If the decision is to continue, the dose of the vaccine needs to be appropriately reduced to lessen the risk of a subsequent systemic reaction.

EFFICACY AND OUTCOMES

Once maintenance dosing is achieved for venom immunotherapy, 80% to 98% of individuals will be protected from systemic symptoms upon sting challenges. Maintenance therapy is generally recommended for 3 to 5 years, with growing evidence that 5 years of treatment provides more lasting benefit. A low risk of systemic reactions to stings (approximately 10%) appears to remain for many years after discontinuing venom immunotherapy. In children who have received venom immunotherapy, the chance of systemic reaction to a sting after discontinuation of immunotherapy is even lower.

The efficacy of immunotherapy for allergic rhinitis has been clearly demonstrated in a number of clinical trials. These studies have shown significant improvements in symptoms, quality of life, medication use, and immunologic parameters. Allergen immunotherapy for allergic rhinitis is also beneficial for at least 3 to 6 years after completion of a 3-year course of treatment.

The efficacy of immunotherapy for asthma has been assessed in many trials, but some studies have been difficult to interpret either because of the use of poor quality allergen extracts or suboptimal study design. The risk/benefit ratio of immunotherapy for asthma must always be considered. Currently, professional societies recommend that patients with asthma and forced expiratory volume in 1 second (FEV_1) values less than 70% should not receive immunotherapy. A Cochrane review in 2004 examined the role of allergen immunotherapy for asthma. This review of 75 trials with 3100 patients found a significant reduction in asthma symptoms and medication use, and an improvement in bronchial hyperreactivity associated with the administration of allergen-specific immunotherapy. The reviewers concluded that immunotherapy is effective in asthma, and commented that one trial found that the size of the benefit was possibly comparable to inhaled corticosteroids.

EVIDENCE-BASED MEDICINE

Moller C, Dreborg S, Ferdousi HA, et al. Pollen immunotherapy reduces the development of asthma in children with seasonal rhinoconjunctivitis (the PAT-Study). *J Allergy Clin Immunol.* 2002;109:251.

This study evaluates the use of immunotherapy versus placebo in 206 children, 6 to 14 years of age, with only allergic rhinitis. The children were treated for 3 years with grass and/or birch extract depending on their sensitivities. After 3 years of immunotherapy, 19 patients developed asthma; 60 did not. In the placebo arm, 32 children developed asthma over 3 years, whereas 40 did not. The odds ratio for developing asthma in those receiving placebo was 2.5 times greater than that for children treated with allergen immunotherapy. This study was the first to demonstrate clearly that allergy immunotherapy may prevent or delay the onset of asthma in children with allergic rhinitis.

Golden DBK, Kagey-Sobotka A, Norman PS, et al. Outcomes of allergy to insect stings in children, with and without venom immunotherapy. *N Engl J Med.* 2004;351:668.

This study by Golden and colleagues evaluated the long-term outcomes of venom immunotherapy in 512 sensitized children. The mean follow-up was 18 years with a mean duration of immunotherapy of 3.5 years. The rate of systemic reactions after being restung was significantly greater among patients not treated with immunotherapy (17%) compared to those treated with venom immunotherapy (3%). In those treated with immunotherapy who only had skin manifestations prior to therapy, none had systemic reactions when restung.

CONCLUSION

Allergen immunotherapy has been a valuable tool in treating allergic rhinitis, asthma, and stinging insect hypersensitivity for decades. Although newer pharmacologic agents continue to become available, immunotherapy is still the only available treatment that alters the natural course of allergic diseases. Even though there are some risks, these can be minimized when immunotherapy is given in an appropriate environment to carefully selected patients. Recent guidelines have been established to further reduce the risks by establishing a universal system of reporting dilutions and establishing appropriate dosing. Despite a large body of evidence demonstrating the positive therapeutic benefits of immunotherapy, only 3 million patients in the United States are receiving immunotherapy out of a potential 40 to 50 million allergic patients, many of whom could benefit from this therapy. Newer therapies, such as anti-IgE (omalizumab), when used with immunotherapy, may improve the efficacy and safety profile of immunotherapy in the future. In addition, newer forms of immunotherapy such as T-cell peptides or immunostimulating sequences of DNA containing CpG motifs combined with allergens are currently under investigation.

BIBLIOGRAPHY

Aaronson DW, Gandhi TK. Incorrect allergy injections: allergists' experiences and recommendations for prevention. *J Allergy Clin Immunol.* 2004;113:117.

Abramson MJ, Puy RM, Weiner JM. Allergen immunotherapy for asthma. *Cochrane Database Syst Rev.* 2003;(4):CD001186.

Amin HS, Liss GM, Berstein DI. Evaluation of near-fatal reactions to allergen immunotherapy injections. *J Allergy Clin Immunol.* 2006;117:169.

Bernstein DI, Wanner M, Borrish L, et al. Twelve-year survey of fatal reactions to allergen injections and skin testing: 1990–2001. *J Allergy Clin Immunol.* 2004;113:1129.

Golden DBK, Kagey-Sobotka A, Norman PS, et al. Outcomes of allergy to insect stings in children, with and without venom immunotherapy. *N Engl J Med.* 2004;351:668.

Li JT, Lockey IL, Bernstein JM, et al. Allergen immunotherapy: a practice parameter. *Ann Allergy Asthma Immunol.* 2003;90:1.

Lieberman P, Kemp SF, Oppenheimer J, et al. The diagnosis and management of anaphylaxis: an updated practice parameter. *J Allergy Clin Immunol.* 2005;115:S483.

Moller C, Dreborg S, Ferdousi HA, et al. Pollen immunotherapy reduces the development of asthma in children with seasonal rhinoconjunctivitis (the PAT-Study). *J Allergy Clin Immunol.* 2002;109:251.

Polos R, Al-Delaimy W, Russo C, et al. Greater risk of incident asthma cases in adults with allergic rhinitis and effect of allergen immunotherapy; a retrospective cohort study. *Respir Res.* 2005;6:153.

Ross RN, Nelson HS, Finegold I. Effectiveness of specific immunotherapy in the treatment of asthma: a meta-analysis of prospective, randomized, double-blind, placebo-controlled studies. *Clin Ther.* 2000;22:329.

Ross RN, Nelson HS, Finegold I. Effectiveness of specific immunotherapy in the treatment of allergic rhinitis: an analysis of randomized, prospective, single- or double-blind, placebo-controlled studies. *Clin Ther.* 2000;22:342.

Till SJ, Francis JN, Nouri-Aria K, et al. Mechanisms of immunotherapy. *J Allergy Clin Immunol.* 2004;113:1025.

Anaphylaxis and Its Management

Sharon E. Leonard, MD and Lawrence Schwartz, MD, PhD

DEFINITION

Charles Richet and Paul Portier in 1902 coined the term *anaphylaxis* after observing experimental dogs die after repeated injections with sea anemone toxin. They were attempting to induce protection from the toxin (prophylaxis) but paradoxically produced the opposite effect. Since that time, pathophysiologic mechanisms and therapeutic regimens have become better understood. Nevertheless, more precise diagnostic tools along with interventions that reduce risk and treat serious manifestations are needed for anaphylaxis.

Because anaphylaxis comprises a constellation of signs and symptoms and has multiple causes, a precise and universally accepted definition has been elusive. Confusion arises because systemic reactions can be mild, moderate, or severe; and some clinicians reserve the term for severe reactions, whereas others use it to include milder cases. Furthermore, anaphylaxis can be localized or isolated to a particular organ system (e.g., the skin, the latter referred to as cutaneous anaphylaxis). Most authorities agree that a good working definition of systemic anaphylaxis should include the acute onset of significant symptoms and signs of either respiratory difficulty, hemodynamic changes, or both that may occur in conjunction with involvement of skin (urticaria and angioedema) and other mucosal sites (e.g., gastrointestinal). In terms of pathophysiology, anaphylaxis can be defined as a form of immediate hypersensitivity arising when mast cells and/or basophils are provoked to secrete mediators with potent vasoactive and smooth muscle contractile activities that evoke a systemic response. The systemic response can involve one or more principal targets, including the cardiovascular, cutaneous, respiratory, and gastrointestinal systems, sites where mast cells are most abundant.

The terms *anaphylactic* and *anaphylactoid,* respectively, attempt to distinguish between mast cell activation initiated by allergen and IgE, classical immediate hypersensitivity, versus those that initiate mast cell activation by alternative pathways. For example, foods and venoms are common causes of allergen-to-IgE-to-FcεRI-mediated mast cell activation, whereas radiocontrast media, vancomycin, aspirin, and natural products (C3a, C5a, Substance P) activate independently of the IgE-to-FcεRI pathway. Furthermore, allergen-mediated anaphylaxis requires a prior exposure to the allergen that leads to IgE production and then mast cell sensitization. In contrast, anaphylactoid reactions can occur on the first exposure to an offending agent. The manifestations are clinically indistinguishable because the mediators elicited from the mast cells by these two pathways overlap extensively. Therefore, acute therapies are similar. However, understanding differences in causation will impact therapeutic interventions aimed at preventing future attacks.

PATHOPHYSIOLOGY

Cells

Mast cells and basophils are the principal cells involved in anaphylactic reactions, although other cells, including eosinophils, monocytes, and epithelial cells, may also participate and thereby affect the intensity, duration, or character of the reaction. In classic anaphylaxis, an allergen exposure must lead to sensitization before an immediate hypersensitivity reaction can occur. This process, which takes 1 to 2 weeks, involves antigen processing by antigen-presenting cells, which then present peptide antigens to TH2 cells that nurture and instruct allergen-specific B cells to switch from production of IgM or IgG to IgE. Consequently, anaphylaxis does not occur on first exposure to an allergen but may occur after subsequent exposures.

Sensitized mast cells and basophils are armed with allergen-specific IgE that binds to its high-affinity cell-surface receptor, FcεRI. Activation occurs after multivalent allergens cross-link IgE and thereby aggregates FcεRI, resulting in mediator release from the mast cell. Monovalent antigens fail to elicit mediator release because they bind IgE molecules without cross-linking them.

Mediators

Mediators released by mast cells and basophils include preformed mediators stored in secretory granules, newly generated products of arachidonic acid, and an array of cytokines and chemokines. Histamine is the sole biogenic amine stored in all granules of human mast cells and human basophils and is responsible for many of the signs and symptoms associated with systemic anaphylaxis. When released, it diffuses freely and interacts with H1, H2, H3, and H4 receptors. Stimulation of H1 receptors, found on endothelial cells, smooth muscle cells, and sensory nerves, leads to bronchial and gastrointestinal smooth muscle contraction, vascular smooth muscle relaxation, increased permeability of postcapillary venules, coronary artery vasoconstriction, and pruritus. In the central nervous system (CNS), blocking H1 receptors appears to cause drowsiness. H2 receptors reside on gastric parietal cells and at lower levels on inflammatory cells, bronchial epithelium, endothelium, and in the CNS. H2-receptor-mediated increased acid production in the stomach, albeit transient, may occur during systemic anaphylaxis, but it is more likely to become clinically significant when histamine levels are chronically elevated, as observed in patients with systemic mastocytosis. H3 receptors are found primarily on cells in the CNS. H4 receptors are found on hematopoietic cells, such as mast cells, basophils, and eosinophils, and they may modulate certain aspects of inflammation, such as eosinophil recruitment.

Prostaglandin D_2 (PGD_2) is the principal cyclooxygenase (COX)-catalyzed product of arachidonic acid secreted by activated mast cells but not basophils. Both COX-1 and COX-2 are involved in PGD_2 production by mast cells. Consequently, a nonselective COX inhibitor might be better than a selective one at blocking PGD_2-mediated responses during anaphylaxis. Furthermore, the leukotriene C_4 is the principal 5-lipoxygenase-catalyzed product released by both mast cells and basophils after its formation from arachidonic acid. LTC_4 and its bioactive metabolites, LTD_4 and LTE_4, bind to $CysLT_1$ (bronchial smooth muscle, epithelial and endothelial cells, leukocytes) and $CysLT_2$ (vascular smooth muscle, endothelial and epithelial cells, leukocytes, heart muscle), both G-protein-coupled receptors, causing bronchoconstriction, mucus secretion, eosinophil recruitment, vasopermeability, diminished cardiac contractility, vasoconstriction of coronary and peripheral arteries, and vasodilation of venules. Antagonists of CysLT1 (montelukast, zafirlukast) and a 5-lipoxygenase inhibitor (zileuton) are currently available on the market.

Mast cells also are the sole or principal source of heparin proteoglycan and certain proteases. All have β-tryptase in their secretory granules. One subset, called MC_{TC} cells, also stores chymase, mast cell carboxypeptidase, and cathepsin G (like neutrophils and monocytes)

in their secretory granules and expresses CD88 (C5aR) on their surface. The other subset has β-tryptase without the other proteases in their secretory granules and no CD88, and they are called MC_T cells. Mature β-tryptase is released from secretory granules by activated mast cells; levels in serum serve as a clinical marker for mast cell activation. In contrast, precursor forms of α- and β-tryptases (protryptases) are spontaneously secreted by mast cells at rest; levels in serum serve as a clinical marker of the total body burden of mast cells. Current immunoassays for tryptase measure either the mature β-tryptase, or total tryptase (mature + pro forms of tryptase). Basophils express small amounts of tryptase and are deficient in the other proteases, but they also express CD88.

Cytokines (tumor necrosis factor alpha [TNF-α], IL-4, 5, 6, 8, 13 and 16, granulocyte-macrophage colony-stimulating factor [GM-CSF], bFGF, VEGF) and chemokines (IL-8, monocyte chemotactic protein-1, monocyte inflammatory protein-1α) represent another dimension of the mediators released by mast cells and, to a lesser extent, basophils. Although not produced only by these cell types, their delayed secretion after cell activation (hours to days) augment and extend the vasoactive and inflammatory potential of such cells and may impact the severity and duration of anaphylaxis. As selective antagonists of the relevant cytokines and chemokines become available and are tested for therapeutic benefits, their roles in the pathogenesis of anaphylaxis will be better understood.

ETIOLOGY

The most common allergens causing systemic anaphylactic reactions include drugs, insect venoms, foods, radiocontrast media, allergen immunotherapy injections, and latex. Although known causes can be identified in the majority of cases, between 25% and 35% are idiopathic. Most allergens are typically proteins or glycoproteins that serve as complete antigens, capable of eliciting immediate hypersensitivity reactions in a sensitized subject without further processing. The protease activity of some allergens may facilitate their penetration at mucosal sights. In contrast to complete antigens, most drugs act as haptens. They become covalently linked to self-proteins in the circulation, in tissues, or on cells, emerging as multivalent allergens.

Foods

Food is the leading known cause of anaphylactic reactions. Most cases of food-induced anaphylaxis in children occur through egg, peanut, cow's milk, wheat or soy, whereas peanuts, tree nuts, and seafood account for most reactions in adults. Peanut allergy has doubled in prevalence over the past two decades in the United States and Europe but is uncommon in Asia. Apparently, the roasted forms used in the United States exhibit increased allergenicity, and topical ointments containing peanut oil used in Europe increase sensitization. Reactions to allergens in seeds such as sesame seem to be growing in importance, and a variety of different foods have proven to be important allergens in specific individuals. Food-induced reactions typically occur after a sensitive individual ingests that food, but they may also occur when a sensitive subject is kissed by someone who has recently ingested the food allergen.

Hypersensitivity to fresh fruits most commonly manifests itself as oral allergy syndrome (OAS), a form of contact urticaria that occurs within minutes of ingestion and presents as itching, burning, and swelling of lips, tongue, roof of the mouth, or throat. Rarely do these reactions progress to systemic anaphylaxis. Many of these sensitivities are associated with cross-reactivities between food and pollen allergens (e.g., melon with ragweed pollen; peach and apple with birch pollen). Also, the food epitopes associated with this syndrome are typically conformational (rather than linear), and thus they are more easily destroyed by heating, protease degradation, and acid denaturation.

Drugs

A myriad of drugs are known to be responsible for anaphylaxis. Most drugs act as haptens and become covalently linked to self-proteins in the circulation, in tissues, or on cells, emerging as multivalent allergens. Penicillin allergy is reported in 10% of the population, but in actuality up to 90% of those patients do not have specific IgE and could use penicillin as safely as the general population. Approximately 1% to 8% of patients with penicillin-specific IgE antibodies are thought to develop an immediate-type hypersensitivity to cephalosporins. Aztreonam, in contrast, lacks these cross-reactive epitopes and may be safely used in penicillin-allergic patients.

Radiocontrast media (RCM), narcotics, and vancomycin are common causes of anaphylactoid reactions. Low ionic strength radiocontrast media are less likely than high ionic strength varieties to elicit a systemic reaction. Vancomycin produces a mast cell activation event known as red man syndrome, typically involving flushing without cardiovascular compromise, and it usually can be avoided by reducing the rate of administration of the antibiotic. In patients with systemic mastocytosis, these agents must be used cautiously, if at all, because their increased mast cell burden results in increased mediator release.

Aspirin hypersensitivity typically manifests as either a respiratory or a cardiovascular reaction, although sometimes overlap is observed. Respiratory reactions include bronchospasm, nasal congestion, and rhinorrhea and may extend beyond the respiratory tract to include abdominal cramping, watery diarrhea, and urticaria. Cardiovascular reactions, identical clinically to allergen-induced systemic anaphylaxis and shock, also can occur. In most cases such reactions appear to be pharmacologically (not IgE) mediated, and in sensitive subjects they can occur to any of the COX-1 inhibitors. Although COX inhibitors may shunt arachidonic acid metabolism to the lipoxygenase pathway, a mechanism to explain mast cell activation has not yet emerged. COX-2-selective inhibitors appear to be relatively safe in aspirin-sensitive asthmatics. They also are less likely to cause cardiovascular collapse but are contraindicated in this subgroup of patients. Less commonly, sensitivity occurs to only one of the drugs within this class and is due to IgE against an associated unique chemical moiety.

Insects

Insect sting anaphylaxis is primarily caused by the Hymenoptera order that includes the families Apidae (honeybees, bumblebees), Vespidae (hornets, yellow jackets, paper wasps) and Formicidae (fire ants). Cross-reactivity within families is high but low between families. Furthermore, cross-reactivity explains why a person may exhibit an anaphylactic reaction on the first exposure to one insect's sting when previously exposed to a different one. In contrast to stinging insects, allergens from biting insects of the Diptera order (mosquitoes, gnats, midges, true flies) are salivary in origin and do not cross-react with Hymenoptera venom allergens. Anaphylaxis to these salivary proteins appears to be uncommon, but precise epidemiologic data is problematic because people are often unaware of an ongoing mosquito bite, and commercial diagnostic reagents of high quality are not yet available.

Latex

Latex allergens are derived from the rubber tree, *Hevea brasiliensis*. Irritant dermatitis is the most frequent contact reaction and does not involve acquired immunity. Contact hypersensitivity results from cell-mediated immunity to haptenic chemicals added to latex during processing and produces a poison ivy–like local reaction. In contrast, immediate hypersensitivity occurs when IgE is made against the water-soluble, heat-stable, membrane-bound proteins naturally found in this plant-derived product. Cutaneous (elastic materials), mucosal or intravascular (catheters), oral (balloon), or inhaled (powdered latex gloves) routes of exposure have been well documented. IgE-mediated cross-reactivities between latex proteins with allergens in certain fresh foods such as banana, chestnut, avocado, kiwi, peach, bell pepper, and tomato have been reported and may necessitate avoidance of these foods.

Miscellaneous

Although foods, drugs, insects, and latex are the most common known causes of anaphylaxis, exercise-induced, seminal fluid–induced, and progesterone-induced are rare causes worth mentioning. Exercise-induced anaphylaxis is a form of physical allergy resulting from activation of mast cells. It can occur after mild to vigorous exercise and is often associated with ingestion of a specific food or medication. In such patients, exercise is not recommended 1 hour before or within 4 hours after eating. Seminal fluid has induced anaphylaxis by IgE to a specific protein in seminal plasma, spermatozoa, and exogenous allergens transferred through semen. Fertility is intrinsically unaffected and can be achieved with excellent success via in vitro methods. Finally, progesterone-induced anaphylaxis is a cyclic premenstrual reaction to progesterone produced during the luteal phase of a woman's menstrual cycle with a variety of presentations, including erythema multiforme, eczema, urticaria, angioedema, and anaphylaxis.

EPIDEMIOLOGY

Overall Incidence

Because of the lack of a precise definition, underreporting, and misdiagnosis, the annual incidence and prevalence of those at risk for anaphylaxis is difficult to assess accurately. One estimate in the United States attributes approximately 1500 to 2000 deaths per year from systemic anaphylaxis. Nonfatal cases are much more common, estimated to occur at an incidence of 10 to 100 cases per 100,000 person-years. Furthermore, between 1% and 15% of the U.S. population may be at risk for anaphylaxis from foods, drugs, latex, or insect stings.

Foods

About a third of all anaphylactic reactions treated in U.S. emergency departments are food induced and account for about 100 deaths per year. Food allergy is found in about 6% of children and 3% of adults, and consequently these individuals are at risk for food-induced anaphylaxis. Sensitivities to peanut, tree nuts, and seafood are typically lifelong, whereas most children lose sensitivities to cow's milk, egg, wheat, and soy by 5 years of age. About 20% of children lose peanut sensitivity by school age. However, a small portion will regain the sensitivity later in life, particularly if they continue to avoid it.

Drugs

Drugs are the second most common known cause of anaphylaxis, occurring at a rate of 1 per 3000 hospitalized patients. β-Lactam antibiotics and radiocontrast media provoke most such events, but the list of offending agents is lengthy and continues to increase. Furthermore, the risk of drug-induced anaphylaxis increases with age, which is most likely related to the higher likelihood of multiple drug use. During general anesthesia, systemic anaphylactic reactions occur with a frequency of about 1 in 3500, and muscle relaxants, latex, and induction drugs are the three classes of agents most commonly implicated.

Insects

Systemic allergic reactions to insect stings are reported by 0.4% to 3% of individuals. The incidence of hymenoptera venom allergy in children is approximately 0.4% to 0.8% with clinical features that usually range from urticaria to anaphylaxis.

There is a 2:1 male-to-female ratio that probably reflects relative exposure. Annually, about 45 deaths are attributed to insect stings in the United States. Approximately half of the fatal reactions occur in individuals with no prior history of allergic reactions to stings. Many more men than women die from insect sting reactions, and greater than 80% of the deaths from insect stings occur in persons older than 40 years.

Latex

The incidence of latex allergy dramatically increased when the widespread use of contact precautions was implemented throughout health care. Estimates of the prevalence of latex hypersensitivity range from 1% to 6% in the general population and about 10% among regularly exposed health care workers. Other populations at risk include those with neural tube defects, congenital urinary tract disorders, and others who have undergone multiple surgical procedures. However, the incidence of latex-induced anaphylaxis now appears to have declined dramatically with the elimination of powdered latex gloves, better recognition of the condition, and the availability of latex-free paraphernalia at most hospitals.

DIAGNOSIS AND DIFFERENTIAL DIAGNOSIS

Signs and Symptoms

Systemic anaphylaxis may include any combination of common signs and symptoms. In the acute event, the initial diagnosis is based on clinical observations and a history of exposure to an offending agent. Cutaneous manifestations of anaphylaxis, including urticaria and angioedema, are by far the most common symptoms, occurring in greater than 90% of cases. The respiratory and cardiovascular systems are involved less frequently than the skin, but they are responsible for producing signs and symptoms that are clinically more recognized as systemic anaphylaxis. Dyspnea, wheezing, upper airway obstruction from edema, dizziness, syncope, and hypotension are symptoms associated with severe reactions. Gastrointestinal manifestations, such as nausea, vomiting, diarrhea, and abdominal pain, also affect about a third of patients. Headache, rhinitis, substernal pain, pruritus, and seizure occur less frequently.

Time Course

Symptom onset varies widely but generally occurs within seconds or minutes of exposure. Anaphylaxis can be protracted, lasting for more than 24 hours, or recur after initial resolution. The incidence of biphasic reactions is estimated to be up to 20%, occurring most commonly with food. Manifestations can be identical, worse, or less severe than the initial phase, and fatalities have occurred. Most episodes occur within the first 8 hours after resolution of the first event, but recurrences have been recorded as late as 72 hours after. There is no consistent clinical presentation that predicts the recurrence of symptoms, and the cause of biphasic reactions is unknown. Clinical importance relates to the length of time patients should be observed after successful treatment of the initial reaction; recommendations have ranged from 2 to 24 hours.

Laboratory Diagnosis

Anaphylaxis can be precisely confirmed in the laboratory by demonstrating antigen-specific IgE (sensitization) and an elevated level of mast cell mediators in serum or plasma (mast cell activation) (Table 42–1). Skin testing or in vitro measurements of antigen-specific IgE should be delayed for at least 2 weeks after the precipitating event to prevent false-negative results. An increased level of mature β-tryptase in serum, which peaks 15 to 60 minutes after the onset of anaphylaxis and then declines with a half-life of about 2 hours (normal levels being undetectable), indicates that mast cell activation occurred. Alternatively, a significant increase in total tryptase levels during the acute event compared to a baseline level (which can be obtained either before, or more than 24 hours after signs and symptoms have resolved) can also be used. In systemic anaphylaxis induced experimentally by an insect sting, the increased serum level of mature tryptase correlates closely with the drop in mean arterial pressure, indicating that the magnitude of mast cell activation is a primary determinant of clinical severity. Although an elevated serum mature tryptase level may be useful for distinguishing anaphylaxis from other conditions in the differential, some cases of putative anaphylaxis, particularly after food ingestion, are not associated with an elevated level of mature tryptase. This observation raises questions of

Table 42–1. Laboratory tests in the differential diagnosis of anaphylaxis.

Test	Comment
Serum or plasma tryptase	Mature β-tryptase or total tryptase in either serum or plasma peak 15–60 min after the onset of anaphylaxis and then decline with a $t_{1/2}$ of ~2 h. Comparing acute and baseline levels improve sensitivity and specificity.
Plasma histamine	Histamine in plasma peaks 5–10 min after symptom onset and declines to baseline by 10–30 min. Histamine may be released ex vivo by passing basophils in blood through a small-bore needle under vacuum or when blood clots.
24-h urinary histamine or histamine metabolites (methylhistamine, methylimidazole acetic acid)	May be elevated in the urine for up to 24 h after symptom onset, but histamine-containing foods and histamine-producing bacteria may be problematic.
Plasma-free metanephrine	Elevated in pheochromocytoma, not systemic anaphylaxis.
Urinary vanillylmandelic acid	Elevated in pheochromocytoma, not systemic anaphylaxis.
Serum serotonin	Elevated in carcinoid syndrome, not systemic anaphylaxis.
Urinary 5-hydroxyindoleacetic acid	Elevated in carcinoid syndrome, not systemic anaphylaxis.
Serum vasointestinal polypeptide hormone panel: pancreastatin, vasoactive intestinal peptide, substance P, neurokinin	To rule out gastrointestinal tumors or medullary carcinoma of the thyroid, which can secrete these vasoactive mediators.

whether there are anaphylactic pathways that bypass mast cells, perhaps involving basophil activation.

Plasma histamine levels rise more rapidly than those of mature tryptase, 5 to 10 minutes after symptom onset, and remain elevated for a very limited period of time, usually only 15 to 30 minutes. Thus it is usually less useful than serum tryptase because most patients are seen after peak histamine levels have declined to baseline. Urinary histamine or methylhistamine levels also may reflect overall levels of released histamine but are affected by ingested histamine-containing foods, histamine-producing mucosal bacteria, and variability in histamine metabolism.

Differential Diagnosis

Anaphylaxis should be distinguished from a variety of disorders with overlapping presentations. Vasovagal syncope is the most common condition that mimics anaphylaxis. The presence of bradycardia and lack of cutaneous symptoms such as urticaria, pruritus, and angioedema during a vasovagal event helps distinguish it from anaphylaxis. However, bradycardia uncommonly occurs during anaphylaxis, possibly indicating underlying coronary artery disease or due to a cardioinhibitory reflex. Flushing disorders such as carcinoid syndrome and pheochromocytoma can be confused with anaphylaxis but are not typically associated with urticaria or hypotension. Determining serum serotonin, urinary 5-hydroxyindole acetic acid, catecholamines, and vanillylmandelic acid levels confirm the diagnosis of these disorders.

Scombroidosis presents with flushing, palpitations, headache, and gastrointestinal symptoms and occurs within 5 to 90 minutes of ingesting histamine in poorly stored fish. Signs and symptoms can last several hours depending on the amount of histamine ingested. It usually responds to histamine blockers but occasionally requires epinephrine and intravenous (IV) fluids.

Acute attacks of hereditary and acquired angioedema due to C1 esterase inhibitor deficiency are not associated with pruritic urticaria, and they persist longer than attacks of anaphylaxis. Shock due to complement activation by contaminated hemodialysis tubing, without involving mast cell activation, also has been reported. Acute serum sickness, various cell activation syndromes, endotoxin-mediated septic shock, and superantigen-mediated toxic shock syndromes present with fever, which is not characteristic of anaphylaxis by itself. Also, hypoglycemia, seizure, and primary pulmonary or cardiac events present with similar symptoms. Nonorganic diseases such as panic attacks and vocal cord dysfunction can be a challenge to distinguish from anaphylaxis, especially by history alone, but nevertheless must be considered.

Systemic mastocytosis is an important condition to consider in the differential diagnosis of anaphylaxis. In adults, a somatic activating mutation in the gene for Kit in mast cell progenitors results in an excessive body burden of mast cells. In children with this disorder the disease may regress spontaneously. Patients with too many mast cells are at increased risk for anaphylaxis, and anaphylaxis may be a presenting manifestation of systemic mastocytosis. For example, anaphylaxis to an insect sting, particularly in the absence of venom-specific IgE (due to direct mast cell agonists), should raise the possibility of systemic mastocytosis. Diagnostic tests for systemic mastocytosis might include a biopsy of a skin lesion suspected to be urticaria pigmentosa, a bone marrow biopsy stained for mast cells (antitryptase immunohistochemistry being most sensitive), detection of mast cells in the bone marrow aspirate by flow cytometry that express surface CD2 and CD25, and an elevated serum level (20 ng/mL or more) of total tryptase (mature plus pro forms of tryptase) during a nonacute interval.

TREATMENT

Acute

Fatal outcomes in anaphylaxis are principally due to either airway constriction or hypotension. Accordingly, the acute treatment of systemic anaphylaxis requires that airway patency, blood pressure, and cardiac status be assessed (Fig. 42–1) (Table 42–2). Oxygen should be administered and an airway established. Epinephrine, the most critical drug to administer, should be immediately injected intramuscularly (IM) into the thigh for any signs of airway compromise. The dose using 1:1000 concentration is 0.2 to 0.5 mg for adults and 0.01 mg/kg up to 0.3 mg for children. The dose may be repeated every 10 to 20 minutes. Early use is associated with improved outcomes. Patients exhibiting signs and symptoms of hypotension should immediately assume the Trendelenburg position to prevent progression to anaphylactic shock and the so-called empty ventricle syndrome, and then they should receive epinephrine. Most hypotensive anaphylactic deaths are preceded by syncope occurring in the sitting or upright position. Assuming the Trendelenburg position, even without the administration of epinephrine, is likely to abort any life-threatening shock from occurring.

Epinephrine relaxes bronchial smooth muscle and improves vasomotor tone and vasopermeability, thereby counteracting bronchospasm, hypotension, and tissue edema. However, the benefits of epinephrine need to be weighed against its disadvantages in elderly patients and in those with cerebrovascular disease, coronary artery disease, hypertension, diabetes, hyperthyroidism, cardiomyopathy, and narrow-angle glaucoma, where it can precipitate myocardial infarction, arrhythmias, stroke, and pulmonary edema. Despite these relative contraindications, there are no absolute contraindications in administering epinephrine for systemic anaphylaxis. The route of administration should be IM into the

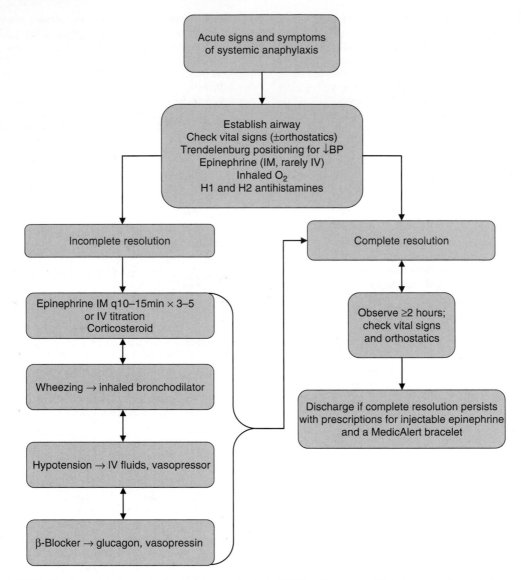

Figure 42-1. Acute management of systemic anaphylaxis. BP, blood pressure; IM, intramuscular; IV, intravenous; O_2, oxygen.

lateral midthird of the thigh to obtain good systemic distribution. IM administration reaches peak serum concentration in less than 10 minutes versus around 30 minutes for subcutaneous injections. IV administration of 1 mg/100 mL solution, titrated clinically at 30 to 100 mL/hour, should only be considered in a medical facility with appropriate equipment and expertise for administration and monitoring. It should be reserved for refractory anaphylaxis or circulatory collapse because of the risk of serious complications.

Other drugs used to treat anaphylaxis include antihistamines, prednisone, volume expanders, and vasopressors.

Parenteral administration of H1 receptor (diphenhydramine, 1 to 2 mg/kg up to 50 mg) and H2 receptor (ranitidine, 300 mg IV over 5 minutes) antihistamines may prevent progression of some of the signs and symptoms, particularly urticaria and pruritus, but are not likely to reverse hypotension or tissue edema. Prednisone (20 mg orally), Solu-Medrol (40 mg IV), or a comparably potent corticosteroid may reduce the risk of protracted or the late phase of biphasic anaphylaxis but is unlikely to be of benefit acutely. An aerosolized β-agonist might attenuate bronchospasm not responding to parenteral epinephrine. Volume expanders should be

Table 42–2. Drugs and other agents used to treat anaphylaxis.

Drug/Agent	Dose and Route of Administration	Comment
Epinephrine (1:1000)	0.3–0.5 mg IM (adult); 0.01 mg/kg IM (child)	Initial drug of choice; should be given immediately; may repeat q10–15min
	0.1–1.0 mg epinephrine in 10 mL normal saline IV bolus	If no response to IM administration and patient in shock with cardiovascular collapse
	1 mg/100 mL at 30–100 mL/h IV	Delivered with a calibrated pump and titrated to blood pressure in an emergency department or intensive care setting
Antihistamines		
Diphenhydramine	25–50 mg IM or IV (adult); 12.5–25 mg PO, IM, or IV (child)	Route of administration depends on severity of episode
Ranitidine	50 mg (adults) or 2–4 mg/kg (child) IV	Other H2 receptor antihistamines also acceptable. Cimetidine administered too rapidly is associated with hypotension
Corticosteroids		
Hydrocortisone	0.1–1 g IV or IM (adult); 10–100 mg IV (child)	Precise dose not established; for milder episodes, oral prednisone, 30–60 mg.
Methylprednisolone	40–125 mg IV	As above.
Drugs for Resistant Bronchospasm		
Aerosolized β-agonist (albuterol, metaproterenol)	0.25–0.5 mg in MDI or in 1.5–2 mL saline for nebulization as needed	Useful for bronchospasm not responding to epinephrine.
Aminophylline	Dose as for asthma	Rarely indicated for recalcitrant bronchospasm; β-adrenergic agonist is drug of choice.
Volume Expanders		
Crystalloids (normal saline or Ringer's lactate)	1000–2000 mL IV over 15–60 min (adults); 30 mL/kg in first hour (child)	Rate of administration titrated against blood pressure response for IV volume expanders; after initial infusion, further administration requires tertiary care monitoring; in patients who are β-adrenergic receptor blocked, larger amounts may be needed.
Colloids (hydroxyethyl starch)	500 mL IV over 15–30 min (adult)	
Dopamine	2–20 µg/kg/min IV titrated against blood pressure	Dopamine is probably the drug of choice; the rate of infusion should be titered against the blood pressure response; continued infusion requires intensive care monitoring.
Drugs Used in Patients Who Are β-Blocked		
Glucagon	1–5 mg IV push → 5–15 µg/min IV	Glucagon is probably the drug of choice, but studies are anecdotal. Titrate continuous infusion against blood pressure.
Vasopressin	10–40 IU IV or IM, and/or 0.01–0.04 IU/min IV	Vasopressin may facilitate effects of epinephrine as well as reverse shock by itself.
Atropine sulfate	0.3–0.5 mg IV; repeat as needed q10min to a maximum of 2 mg (adult)	Atropine is useful to reverse paradoxical bradycardia in the setting of hypotensive anaphylaxis.
Ipratropium		Ipratropium might be considered as an alternative or added to an inhaled β2-adrenergic agonist for wheezing.

IM, intramuscular; IV, intravenous; MDI, metered-dose inhaler; PO, by mouth.

administered for persistent hypotension and the rate titrated against blood pressure response. If hypotension persists despite Trendelenburg positioning, epinephrine, and volume expanders, dopamine should be initiated.

Patients taking β-blockers are more likely to experience severe anaphylaxis characterized by paradoxical bradycardia, profound hypotension, and severe bronchospasm because the actions of epinephrine released naturally are blocked. Furthermore, they are often resistant to administered epinephrine. Glucagon administered at the initial dose of 1 to 5 mg IV followed by infusion of 5 to 15 µg/minute titrated against blood pressure should then be considered. Glucagon increases cyclic adenosine monophosphate (cAMP), which increases cardiac output. Vasopressin (10 to 40 IU IM or IV or 0.01 to 0.04 IU/minute IV) also should be considered in epinephrine-resistant hypotensive anaphylactic shock. Atropine sulfate (0.3 to 0.5 mg IV) should be considered if bradycardia is associated with hypotension. Ipratropium might be considered as an alternative to or added to inhaled β-adrenergics for wheezing.

Prevention

Patients at greatest risk for anaphylaxis are those who already have experienced an anaphylactic reaction. An auto-injectable epinephrine device (Epi-Pen, Epi-Pen Jr, or Twinject) should be prescribed and available at all times. Patient compliance with these lifesaving devices is suboptimal secondary to lack of knowledge about anaphylaxis and the proper instruction about use of the device. A demonstration using a training device should accompany every prescription. Furthermore, the patient should be instructed to check the expiration date frequently and keep the device at room temperature. Temperatures at either extreme will affect epinephrine stability and cause the solution to become yellow or cloudy. MedicAlert jewelry, available on the Internet, also should be recommended. Finally, a referral to an allergist is recommended for further evaluation and treatment options.

In subjects with recurrent anaphylaxis, prophylactic use of H1 and H2 receptor antihistamines appears to be beneficial. A leukotriene antagonist and/or COX inhibitor may provide additional benefit but have not been systematically studied. Finally, cyclosporin A (3 to 5 mg/kg) might be considered in difficult cases of recurrent anaphylaxis because of its ability to inhibit mast cell activation in vitro and cutaneous mast cell activation (urticaria) in vivo. Whether corticosteroids, which do not inhibit mast cell activation in vitro, or immediate skin test responses to allergens in vivo provide a major benefit in most patients with recurrent anaphylaxis is debatable.

Specific anaphylactic syndromes have unique considerations. Food-allergic subjects are asked to avoid the offending agent. Education about how to read food labels and avoid exposure in the community is essential. Referral to the Food Allergy Network is also recommended. A school action plan should be put in place for all children. Definitive treatment such as immunotherapy is not available currently, but trials are now being conducted for certain foods such as peanuts, milk, and eggs. Anti-IgE therapy to reduce sensitivity is another therapy being evaluated experimentally.

Radiocontrast media reactions can be prevented or attenuated by pretreatment with prednisone, 50 mg, given at 13, 7, and 1 hour prior, and 50 mg of diphenhydramine and 300 mg ranitidine orally or IV 1 hour prior. Administration of 25 mg of ephedrine orally 1 hour prior may provide a small additional benefit. In general, patients who are sensitive to an antibiotic need to avoid it. However, desensitization protocols for many patients with IgE-mediated drug allergies are available. Desensitization protocols also exist for non-IgE-dependent aspirin-sensitive patients, and they are particularly effective for those with asthma and nasal polyps. In both cases, desensitization lasts for as long as the drug is continuously/regularly administered; in contrast to immunotherapy, once the drug has cleared, sensitivity is likely to return.

Venom immunotherapy is recommended for anaphylaxis associated with hymenoptera stings. In children and adults, venom immunotherapy is safe and 95% or more effective at attenuating clinically significant reactions to future stings. In children, there is also a significantly lower risk of systemic reactions to stings even 10 to 20 years after treatment is stopped, which seems to be greater than the temporal benefit seen in adults.

Systemic mastocytosis patients, in addition to prophylactic pharmacologic measures, should avoid using direct mast cell agonists such as codeine, morphine, and vancomycin. Women who experience seminal fluid-induced anaphylaxis should have their male partner wear a condom. Desensitization protocols are also available at some centers. Progesterone-induced anaphylaxis may respond to the luteinizing hormone-releasing hormone analog Lupron or to oophorectomy. Finally, with idiopathic anaphylaxis, alternate-day corticosteroids or cyclosporin A are therapeutic options to consider.

EVIDENCE-BASED MEDICINE AND FUTURE DIRECTIONS

Because anaphylaxis is a life-threatening condition, ethical limitations impede systematic or provocation studies. Consequently, human data on the safety and efficacy of pharmacological treatments for anaphylaxis are limited. Management guidelines, which emphasize a central role for epinephrine, are based largely on expert opinion and noncontrolled studies. Reactions can spontaneously resolve with endogenous compensatory responses, but failure to use adrenaline has been considered a major factor contributing to lethal outcomes. Ongoing and future research will provide more precise diagnostic tools that also delineate different pathways of anaphylaxis, indicating which cell types and biochemical pathways are involved. The factors that increase risk for an anaphylactic response will be better understood. Consequently, interventions that reduce anaphylactic risk, including more effective and long-lasting desensitization therapies, and more effectively reverse the signs and symptoms of this potentially fatal disorder will be developed.

BIBLIOGRAPHY

AAAAI Board of Directors Position Statement. Anaphylaxis in schools and other child-care settings. *J Allergy Clin Immunol.* 1998;102:173.

Brown SG, Blackman KE, Stenlake V, et al. Insect sting anaphylaxis; prospective evaluation of treatment with intravenous adrenaline and volume resuscitation. *Emerg Med J.* 2004;21:149.

Chiu AM. Anaphylaxis: drug allergy, insect stings, and latex. *Immunol Allergy Clin North Am.* 2005;25:389.

Golden DB. Stinging insect allergy. *Am Fam Physician.* 2005;67:2541.

Joint Task Force on Practice Parameters, Asthma and Immunology American Academy of Allergy, Asthma and Immunology American College of Allergy, and Asthma and Immunology. Joint Council of Allergy. The diagnosis and management of anaphylaxis: an updated practice parameter. *J Allergy Clin Immunol.* 2005;115:S483.

Lieberman P. Anaphylaxis. *Med Clin North Am.* 2006;90:77.

Neugut A, Ghatak A, Miller R. Anaphylaxis in the United States: an investigation into its epidemiology. *Arch Intern Med.* 2001;161:15.

Pons L, Palmer K, Burks W. Towards immunotherapy for peanut allergy. *Curr Opin Allergy Clin Immunol.* 2005;5:558.

Pumphrey RS. Fatal posture in anaphylactic shock. *J Allergy Clin Immunol.* 2003;112:451.

Sampson HA, Munoz-Furlong A, Campbell RL, et al. Second symposium on the definition and management of anaphylaxis: summary report—Second National Institute of Allergy and Infectious Disease/Food Allergy and Anaphylaxis Network symposium. *J Allergy Clin Immunol.* 2006;117:391.

Schwartz LB. Diagnostic value of tryptase in anaphylaxis and mastocytosis. In: Akin C, ed. *Immunology and Allergy Clinics.* New York: Elsevier. In press.

Sicherer SH, Leung DY. Advances in allergic skin disease, anaphylaxis, and hypersensitivity reactions to foods, drugs, and insects. *J Allergy Clin Immunol.* 2005;116:153.

Simons FER, Gu X, Simons K. Epinephrine absorption in adults: intramuscular versus subcutaneous injection. *J Allergy Clin Immunol.* 2001;108:871.

Thomas M, Crawford I. Best evidence topic report. Glucagon infusion in refractory anaphylactic shock in patients on beta-blockers. *Emerg Med J.* 2005;22:272.

Index

Note: Page numbers followed by a *t* or *f* indicate that the entry is included in a table or figure.

management of, 90
pathogenesis of, 89
peau d'orange from, 90*f*
prognosis for, 90
colloids, 369*t*
combined T- and B-cell
immunodeficiencies,
phenotypes of, 280*t*
common variable immunodeficiency
(CVID), 270
clinical manifestations of, 270–271
treatment for, 271
complement activation
classical pathways and, 209*f*
inhibitors/regulators of, 211*t*
late steps of, 210*f*
MAC and, 210*f*
complement deficiencies, 275–277
definition of, 275
laboratory evaluation of, 276
treatment for, 277
complement fragments, biologic
properties of, 206, 210*t*
complement receptors, 211*t*
complement system, 2, 206–214
clinical associations for, 208–210
evidence based medicine for, 213 214
pathways of, 206
physiologic activities of, 206, 208*t*
proteins of, 207*t*, 213
complement therapeutics, in clinical
practice, 212–213
complementarity-determining regions
(CDRs), 4
complementary/alternative medicine
(CAM)
for allergic rhinoconjunctivitis,
303–304
for allergic/asthmatic disease, 299–309
for asthma, 302–303
definition of, 299
domains of, 300*f*
epidemiology of patient use of,
300–301
ethical/legal issues with, 304–308
evidence-based medicine for, 308–309
liability risks for physicians, 308
patient identification using, 300–302
patient screening for, 302
rationale for use of, 301
side effects of, 304–306
study methodologies for, 300
concha bullosa, 48*f*
congenital neutropenia, 284–285
conjunctivitis, 22
differential diagnosis of, 23*t*
conjunctivorhinitis, 21
constructing combination regimens, for
HIV infection, 294

contact dermatitis. *See also* allergic
contact dermatitis
of eyelids, 27
contact sensitivity, of ear, 74
contact urticaria
clinical symptoms of, 91
definition of, 91
diagnosis of, 91–92
management of, 92
pathogenesis of, 91
prognosis for, 92
COPD. *See* chronic obstructive
pulmonary disease
corticosteroid therapy, systemic, 335–342
chemical structure of, 336*f*–337*f*
pharmacokinetics of, 335–338
corticosteroids
for hypersensitivity pneumonitis, 188
inhaled, 159, 160*t*
oral, 159
suggested dosage for, 169*t*
Cottonwood pollen, 36*t*
cough
allergic diseases and, 78–83
allergic rhinitis and, 78–79
American College of Chest Physicians'
Evidence-Based Clinical Practice
Guidelines for, 78
asthma and, 80–81
causes of, 78, 79*t*
definition of, 78
evidence-based medicine for, 83
GERD and, 81
infectious rhinitis and, 80
nonasthmatic, 168
symptomatic treatment of, 81
treatment approaches to, 82*t*
cromolyn sodium, 159, 160*t*
CRS. *See* chronic rhinosinusitis
Cryptococcus albidus, 179*t*
Cryptostroma corticale, 179*t*
crystalloids, 369*t*
cutaneous infections, superantigens and,
96–97
CVID. *See* common variable
immunodeficiency
cyclosporine, 180*t*
Cynodon dactylon, 35*t*, 36*t*
cyproheptadine, 321
cystic fibrosis, 168–169
cytokines, 58

D

Dactyis glomerata, 35*t*
Dactylis glomerata, 35*t*
darunavir, 293*t*
daytime somnolence, fatigue and, 59*f*
delavirdine, 292*t*
delayed pressure urticaria

clinical symptoms of, 89
definition of, 89
diagnosis of, 89
management of, 89
pathogenesis of, 89
prognosis for, 89
standardized pressure test for, 90*f*
DEPs. *See* diesel exhaust particles
dermatophytid reaction, 74
dermographic urticaria, 88–89
clinical photo of, 89*f*
clinical symptoms of, 89
definition of, 88–89
diagnosis of, 89
management of, 89
pathogenesis of, 88–89
DES. *See* dry-eye syndrome
desloratadine, 322, 326
desonide, 102*t*
desoximetasone, 102*t*
dexamethasone, chemical structure of,
336*f*
DGS. *See* DiGeorge syndrome
didanosine, 292*t*
diesel exhaust particles (DEPs), 250
dietary guidelines, 311
dietary history, medical history and, 14
diflorasone diacetate, 102*t*
DiGeorge syndrome (DGS), 277–278
clinical manifestations of, 277–278
diphenhydramine, 321, 369*t*
direct antigen inhalation challenge, for
hypersensitivity
pneumonitis, 187
dopamine, 369*t*
drug allergies, 236–246
classification of, 236, 239*f*
clinical assessment of, 238
definition of, 236
desensitization for, 240
diagnosis of, 238–240
evidence-based medicine for,
243–245
management of, 240–243
medical history and, 13
recent advances in, 245
skin testing for, 238–239
drug incidence, of anaphylaxis, 365
drug reaction
type A, 236
type B, 236
drug sources, of anaphylaxis, 364
dry powder inhalers, 331, 331*t*
dry-eye syndrome (DES), 26–27
dual-asthmatic response, 153*f*
Duncan syndrome, 284
dust mites
avoidance measures for, 316*t*
background on, 315